Contributors

Abha Rani Sinha
Principal cum Superintendent and Professor
Department of Obstetrics and Gynecology
Sri Krishna Medical College
Muzaffarpur, Bihar, India

Ajit Kumar Nayak
Professor and Head
Department of Obstetrics and Gynecology
Fakir Mohan Medical College and Hospital
Balasore, Odisha, India

Akanksha Gupta
Senior Resident
Department of Obstetrics and Gynecology
All India Institute of Medical Sciences
New Delhi, India

Alka Pandey
Professor
Department of Obstetrics and Gynecology
Lord Buddha Koshi Medical College and Hospital
Saharsa, Bihar, India
Vice President, FOGSI (2022–2023)

Ankita Chonla
Senior Resident
Department of Obstetrics and Gynecology
Maulana Azad Medical College and
Lok Nayak Hospital
New Delhi, India

Archana Baser
Head of Unit
Akash Hospital
Indore, Madhya Pradesh, India

Aruna Nigam
Professor and Head
Department of Obstetrics and Gynecology
Hamdard Institute of Medical Sciences
and Research
Jamia Hamdard, New Delhi, India

Ashis Kumar Mukhopadhyay
Professor and Unit Chief
Department of Obstetrics and Gynecology
Chittaranjan Seva Sadan College of Obstetrics
Gynecology and Child Health
Kolkata, West Bengal, India

Ashwin Shetty
Consultant
Department of Obstetrics and Gynecology
Sir HN Reliance Foundation Hospital
Mumbai, Maharashtra, India

Aswath Kumar
Professor
Department of Gynecology
Jubilee Mission Medical College
Thrissur, Kerala, India

Bharti Maheshwari
Professor and Head
Department of Obstetrics and
Gynecology and IVF
Muzaffarnagar Medical College
Meerut, Uttar Pradesh, India

Bhawana Tiwary
Assistant Professor
Department of Reproductive Medicine
Indira Gandhi Institute of Medical Sciences
Patna, Bihar, India

Chanchal Singh
Lead Consultant
Department of Fetal Medicine
Madhukar Rainbow Children's Hospital
and BirthRight
Rainbow Hospitals
New Delhi, India

Contributors

Charmila Ayyavoo
Director
Aditi Hospital and Parvathy Ayyavoo
Fertility Centre
Trichy, Tamil Nadu, India

Chinmayee Ratha
Director
Resolution Fetal Medicine Center
Hyderabad, Telangana, India

Darryl Gibson Edwin
Resident
Department of Obstetrics and Gynecology
Maharishi Markandeshwar Institute of Medical Sciences and Research
Mullana, Ambala, Haryana, India

Deepa Lokwani Masand
Senior Professor and HOU
Department of Obstetrics and Gynecology
Jaipur National University Institute
of Medical Sciences and Research Centre
Jaipur, Rajasthan, India
President, National Association for Reproductive and Child Health Care of India (NARCHI)

Deepali Kale
Associate Professor
Department of Obstetrics and Gynecology
Seth GS Medical College, KEM Hospital
and Nowrosjee Wadia Maternity Hospital
Mumbai, Maharashtra, India

Deepika Kashyap
Senior Resident
Department of Obstetrics and Gynecology
All India Institute of Medical Sciences
New Delhi, India

Deval Rishi Pandit
Intern
Kasturba Medical College (MAHE)
Mangaluru, Karnataka, India

Fessy Louis T
Professor and Head
Department of Reproductive Medicine and Surgery
Amrita Institute of Medical Sciences
Kochi, Kerala, India

Hafizur Rahman
Former Additional Professor and Head
Department of Obstetrics and Gynecology
All India Institute of Medical Sciences
Nadia, West Bengal, India
Governing Council Member, Indian College of Obstetricians and Gynaecologists (ICOG)
Hony Secretary, The Gangtok OB-GYN Society

Haresh U Doshi
Professor and Head
Department of Obstetrics and Gynecology
GCS Medical College, Hospital and Research Center
Ahmedabad, Gujarat, India

Hem Kanta Sarma
Professor and Head
Department of Obstetrics and Gynecology
Jorhat Medical College
Jorhat, Assam, India

Indu Lata
Professor
Department of Maternal and Reproductive Health
Sanjay Gandhi Postgraduate Institute of Medical Sciences
Lucknow, Uttar Pradesh, India

Jai Bhagwan Sharma
Professor
Department of Obstetrics and Gynecology
All India Institute of Medical Sciences
New Delhi, India

Jaya Chawla
Fellow, Maternal Fetal Medicine (AIIMS)
Professor
Department of Obstetrics and Gynecology
Atal Bihari Vajpayee Institute of Medical Sciences
and Dr Ram Manohar Lohia Hospital
New Delhi, India

Juhi Bharti
Additional Professor
Department of Obstetrics and Gynecology
All India Institute of Medical Sciences
New Delhi, India

Jyotsna S Dwivedi
Assistant Professor
Department of Obstetrics and Gynecology
Seth GS Medical College, KEM Hospital
and Nowrosjee Wadia Maternity Hospital
Mumbai, Maharashtra, India

Jyotsna Suri
Professor and Consultant
Department of Obstetrics and Gynecology
Vardhman Mahavir Medical College
and Safdarjung Hospital
New Delhi, India

K Aparna Sharma
Professor
Department of Obstetrics and Gynecology
All India Institute of Medical Sciences
New Delhi, India

K Deepthi D Nair
Assistant Professor
Department of Obstetrics and Gynecology
Jubilee Mission Medical College Hospital
and Research Institute
Thrissur, Kerala, India

Kasturi V Donimath
Professor and Head
Department of Obstetrics and Gynecology
Karnataka Institute of Medical Sciences
Hubballi, Karnataka, India

Kausha Shah
Consultant Obstetrician and Gynecologist
Unit Head
Bharat Ratna Dr Babasaheb Ambedkar
Municipal General Hospital
Shatabdi and KK Specialty Hospitals
Mumbai, Maharashtra, India

Kiran Pandey
Professor
Government Medical College
Jalaun, Uttar Pradesh, India
Professor and Former Head
Department of Obstetrics and Gynecology
GSVM Medical College, Kanpur
Chairperson, Medical Education Committee
FOGSI (2022–2025)
ICOG Governing Council Member (2023–2025)

Krutika Ramdin
Senior Resident
HBT Medical College and Dr RN Cooper Hospital
Mumbai, Maharashtra, India

Latika Chawla
Consultant Gynecologist and
Endoscopic Surgeon
Endometriosis Excision Surgeon
Surya and Criticare Hospitals
Mumbai, Maharashtra, India

Leena Wadhwa
Professor and IVF In-charge
Department of Obstetrics and Gynecology
ESI-PGIMSR and Model Hospital
New Delhi, India

Madhavi M Gupta
Director–Professor
Department of Obstetrics and Gynecology
Maulana Azad Medical College and
Lok Nayak Hospital
New Delhi, India

Mala Srivastava
Head of Gyne-Oncology Unit
Senior Consultant and Professor
Ganga Ram Institute of Postgraduate Medicine
and Research (GRIPMER)
Department of Endoscopic and Robotic Surgeon
Sir Ganga Ram Hospital
New Delhi, India

Mukta Agarwal
Professor
Department of Obstetrics and Gynecology
All India Institute of Medical Sciences
Patna, Bihar, India

Neha Mishra
Assistant Professor
Department of Obstetrics and Gynecology
Atal Bihari Vajpayee Institute of Medical Sciences
and Dr Ram Manohar Lohia Hospital
New Delhi, India

Niharika Dhiman
Professor
Department of Obsterics and Gynecology
Maulana Azad Medical College and
Lok Nayak Hospital
New Delhi, India

Contributors

Nilanchali Singh
Assistant Professor
Department of Obstetrics and Gynecology
All India Institute of Medical Sciences
New Delhi, India

Nisha
Senior Resident
Department of Obstetrics and Gynecology
All India Institute of Medical Sciences
New Delhi, India

Panchanan Das
Professor
Department of Obstetrics and Gynecology
Gauhati Medical College and Hospital
Guwahati, Assam, India

Pavika Lal
Associate Professor
Department of Obstetrics and Gynecology
GSVM Medical College
Kanpur, Uttar Pradesh, India

Pikee Saxena
Director Professor
Department of Obstetrics and Gynecology
Lady Hardinge Medical College and
Smt Sucheta Kriplani Hospital
New Delhi, India

Pooja Sharma
Senior Resident
Department of Obstetrics and Gynecology
University College of Medical Sciences
and Guru Teg Bahadur Hospital
New Delhi, India

Pratik Tambe
ART Consultant and Gynec Endoscopic Surgeon
Department of Obstetrics and Gynecology
Ashirwad IVF
Mumbai, Maharashtra, India
Chairperson, AMOGS Endocrinology
Committee (2020–2024)
Governing Council Member, ICOG (2020–2025)
Chairperson, FOGSI Endocrinology
Committee (2017–2019)

Pushpa Junghare
Professor and Head
Department of Obstetrics and Gynecology
Dr Panjabrao Deshmukh Memorial
Medical College
Amravati, Maharashtra, India

Radhika MS
Resident
Department of Obstetrics and Gynecology
KC General Hospital
Bengaluru, Karnataka, India

Reena Wani
Head
Department of Obstetrics and Gynecology
HBT Medical College and Dr RN Cooper Hospital
Mumbai, Maharashtra, India

Richa Vatsa
Associate Professor
Department of Obstetrics and Gynecology
All India Institute of Medical Sciences
New Delhi, India

Ruby Bhatia
Professor and Head
Department of Obstetrics and Gynecology
Maharishi Markandeshwar Institute of Medical
Sciences and Research
Mullana, Ambala, Haryana, India

Sandhya Jain
Professor
Department of Obstetrics and Gynecology
University College of Medical Sciences
and Guru Teg Bahadur Hospital
New Delhi, India

Sanjum Yasmin Malik
Senior Resident
Department of Obstetrics and Gynecology
Maharishi Markandeshwar Institute of Medical
Sciences and Research
Mullana, Ambala, Haryana, India

Sarita Bhalerao
Consultant Obstetrician and Gynecologist
Bhatia, Saifee, Reliance HNH, and
Breach Candy Hospitals
Mumbai, Maharashtra, India
Secretary Elect, ICOG

Saroj Rajan
Senior Resident (Academics)
Department of Obstetrics and Gynecology
All India Institute of Medical Sciences
New Delhi, India

Sayanti Paul
Assistant Professor
Department of Obstetrics and Gynecology
All India Institute of Medical Sciences
Nadia, West Bengal, India

Seema Grover
Professor and Head
Department of Obstetrics and Gynecology
Guru Gobind Singh Medical College
Faridkot, Punjab, India

Seema Singhal
Additional Professor
Department of Obstetrics and Gynecology
All India Institute of Medical Sciences
New Delhi, India

Sharda Patra
Director–Professor
Department of Obstetrics and Gynecology
Lady Hardinge Medical College and
Smt Sucheta Kriplani Hospital
New Delhi, India

Sheela Mane
Professor
Department of Obstetrics and Gynecology
KC General Hospital
Bengaluru, Karnataka, India

Shikha Seth
Professor and Head
Department of Obstetrics and Gynecology
All India Institute of Medical Sciences
Gorakhpur, Uttar Pradesh, India

Shobha N Gudi
Professor and Head
Department of Obstetrics and Gynecology
St Philomena's Hospital
Bengaluru, Karnataka, India

Shreshtha Gupta
Associate Professor
Department of Obsterics and Gynecology
Maulana Azad Medical College and
Lok Nayak Hospital
New Delhi, India

Shristi Jaiswal
Assistant Professor
Department of Obstetrics and Gynecology
All India Institute of Medical Sciences
Gorakhpur, Uttar Pradesh, India

Shweta Prasad
Senior Resident
Department of Obstetrics and Gynecology
Lady Hardinge Medical College and
Smt Sucheta Kriplani Hospital
New Delhi, India

Sneh Yadav
Postgraduate Student
Department of Obstetrics and Gynecology
ESI-PGIMSR and Model Hospital
New Delhi, India

Sneha Bhuyar
AMOGS Chairperson, Medical Disorders
Committee (2022–2024)
IMA State Chairperson for Mission Pink Health
President, IMA Yavatmal

Suchandana Dasgupta
Senior Resident
Department of Obstetrics and Gynecology
Vardhman Mahavir Medical College
and Safdarjung Hospital
New Delhi, India

Supriya Kumari
Senior Resident
Department of Obstetrics and Gynecology
All India Institute of Medical Sciences
New Delhi, India

Vandana Agarwal
Assistant Professor
Department of Obstetrics and Gynecology
Atal Bihari Vajpayee Institute of Medical Sciences and Dr Ram Manohar Lohia Hospital
New Delhi, India

Vanisha Anand
Assistant Professor
Department of Obstetrics and Gynecology
Maharishi Markandeshwar Institute of Medical Sciences and Research
Mullana, Ambala, Haryana, India

Vidushi Tewari
Assistant Professor
Department of Obstetrics and Gynecology
Maharishi Markandeshwar Institute of Medical Sciences and Research
Mullana, Ambala, Haryana, India

Vidya A Thobbi
Professor and Head
Department of Obstetrics and Gynecology
Al-Ameen Medical College Hospital
Bijapur, Karnataka, India
President, KSOGA

Vinita Sinha
Assistant Professor
Department of Obstetrics and Gynecology
Nalanda Medical College and Hospital
Patna, Bihar, India

Vrunda Appannagari
Associate Consultant
Department of Fetal Medicine
Madhukar Rainbow Children's Hospital and BirthRight
Rainbow Hospitals
New Delhi, India

Zeba Khanam
Assistant Professor
Department of Obstetrics and Gynecology
Hamdard Institute of Medical Sciences and Research
Jamia Hamdard, New Delhi, India

Foreword

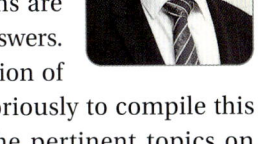

It gives me immense pride in writing the foreword for this book, *OSCE in Obstetrics & Gynecology.* I am confident this book will be a huge boon for the students as it is a one-of-a-kind textbook on this relatively new pattern of examination.

OSCE, i.e., Objectively Structured Clinical Examination questions are different in format from the traditional theory-based questions and answers. This pattern of examination mainly tests a student's clinical application of knowledge. Professor Ashok Kumar and his team have worked laboriously to compile this book. It is a very comprehensive textbook spanning almost all the pertinent topics on Obstetrics as well as Gynecology.

This textbook is in accord with the motto of FOGSI which is dissemination of updated knowledge and education in the ever-expanding science of Obstetrics and Gynecology. It is a unique bank of practically based OSCE questions and answers based on the latest clinical guidelines which contains elaborative information in a very reader-friendly colorful layout.

I am sure our students will enjoy reading this book and appear in their examinations with confidence and clarity.

Hrishikesh D Pai
President, FOGSI (2022–2023)

Foreword

It is a pleasure to have been asked to pen the foreword for this book, *OSCE in Obstetrics & Gynecology*. On behalf of the Indian College of Obstetricians & Gynecologists (ICOG), the academic wing of FOGSI, I congratulate all contributors. Just like medicine, the pattern of conducting examinations has also evolved with time. Objectively Structured Clinical Examination (OSCE) questions are the latest format of testing a student's clinical application of knowledge.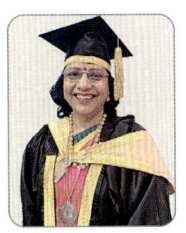

I endorse this book with great pride as it is one of the very few textbooks based purely on the OSCE format of questions and answers. It is a very well-designed book targeted mainly for undergraduate as well as postgraduate students to guide them during their preparation. The chapters are written in a comprehensive, yet lucid style. The 49 chapters comprise of clinically relevant questions along with a plethora of image-based questions, color plates of instruments, specimens, and radiology pictures.

The esteemed authors from across the nation have poured their hard work into drafting each chapter with updated and precise content using their vast knowledge and experience. I am confident that this textbook will be a great asset to the undergraduate as well as postgraduate aspirants in enhancing their knowledge towards academic excellence.

Laxmi Shrikhande
Chairperson, ICOG (2022–2023)

Preface

Various Entrance and Exit examinations process has evolved with time. Now OSCE (Objectively Structured Clinical Examination) is accepted as a standard tool of examination for both the undergraduate as well as postgraduate examinations. However, there is a dearth of standard textbooks based on this relatively new pattern of examination, to guide students.

This paucity of a comprehensive textbook on OSCE has inspired the genesis of this book. It is a unique amalgamation of the endeavors of our country's esteemed faculty from across the nation. It comprises of various chapters spanning a wide array of topics of both obstetrics as well as gynecology. The contributors in their specific field of expertise have worked laboriously and each chapter has been designed systematically and each station has been formulated to provide practically relevant and important questions along with their answers. The authors have used their wide array of knowledge and vast experience as clinicians and teachers to formulate the questions in a manner which would be accepted globally. OSCE questions based on history taking, clinical examination, investigations, management, and counseling have been included. The principles of patient management are in accordance with the standard clinical guidelines. Images and photographs have been included amply as they comprise an essential component of this new pattern of examination and students are expected to identify them. References for additional reading have also been provided.

This book has been primarily written for undergraduate and postgraduate students to guide them in their preparation for their professional examinations. However, it will be a very handy and informative bank of knowledge, especially on the practical and clinical aspects of obstetrics and gynecology for all practitioners as well.

We hope this book serves its purpose of guiding the students to help them ace their OSCE with ease and confidence.

Happy Learning

Ashok Kumar
Vandana Agarwal

Acknowledgments

At the outset, we would like to extend our sincere gratitude to President, FOGSI, Dr Hrishikesh D Pai and ICOG, Chairperson, Dr Laxmi Shrikhande for giving us the responsibility of one of its kind books on OSCE Stations. We thank them for their continuous guidance and support.

The completion of this textbook has been possible owing to the hard work of numerous teachers across the country. First and foremost, we would like to acknowledge and express our thanks to all the esteemed authors who have carved out time and contributed so meticulously.

We would like to thank Dr Nidhi Dahiya, Atal Bihari Vajpayee Institute of Medical Sciences and Dr Ram Manohar Lohia Hospital, New Delhi, India, for helping us throughout the process of compiling this book.

We would also like to extend our gratitude to Shri Jitendar P Vij (Group Chairman), Mr Ankit Vij (Managing Director), and MS Mani (Group President), Ms Chetna Malhotra (Senior Director—Professional Publishing, Marketing and Business Development), and Ms Himani Pandey (Development Editor), for their help and assistance in completing the project within the time frame.

Ashok Kumar
Vandana Agarwal

Contents

SECTION 1
OBSTETRICS

1. **Physiological Changes During Pregnancy** 3
   Abha Rani Sinha, Vinita Sinha, Bhawana Tiwary

2. **Fetal Skull and Maternal Pelvis** 15
   Alka Pandey

3. **Ultrasound in First and Second Trimester** 47
   Archana Baser

4. **First Trimester Screening and Ultrasound Markers** 66
   Chinmayee Ratha

5. **Congenital Malformations in Fetus** 73
   Chanchal Singh, Vrunda Appannagari

6. **Labor** 88
   Hem Kanta Sarma

7. **Abnormal Labor** 101
   Pratik Tambe, Deepali Kale, Jyotsna S Dwivedi

8. **Preterm Labor** 127
   Haresh U Doshi

9. **Hyperemesis Gravidarum** 137
   Bharti Maheshwari

10. **Anemia in Pregnancy** 143
    Kiran Pandey, Pavika Lal

11. **Hypertensive Disorders in Pregnancy** 156
    Charmila Ayyavoo

12. **Heart Disease in Pregnancy** 170
    Deepa Lokwani Masand

13. **Hyperglycemia in Pregnancy** 186
    Hafizur Rahman, Vandana Agarwal, Sayanti Paul

14. **Rh-Negative Pregnancy** 196
    K Deepthi D Nair

15. **Multiple Pregnancy** 209
    Mala Srivastava

16. **Liver Disease in Pregnancy** 220
    Sarita Bhalerao, Latika Chawla, Ashwin Shetty, Kausha Shah

17. **HIV in Pregnancy** 226
    Sheela Mane, Radhika MS

18. **Fetal Growth Restriction** 233
    Pushpa Junghare

19. **Antepartum Hemorrhage** 244
    Jaya Chawla

20. **Pregnancy beyond Expected Date of Delivery** 257
    Indu Lata

21. **Postpartum Hemorrhage** 269
    *Ruby Bhatia, Sanjum Yasmin Malik, Vidushi Tewari, Vanisha Anand,
    Darryl Gibson Edwin*

22. **Obstetric Critical Care** 302
    Jyotsna Suri, Suchandana Dasgupta

23. **Maternal and Neonatal Health Programs** 319
    Aruna Nigam, Zeba Khanam

24. **Abortion** 330
    Shobha N Gudi

25. **Recurrent Pregnancy Loss (I)** 344
    K Aparna Sharma, Richa Vatsa

26. **Recurrent Pregnancy Loss (II)** 352
    Sneha Bhuyar

27. **Bad Obstetric History** 358
    Juhi Bharti, Supriya Kumari, Akanksha Gupta

28. **Contraception** 365
    Pikee Saxena, Shweta Prasad

SECTION 2
GYNECOLOGY

29. **Pediatric and Adolescent Gynecology** 387
    Mukta Agarwal

30. **Abnormal Uterine Bleeding** 395
    Sharda Patra

31. **Endometriosis (I)** 407
    Ashis Kumar Mukhopadhyay

32. **Endometriosis (II)** 416
    Juhi Bharti, Vandana Agarwal

33. **Ectopic Pregnancy** 422
    Sandhya Jain, Pooja Sharma

34. **Uterine Fibroid** 433
    Jai Bhagwan Sharma, Richa Vatsa

35. **Genitourinary Infections and STDs** 444
    Niharika Dhiman, Shreshtha Gupta

36. **Pelvic Inflammatory Disease** 454
    Leena Wadhwa, Sneh Yadav, Deval Rishi Pandit

37. **Polycystic Ovarian Syndrome** 469
    Seema Grover

38. **Pelvic Organ Prolapse (I)** 479
    Panchanan Das

39. **Pelvic Organ Prolapse (II)** 488
    Reena Wani, Krutika Ramdin

40. **Reproductive Medicine and Surgery** 501
    Fessy Louis T

41. **Amenorrhea** 517
    Vidya A Thobbi

42. **Endometrial Carcinoma** 526
    Seema Singhal, Saroj Rajan

43. **Cervical Carcinoma** 537
    Kasturi V Donimath

44. **Gestational Trophoblastic Neoplasia** 550
    Neha Mishra

45. **Hysterectomy** 566
    Nilanchali Singh, Nisha, Deepika Kashyap

46. **Menopause** 575
    Madhavi M Gupta, Ankita Chonla

47. **Urinary Incontinence and Vesicovaginal Fistula** 581
    Ajit Kumar Nayak

48. **Gynecological Endoscopy** 591
    Aswath Kumar

49. **Infertility** 597
    Shikha Seth, Shristi Jaiswal

Index *621*

SECTION 1

Obstetrics

1. **Physiological Changes During Pregnancy**
   Abha Rani Sinha, Vinita Sinha, Bhawana Tiwary
2. **Fetal Skull and Maternal Pelvis**
   Alka Pandey
3. **Ultrasound in First and Second Trimester**
   Archana Baser
4. **First Trimester Screening and Ultrasound Markers**
   Chinmayee Ratha
5. **Congenital Malformations in Fetus**
   Chanchal Singh, Vrunda Appannagari
6. **Labor**
   Hem Kanta Sarma
7. **Abnormal Labor**
   Pratik Tambe, Deepali Kale, Jyotsna S Dwivedi
8. **Preterm Labor**
   Haresh U Doshi
9. **Hyperemesis Gravidarum**
   Bharti Maheshwari
10. **Anemia in Pregnancy**
    Kiran Pandey, Pavika Lal
11. **Hypertensive Disorders in Pregnancy**
    Charmila Ayyavoo
12. **Heart Disease in Pregnancy**
    Deepa Lokwani Masand
13. **Hyperglycemia in Pregnancy**
    Hafizur Rahman, Vandana Agarwal, Sayanti Paul
14. **Rh-Negative Pregnancy**
    K Deepthi D Nair
15. **Multiple Pregnancy**
    Mala Srivastava
16. **Liver Disease in Pregnancy**
    Sarita Bhalerao, Latika Chawla, Ashwin Shetty, Kausha Shah
17. **HIV in Pregnancy**
    Sheela Mane, Radhika MS
18. **Fetal Growth Restriction**
    Pushpa Junghare
19. **Antepartum Hemorrhage**
    Jaya Chawla
20. **Pregnancy beyond Expected Date of Delivery**
    Indu Lata
21. **Postpartum Hemorrhage**
    Ruby Bhatia, Sanjum Yasmin Malik, Vidushi Tewari, Vanisha Anand, Darryl Gibson Edwin
22. **Obstetric Critical Care**
    Jyotsna Suri, Suchandana Dasgupta
23. **Maternal and Neonatal Health Programs**
    Aruna Nigam, Zeba Khanam
24. **Abortion**
    Shobha N Gudi
25. **Recurrent Pregnancy Loss (I)**
    K Aparna Sharma, Richa Vatsa
26. **Recurrent Pregnancy Loss (II)**
    Sneha Bhuyar
27. **Bad Obstetric History**
    Juhi Bharti, Supriya Kumari, Akanksha Gupta
28. **Contraception**
    Pikee Saxena, Shweta Prasad

CHAPTER 1
Physiological Changes During Pregnancy

Abha Rani Sinha, Vinita Sinha, Bhawana Tiwary

OSCE 1.

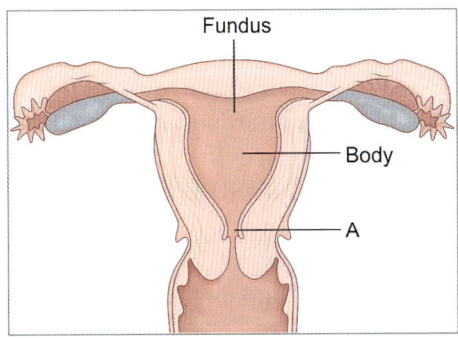

1. Label the point A.
2. What is the length of A in nonpregnant woman?
3. Name the structure that it forms in pregnancy?
4. Mention any two importance of lower uterine segment in pregnancy?

Ans.

1. Point A—uterine isthmus.
2. Length in nonpregnant state is 0.5 cm.
3. The uterine isthmus forms lower uterine segment in pregnancy.
4. Importance of lower uterine segment in pregnancy:
   - Cesarean section is performed at this site.
   - Implantation of placenta here is known as placenta previa.

OSCE 2.

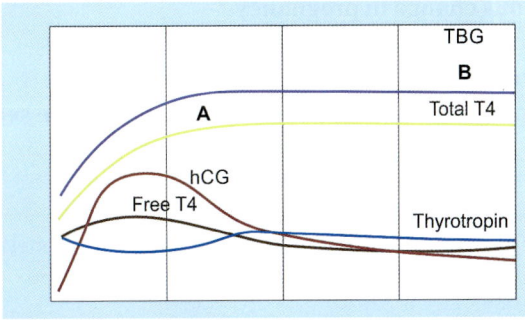

Section 1: Obstetrics

1. Label points A, B.
2. Mention four changes in thyroid gland in pregnancy.
3. Mention any two fetal complications due to deficiency of hormone B.
4. What is the normal range of thyroid stimulating hormone in pregnant women in the three trimesters?
5. Mention changes in T3 and T4 concentration in pregnancy.

Ans.

1. A—hCG, B—total T4.
2. Four changes in thyroid gland:
   a. Hyperplasia of thyroid gland
   b. TSH level declines in first trimester.
   c. TBG level increases and reaches zenith at 20 weeks.
   d. TSH receptors are cross-stimulated by massive quantities of hCG.
3. IUGR, fetal hypothyroidism, stillbirth, abortion, and mental retardation.
4. Normal range of TSH (FOGSI) in Pregnancy
   a. *Pregnancy in first trimester:* Up to 2.5 mIU/L
   b. *Second trimester:* Up to 3 mIU/L
   c. *Third trimester:* Up to 3 mIU/L
5. Elevated TBG level increases total T3 and total T4 concentration but does not affect free T3 and T4.

OSCE 3.

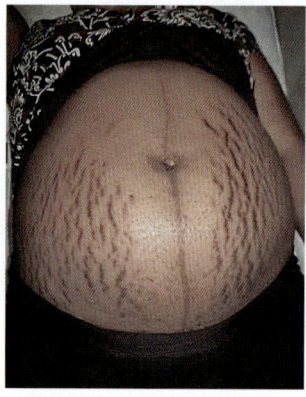

1. Identify the cutaneous change in pregnancy.
2. Name two other cutaneous changes in pregnancy.
3. What is the hormone responsible for these changes?
4. Name any two nonpregnant conditions in which striae can be seen.

Ans.

1. Linea nigra with striae gravidarum.
2. Pregnancy mask (chloasma), spider angioma, Linea nigra, striae gravidarum, breast changes, palmar erythema.

Chapter 1: Physiological Changes During Pregnancy

3. Melanocyte-stimulating hormone (Estrogen and progesterone also have MSH effect).
4. Obesity and Cushing's syndrome.

OSCE 4.

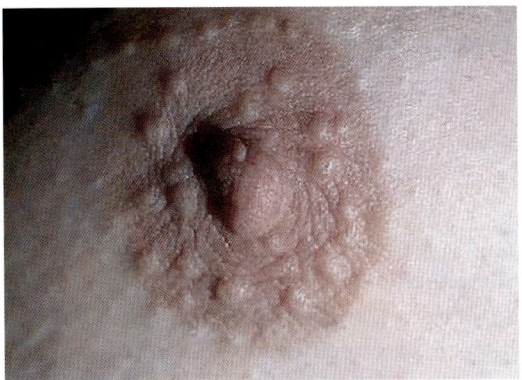

1. Identify the changes in breast during pregnancy.
2. What are modified sebaceous glands of breast called?
3. What is the function of these sebaceous glands?
4. When does colostrum first appear in pregnancy?

Ans.
1. Increase in size of breast, hyperpigmentation of nipple areola complex, Montgomery tubercles, secondary areola.
2. Montogomery tubercles.
3. Their secretion keeps nipple and areola moist and healthy.
4. At 12 weeks.

OSCE 5.
1. What is the normal creatinine level in pregnancy?
2. Give two reasons why GFR increases in pregnancy?
3. Why does nocturia occur in pregnancy?
4. Give three reasons for right urethral dilatation more than left in pregnancy.

Ans.
1. <0.9 mg/dL
2. a. Hypervolemia-induced hemodilution.
   b. Increased renal plasma flow.
3. During day pregnant women accumulate water as edema. At night in recumbent position, this is mobilized with diuresis.
4. a. Cushioning provided to the left ureter by sigmoid colon.
   b. Dextrorotation of uterus compressing right ureter.
   c. Markedly dilated right ovarian vein complex lying over right ureter.
   d. Markedly dilated right ovarian vein complex lying over right ureter.

OSCE 6.

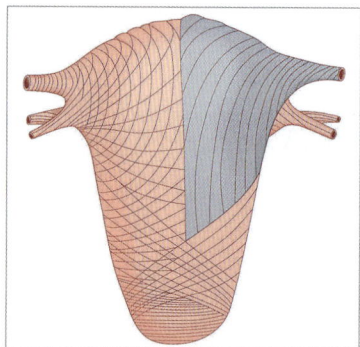

1. What is this specific arrangement of uterine musculature called?
2. What is the advantage of this arrangement of muscle fibers?
3. Mention the three different arrangements of uterine musculature in pregnancy.

Ans.

1. Pinard's living ligature.
2. Prevention of PPH.
3. Uterine musculature is arranged in three strata:
   a. Outer hood-like layer which arches over fundus and extends into various ligaments.
   b. Middle layer is dense network of muscles fibers perforated in all directions by blood vessel.
   c. Internal layer with sphincter-like fibers around fallopian tube and cervical os.

OSCE 7.

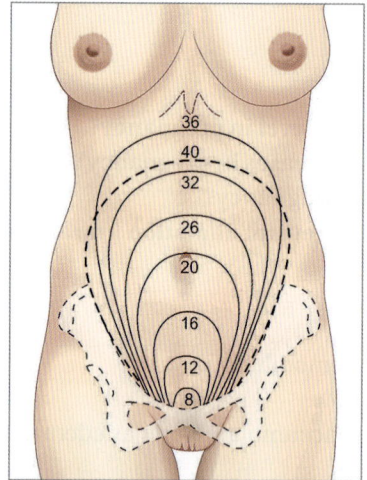

1. When is uterus palpable per abdominally?
2. What is the rate of increment of symphysiofundal height and abdominal girth?
3. Name two conditions in which symphysiofundal height is more than period of gestation?

Ans.
1. At 12 weeks.
2. *Rate of increment:* Symphysiofundal height after 24 weeks the SFH measured in cm corresponds to weeks of pregnancy up to 36 weeks with +/− 2 cm. Abdominal girth 1 cm per week in 2nd trimester and up to 36 weeks.
3. Wrong LMP, macrosomia, hydatidiform mole, polyhydramnios, multiple pregnancy, concealed accidental hemorrhage, pelvic tumor.

OSCE 8.

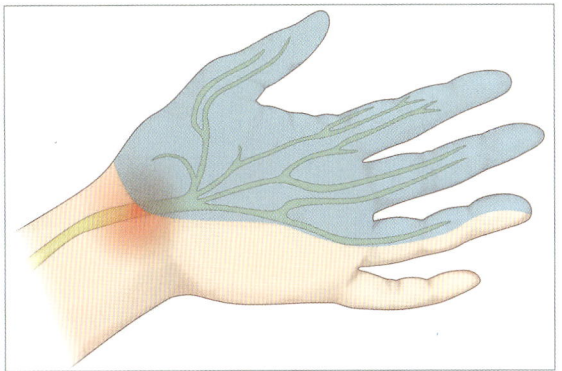

1. Identify this ailment of pregnancy.
2. Name the nerve involved in this condition.
3. What will be the presenting complain?

Ans.
1. Carpel tunnel syndrome.
2. Median nerve.
3. Numbness, pain, paresthesia in hands and arms in thumb, index, and middle finger and partly in ring finger.

OSCE 9.

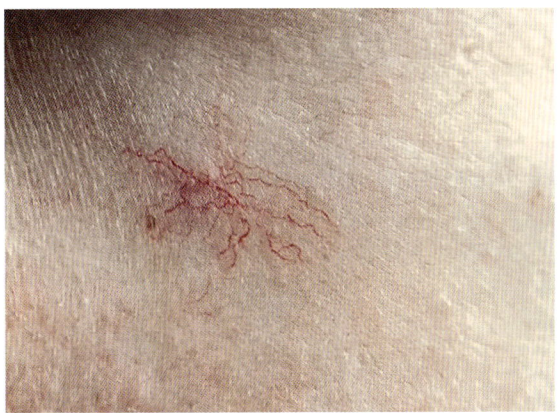

Section 1: Obstetrics

A primigravida comes to ANC OPD during her first trimester. She complains of having these red patches on her chest. She is afebrile and does not have any other complain.
1. Identify this lesion.
2. Mention the hormone responsible for these lesions.
3. Name any two nonpregnant conditions in which similar lesions can be seen.
4. Do these lesions leave any scar? (yes/no)

Ans.

1. Spider angioma.
2. Estrogen.
3. Liver cirrhosis, thyrotoxicosis, rheumatoid arthritis.
4. No.

OSCE 10.

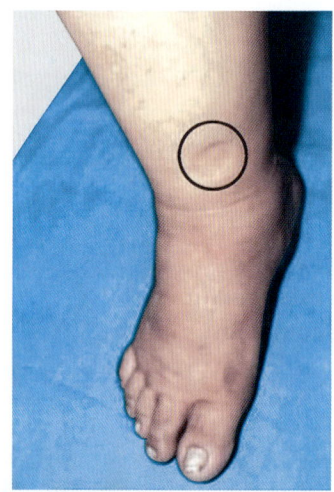

1. Identify this condition in pregnancy.
2. What are the causes for this condition in pregnancy?
3. How will you differentiate between physiological and pathological edema in pregnancy?

Ans.

1. Edema in pregnancy.
2. a. Physiological.
   b. *Pathological:* Pre-eclampsia, severe anemia, heart failure, nephrotic syndrome.
3. Physiological edema is usually bilateral, subsides on rest alone with limb elevation, and is not associated with any other feature of pre-eclampsia or proteinuria.

OSCE 11.

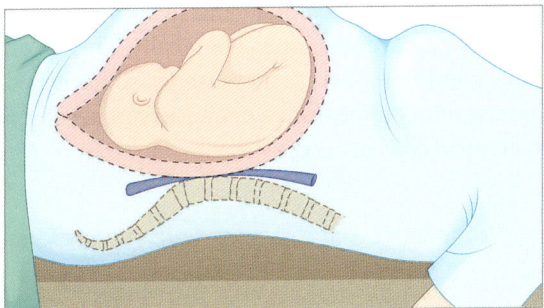

1. What could be the possible diagnosis?
2. What is the underlying physiology for this condition?
3. What are the symptoms of this syndrome?

Ans.

1. Supine hypotension syndrome.
2. When gravid uterus produces compression effect on inferior vena cava and aorta (aortocaval), when patient lies in supine position. This leads to decreased venous return to heart.
3. Hypotension, tachycardia, syncope, vomiting, dizziness, sweating.

OSCE 12.

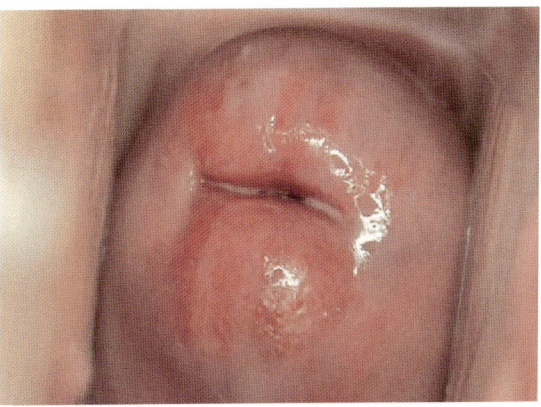

1. Identify the picture in pregnancy.
2. Mention four cervical changes occurring in pregnancy.
3. What is ferning?
4. Why is pap test evaluation difficult in pregnancy?

Ans.

1. Cervical eversion of pregnancy.
2. Increased vascularity, increased edema, hypertrophy and hyperplasia of cervical gland, eversion.

3. Due to the effect of progesterone, cervical mucus when spread and dried on a glass slide, shows poor crystallization termed "beading" and in some due to amniotic fluid leakage arborization of ice-like crystals are seen microscopically. This is called "ferning".
4. Due to hyperestrogenic condition, there is increased vascularity, edema and hypertrophy, hyperplasia and hypersecretory appearance of endocervical cells, which makes it difficult to differentiate from atypical cells of cervix.

OSCE 13.

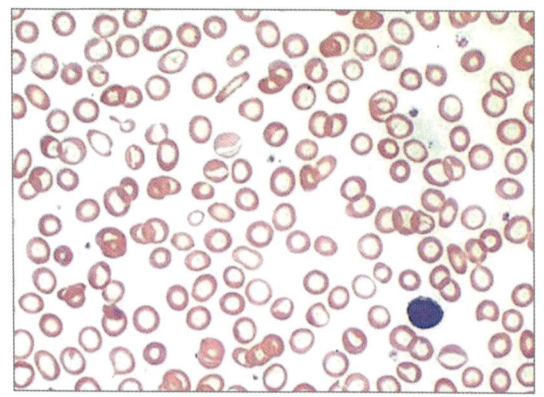

(Hb 8.4 g/dL, MCV 70, MCH 24, MCHC 28, HCT 28)

1. Identify the peripheral blood smear.
2. Mention any two causes of this peripheral smear.
3. Mention any two reasons for physiological anemia of pregnancy.
4. What is the WHO cut-off for anemia in pregnancy?

Ans.

1. Hypochromic microcytic anemia.
2. Iron deficiency anemia, thalassemia.
3. Hemodilution in pregnancy, negative iron balance.
4. *WHO cut-off for anemia in pregnancy:* Hb <11 g/dL.

OSCE 14.

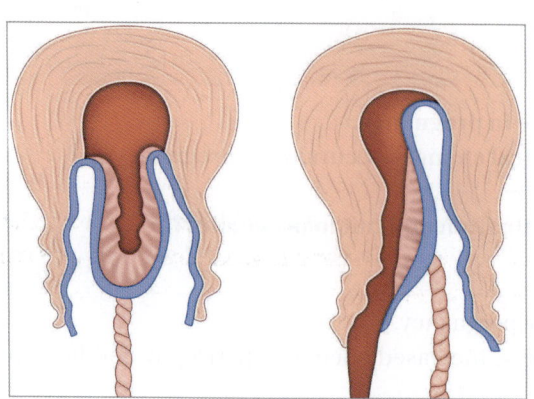

1. Identify the process.
2. What is the normal site for attachment of placenta?
3. Mention four structural abnormalities of placenta.
4. What are the two methods of placental separation?
5. What is the plane of cleavage of placental separation?

Ans.

1. Fundal attachment
2. Anterior and posterior walls.
3. Spuriata, bilobate, succenturiate, extrachorialis (circumvallate, circummarginate), velamentous cord insertion.
4. Schultz method, Duncan method.
5. Through decidua spongiosa.

OSCE 15.

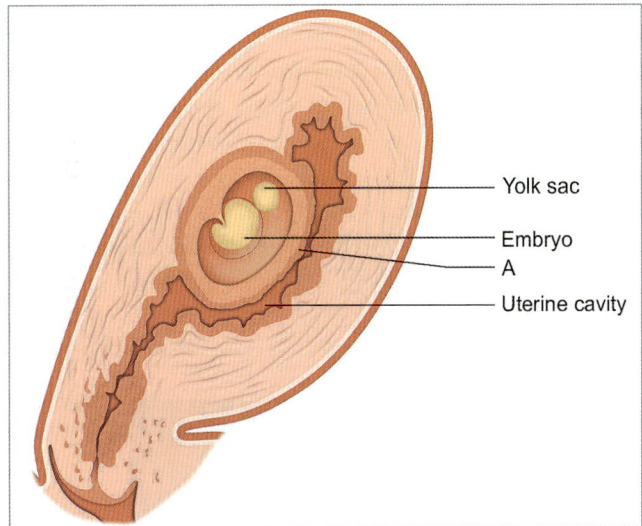

1. Identify layer A of pregnant uterus.
2. Name the four types of decidua.
3. What is Nitabuch's layer?
4. Name two components of zona functionalis.

Ans.

1. Decidua Capsularis
2. Decidua basalis, Decidua parietalis, Decidua capsularis, and Decidua vera
3. It is a zone of fibrinoid degeneration where trophoblasts meet the decidua basalis.
4. Zona functionalis, Zona basalis

Section 1: Obstetrics

OSCE 16.

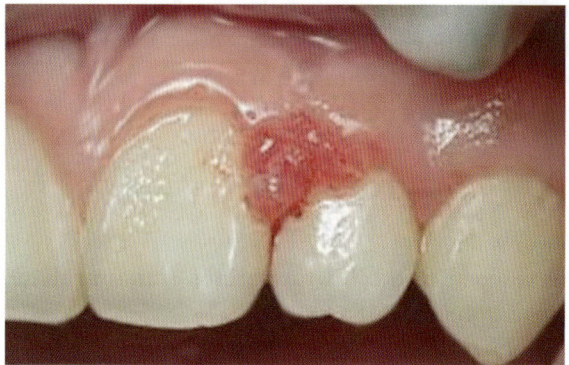

1. Identify this condition.
2. Which vitamin supplementation can prevent this condition from occurring in pregnancy?
3. What is Epulis gravidarum?
4. What is the usual course of Epulis gravidarum?

Ans.

1. Gingivitis of pregnancy
2. Vitamin C
3. Epulis gravidarum is a tumor-like enlargement of gingival or alveolar mucosa which generally occurs in the second or third trimester.
4. It usually regresses 1–2 months after delivery.

OSCE 17.

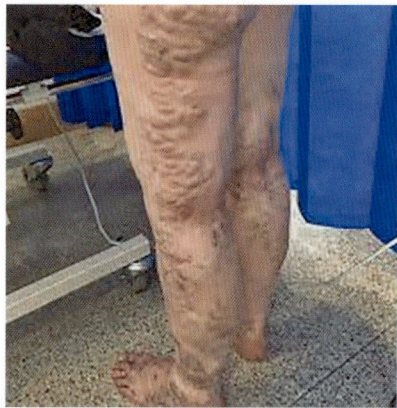

1. Identify this condition.
2. What causes the increased incidence of this condition in pregnancy?

Ans.

1. Varicose veins.

2. Increased level of progesterone in pregnancy causes dilatation of blood vessels wall and decreased valve function. Moreover, increased blood volume also increases the likelihood of varicose veins in pregnancy.

OSCE 18.

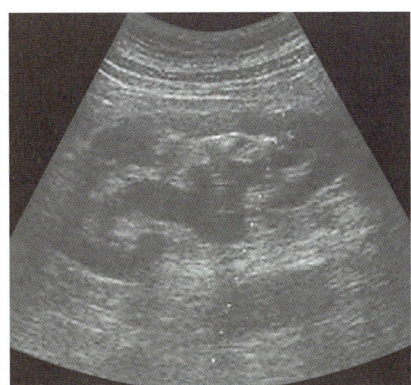

1. Identify this ultrasound image.
2. What happens to size of kidney in pregnancy and by how much is this change?
3. What is asymptomatic bacteriuria of pregnancy?
4. By what percentage GFR (Glomerular Filtration Rate) increase in pregnancy?

Ans.

1. Dilated pelvicalyceal system
2. Each kidney increases in length by 1-1.5 cm in pregnancy along with a concomitant increase in its weight.
3. Asymptomatic bacteriuria is defined as a quantitative count of >10⁸ colony forming units/liter in the absence of symptoms.
4. 50% increase in GFR occurs in pregnancy.

OSCE 19.

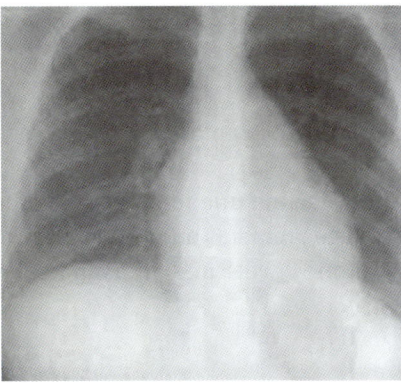

1. What is the finding being depicted in the above chest X-ray taken in pregnancy?
2. By how much does the cardiac capacity change in pregnancy?

3. By what percentage size of heart change in pregnancy?
4. Mention the changes in cardiac output and heart rate in pregnancy.

Ans.

1. Apparent cardiomegaly on chest X-ray as the heart is displaced upwards and to the left with rotation on its long axis.
2. Cardiac capacity increases by 70–80 mL in pregnancy.
3. Size of heart increases by 12% in pregnancy.
4. Cardiac output increases by 30–35% and heart rate increases by 20% in pregnancy over nonpregnant levels.

OSCE 20.

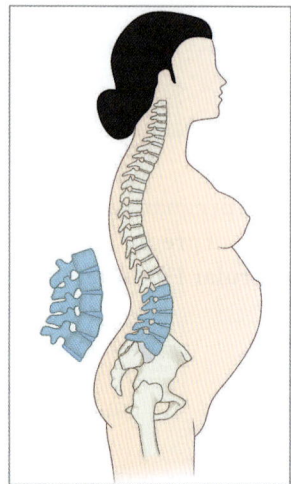

1. Identify this posture in pregnancy.
2. What causes this postural change in pregnancy?
3. Mention the changes in calcium metabolism in pregnancy.
4. What change occurs in parathyroid hormone and phosphate in pregnancy?

Ans.

1. Lordosis of pregnancy.
2. It occurs due to progressive increase in anterior convexity of the lumbar spine, preserving center of gravity.
3. Maternal total calcium levels decline due to decreased albumin bound concentration. The serum ionized level, however, remains unchanged.
4. Maternal parathyroid hormone levels and phosphate levels remain unchanged in pregnancy.

CHAPTER 2

Fetal Skull and Maternal Pelvis

Alka Pandey

OSCE 1.
1. What are the boundaries of fetal vertex?
2. Name the sutures present in fetal skull.
3. How do you differentiate between anterior and posterior fontanelle?
4. How many bones are present in fetal skull?
5. Where is the vacuum cup applied on the fetal skull?

Ans.

1. Vertex is a quadrangular area bounded anteriorly by the bregma and coronal sutures behind by the lambda and lambdoid sutures and laterally by lines passing through the parietal eminences.

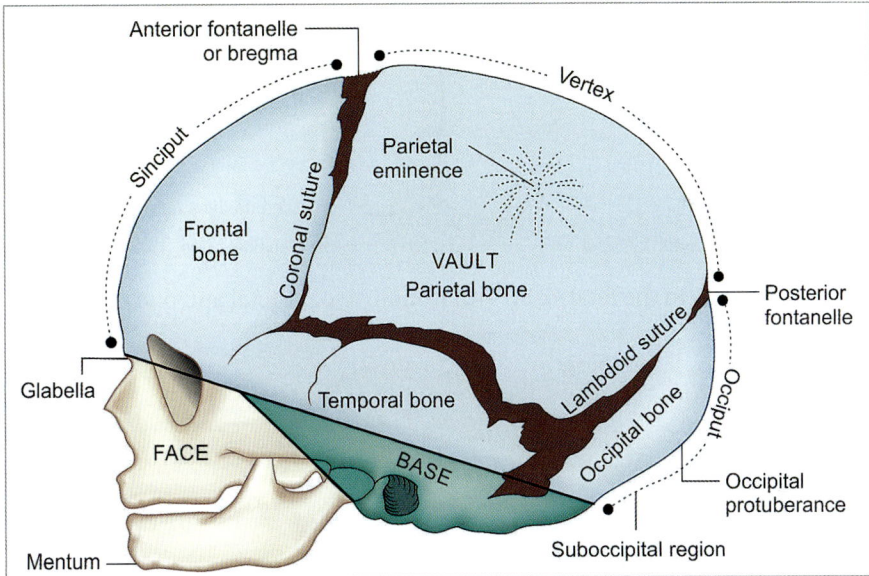

2. Sutures names:
   - The sagittal or longitudinal suture
   - The coronal sutures
   - The frontal suture
   - The lambdoid sutures

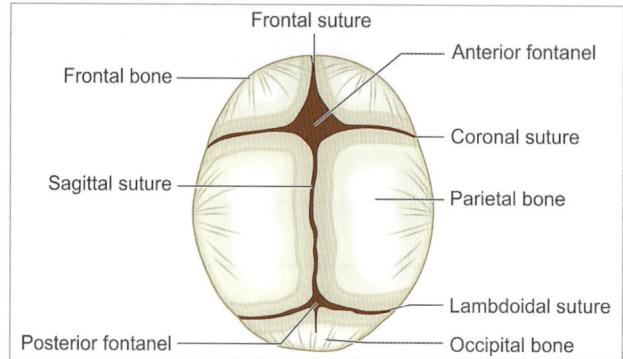

3. a. *Anterior fontanelle:* It is formed by joining of the four sutures in the midplane. The sutures are anteriorly frontal, posteriorly sagittal and on either side coronal. Its anteroposterior and transverse diameter are 3 cm. The floor is formed by a membrane which ossifies at 18 months after birth.
   b. *Posterior fontanelle:* Formed by junction of three sutures, anteriorly sagittal suture and lambdoid sutures on either side. It is triangular in shape and measures 1.2 × 1.2 cm. Its floor becomes bony at term.

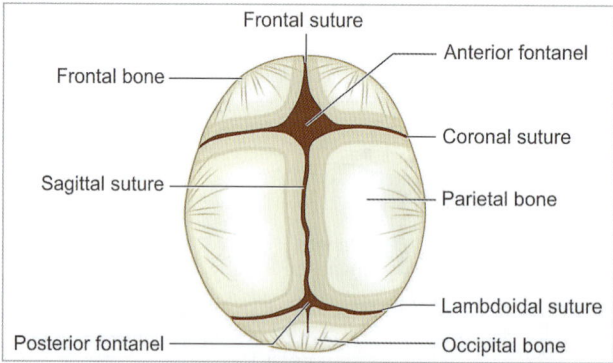

4. There are five bones in the fetal skull. Two frontal, two parietal and one occipital.

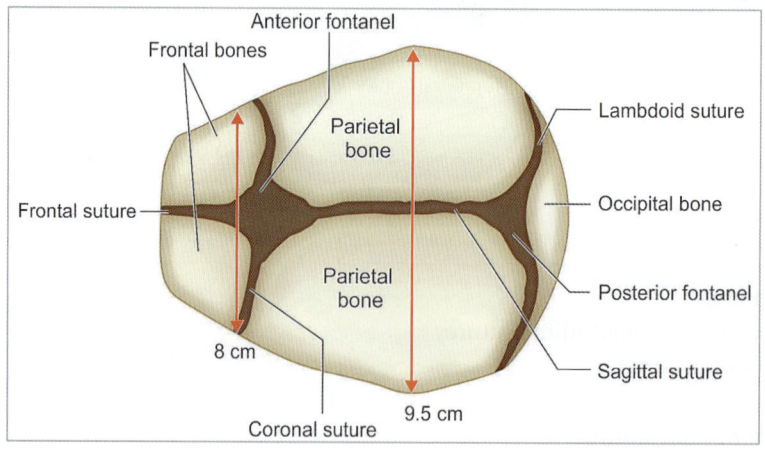

5. The vacuum cup is applied midsagittal about 6 cm from the center of the anterior fontanelle or 3 cm in front of posterior fontanelle.

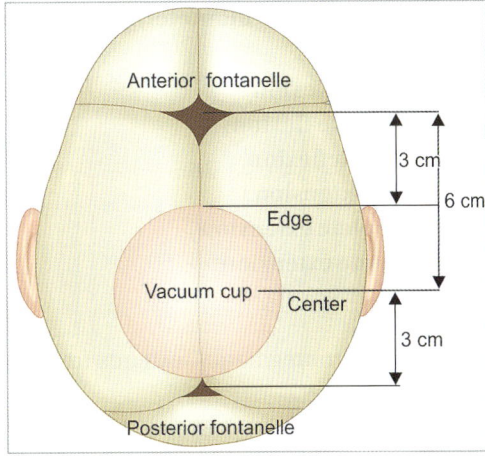

OSCE 2.

1. **Name and give the diameters of the followings:**
   - **Biparietal diameter**
   - **Bitemporal**
   - **Bimastoid**
   - **Super subparietal diameter**
   - **Smallest circumference of the fetal skull**

Ans.

1. In the suboccipitobregmatic plane, the circumference of the head is 32–34 cm:

Transverse diameters of the fetal skull.		
Biparietal diameter	9.5 cm	Between the 2 parietal eminences
Bitemporal diameter	8.5 cm	
Bimastoid diameter	7.5 cm	Between the 2 mastoid processes (Not reducible nor destroyable even by destructive procedures
Supra-subparietal	8.25–9 cm	Asynclitic head

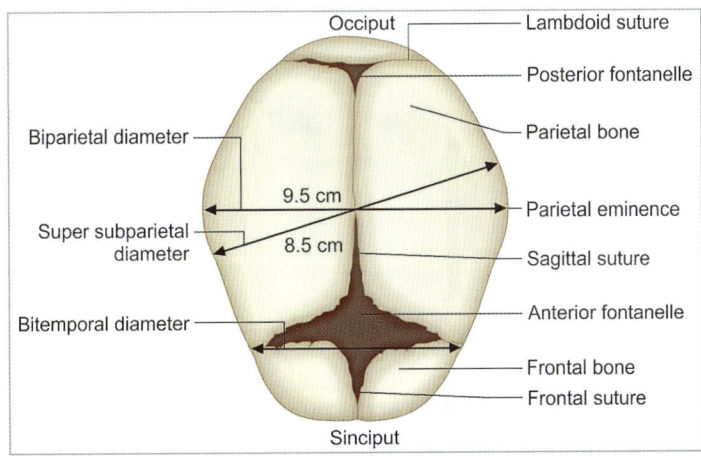

OSCE 3. Name the diameter, presentation, and measurement of the head in different attitudes:
1. Complete flexion
2. Incomplete flexion
3. Marked deflexion
4. Partial extension
5. Incomplete extension
6. Complete extension

Ans.

1. Suboccipitobregmatic—extends from the nape of the neck to the center of the bregma—9.5 cm, vertex.
2. Suboccipitofrontal—extends from the nape of the neck to the anterior end of the anterior fontanel or center of the sinciput—10 cm, vertex.
3. Occipitofrontal—extends from the occipital eminence to the root of the nose (glabella)—11.5 cm.
4. Mentovertical—extends from the midpoint of the chin to the highest point on sagittal suture—14 cm, brow.
5. Submentovertical—extends from junction of floor of the mouth and neck to the highest point on the sagittal suture—11.5 cm, face.
6. Submentobregmatic—extends from junction of floor of the mouth and neck to the center of the bregma—9.5 cm, face.

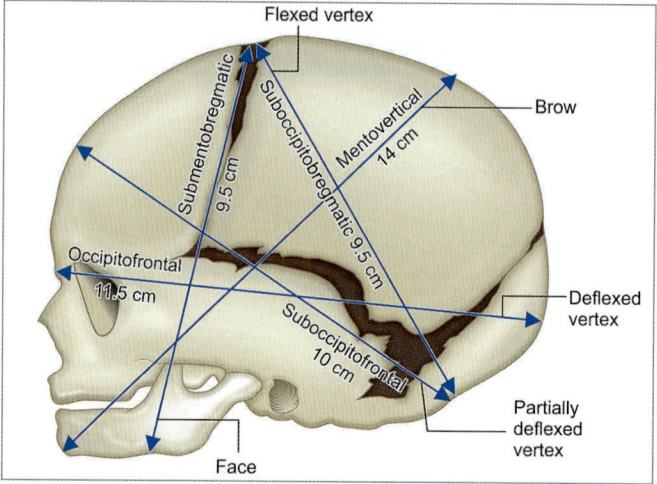

OSCE 4.
1. What is moulding?
2. What are the types of moulding?
3. Is moulding normal?
4. What is the effect of severe moulding of the fetal head?
5. How long does moulding persist after birth?

Ans.

1. Alteration in the shape of forecoming head while passing through resistant birth passage during labor causing compression of engaging diameter of the head with corresponding elongation of the diameter at right angle.

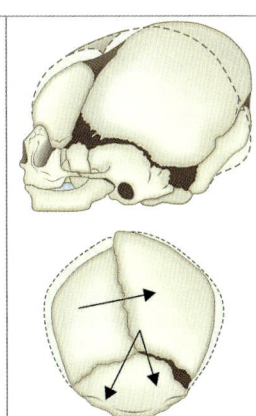

Moulding....
- Reshaping of the fetal skull:
  - Obliteration of the sutures
  - Overlapping of the bones of the vault:
    × One parietal bone overlaps the other
    × Both overlap the occipital bone
- It accounts for diminution of the biparietal diameter and suboccipitobregmatic diameters by 0.5–1 cm or even more

2. Types of moulding:
   - Sutures apposed—degree 1
   - Sutures overlapped but—reducible—degree 2
   - Sutures overlapped—irreducible—degree 3

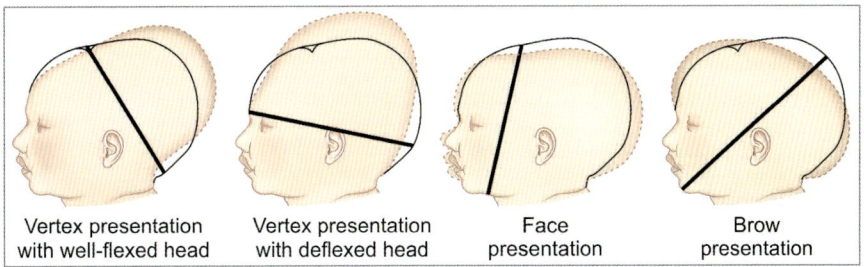

| Vertex presentation with well-flexed head | Vertex presentation with deflexed head | Face presentation | Brow presentation |

3. Slight moulding is beneficial as it enables the head to pass more easily through the birth canal.
4. Extreme degree of moulding in severe disproportion may lead to tear of tentorium cerebelli or subdural hemorrhage.
5. Moulding disappears in few hours after birth

OSCE 5.
1. **What is caput?**
2. **What is the importance of caput?**
3. **How long does it persist?**
4. **What is the treatment?**
5. **What is the difference between caput and cephalohematoma?**

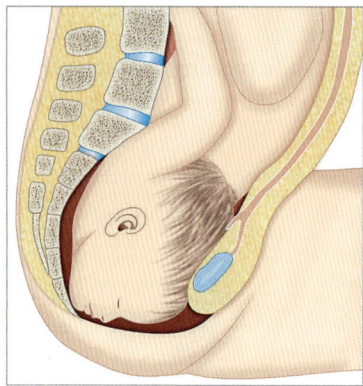
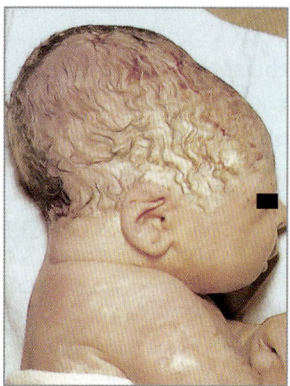

Ans.

1. Stagnation of fluid in the layers of the scalp beneath the girdle of contact gives rise to a swelling known as caput.
2. Static position of the head for long period of time causes it. It gives an idea about the position of head and degree of flexion achieved in the pelvis in left position the caput is situated on right parietal bone and vice versa. With increasing flexion, the caput is placed more posteriorly.
3. Caput disappears spontaneously within 24 hours after birth.
4. It is harmless and needs no treatment.
5. Caput is not limited by suture line and is present at birth. Cephalohematoma is not present at birth, it slowly appears after 12–24 hours. Cephalohematoma is limited by the suture line of the skull as the pericranium is fixed to the margins of the bone. cephalohematoma takes 6–8 weeks to resolve whereas caput disappears in few days.

OSCE 6.

1. Identify this condition.
2. What are the risk factors for this condition?
3. It is common in which gender?
4. How is it diagnosed?
5. What is prevention and management?

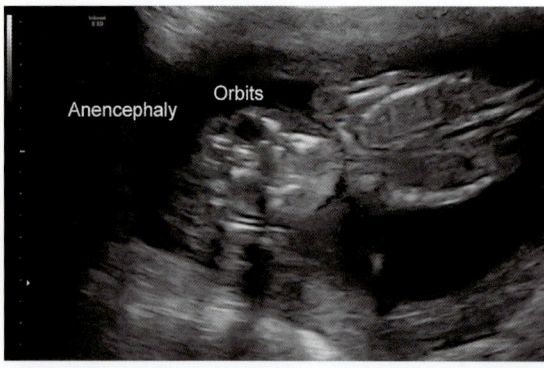
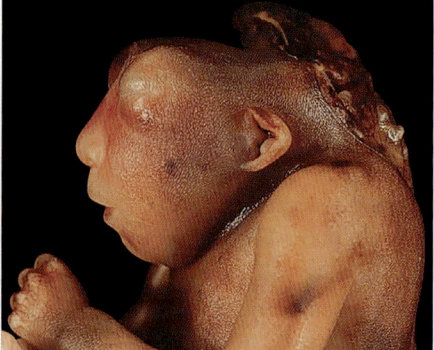

Chapter 2: Fetal Skull and Maternal Pelvis

Ans.
1. This is anencephaly. This results from deficient development of vault of the skull and brain tissue.
2. Risk factors:
   - Folic acid (vitamin B_9) deficiency before and during pregnancy.
   - High heat exposure during pregnancy, such as having a fever or using a hot tub or sauna.
   - Certain medications that treat seizures, migraine headaches and bipolar disorder.
   - Opioid use during pregnancy.
3. 70% of anencephalic fetuses are females.
4. Anencephaly may be diagnosed during pregnancy through a routine ultrasound or blood screening. Pregnancies involving anencephaly produce high levels of a specific fetal protein called alpha-fetoprotein.
5. *Prevention and management:* It is not always possible to prevent anencephaly. 400 mcg of folic acid daily may reduce the chances of anencephaly. If diagnosed before 20 weeks the pregnancy should be terminated.

OSCE 7.
1. **What is this condition?**
2. **What findings are there on USG?**
3. **What are the causes?**
4. **How do you diagnose it clinically?**
5. **What is the prognosis?**

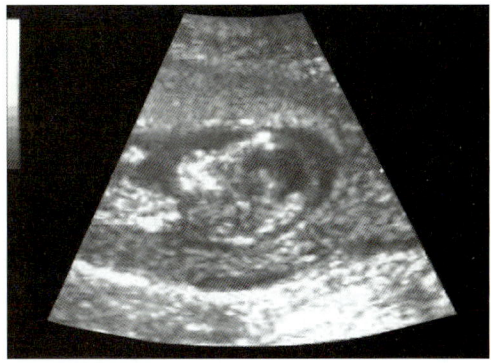

Ans.
1. This is hydrocephalus

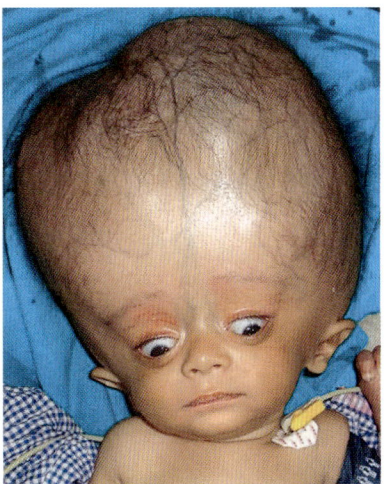

2. On USG, a diameter ≥15 mm confirms a diagnosis of fetal hydrocephalus, but lateral ventricular diameters of between 10 and 14 mm should also arouse suspicion of fetal hydrocephalus. Vault bones are thinner. A separation of 3 mm or more of the choroid plexus from the ventricular wall is another indication of hydrocephalus/ventriculomegaly. Lateral and third ventricles are dilated with marked thinning of cerebral cortex.
3. Hydrocephalus may be congenital or acquired. The most common causes of *congenital hydrocephalus* are:
   - Spina bifida and other brain and spinal cord (neural tube) defects.
   - A narrowing of the small passage between the third and fourth ventricles of brain (aqueductal stenosis).
   - Complications of premature birth, such as bleeding within ventricles.
   - Infections during pregnancy, such as rubella, can cause inflammation in fetal brain tissue.
   - *Acquired hydrocephalus may be due to* head trauma, stroke, brain, or spinal cord tumors.
4. On per abdomen examination, head is bigger in size which does not engage even on pushing. During labor on internal examination, gaping sutures and fontanels are felt. There is crackling sensation on pressing the head.
5. Fetal outlook is extremely poor except in mild variety. Maternal prognosis is good.

OSCE 8.
1. Name the types of parent female pelvis.
2. Enumerate the anatomical features of gynecoid pelvis.
3. Enumerate the anatomical features of anthropoid pelvis.
4. Enumerate the anatomical features of android pelvis.
5. Enumerate the anatomical features of platypelloid pelvis.

Ans.

1.

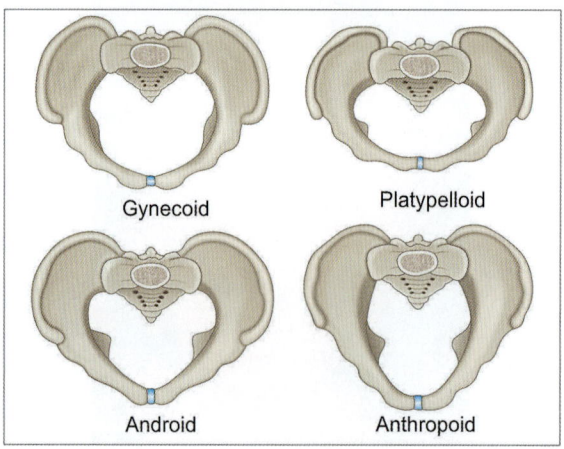

2.

Feature	Gynecoid
Brim	Round
For pelvis	Generous
Side walls	Straight
Ischial spine	Not prominent (blunt)
Subpubic angle	90
Incidence	50%

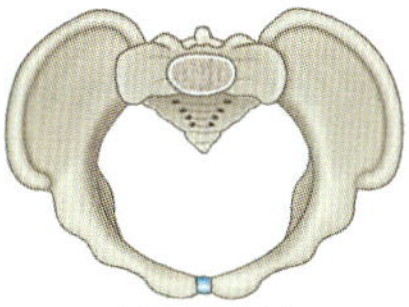

Gynecoid

3.

Feature	Android
Brim	Heart-shaped/ triangular
For pelvis	Narrow
Side walls	Convergent
Ischial spine	Prominent
Subpubic angle	<90
Incidence	20%

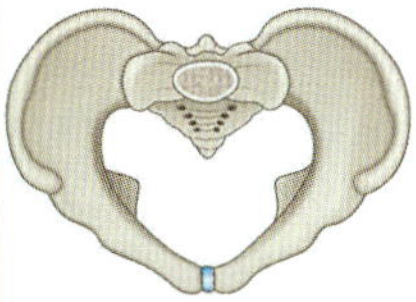

Android

4.

Feature	Anthropoid
Brim	Long oval
For pelvis	Narrow
Side walls	Divergent
Ischial spine	Not prominent
Subpubic angle	>90
Incidence	25%

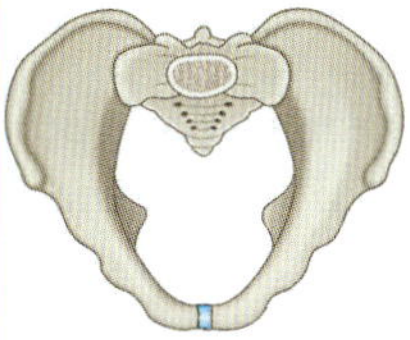

Anthropoid

5.

Feature	Platypelloid
Brim	Flat (kidney)
For pelvis	Wide
Side walls	Divergent
Ischial spine	Not prominent
Subpubic angle	>90
Incidence	5%

Platypelloid

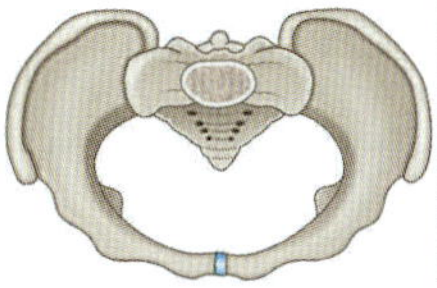

OSCE 9.

1. What is ischial spine?
2. What is the plane of ischial spine?
3. What are the different stations of fetal head?
4. Enumerate the importance of ischial spine.

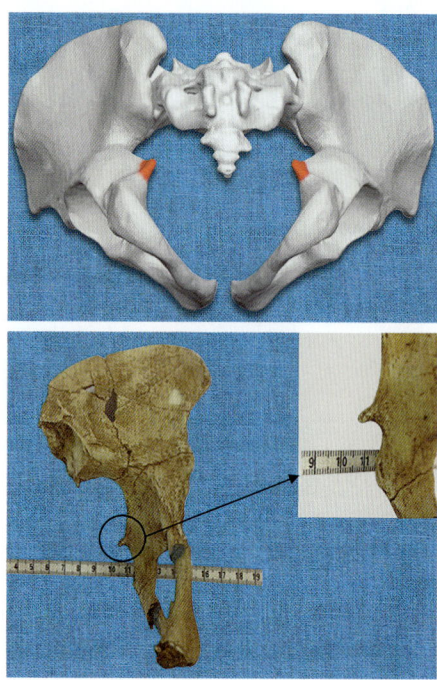

Ans.

1. The ischial spine is a sharp bony prominence found on the ramus of the ischium. It sits between the greater and lesser sciatic notches, at the level of the lower border of the acetabulum.
2. Level 0 is the "plane of ischial spines", defined by the imaginary line that joins the two ischial spines.

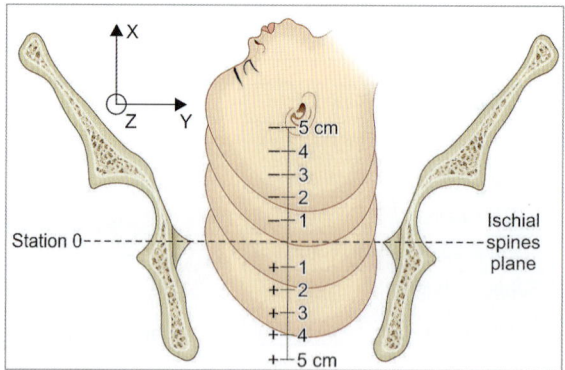

3. The maternal pelvis is divided into 11 levels, from −5 cm to +5 cm, in a coronal plane.
4. If the top of the head is located 1 cm beyond this plane at Level 0, the station is +1 cm.

> **At the level of the ischial spine.**
> - The plane of obstetric outlet (plane of the least pelvic dimensions)
> - The levator ani muscles
> - The obstetric axis of the pelvis changes its direction
> - The head is considered engaged when the vault is felt vaginally at or below this level
> - Internal rotation of the head occurs when the occiput is at this level
> - Forceps is applied only when the head at this level (mid forceps) or below it (low and outlet forceps)
> - Pudendal nerve block is carried out at this level
> - Normal level of the external os of the cervix

OSCE 10.
1. **What is false pelvis?**
2. **What is the inclination of pelvis?**
3. **What is sacral angle?**
4. **Enumerate bony landmarks on the brim of the pelvis separating the two pelvis from the false pelvis.**
5. **Name the anteroposterior diameters of pelvic brim.**

Ans.

1. The false pelvis is formed by the iliac portions of the innominate bone and is limited above by the iliac crest. Its boundaries are posteriorly lumbar vertebrae, laterally iliac fossa, and anteriorly anterior abdominal wall.

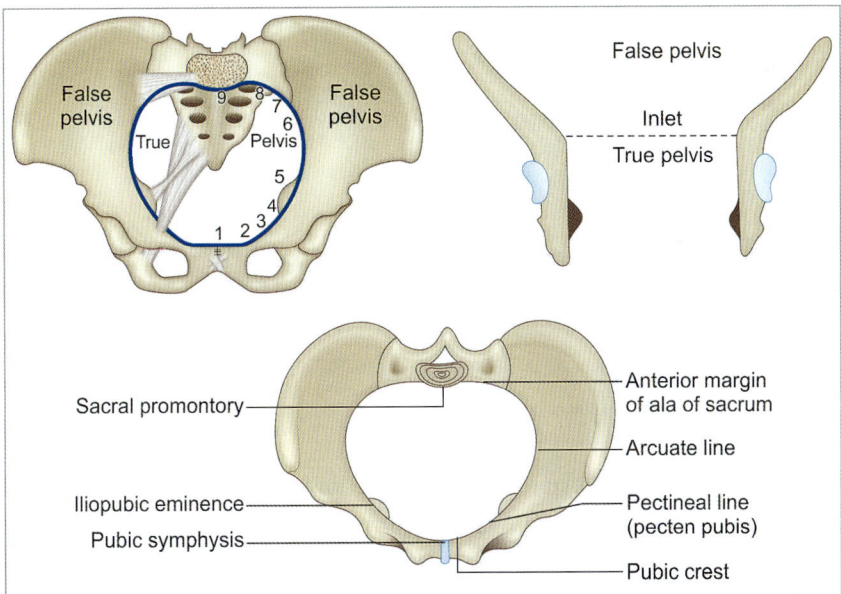

2. In the erect posture, the plane of the pelvic inlet makes an angle of 55 degree with the horizontal and is called angle of inclination.
3. A sacral angle is the angle formed by the true conjugate with the first two pieces of the sacrum.

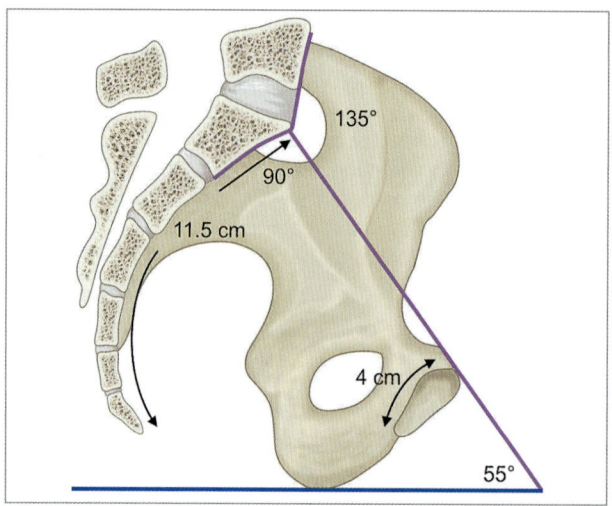

4. True conjugate (obstetrical conjugate), the distance between the midpoint of the sacral promontory to the inner margin of the upper border of symphysis pubis—11 cm. Obstetric conjugate is the distance between the midpoint of sacral promontory to prominent bony projection in the midline on the inner surface of symphysis pubis—10 cm.

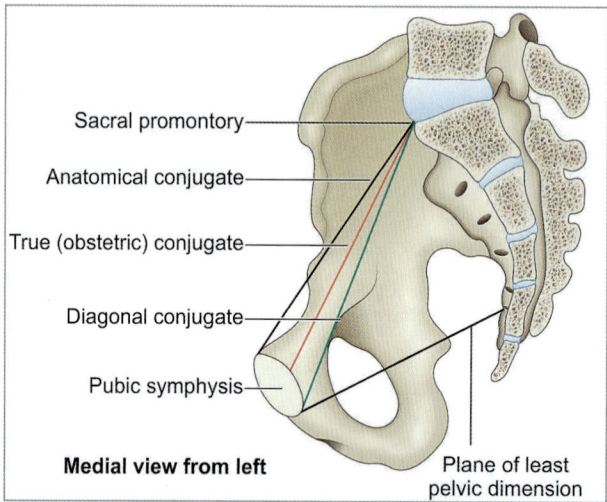

5. a. Diagonal conjugate the distance between the lower border of symphysis pubis to the midpoint on the sacral promontory—12 cm.
   b. Obstetric conjugate is computed by subtracting 1.5-2 cm from the diagonal conjugate.

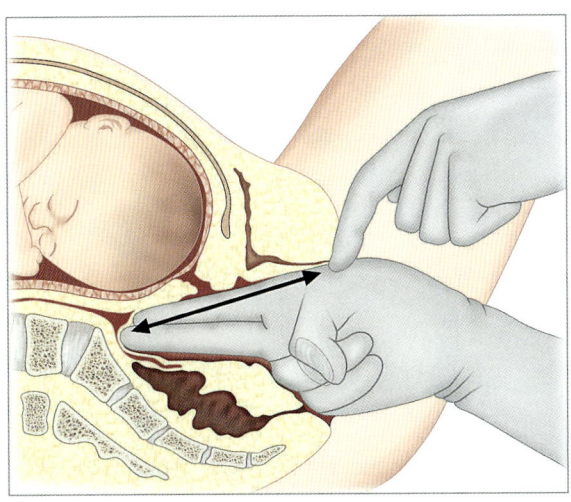

> **OSCE 11.**
> 1. What is the longest diameter of pelvic inlet?
> 2. What is the extent of oblique diameters?
> 3. What is the axis of pelvic inlet?
> 4. What is sacrocotyloid diameter?
> 5. What is curve of Carus and obstetrical pelvis axis?

> **Ans.**

1. The longest diameter is transverse diameter—13 cm.
2. There are two oblique diameters, right and left. Each one extends from one sacroiliac joint to the opposite iliopubic eminence and measures 12 cm.
3. Axis is a mid-perpendicular line drawn to the plane of the pelvic inlet. Its direction is downwards and backwards.
4. Sacrocotyloid diameter is the distance between the midpoint of the sacral promontory to iliopubic eminence.
5. The curve of Carus is formed by joining the axes of inlet, cavity, and outlet. It is uniformly curved. The fetus does not traverse this path.

   Obstetrical pelvic axis: It is through this axis that the fetus negotiates the pelvis. Its direction is first downwards and backwards up to level of ischial spines and then directed forwards.

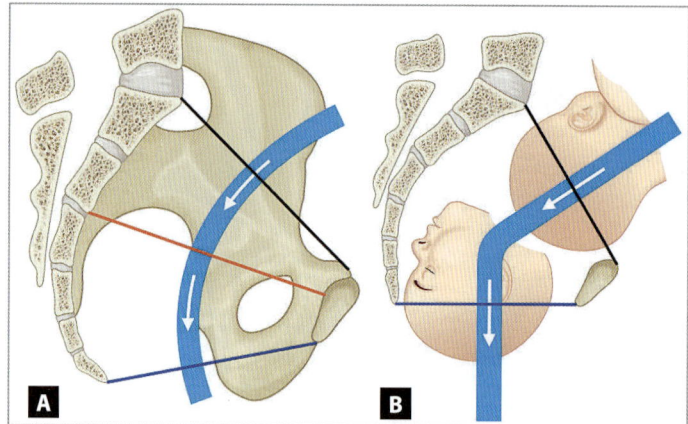

Pelvic axis—(A) Axes of inlet, cavity and outlet are shown by arrows drawn perpendicular to the planes. The shaded area over the axes is the anatomical pelvic axis (curve of Carus); (B) Obstetric pelvic axis—as shown by the shaded area is directed downward and backward up to ischial spines and then directed forward.

OSCE 12.

1. **What are the boundaries of obstetrical outlet?**
2. **What is the plane of least pelvic dimension?**
3. **What is interspinous diameter?**
4. **What is AP diameter of obstetrical outlet?**

Ans.

1. Obstetrical outlet is bounded above by the plane of least pelvic dimensions and below by anatomical outlet.
2. Plane of least pelvic dimension extends from the lower border of symphysis pubis to tip of ischial spine and posteriorly to meet the tip of the fifth sacral vertebra.
3. Interspinous diameter is the distance between the tip of two ischial spines—10.5 cm.
4. Anteroposterior diameter of obstetric outlet extends from inferior border of symphysis pubis to the tip of sacrum.

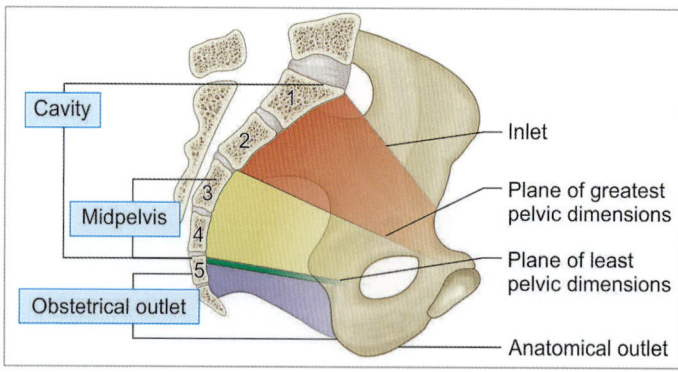

Chapter 2: Fetal Skull and Maternal Pelvis

OSCE 13.
1. Describe the boundaries of anatomical outlet.
2. What is the AP diameter of anatomical outlet?
3. What is transverse diameter of outlet?
4. What is subpublic angle?
5. What is waste space of Morris?

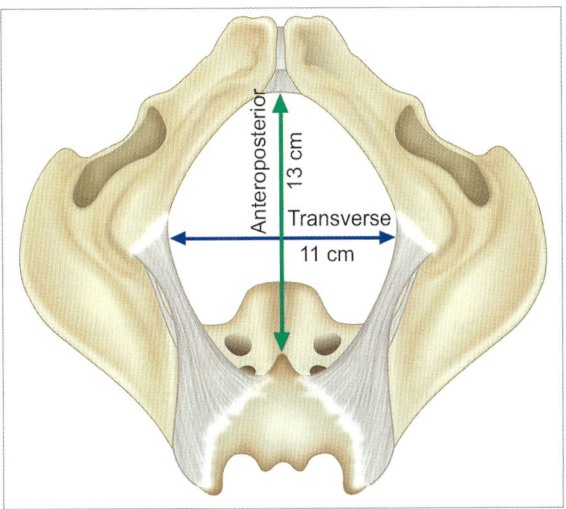

Ans.

1. Anatomical outlet is bounded in front by the lower border symphysis pubis, laterally by the ischiopubic rami, ischial tuberosity and sacrotuberous ligament and posteriorly by tip of coccyx.

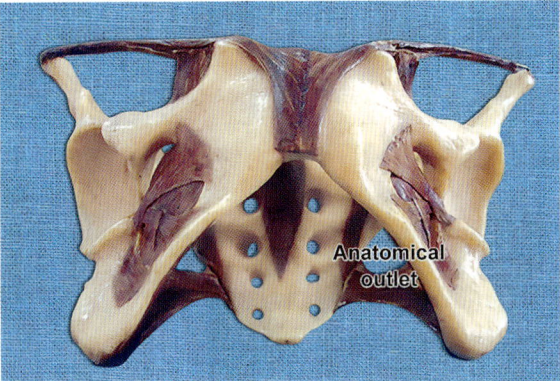

2. AP diameter extends from the lower border of symphysis pubis to the tip of coccyx. It measures 13 cm with the coccyx pushed back by the head. With the coccyx in normal position, the measurement is 2.5 cm less.
3. Transverse diameter of outlet measures—11 cm between inner borders of ischial tuberosities.

4. Subpubic angle is formed by the approximation of the two descending pubic rami. In normal female pelvis it measures 85 degrees.

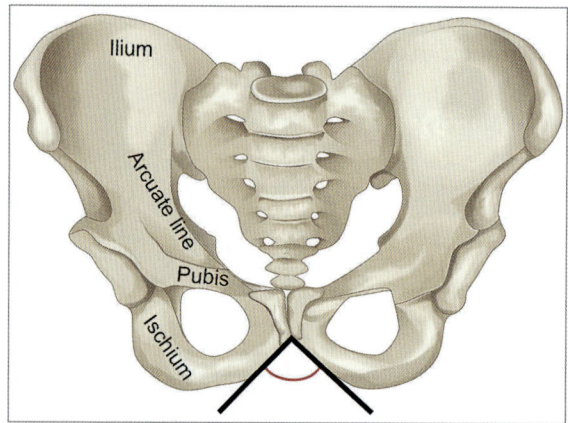

5. When a round disk of 9.3 cm diameter is placed under the pubic arch, the distance between the symphysis pubis and the circumference of the disk is measured. This measurement is the waste space of Morris and should not exceed 1 cm in a normal pelvis.

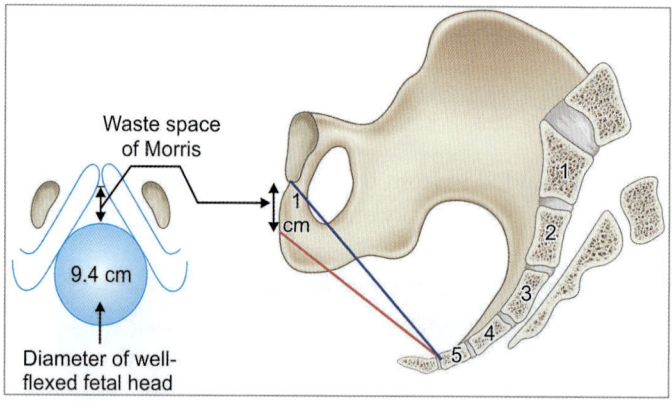

OSCE 14.
1. In normal labor which position of the head is the most common?
2. What is asynclitism?
3. What are the principal movements in labor?
4. Restitution is the opposite of which movement?
5. External rotation occurs in which direction?

Ans.
1. Left occipitoanterior is the most common position in normal labor. Due to lateral inclination of the head, the sagittal suture does not strictly correspond with the available transverse diameter of the inlet. It is either deflected anteriorly towards the symphysis pubis or posteriorly toward the sacral promontory.

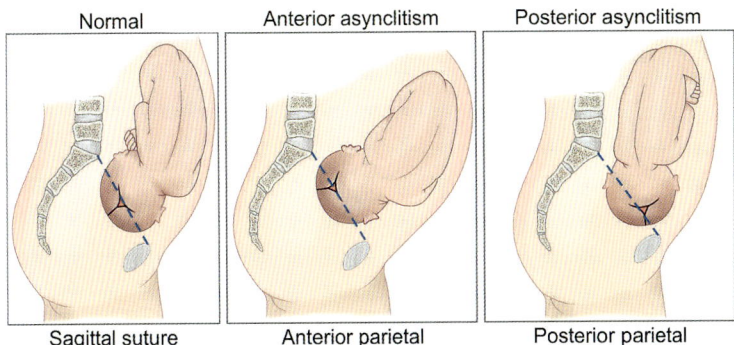

2. When the sagittal suture lies anteriorly, the posterior parietal bone becomes the leading presenting path and is called posterior asynclitism. This is more frequent in primigravida because of good uterine tone and tight abdominal wall. When the sagittal suture lies more posteriorly, then the anterior bone presents, and this is anterior asynclitism more common in multigravida.

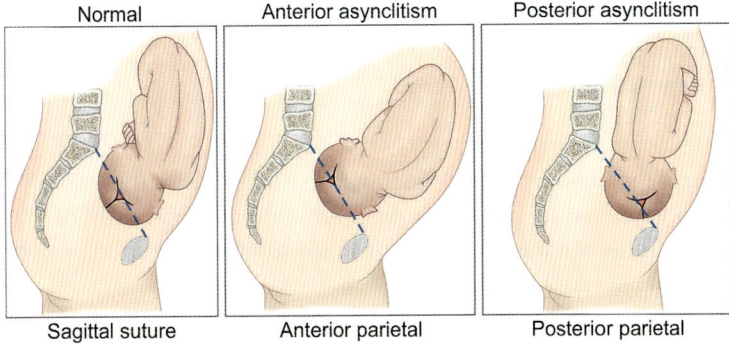

3. The principal movements in labor are engagement, descent, flexion, internal rotation, crowning, extension, restitution, external rotation, and expulsion of the trunk.

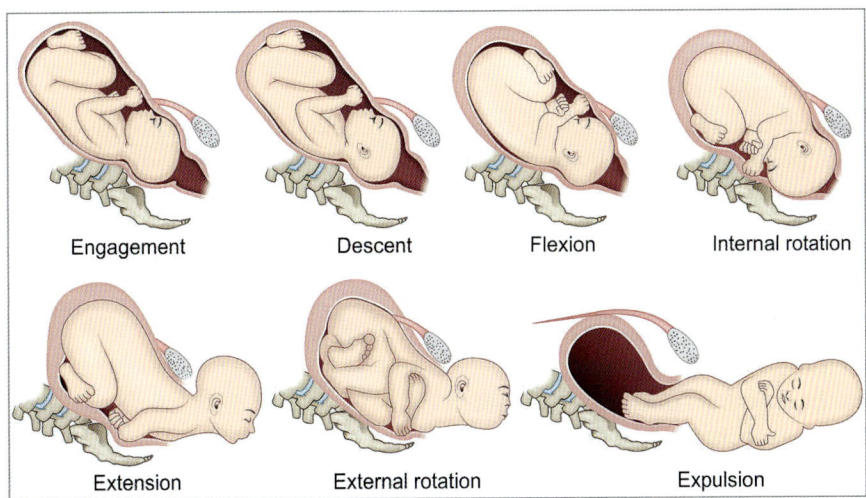

4. Restitution is opposite to internal rotation.
5. External rotation occurs in same direction as that of restitution.

OSCE 15.

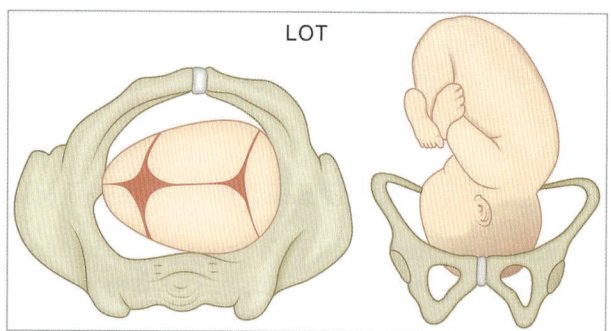

1. What is this condition?
2. What is deep transverse arrest?
3. What are the causes?
4. What is the management?
5. What are the causes of unengaged head?

Ans.

1. Sagittal suture of the head is lying in the transverse diameter of the pelvis.
2. Sagittal suture is placed in transverse bispinous diameter and there is no progress in descent of the head even after 1/2–1 hour following full dilatation of the cervix. This is known as deep transverse arrest.
3. Causes of deep transverse arrest are (a) faulty pelvic architecture such as prominent ischial spine, flat sacrum and convergent side walls (b) deflexion of the head (c) weak uterine contraction.
4. Vaginal delivery is not safe in inadequate pelvis or big baby, therefore cesarean section is recommended. Where vaginal delivery is considered safe, ventouse delivery, manual rotation and application of forceps, forceps rotation and delivery with Kielland in the hands of an expert can be done.
5. Causes of unengaged head at term are deflexed head, cephalopelvic disproportion, polyhydramnios, hydrocephalus, placenta previa, pelvic tumors, high pelvic inclination.

OSCE 16. In case of occipitoposterior position, what happens if there is:
1. Long anterior rotation of occiput.
2. When there is short anterior rotation?
3. When there is nonrotation?
4. When there is short posterior rotation?
5. What is the mechanism of face to pubis delivery?
6. Why there are more chances of injury in occipitosacral position?

Ans.

1. Diameter of engagement is oblique diameter, engaging diameter of head is occipitofrontal 11.5 cm or suboccipitofrontal 10 cm. With good uterine contraction and favorable pelvis there is increasing flexion with engagement and descent.
2. This is followed by long anterior internal rotation of occiput 3/8th of circle. There is simultaneously rotation of anterior shoulder through 2/8th of circle. Head is delivered by extension followed by restitution and external rotation. In case of mild deflexion of the head, anterior rotation of occiput through 1/8th of a circle occurs and the head goes into deep transverse arrest.

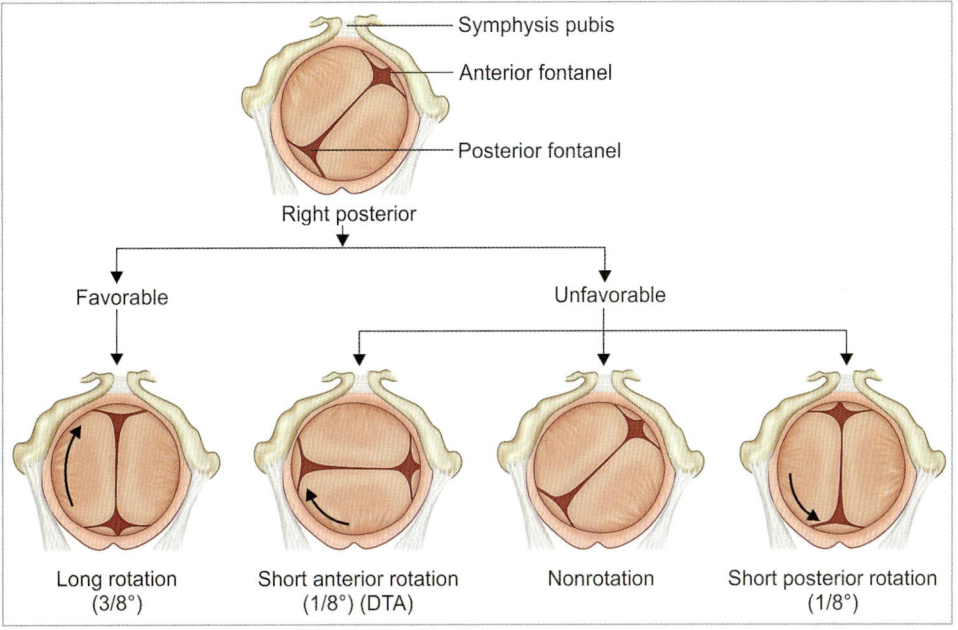

3. In cases of moderate deflexion there is nonrotation of occiput and the head is in persistent occipitoposterior position.
4. In cases of severe deflexion, there is posterior rotation of occiput leading to occipitosacral position. In spacious gynecoid or anthropoid face to pubis delivery occurs or there may be arrest of labor.
5. Mechanism of face of pubis delivery, there is descent until the root of the nose hinges under symphysis pubis. Flexion occurs releasing successively the brow vertex and occiput out of the stretched perineum and the face is born by extension. Restitution and external rotation follow.
6. There are more chances of perineal injuries because of wide biparietal diameter 9.5 cm stretches the perineum and occipitofrontal diameter emerges out of the introitus.

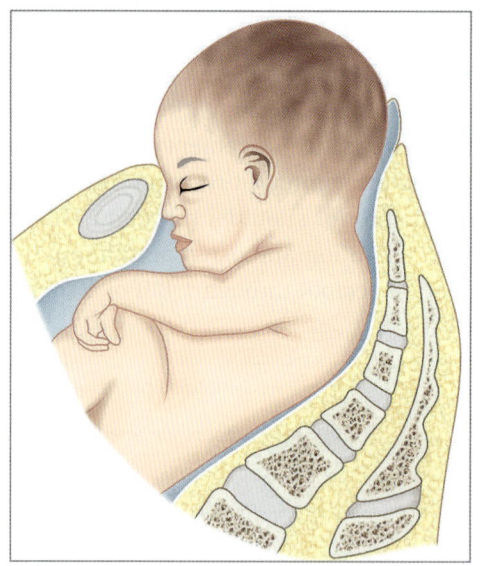

OSCE 17.

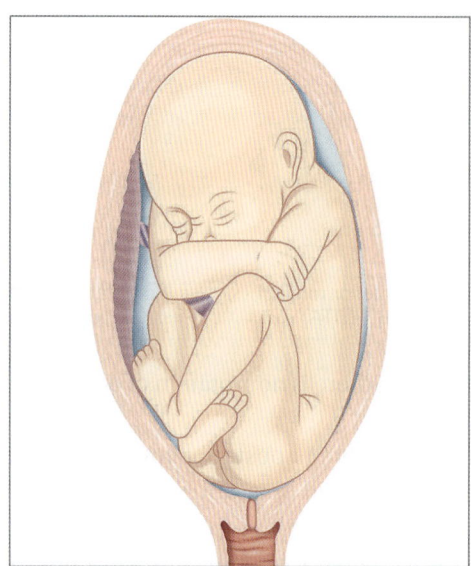

1. What is this position, what are the principal movements which occur at buttocks?
2. What are the principal movements which take place at the shoulder?
3. Where are the principal movements which occur at head?
4. What are the methods employed for delivering the after coming head?

Ans.

1. This position is breech.
   Mechanism of labor in breech:

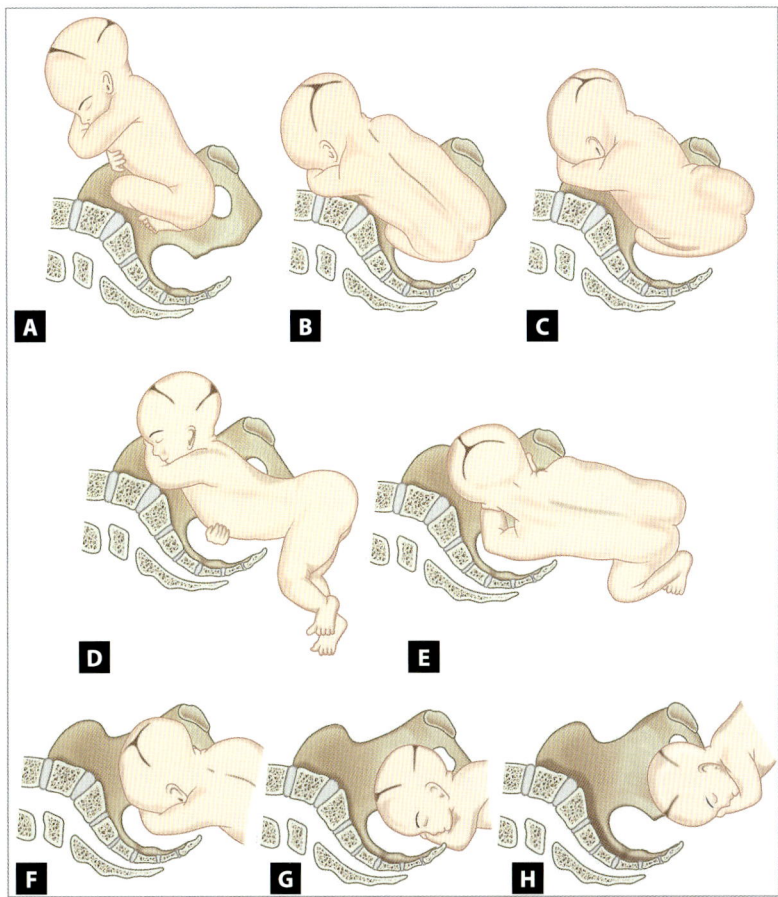

- The diameter of engagement of buttock is one of the oblique diameters of the inlet. The engaging diameter is bitrochanteric 10 cm with the sacrum directed toward the iliopubic eminence. When the diameter passes through the pelvic brim, the breech is engaged.
- Descent of the buttocks occurs until the anterior buttock touches the pelvic floor.
- Internal rotation of the anterior buttock occurs through 1/8th of a circle placing it behind the symphysis pubis.
- Further descent with lateral flexion of the trunk occurs until the anterior hip hinges under the symphysis pubis which is released first followed by the posterior hip.
- Delivery of the trunk and the lower limbs follow.
- Restitution occurs so that the buttocks occupy the original position as during engagement in oblique diameter.
- Bisacromial diameter 12 cm engages in the same oblique diameter as that occupied by the buttocks at brim soon after the delivery of the breech.
- Descent occurs with internal rotation of the shoulders bringing the shoulder to lie in the anteroposterior diameter of the pelvic outlet. The trunk simultaneously rotates externally through 1/8th of a circle.

2. a. Delivery of the posterior shoulder followed by the anterior one is completed by anterior flexion of the delivered trunk.
   b. Restitution and external rotation untwisting of the trunk occurs putting the anterior shoulder towards the right thigh in LSA and left thigh in RSA.
   c. External rotation of the shoulder occurs in the same direction because of internal rotation of the occiput through 1/8th of circle anteriorly. The fetal trunk is now positioned as dorsoanterior.
   d. Engagement of the head occurs either through the opposite oblique diameter as that occupied by the buttocks or through the transverse diameter the engaging diameter of the head is suboccipitofrontal 10 cm.
   e. Descent with increasing flexion occurs.
   f. Internal rotation of the occiput occurs anteriorly through 1/8th or 2/8th of a circle placing the occiput behind the symphysis pubis.
   g. Further descent occurs until the subocciput hinges under the symphysis pubis.
   h. Head is born by flexion chin mouth, nose, forehead, vertex, and occiput appearing successively. The expulsion of the head from the pelvic cavity depends entirely upon the bearing down efforts and not at all on uterine contraction.
3. Delivery of the head:
   Burns–Marshall method: The baby is allowed to hang by its own weight. The assistant gives suprapubic pressure in a downwards and backwards direction to promote flexion of the head.

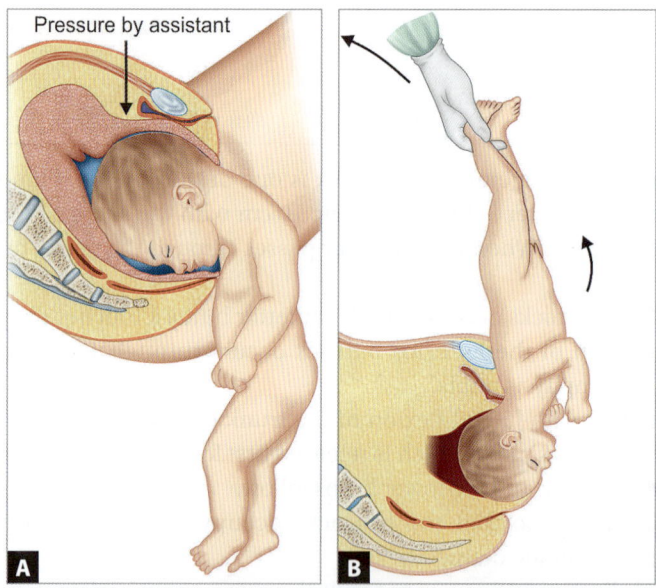

(A) Delivery of aftercoming head by Burns-Marshall method;
(B) Continuation of the Burns-Marshall method.

As the nape of the neck is visible under pubic arch the ankle of the baby is held with a finger of the right hand in between the two ankles. A steady traction is maintained and the trunk is swung upwards and forwards towards the mother's abdomen while the left hand guards the perineum and successively the face and brow are born.

Forceps delivery—when the occiput lies against the back of symphysis pubis, the leg of child is raised by the assistant to facilitate introduction of the blades from below. The pull of the forceps follows the axis of the birth canal. The head should be delivered slowly.

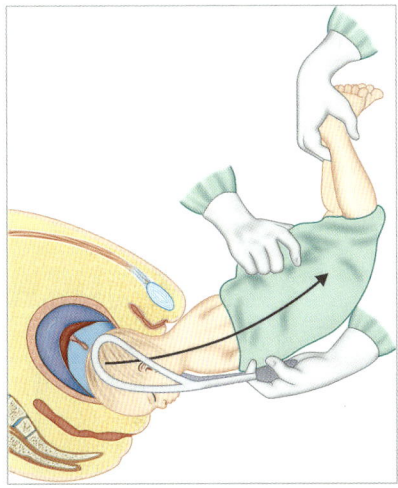

4. The baby is placed on the supinated left forearm with the limbs hanging on either side, the middle and the index fingers of the left hand are placed over the malar bone on either sides, this maintains flexion of head.

The ring and little fingers of pronated right hand are placed on the child's right shoulder, index finger is placed on the left shoulder and the middle finger is placed on the suboccipital region, traction is now given downwards and backwards, till the nape of the neck is visible under the public arch. The assistant gives suprapubic pressure during this period to maintain flexion.

Thereafter the fetus is carried in upwards and forwards direction towards the mother's abdomen releasing the face brow and lastly the trunk is depressed to release the occiput and vertex.

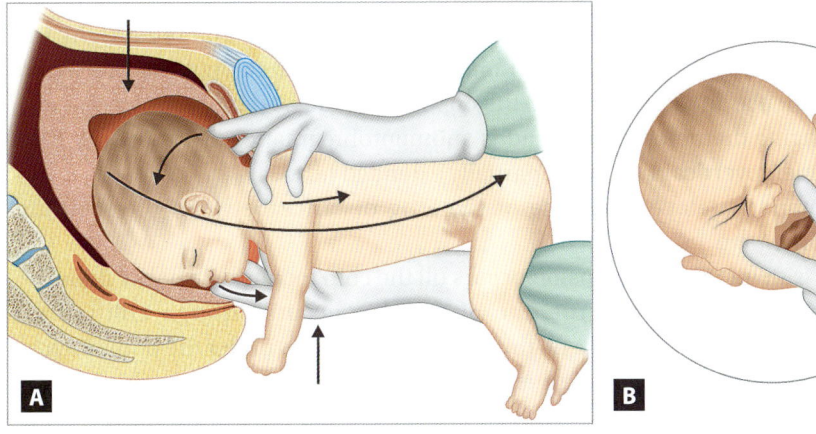

OSCE 18.

1. Describe the mechanism of labor in mentoanterior position.
2. What are the pelvic findings of face presentation?
3. What is the clinical course of labor in mentoanterior position?
4. Do you expect normal delivery in mentoposterior position?

Mechanism of mentoanterior position

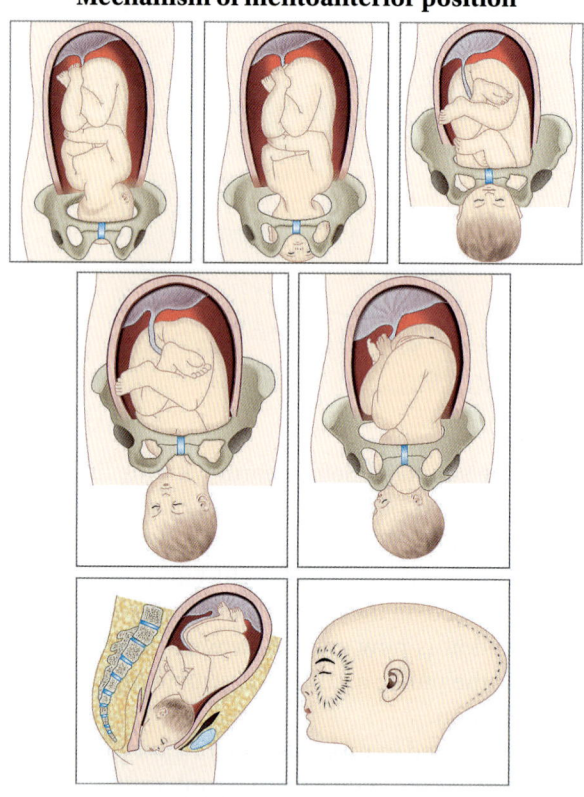

Ans.

1. *Engagement:* The diameter of engagement is the oblique diameter right in LMA (left mentoanterior), left in RMA (right mentoanterior) with the mentum related to one iliopubic eminence and the glabella to the opposite sacroiliac joint.

   The engaging diameter of the head is submentobregmatic 9.5 cm in fully extended head or submentovertical 11.5 cm in partially extended head.

   Engagement is delayed because of the long distance between the mentum and biparietal plane 7 cm.

   Descent with increasing extension occurs till the chin touches the pelvic floor.

   Internal rotation—internal rotation of the chin occurs through 1/8th of a circle anteriorly. Further descent occurs till the submentum hinges under the pubis arch.

   Delivery of the head—the head is born by flexion delivering the chin, face, brow, vertex and lastly the occiput.

The diameter distending the vulval outlet is submentovertical 11.5 cm. Restitution occurs through 1/8th of a circle opposite to the direction of internal rotation. External rotation occurs further 1/8th circle to the same side of restitution.

2. Vaginal examination reveals the mouth with hard alveolar margins, nose, malar eminence, supraorbital ridges and the mentum.

In early labor because of high head and sausage shaped bag of membranes, the parts are not clearly defined. In late labor, the parts are often obscured due to edema. It is often confused with breech presentation.

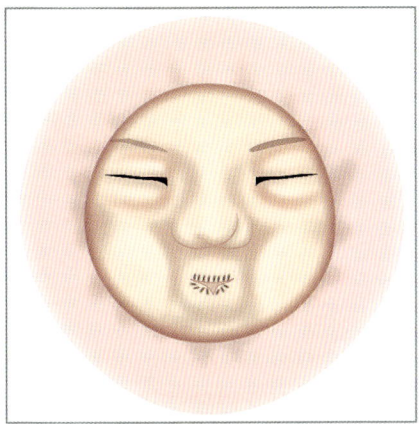

The distinguishing features are:
- The mouth and the malar eminences are not in a line but in breech, the anus and the ischial tuberosities are in one line.
- Sucking effect of mouth.
- Hard alveolar margins
- Absence of meconium staining of the examination finger.

In spite of the fact that the engaging diameter of the head in flexed vertex and the extended face presentation is the same 9.5 cm the clinical course of the latter is adversely affected because of the following.
- Irregular face ill fits with the lower uterine segment the poor ball valve action results in formation of elongated bag of membranes which is likely to rupture early.

3. Chance of cord prolapse is more.

Delay of labor in all the stages is common. The causes are (a) weak uterine contraction (b) absence of moulding of the facial bones (c) delayed engagement—the distance between the biparietal plane to chin is 7 cm and to occiput is only 3 cm (d) late internal rotation and (e) arrest and at times insuperable obstruction if mentoposterior fails to rotate anteriorly.

Chances of damage to the perineum is more because wide biparietal diameter 9.5 cm stretches the perineum and submentovertical diameter 11.5 cm emerges out of the introitus.

4. In persistent mentoposterior position normal delivery is not possible.

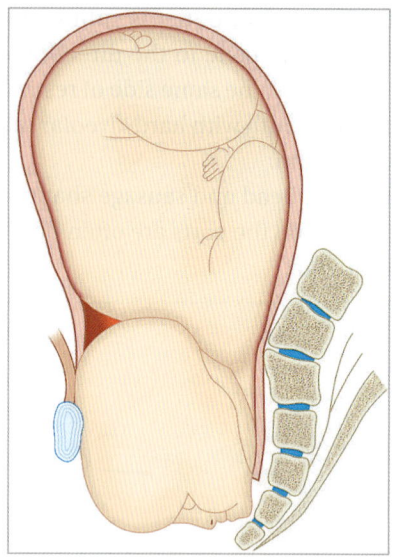

OSCE 19.

1. What is the engaging diameter of the head in brow presentation?
2. How is the position confirmed in brow presentation?
3. Can it be delivered vaginally?
4. In transverse lie what maneuver after 38 weeks can be tried to make the presentation cephalic?
5. What are causes of unengaged head at term?

Ans.

1. The engaging diameter of the head is mentovertical—14 cm.
2. The position is confirmed on vaginal examination by palpating supraorbital ridges and anterior fontanelle.
3. There is no mechanism of labor in an average size baby with normal pelvis in brow position.

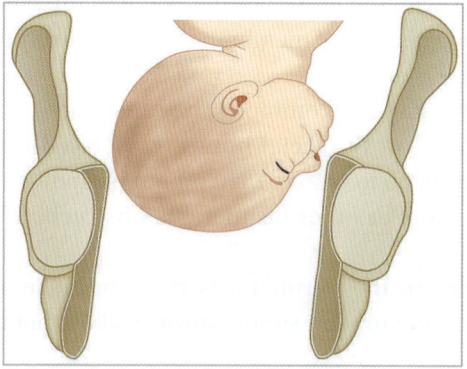

Brow presentation.

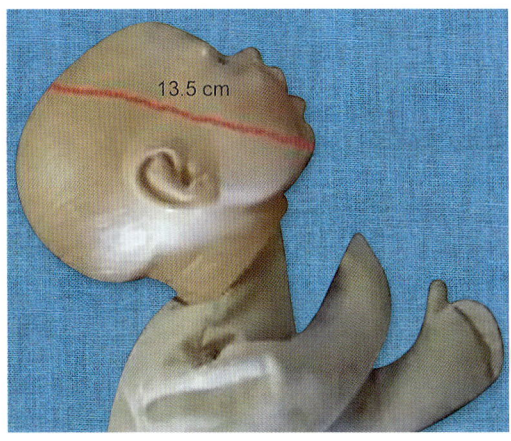

Mentovertical diameter
- Diameter extending from the chin to furthest point of vertex
- Measures 13 cm
- Largest anteroposterior diameter
- Head is partially extended
- Associated with brow presentation

4. External cephalic version can be done to convert transverse lie to cephalic in transverse lie.

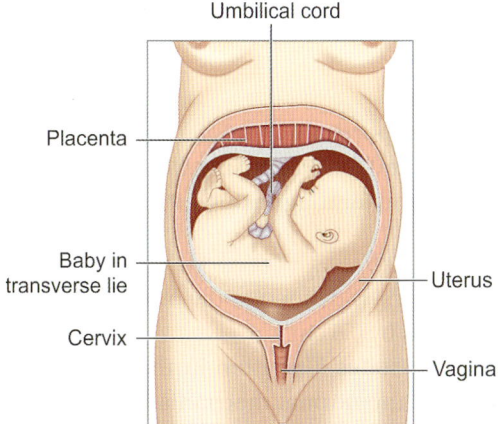

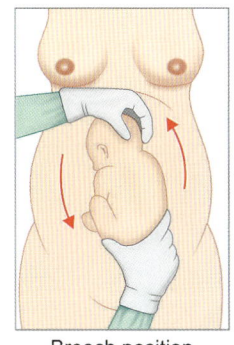
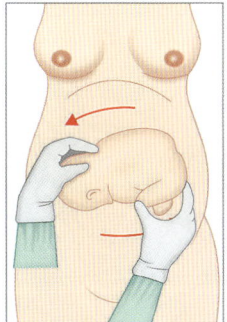
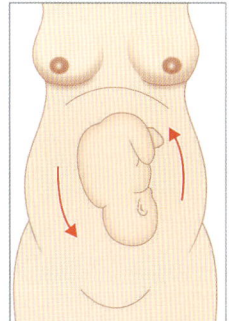

5. Common causes of unengaged head at term are: Deflexed head, cephalopelvic disproportion, polyhydramnios, hydrocephalus, placenta previa, pelvic tumors, high pelvic inclination.

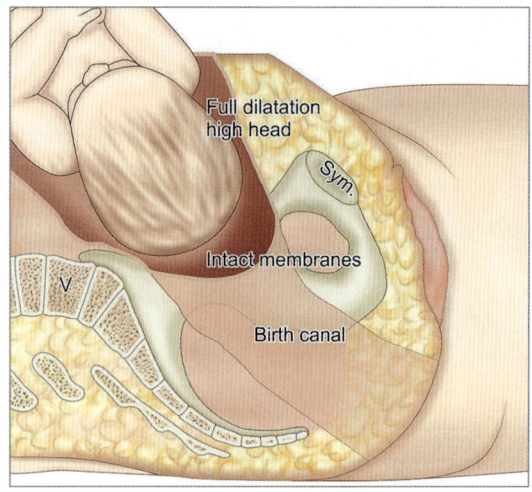

OSCE 20.
1. What is contracted pelvis?
2. How would you assess pelvis?
3. What is cephalopelvic disproportion?
4. What is the abdominal method for diagnosing CPD?
5. What is the combined method for diagnosing CPD?

Ans.

1. Anatomically, contracted pelvis is defined as the one where the essential diameter of one or more planes are shortened by 0.5 cm.

   The obstetric definition states alteration in the size and or shape of the pelvis of sufficient degree as to alter the normal mechanism of labor in an average size baby is contracted pelvis.

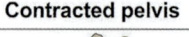

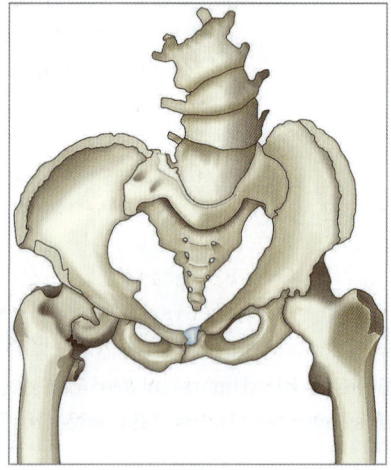

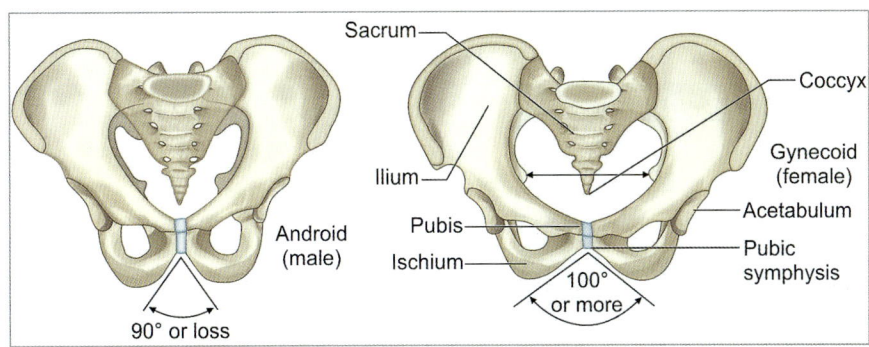

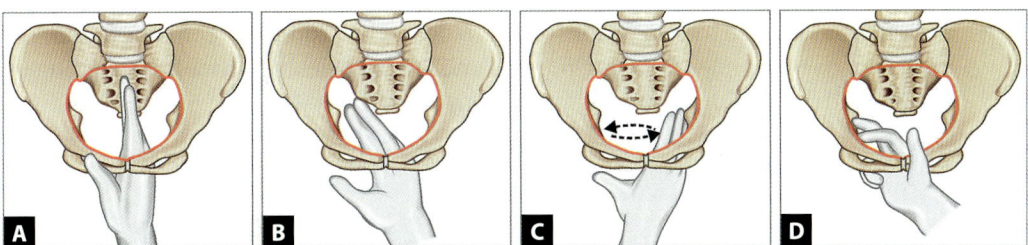

(A) Sacrum; (B) Sacrospinous notch; (C) Ischial spine; (D) Iliopectirneal lines.

2. Assessment of pelvis is done after 37th week or at the beginning of labor.

Patient lies in dorsal position after emptying the bladder. With full aseptic and antiseptic measures internal examination is done.

Sacrum: The sacrum may be smooth, short and well curved and the sacral promontory usually cannot be reached, or the sacrum may be long or straight

Sacrosciatic notch: The notch is sufficiently wide so that two finger can be easily placed over the sacrospinous ligament covering the notch.

Ischial spines: Spines are difficult to palpate. They may be prominent and encroach the cavity thereby diminishing the available space in the midpelvis.

- *Iliopectineal lines:* Any breaking suggests narrow forepelvis.
- *Sidewalls:* Normally they are parallel or divergent. They may be convergent.
- *Posterior surface of the symphysis pubis:* It normally forms a smooth rounded curve. Presence of angulation or breaking suggests abnormality.
- *Sacrococcygeal joint:* Its mobility is noted
- *Pubic arch:* Normally, the pubic arch is rounded and should accommodate the palmar aspect of two fingers.
- *Diagonal conjugate:* In normal pelvis, it is difficult to feel the sacral promontory.
- In order to reach the promontory, the elbow and the wrist are to be depressed sufficiently while the fingers are mobilized in upward direction. The point at which the bone recedes from the finger is the sacral promontory.
- The fingers are then moved under the symphysis pubis and a marking is placed over the gloved index finger by the index finger of left hand.

- Internal finger are removed and distance between the marking and tip of middle finger gives the measurement of diagonal conjugate

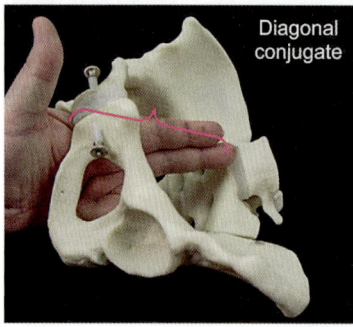
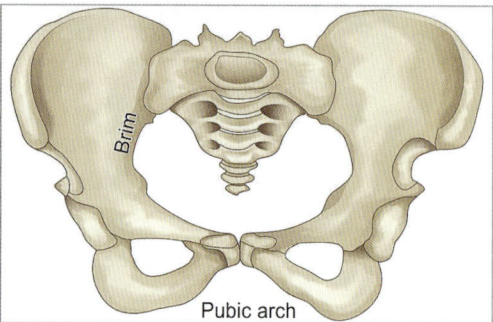

- *Subpubic angle:* The inferior pubic rami are defined and in female the angle roughly corresponds to the fully abducted thumbs and index finger. In narrow angle, it roughly corresponds to the fully abducted middle and index fingers.

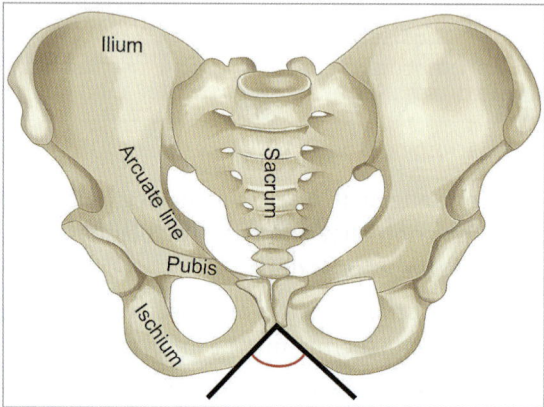

- *Transverse diameter of the outlet:* It is measured by placing the knuckles of the first interphalangeal joint or knuckles of the clinched fist between the two ischial tuberosities normally it accommodates four knuckles.

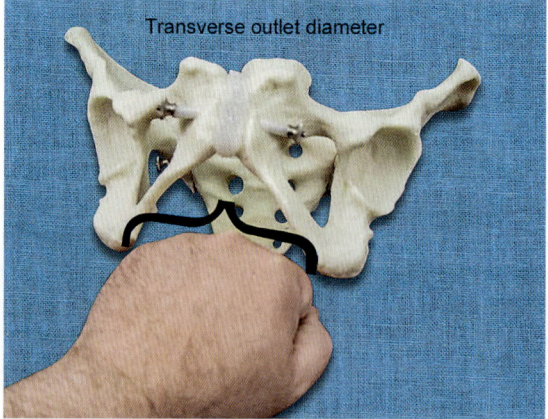

- *Anteroposterior diameter of the outlet:* The distance between the inferior margin of the symphysis pubis and the skin over the sacrococcygeal joint can be measured either with the method employed for diagonal conjugate or by external calipers.

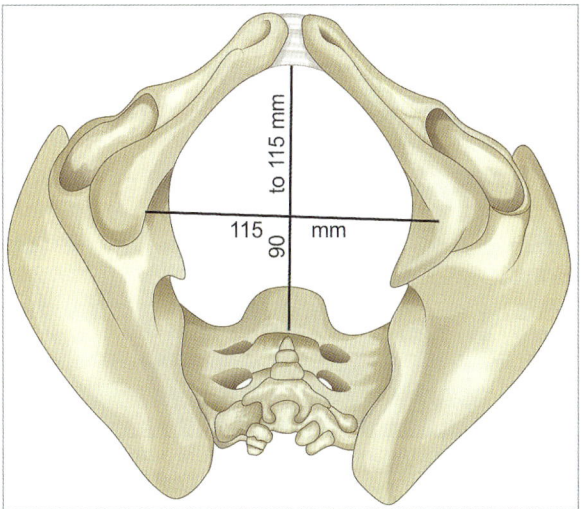

3. The disparity in the relation between the head and the pelvis is called cephalopelvic disproportion.

    Abdominal method of diagnosing CPD—the patient is placed in dorsal position with the thighs slightly flexed and separated.

    The head is grasped by the left hand. Two fingers of the right hand are placed above the symphysis pubis thus keeping the inner surface of the finger in line with the anterior surface of the symphysis pubis to note the degree of overlapping if any, when the head is pushed downwards and backward.

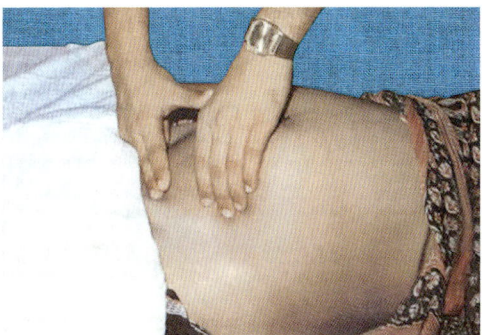

4. *Abdominovaginal method (Muller–Munro Kerr):* This bimanual method is superior to the abdominal method as the pelvic assessment can be done simultaneously abdominally and vaginally.

    Muller introduced the method by placing the vaginal fingertips at the level of ischial spines to note the descent of the head. Munro Kerr added placement of the thumb over the symphysis pubis to note the degree of overlapping. Bladder and bowel must be emptied.

5. The patient is placed in lithotomy position and the internal examination is done taking all aseptic precautions. Two fingers of the right hand are introduced into the vagina with the fingertips placed at the level of ischial spines and thumb is placed over the symphysis pubis. The head is caught by the left hand and is pushed in downward and backward direction into the pelvis.

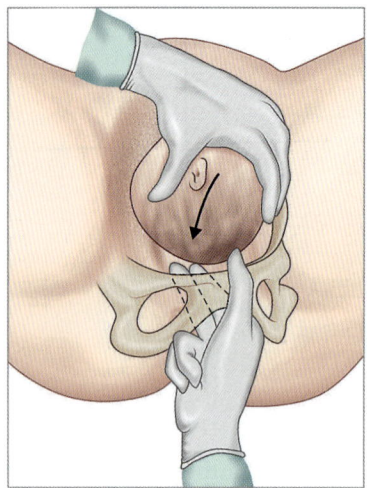

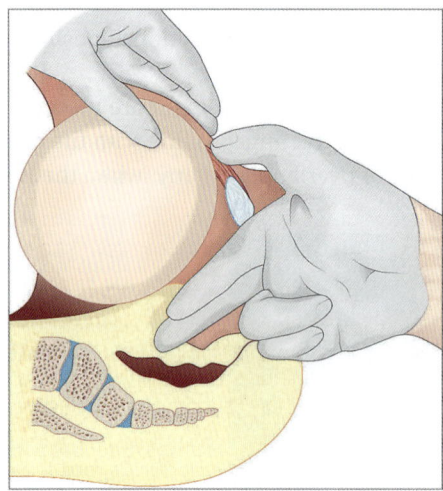

Cephalopelvic disproportion tests

Muller-Kerr's method:
- It is more valuable in detection of the degree of disproportion
- The patient evacuates her bladder and rectum
- The patient is placed in the dorsal position
- The left hand pushes the head into the pelvis and vaginal examination is done by the right hand while its thumb is placed over the symphysis to detect disproportion

Conclusion
- The head can be pushed down up to the level of ischial spines and there is no overlapping of parietal bone over the symphysis pubis—no disproportion.
- The head can be pushed down a little but not up to the level of ischial spines and there is slight overlapping of the parietal bone—slight or moderate disproportion.
- The head cannot be pushed down and instead the parietal bone overhangs the symphysis pubis displacing the thumbs—severe disproportion.

CHAPTER 3

Ultrasound in First and Second Trimester

Archana Baser

OSCE 1.

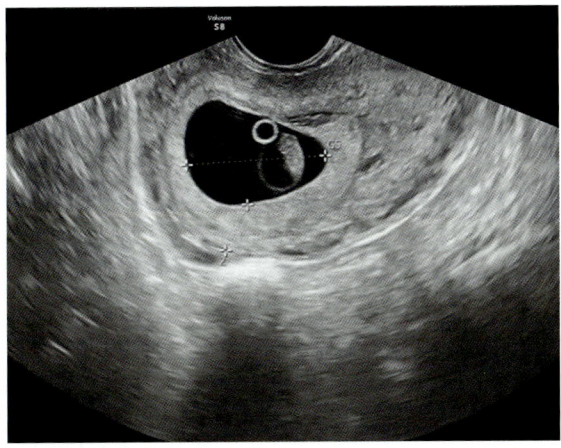

1. Identify the picture. What are the key structures seen?
2. What is the aim of an early pregnancy scan?
3. Till what gestational age dating can be done and what is the most accurate parameter for dating?
4. Discuss the discriminatory zone of β-hCG in TAS and TVS scan.

Ans.

1. Early pregnancy scan/viability scan.
   Key structures seen are:
   - Adequate decidual reaction
   - Gestational sac
   - Yolk sac
   - Amnion
   - Embryo
2. *Aims of early pregnancy scan:*
   - Determination of location of pregnancy (intrauterine or extrauterine)
   - Determination of fetal number
   - Presence or absence of cardiac activity
   - Calculation of gestational age.

3. Dating can be done till the 13 weeks period of gestation and the most accurate parameter for dating is CRL measurement.
4. The discriminatory zone/or critical value of serum β-hCG for detection of intrauterine pregnancy by transabdominal sonography is 6500 mIU/mL and for transvaginal sonography is 1,500 mIU/mL.

OSCE 2.

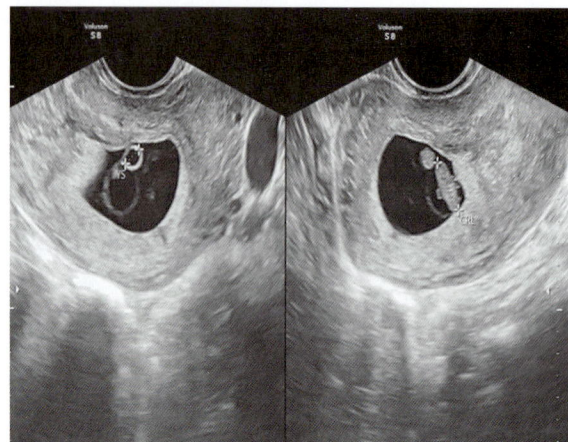

1. What is a double decidual sign?
2. What is the critical landmark for identifying a true gestational sac?
3. What is a double bleb sign?
4. At what gestational age is a gestational sac, yolk sac, fetal pole, and cardiac activity evident in TVS scan?
5. At what MSD (mean sac diameter) is a yolk sac and embryo with cardiac activity evident by TVS scan?

Ans.

1. Double decidual sac sign is a sonographic feature seen in normal intrauterine pregnancy depicting appearance of two concentric echogenic rims of which outer ring is *decidua parietalis* and inner ring is *decidua capsularis*.
2. The critical landmark for identifying a true gestational sac is the presence of Yolk sac.
3. Double bleb sign is a sonographic feature showing a Yolk sac and Amniotic sac in the gestational sac giving an appearance of two bubbles. The embryonic disk is located in between the two.
4. G sac (gestational sac) seen at 4.5–5 weeks
   - Yolk sac at 5–5.5 weeks
   - Fetal pole at 6 weeks
5. a. Yolk sac at MSD 6 mm
   b. Embryo with CA (cardiac activity) at MSD 12 mm
   c. CA is present in CRL ≥4 mm

OSCE 3.

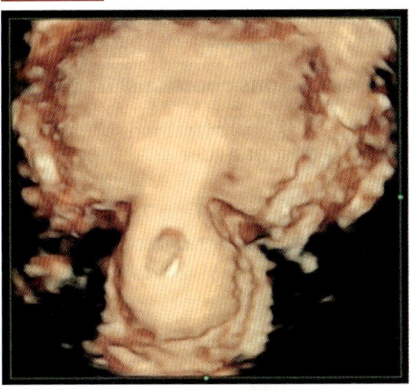
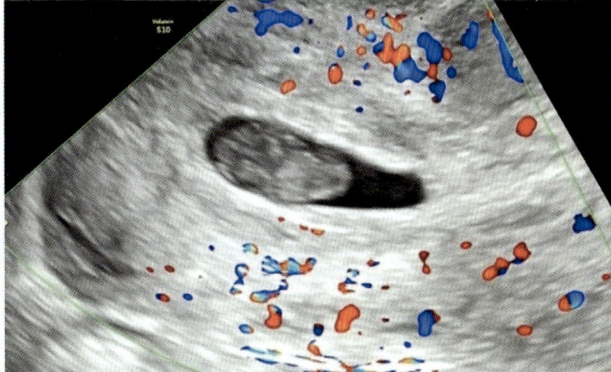

1. Identify the image and comment on it. Enumerate four differential diagnosis of early pregnancy hemorrhage.
2. Enumerate four different types of abortions.
3. How is early pregnancy failure different from missed abortion and an anembryonic pregnancy?
4. What is a sliding sign?

Ans.

1. The above image is suggestive of abortion in progress.

    The differential diagnosis of early pregnancy hemorrhage are:

Obstetrics	Nonobstetric
Implantation bleeding	Cervical polyps
Miscarriages	Cervical erosion
Ectopic pregnancy	Carcinoma cervix
Hydatidiform mole	Anovulatory bleeding

2. The types of abortions are:

Spontaneous	Induced
Threatened abortion	MTP
Inevitable abortion	Septic abortions
Incomplete abortion	
Complete abortion	
Missed abortion	

3. *Early pregnancy failure* is when the pregnancy ends spontaneously such that either the embryo does not appear at all or the cardiac activity does not appear, or there is loss of previously viable embryo.

    Missed abortion is when the cardiac activity in a previous viable embryo/fetus does not appear even when the CRL is greater than 7 mm.

Anembryonic pregnancy or blighted ovum refers to the one in which the gestational sac is seen without the embryo. If on TVS scan, a gestational sac of MSD >25 mm is seen with no identifiable yolk sac or embryo, then it is termed as anembryonic pregnancy.

4. *Sliding sign* is a sonographic feature, that differentiates spontaneous abortions in progress from a cervical ectopic pregnancy. It involves the sliding of products of conception when a slight pressure is applied by the sonographer during TVS. It is absent in cervical pregnancy.

OSCE 4.

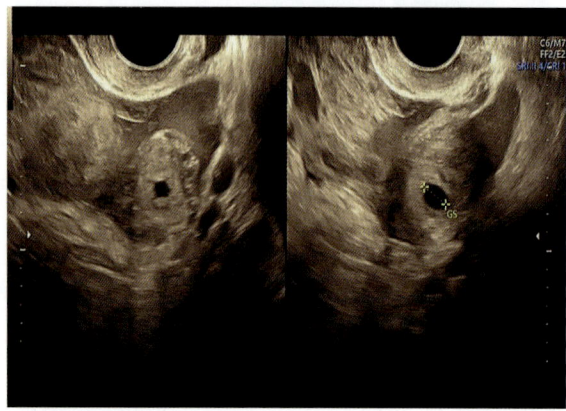

1. What is the image suggestive of?
2. What is Bagel's or Donut sign?
3. Enumerate four sites of ectopic pregnancy.
4. Enumerate four ultrasound features of ectopic pregnancy.
5. Enumerate two criteria for expectant management.

Ans.

1. The image is suggestive of an ectopic pregnancy, with gestational sac seen in the adnexa.
2. Bagel's or Donut sign or Blob sign is a sonographic feature of intact tubal ectopic pregnancy in which a gestational sac is seen in the adnexa surrounded by a hyperechoic ring.
3. The different sites of ectopic pregnancy are:

Tubal (98.3)	Extra tubal site (1.7%)
Ampulla (most common)	Rudimentary horn
Isthmus	Cornual
Infundibulum (fimbrial)	Abdominal
Interstitial	Ovarian
	Cervical
	Cesarean Scar

4. The sonographic features of ectopic pregnancy are:
   • Empty uterine cavity
   • Thickened endometrium

- Pseudogestational sac
- Decidual cast
- Gestational sac in the adnexa with or without cardiac activity
- Ring of fire appearance of the sac, showing increased vascularity in color Doppler
- Blood in the peritoneal cavity

5. Expectant management for Ectopic pregnancy should be done in:
    - Clinically stable patient.
    - Serum β-hCG <1,000 mIU and fall on further tests
    - Only tubal ectopic
    - Diameter of tubal mass not greater than 3.5 cm
    - No signs and symptoms of tubal rupture or hemoperitoneum seen on clinical examination and on TVS.

OSCE 5.

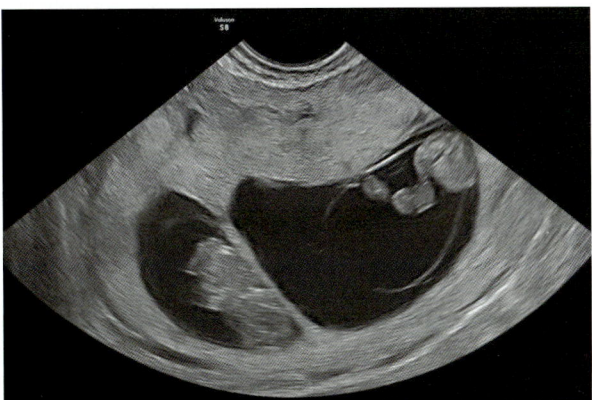

1. Identify the image. What is the optimal time to determine chorionicity?
2. What is Lambda sign and T-sign?
3. Enumerate four important aspects of assessment of multiple pregnancy on an ultrasound.
4. Discuss the types of chorionicity and zygosity in twin gestation.
5. What is the role of ultrasound in appearing twins and vanishing twins?

Ans.

1. Twin gestation—the optimal time to determine chorionicity is 11–14 weeks.
2. *Lambda sign or twin peak* sign refers to the triangular projection of trophoblastic tissue isoechoic with placenta into the intervening membranes from the placental surface corresponding to dichorionic placenta.

    T-sign is when there is absence of Lambda sign. It refers to a thin dividing membrane between two amniotic sacs when there is only one placenta for two gestations. It corresponds to monochorionic placenta.
3. The important and practical aspects on ultrasound are:
    - Total number of gestational sacs

- Total number of amniotic sacs in chorionic cavity
- Total number of Yolk sacs, to diagnose the amnionicity
- Number of placenta
- Chorionic peak sign/Lambda sign, indicative of dichorionicity
- The thickness of intertwin membrane

4. *Chorionicity* refers to placentation

   Zygosity refers to a type of conception.

   The chorion differentiates on day 4 and the Amnion on day 8 after fertilization.

   Dizygotic twins always have dichorionic placenta. Monozygotic depends on the time of division of zygote

Division within 72 hours	Dichorionic diamniotic
Between 4–8 days	Monochorionic diamniotic
Between 8–12 days	Monochorionic monoamniotic
After 13 days	Conjoined twin

5. A diagnostic pitfall in first trimester screening of twins is the appearing twin which is common with monochorionic twins. Ultrasound plays an important role here. Repeat scan should be done for patients with monochorionic twins.

OSCE 6.

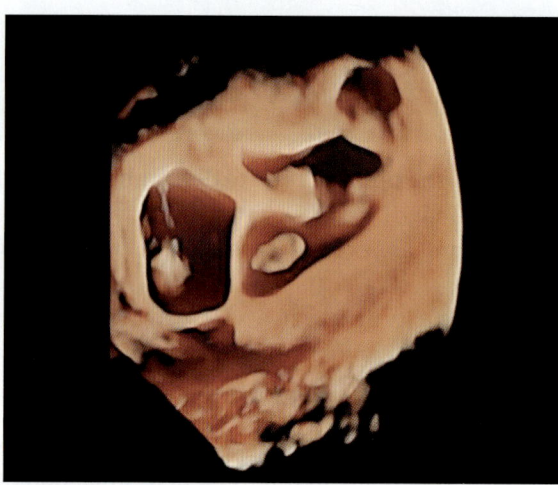

1. What is the order of pregnancy in the above picture?
2. What is Epsilon sign?
3. What sonographic findings determine chorionicity?
4. Enumerate four maternal and four fetal complications associated with multiple gestation.
5. What is the role of ultrasound in multiple pregnancy in second trimester?
6. When and how is embryo reduction done?

Ans.

1. The order of pregnancy in above picture is Quadruplet.
2. Epsilon sign is seen in higher order pregnancy, where three separate gestational sacs meet at a junction of three interfetal membranes (trichorionic triplets)
3. Sonographic findings determining chorionicity are:
    - Total number of gestational sacs
    - Total number of amniotic sacs in chorionic cavity
    - Total number of yolk sacs for diagnosing amnionicity
    - Number of placenta
    - Chorionic peak sign/twin peak sign indicative of dichorionicity
    - The thickness of intertwin membrane
4. *The maternal and fetal complications are:*
    Maternal:
    - Hyperemesis
    - Pre-eclampsia
    - HELLP syndrome
    - Placental abruption
    - Polyhydramnios
    - Placenta previa
    - Gestational diabetes

    Fetal:
    - Vanishing twins
    - Congenital malformations
    - Fetal aneuploidies
    - Single fetal demise
    - Conjoined twins
    - Acardiac twins
    - Twin-to-twin transfusion syndrome
    - Discordant twin
5. *USG importance in second trimester:*
    - To determine chorionicity, if not done in first trimester
    - To assess cervical length to prevent preterm birth
    - To detect congenital malformations which are more common in multiple pregnancy.
    - To detect complications associated with monochorionic placentation.
    - For serial growth assessment, Doppler waveforms, and growth discrepancy.
6. Embryo reduction is done in between 7 and 11 weeks. It can be done transabdominally or transvaginally, with or without anesthesia. It involves injection of potassium chloride (KCl) directly or near the heart under sonographic guidance.

OSCE 7.

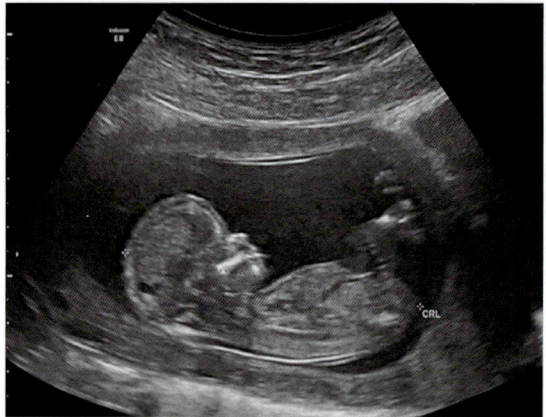

1. What is the timing of first trimester scan and enumerate its advantages?
2. How is first trimester screening for chromosomal abnormalities carried out?
3. What should be the position of fetus while measuring NT?
4. What are the criteria for optimization of NT scan?
5. Enumerate four etiologies of congenital anomalies.

Ans.

1. The timing of the first trimester scan is 11–13.6 weeks.
2. The screening for chromosomal abnormalities is carried out.
3. The position should be a neutral position.
4. *Criteria for NT optimization (AIUM guidelines):*
   - CRL
   - Head
   - Profile face
   - Spine
   - Abdominal transverse view
   - Orbital view and Premaxillary triangle view
   - Visualization of three segments of all 4 limbs, 12 long bones
5. *Etiology of congenital anomalies:*
   - Idiopathic etiology (up to 60%)
   - *Multifactorial (20%):*
     - Neural tube defects—spina bifida, anencephaly
     - Congenital cardiac defects
     - Cleft lip cleft palate
     - Club foot
   - *Genetic (11%):*
     - *Chromosomal disorders (6%):* Trisomy 21, 18, 13
     - *Single gene disorders (5%):*
       - Achondroplasia
       - Neurofibromatosis

- Retinoblastoma
- Marfan's syndrome
- Cystic fibrosis
- Sickle cell disease
- Hemophilia
- DMD
- Fragile X syndrome
	* *Maternal diseases (5%):*
		- Diabetes
		- Epilepsy
	* Infections (2%)
	* Environmental factors (rare 1%)
- *Drugs (rare 1%):*
	* Isotretinoin
	* Alcohol
	* Warfarin
	* Phenytoin
	* Lithium

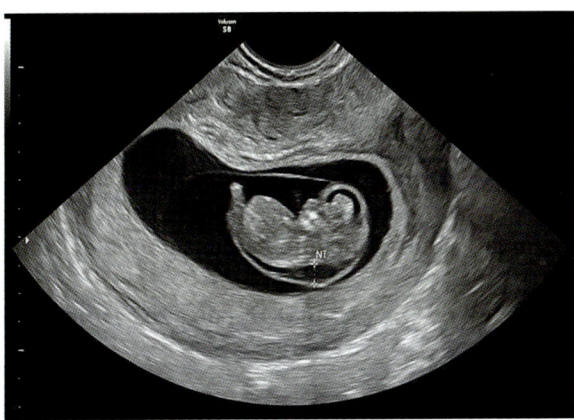

1. What is the ultrasound image suggestive of?
2. What are the advantages of a first trimester scan?
3. What is the significance of raising NT?
4. Enumerate four common anomalies detected in the first trimester scan.
5. What are prenatal tests and enumerate four indications for prenatal diagnosis?

Ans.

1. The image is suggestive of a first trimester scan showing raised nuchal translucency.
2. *Advantages of first trimester scan are:*
   - Timely termination
   - Relatively less complications in termination

- Genetic and chromosomal testing
- Couples with nonlethal and corrected malformations can be offered timely counseling and treatment.
- Less physical and mental trauma to couples
- Cases in which no chromosomal defect is found, proper follow-up and timely delivery with pediatric multispecialty care can be done.

3. Increased NT is a useful marker of chromosomal abnormalities, fetal malformations and genetic syndromes.
4. The common anomalies are:
   - Acrania and Anencephaly
   - Encephalocele
   - Dandy-Walker malformation
   - Open spina bifida
   - Omphalocele
   - Gastroschisis
   - Body stalk anomaly
   - Megacystis
   - Congenital diaphragmatic hernia
   - Congenital heart defects
   - Hydrops fetalis
5. Prenatal tests are performed to diagnose and guide management of the pregnancy, delivery, and neonatal period.
   - *Prenatal methods*

     Noninvasive tests:
     - Ultrasound/dual and quadruple tests
     - Fetal MRI
     - Free-fetal DNA

     Invasive tests:
     - Amniocentesis
     - Chorionic villus sampling
     - Fetal blood sampling
     - Fetal biopsy
     - Fetal surgery

     Indications for prenatal diagnosis:
     - Women at high risk for chromosomal abnormalities, advanced maternal age, previous affected pregnancy, either of the couple is a known carrier of balanced translocation.
     - Family history of a known genetic condition
     - Congenital heart defects
     - Family history of congenital defects like CHD, NTD, renal and CNS anomalies
     - Maternal medical conditions like DM, HTN, autoimmune diseases, hypothyroidism.
     - Abnormal serum screen

- Abnormal or borderline USG findings
- Congenital infections like rubella, CMV, chickenpox, syphilis
- Exposure to smoking, Alcohol, teratogenic drugs like anticonvulsants, oral anti-coagulants, chemotherapeutic drugs
- Multiple gestation.

OSCE 9.

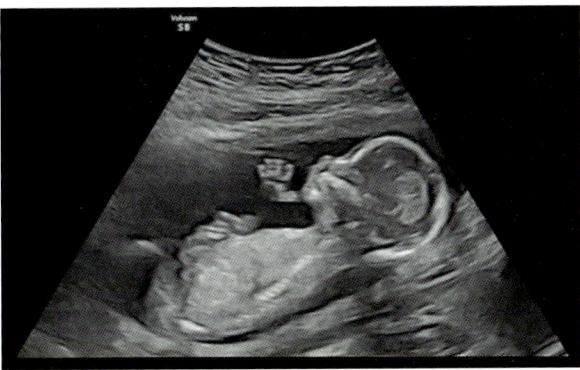

1. What is a TIFFA scan, and at what gestation is it done?
2. What are the factors to be checked during the fetal anomaly scan?
3. Enumerate four second trimester markers for Trisomy 21.
4. Enumerate four common congenital anomalies seen in second trimester scan.
5. Who should be offered mid-trimester anomaly scan?

Ans.

1. TIFFA scan is targeted Imaging for fetal anomalies. It is done around 18–22 weeks.
2. Standard views for the examination of the fetus at mid-trimester anomaly scan are:
    - Skull
    - Brain
    - Face
    - Neck
    - Spine
    - Heart
    - Limbs
    - Abdomen
    - Umbilical cord
    - Thorax
    - Placenta
    - Cervical length
3. Second trimester markers for Trisomy 21 are:
    - Ventriculomegaly
    - Absent or hypoplastic nasal bone
    - Increased nuchal fold thickness

- Intracardiac echogenic focus
- Aberrant right subclavian artery
- Hyperechogenic bowel
- Mild hydronephrosis
- Shortening of Femur or humerus.

4. The common congenital anomalies seen in second trimester are:
   - *NTDs:*
     - Anencephaly
     - Spina bifida
     - Encephalocele
     - Sacrococcygeal teratoma
   - *CNS malformations:*
     - Hydrocephalus
     - Holoprosencephaly
     - Agenesis of corpus callous
     - Septal agenesis
     - Septo optic dysplasia
     - Dandy-Walker malformation
     - Vermian hypoplasia
     - Blake's pouch
     - Arachnoid cyst
   - *Face and Neck:*
     - Cleft lip and palate
     - Macrognathia
     - Microphthalmia
     - Aphasia
     - Hypertelorism
     - Cystic hygroma
     - Hemangioma
     - Lymphangioma
     - Teratoma
   - *Cardiac:*
     - Conotruncal malformations
     - TOF
     - Double outlet right ventricle
     - Truncus arteriosus
     - Transposition of great vessels
   - *GIT:*
     - Tracheoesophageal fistula
     - Duodenal atresia
     - Small bowel obstruction
     - Omphalocele
     - Gastroschisis

5. Every pregnant female should be offered an opportunity for antenatal detection of fetal structural anomalies by a mid-trimester anomaly scan because most of the fetal abnormalities actually occur in the so-called "low-risk" pregnant female.

OSCE 10.

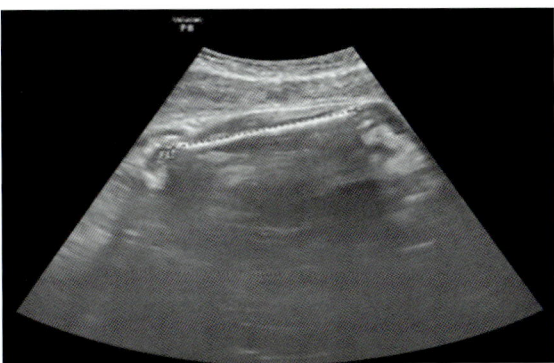

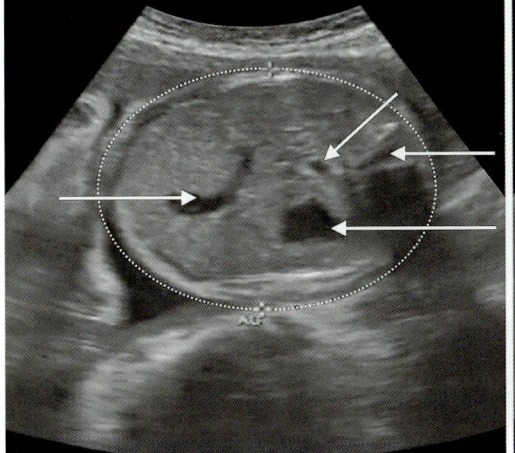
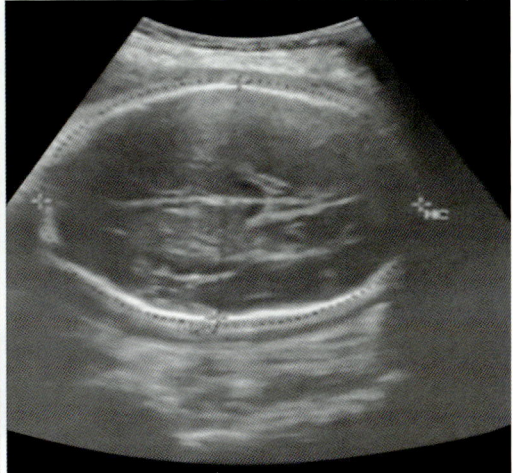

1. What is the above ultrasound image showing?
2. Write the important first trimester measurements.
3. What are the standard biometric measurements of the second trimester?
4. How is fetal weight estimated?
5. How is the gestational age estimated in twin gestation in first trimester?

Ans.

1. The above image shows fetal biometry.
2. The important first trimester measurements are:
   - Mean gestational sac diameter
   - Crown rump length (CRL)
   - Nuchal translucency

3. The standard biometric measurements of second trimester are:
   - Biparietal diameter
   - Head circumference
   - Abdominal circumference
   - Femur length
4. The most important parameter for estimation of fetal weight is abdominal circumference (AC).
   - Various formulas are given for fetal weight estimation, Hadlock and Shepard are commonly used.
   - Fetal weight may vary with race, ethnicity, parity and other environmental and socio-economic factors.
5. In twin pregnancy, CRL of both fetuses is measured and larger CRL is used to assign the gestational age.

OSCE 11.

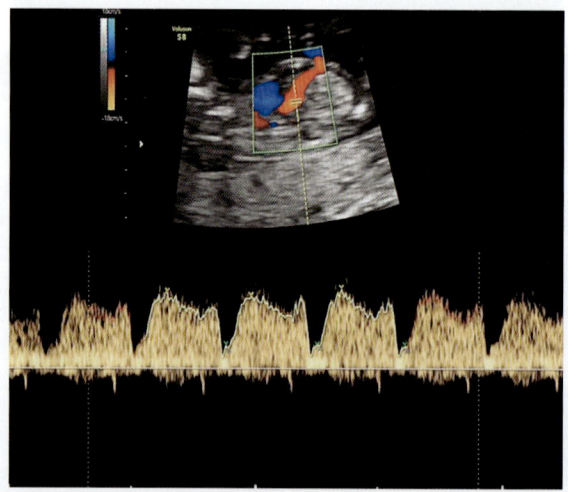

1. **Identify the pulse waveform.**
2. **Write the different forms of fetal arterial dopplers used in ultrasound?**

Ans.

1. The pulse waveform shown is of ductus venosus.
2. The different forms of fetal arterial wave forms is:
   - Ductus venosus
   - Uterine artery
   - Umbilical artery
   - Middle cerebral artery.

OSCE 12.

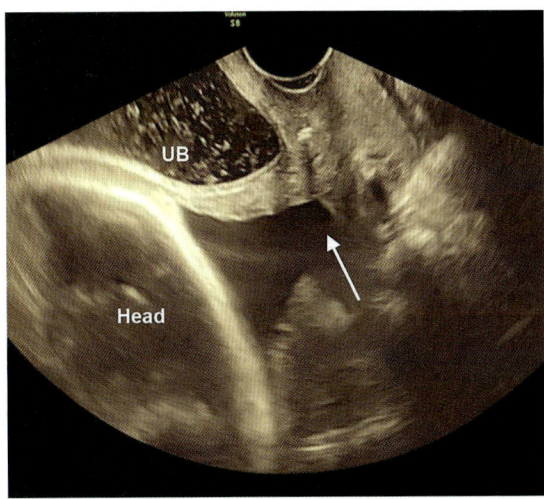

1. Identify the marked structure in the image.
2. What is the gold standard method for assessment of cervical length?
3. What is cervical insufficiency. Enumerate 4 causes?
4. What is funneling of cervix and its importance? What are the different phases of funneling in USG?
5. Enumerate two indications of cerclage.

Ans.

1. The marked stage in the image shows dilated cervix.
2. The Gold standard method for assessment of cervical length is by TVS.
3. Cervical insufficiency is the ability of cervix to retain pregnancy owing to structural and functional defects in the absence of uterine contractions or labor. It is characterized by painless cervical dilation in the second or third trimester with ballooning of the amniotic sac in the vagina, followed by rupture of membranes and expulsion of fetus.

   Etiology of cervical insufficiency are:
   Congenital:
   - Uterine anomalies
   - Isolated developmental weakness

   Acquired:
   - Forcible dilatation during dilatation and curettage
   - Conization of cervix in the past
   - Cauterization of cervix in the past
   - Amputation of cervix or Fothergill's operation in the past
   - Vaginal delivery through not fully dilated cervix
   - Cervical tear

4. Cervical funneling is defined sonographically as the protrusion of Amniotic membranes of >≈5 mm into the internal os as measured along the lateral border of the funnel. The different phases of funneling in USG are T-shaped/Y-shaped/V-shaped/U-shaped.

5. The indications of Cerclage (RCOG 2011) are:
   History indicated:
   - Should be offered to women with 3 or more previous preterm births and or second trimester losses.
   - Should be routinely offered to women with 2 or fewer previous preterm births and or second trimester losses.

   USG indicated:
   - Women with history of 1 or more spontaneous preterm births or mid trimester losses with T, V or U detected on USG or cervical length <≈25 mm before 24 weeks.
   - Not recommended for women without a history of spontaneous preterm delivery or second trimester losses with incidentally detected cervical length <≈25 mm.
   - Not recommended for funneling of cervix in the absence of cervical shortening to <≈25 mm.

OSCE 13.

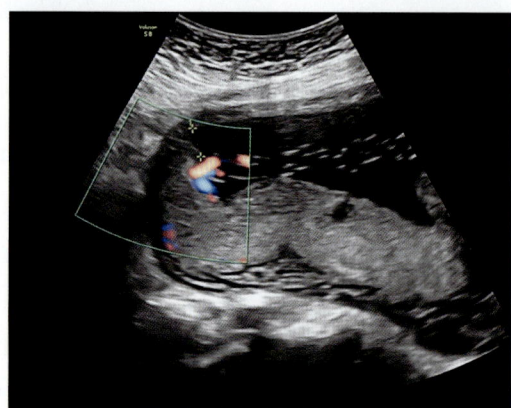

1. Identify the structure in the above ultrasound image and the abnormality seen.
2. Enumerate the types/variants of placenta.
3. Describe the normal ultrasonographic appearance of placenta.
4. How is morbidly adherent placenta seen on ultrasound? What are placental lakes or lacunae?
5. What is the significance of placental size? Enumerate two causes of placental thinning and thickening.

Ans.

1. The structure in the picture is placenta, the abnormality seen is the marginal insertion of the cord.
2. Variants of placenta are:
   According to morphology:
   - Bilobed placenta
   - Succenturiate placenta
   - Circumvallate placenta
   - Placenta membranacea

According to cord insertion:
- Velamentous insertion
- Marginal cord insertion or Battledore placenta

3. Placenta appears discoid in shape.
   - 15–20 cm
   - 3 cm thick
   - 400–600 g at term
   - Present along anterior or posterior uterine walls, some extension to fundus and lateral walls
   - Having uniform intermediate echogenicity
   - Color and power Doppler mode for uteroplacental, fetoplacental circulations and hence placental vascularity
4. The sonographic features of morbidly adherent placenta are:
   - Irregularly shaped multiple placental lacunae (Swiss cheese appearance)
   - Turbulent blood flow on color Doppler through the lacunae
   - Thinning of part of myometrium where placenta is implanted.
   - Loss of retroplacental hypoechoic area
   - Abnormality of serosa—bladder interface
   - Extension of villi into myometrium, serosa, or bladder.
5. Placental size concerns with the midpoint thickness of the organ.

   Placental thinning: It occurs due to vascular deficits. Seen either in systemic, vascular, hematological diseases, SGA fetus, intrauterine infections, chromosomal abnormalities, and severe polyhydramnios.

   Placental thickening: >4 cm
   Heterogeneous—molar pregnancy, triploidy, placental hemorrhage,
   Homogeneous—maternal anemia, hydrops fetalis, in-utero infections, GDM

OSCE 14.

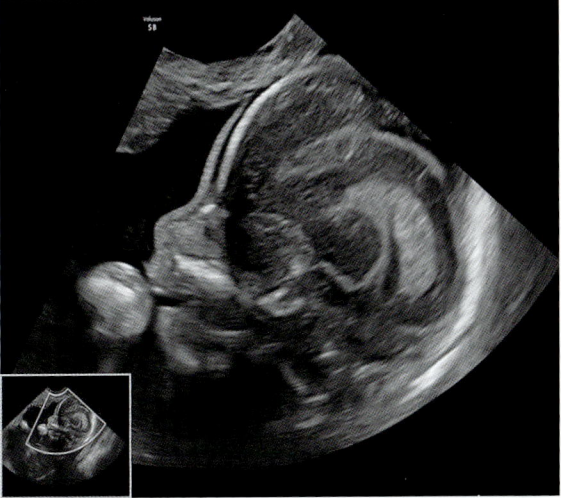

1. Identify the abnormality in the above image.
2. Define the condition.
3. What is the incidence of the above condition?
4. How to assess nasal bone?
5. What is the prognosis of isolated absent/hypoplastic nasal bone fetuses, aneuploidy is ruled out?
6. What is the next step, if hypoplastic nasal bone is evident in first trimester scan?

Ans.

1. The abnormality in the image shows Absent or Hypoplastic nasal bone.
2. Hypoplastic or Absent nasal bone is defined as the absence or ill formed nasal bone in the fetus.
3. 0.5–1.2% of normal fetuses have been found to have a hypoplastic nasal bone on a routine 2nd trimester scan, compared to 43–62% of fetuses with Down syndrome.
4. The ultrasound transducer should be held parallel to the direction of the nose and should be gently tilted from side to side to ensure that the nasal bone is seen separate from the nasal skin. The echogenicity of the nasal bone should be greater than the skin overlying it.
5. Absent or hypoplastic nasal bone occurs in 0.1–1.2% of euploid pregnancies.
6. Next step is to perform a diagnostic test. As the association of hypoplastic nasal bone with chromosomal anomaly is very high. We should directly go for a diagnostic test such as amniocentesis/CVS

OSCE 15.

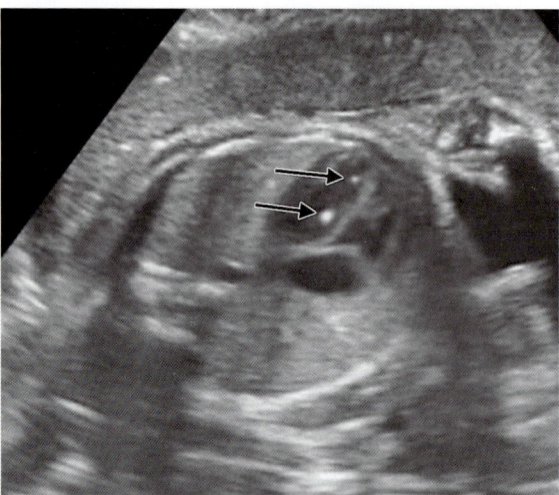

1. Identify the structure and the ultrasound feature in the image.
2. Define the above feature.
3. What is its incidence?
4. State any association of this feature with major cardiac defects.
5. What should be the next step, if this feature is evident on ultrasound?

Ans.

1. Fetal heart with echogenic intracardiac focus
2. Echogenic intracardiac focus
3. 4% pregnancies
4. EIFs are found in approximately 3–5% of pregnancies and are usually benign. They have been associated with fetal chromosome abnormalities, including Down Syndrome. EIF are considered a "soft marker" for Down syndrome, associated with a 1.4–1.8 fold increased risk for Down syndrome when an isolated finding.
5. Complete structural evaluation of fetus. Along with fetal echocardiography.

OSCE 16.

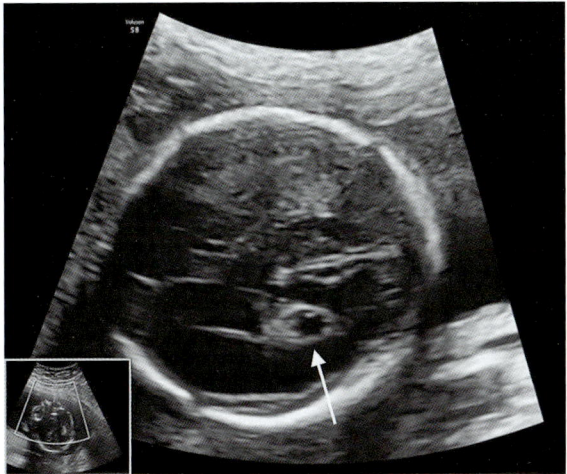

1. Identify the feature in the above image.
2. What is the incidence of this feature?
3. Is there any association with aneuploidy?
4. What should be the next step after this feature is evident on ultrasound?
5. Is there any association of this feature with any type of neurological abnormality?

Ans.

1. Choroid plexus cyst
2. 1–2% normal pregnancies
3. Bilateral choroid plexus cyst is associated with trisomy 18 (Edwards syndrome) and other anomalies such as trisomy 13, 18.
4. A complete neurosonogram, review of biochemical markers and screening test. And if another abnormalities then diagnostic tests such as amniocentesis, CVS.
5. Most CPCs dissapear after delivery. Rarely associated with neurological abnormalities.

CHAPTER 4

First Trimester Screening and Ultrasound Markers

Chinmayee Ratha

OSCE 1. Identify the part highlighted with the arrow in the given picture and answer the questions that follow:

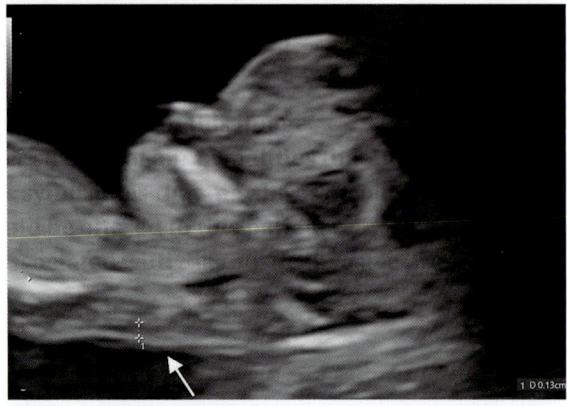

1. What is this region popularly known as?
2. How do we define this parameter?
3. Criteria for an ideal image of this part.
4. What conditions are suspected if this measurement is increased?
5. How do we interpret this marker if the umbilical cord is surrounding the fetal neck?

Ans.
1. Fetal nuchal translucency
2. Nuchal translucency (NT) is the sonographic appearance of a collection of fluid under the skin behind the fetal neck in the first trimester of pregnancy.
3. CRL should be between 45–84 mm
4. Chromosomal abnormalities, cardiac defects, genetic syndromes, infections or it could also be a normal variant.
5. NT is then measured above and below the level of the cord and its average is taken as the final NT.

OSCE 2. Identify the condition and answer the questions that follow:

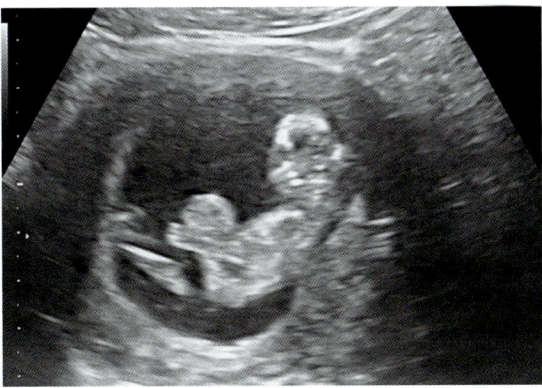

1. Identify the condition.
2. Which chromosomal abnormalities are commonly associated with this condition?
3. When could you consider this normal?
4. How do you classify this condition?
5. What further tests would be advised?

Ans.

1. Exomphalos
2. Trisomy 18 or 13
3. Before completion of 11 weeks—could be physiological herniation of the gut which usually resolves by 11 weeks gestation.
4. Minor—containing bowel, major containing parts of the liver too in addition to bowel, stomach, etc.
5. Chromosomal testing, detailed TIFFA and fetal echo to rule out other associated anomalies, serial growth scans.

OSCE 3. Identify the structure highlighted and answer the following questions:

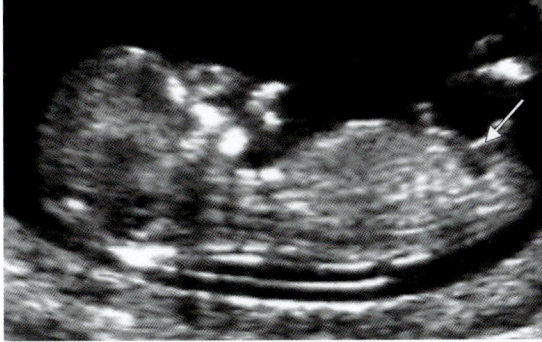

1. Identify the structure.
2. What measurement parameter would you consider as normal?
3. What is the technical name of enlargement of this structure?

Section 1: Obstetrics

4. Which abnormalities are commonly associated with enlargement of this structure?
5. What further tests would be advised?

Ans.

1. Fetal urinary bladder
2. Up to 7 mm is normal in longitudinal diameter in first trimester.
3. Megacystis
4. Chromosomal abnormalities like Down Syndrome, lower urinary tract obstruction, Prune Belly syndrome or it could also be a normal variant.
5. Chromosomal tests, detailed scan for fetal kidneys and ureters and also to rule out other structural anomalies, serial follow-up to look for progressive urinary tract dilatation.

OSCE 4. Observe the following first trimester scan picture carefully and answer the following questions:

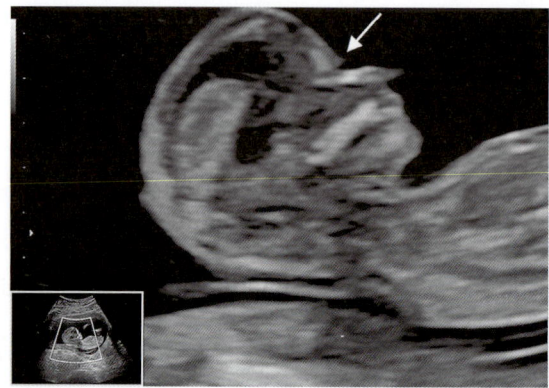

1. Identify the part highlighted with the arrow in the given picture which is a marker for aneuploidies in the first trimester scan.
2. Enumerate two important criteria to diagnose this marker.
3. What conditions do we suspect when this marker is absent?
4. This marker can also be seen in the coronal view of the fetal face in first trimester—True/False.
5. Even if this marker is absent, the fetal outcome may be good—True/False.

Ans.

1. Nasal bone
2. a. Seen in a midsagittal view of the fetal face
   b. Appears as the lower line in an "equals" sign below the skin of the nose—both lines must be seen well and the lower line should be more echogenic to diagnose the presence of nasal bone.
3. Chromosomal abnormalities like Down syndrome may be suspected as it is a marker that helps in screening—please note it is a screening tool, not diagnostic for aneuploidies!
4. True
5. True

OSCE 5. Please see the following first trimester fetal scan picture and answer the questions that follow:

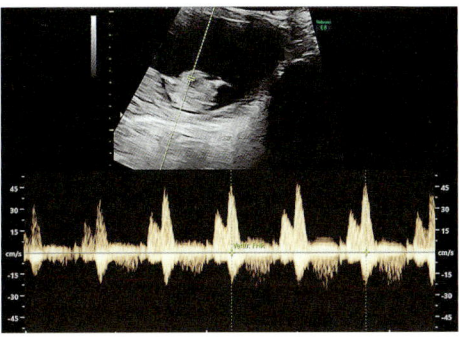

1. Which ultrasound-based marker for aneuploidy is being assessed here?
2. Is this parameter normal or abnormal in the given picture?
3. What parameters will indicate abnormality of this marker?
4. What conditions do we suspect if this parameter is abnormal?
5. What is the follow-up protocol for abnormality in this parameter?

Ans.

1. Tricuspid flows
2. It is normal—there is no regurgitation
3. Bidirectional flow across tricuspid valve with a regurgitant wave seen in ventricular systole showing a jet which occupies more than half of the systole and a maximum speed of 60 cm/s.
4. Chromosomal abnormalities like Down syndrome, cardiac defects, or any form of hyperdynamic circulation. It could be a transient physiological finding too.
5. Counsel based on the combined screening protocol and if all reassuring then recall patient for a detailed TIFFA and echo.

OSCE 6. Please answer the following questions about the coronal section of fetal face in first trimester.

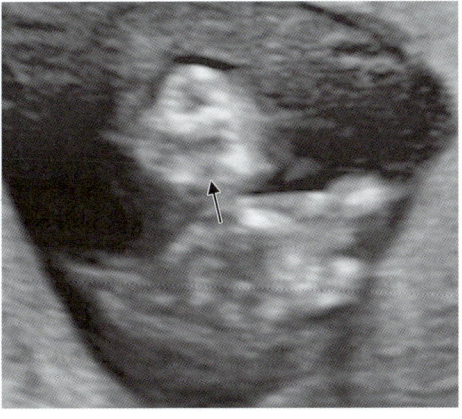

1. What is this marker called?
2. What does it indicate?
3. When is it abnormal?
4. How will you counsel a patient if it is abnormal?
5. What tests will you advise this patient?

Ans.

1. Mandibular gap
2. It is a normal finding and indicates proper development of fetal maxilla.
3. Absent mandibular gap is considered as a marker for micrognathia or severe retrognathia.
4. Possibility of this being familial is explained along with the association of multiple genetic conditions.
5. Detailed TIFFA to rule out any other anomalies, family phenotype assessment to rule out familial cases and for genetic cases, tests can be planned with the geneticist.

OSCE 7. Observe the picture below and answer the questions that follow:

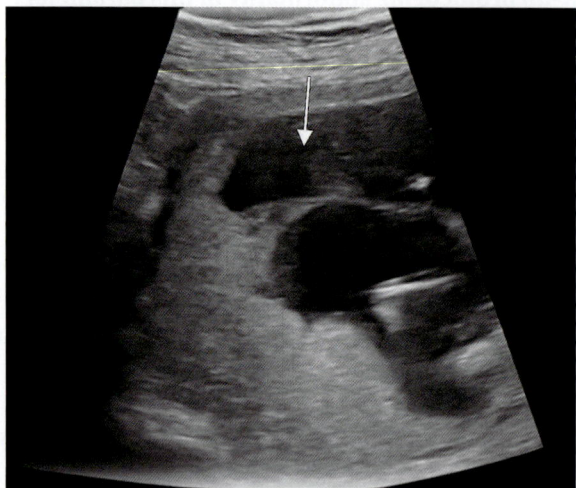

1. Identify the sign.
2. What does it indicate?
3. What is the ideal time frame to assess this sign?
4. If this sign is present and both fetuses have different NT, how is the risk of Down syndrome calculated?
5. If this sign is absent and both fetuses have different NT, how is the risk of Down syndrome calculated?

Ans.

1. Lambda sign
2. Presence of Lambda signs indicate dichorionicity
3. 9–14 weeks

Chapter 4: First Trimester Screening and Ultrasound Markers

4. Both fetuses have separate risks based on their individual NT measurements.
5. Absence of this sign indicates monochorionicity and the average NT is taken to calculate risks of Down syndrome.

OSCE 8. Please see the following first trimester fetal scan picture and answer the questions that follow:

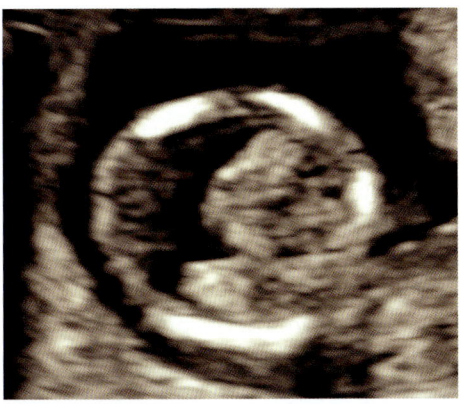

1. Which ultrasound-based marker for aneuploidy is being assessed here?
2. Which aneuploidy is commonly associated with this condition?
3. What are the other structural issues you can expect in this fetus?
4. What further tests will you advise?
5. What is the prognosis of this case?

Ans.

1. Holoprosencephaly
2. Trisomy 13
3. Facial anomalies with midline defects may be present.
4. Chromosomal tests, detailed facial evaluation along with TIFFA, neurosonogram to characterize the brain anomaly.
5. Extremely guarded with a high risk of lethality.

OSCE 9. Note the picture below and answer the questions that follow:

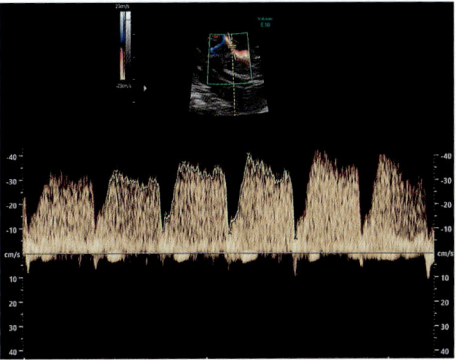

Section 1: Obstetrics

1. Which first trimester marker is depicted in the picture?
2. What kind of blood is carried by this vessel—oxygenated/deoxygenated?
3. What is the size of the pulse wave gate to measure this parameter?
4. This parameter is best tested in a very active fetus—true/false.
5. When is this parameter considered abnormal?

Ans.

1. Ductus venosus
2. Oxygenated blood from the placenta to the fetus.
3. 0.5–1 mm
4. False—DV is measured during periods of fetal quiescence.
5. Abnormal DV is classified as either increased PI or absent or reversed "a" wave. It indicates high risk of chromosomal abnormalities and cardiac disorders in the fetus but rarely it can also have physiological variations.

OSCE 10. Answer the questions that follow the picture.

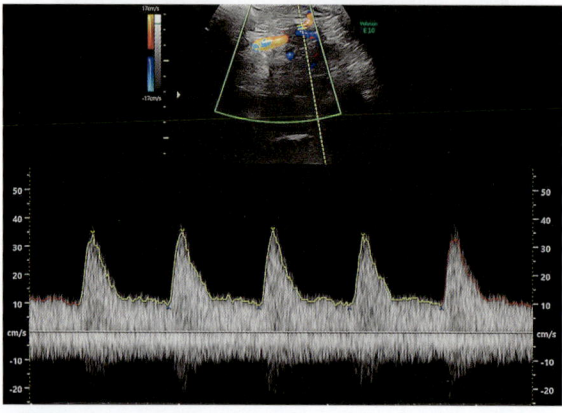

1. Identify the parameter measured.
2. What is the origin of the vessel tested?
3. How is it located during first trimester scan?
4. What is the expected peak systolic velocity (PSV) of this vessel?
5. What does abnormality in this flow pattern indicate?

Ans.

1. Uterine artery
2. It is a branch of the anterior division of the internal iliac artery.
3. It is located lateral to the uterus near the internal cervical os.
4. 60 cm/sec
5. Abnormal uterine artery flows are diagnosed with high mean PI of both sides and indicates high risk for pre-eclampsia in the mother and FGR for the fetus.

CHAPTER 5

Congenital Malformations in Fetus

Chanchal Singh, Vrunda Appannagari

OSCE 1.

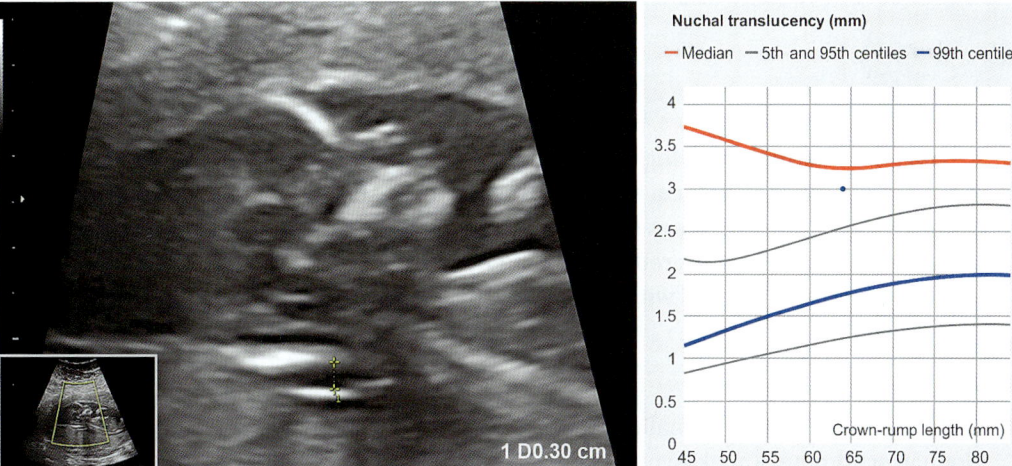

1. Identify two abnormal findings in this image.
2. What is the most common associated chromosomal abnormality?
3. How will you identify it?
4. Fetal karyotype is normal. What is the next best step in management?
5. What percentage of fetuses with NT between 95th–99th centile is likely to be normal?

Ans.

1. a. Absent nasal bone
   b. NT >95th centile
2. Trisomy 21.
3. Chorionic villus sampling or amniocentesis.
4. Early anomaly scan to identify cardiac defects.
5. More than 90% fetuses with NT between 95th–99th centile are likely to be normal.

OSCE 2.

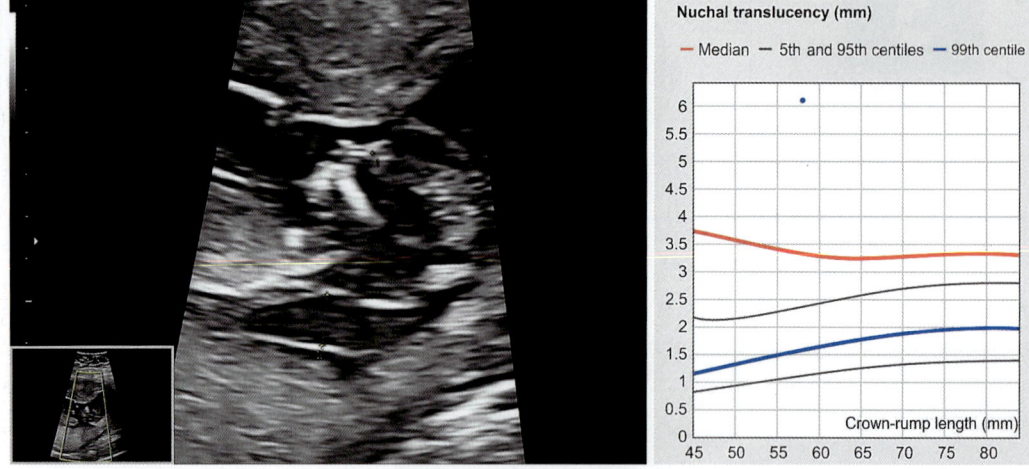

1. Identify the abnormal finding in this image.
2. What are the other structural abnormalities that may be associated with this?
3. Name two genetic syndromes that may be associated with this.
4. What testing should be offered to this patient?
5. What is the risk associated with diagnostic invasive procedures?

Ans.

1. NT >99th centile
2. Cardiac and skeletal abnormalities
3. Noonan syndrome, Kabuki syndrome
4. Diagnostic testing (CVS or amniocentesis)
5. 0.5% risk of miscarriage.

OSCE 3.

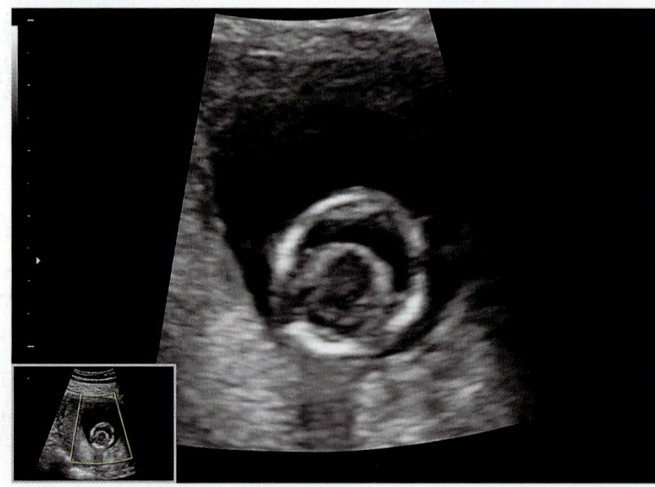

1. Identify the abnormality in this image.
2. What is the most common associated chromosomal abnormality?
3. What is the prognosis?
4. What is the recurrence risk?
5. Name four other structural abnormalities that should always be detected at the first trimester itself.

Ans.

1. Alobar holoprosencephaly
2. 70% of holoprosencephaly is associated with Trisomy 13
3. It is a lethal anomaly and termination of pregnancy should be offered.
4. When associated with trisomy 13, the recurrence risk is 1%.
5. a. Anterior abdominal wall defects
   b. Body stalk anomaly
   c. Acrania
   d. Limb reduction defects

OSCE 4.

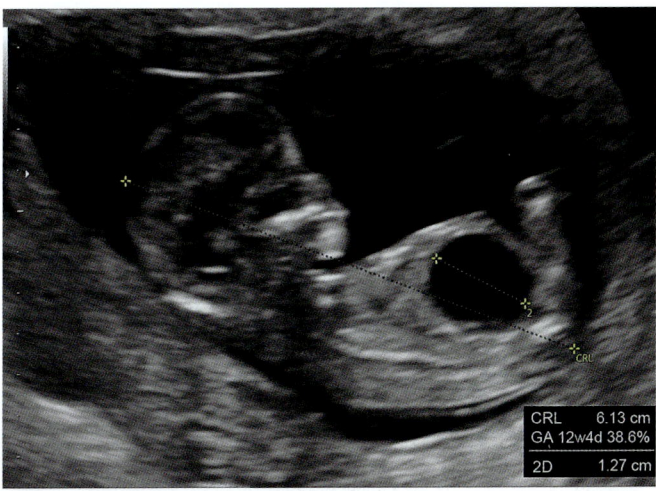

1. Identify the abnormality.
2. Name two differential diagnoses.
3. What percentage is associated with chromosomal abnormalities?
4. Fetal karyotype is normal. What would be the next best step?
5. How is the prognosis of this condition?

Ans.

1. Megacystis.
2. a. Posterior urethral valve
   b. Urethral atresia

3. Mild enlargement of the bladder (7–15 mm) may be associated with chromosomal abnormalities in 25% cases. If the longitudinal measurement is >15 mm, the risk of aneuploidy is 11%.
4. Early anomaly scan at 16–17 weeks.
5. If the fetal karyotype is normal and longitudinal measurement of bladder is 7–15 mm, spontaneous resolution occurs in 90% cases. If measurement is >15 mm, majority of chromosomally normal fetuses will develop obstructive uropathy.

OSCE 5.

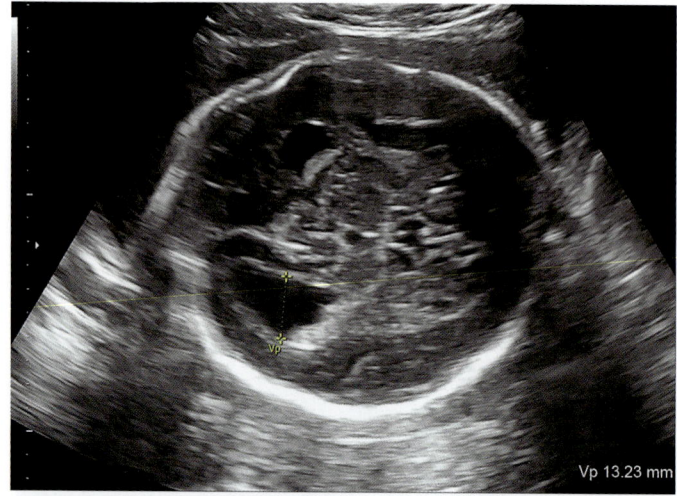

1. Identify the abnormality.
2. Name four possible causes of this finding.
3. How is the severity of ventriculomegaly defined?
4. What is the prognosis in isolated mild ventriculomegaly?
5. The follow-up scan image is given below. What is the diagnosis?

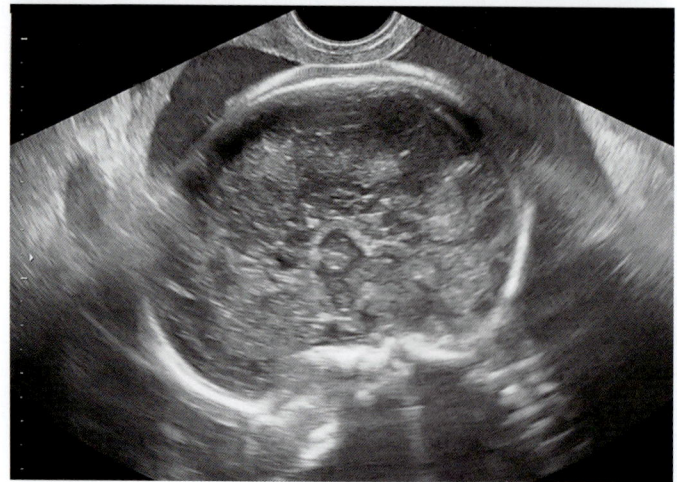

Ans.
1. Mild ventriculomegaly
2. a. Fetal infection
   b. Trisomy 21
   c. Agenesis of corpus callosum
   d. Intracranial hemorrhage
3. Measurement between 10–15 mm is defined as 'mild' and measurements ≥15 mm are defined as severe ventriculomegaly
4. The neurodevelopmental outcome of 'isolated' mild ventriculomegaly is reported to be similar to the general population. It is called 'isolated' only when fetal infection and chromosomal abnormalities have been ruled out on amniocentesis and structural abnormalities have been ruled out on neurosonogram.
5. Agenesis of corpus callosum

OSCE 6. A 32-year-old G2P1L1 with 15 weeks pregnancy is referred in view of high risk for trisomy 21 on triple marker. She gives history of vaginal bleeding off and on since conception. Ultrasound shows a single live fetus growing on 10th centile. Given below is the ultrasound image of the placenta.

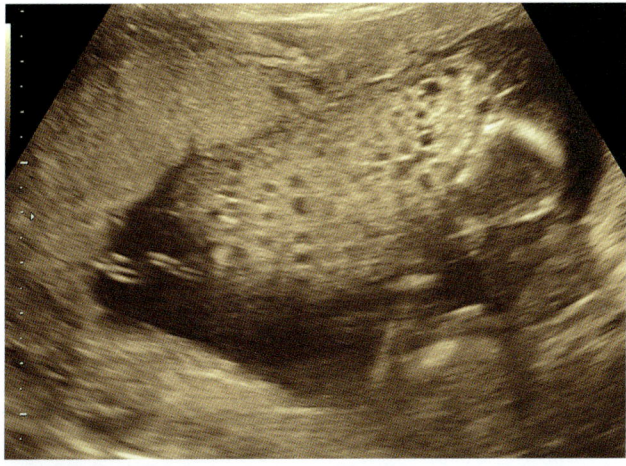

1. What is the likely diagnosis?
2. Which hormone level in the triple marker is likely to be abnormal?
3. Name two obstetric complications associated with this condition.
4. Name two fetal complications associated with this condition.

Ans.
1. Complete hydatidiform mole with a co-existent healthy fetus (CHMCF).
2. Beta-hCG levels will typically be very high giving a high risk for trisomy 21.
3. a. Pre-eclampsia
   b. Persistent gestational trophoblastic disease
4. a. Aneuploidy
   b. Fetal growth restriction

OSCE 7.

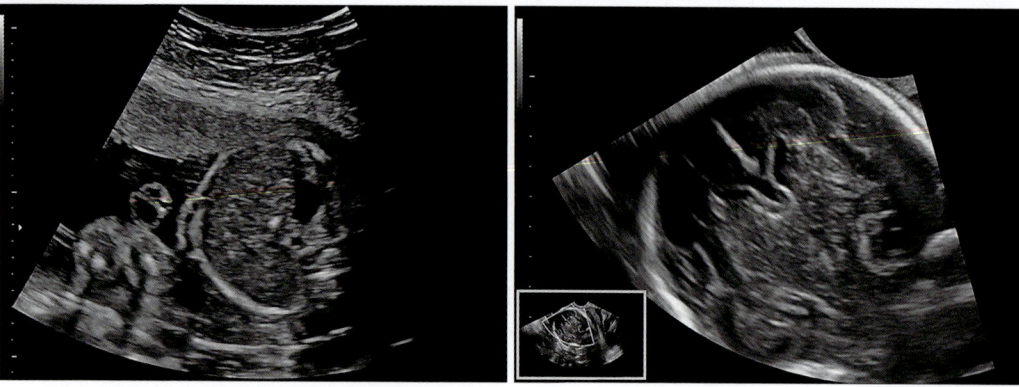

1. Identify the lesions in these images.
2. What is the most likely cause?
3. What is the diagnostic test for this?
4. Name two other pathologies associated with hepatic calcifications.
5. Amniocentesis confirmed fetal infection. Which drug has shown promising results in improving neonatal prognosis in this infection?

Ans.

1. a. Hepatic calcifications
   b. Periventricular calcifications
2. Fetal infection especially fetal CMV infection
3. Amniocentesis for viral PCR on amniotic fluid
4. a. Trisomy 21
   b. Cystic fibrosis
5. Maternal oral Valacyclovir in fetal CMV infection.

OSCE 8.

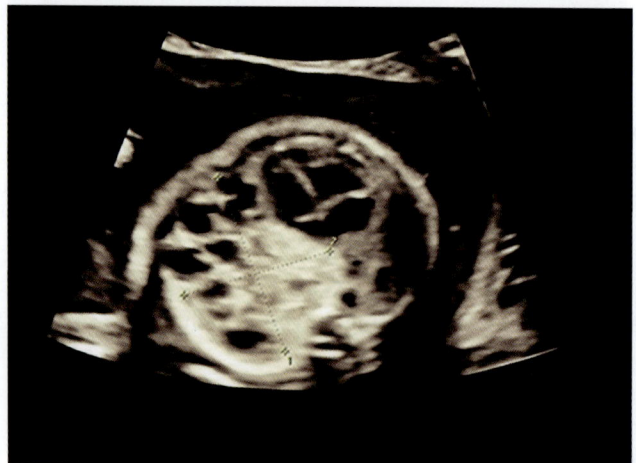

Chapter 5: Congenital Malformations in Fetus

This is the 2D ultrasound image of axial section of fetal thorax showing fetal heart and a large echogenic lesion in the left hemithorax.
1. Identify the abnormality.
2. Name two differential diagnosis and how is each differentiated from this condition?
3. What are the prognostic factors determining prognosis?
4. When if fetal intervention indicted in these lesions?

Ans.

1. Congenital pulmonary adenomatoid malformation (CPAM)
2. a. Bronchopulmonary sequestration—presence of direct feeding vessel from aorta
   b. Congenital diaphragmatic hernia (CDH)—peristalsis in bowel loops in the hemithorax, color Doppler showing hepatic vessels going up into the thorax in the pulled-up liver.
3. CPAM Volume ratio (CVR), presence of dominant cyst >2 cm in size, hydrops.
4. Development of fetal hydrops.

OSCE 9.

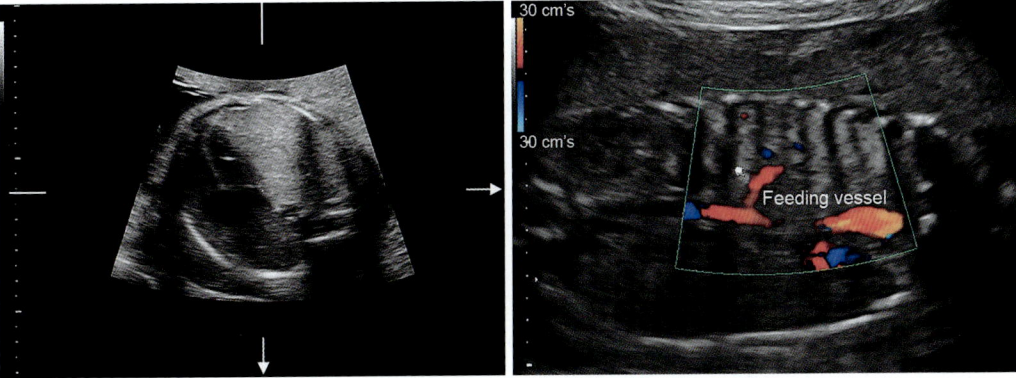

1. Identify the abnormality.
2. How is it identified on ultrasound?
3. Name two differential diagnosis of the intrathoracic variety?
4. What is the prognosis?
5. When is fetal intervention indicated in these lesions?

Ans.

1. Bronchopulmonary sequestration (BPS)
2. It is seen as an echodense triangular area with a direct feeding vessel usually from the descending aorta.
3. a. Congenital pulmonary adenomatoid malformation (CPAM)
   b. Congenital diaphragmatic hernia (CDH)
4. 75% of prenatally diagnosed BPS resolve spontaneously while those associated with hydrops and pleural effusion have poor prognosis.
5. a. Thoracoamniotic shunt if large pleural effusion develops before 30 weeks.
   b. Ablation of feeding vessel if fetal hydrops develops.

OSCE 10.

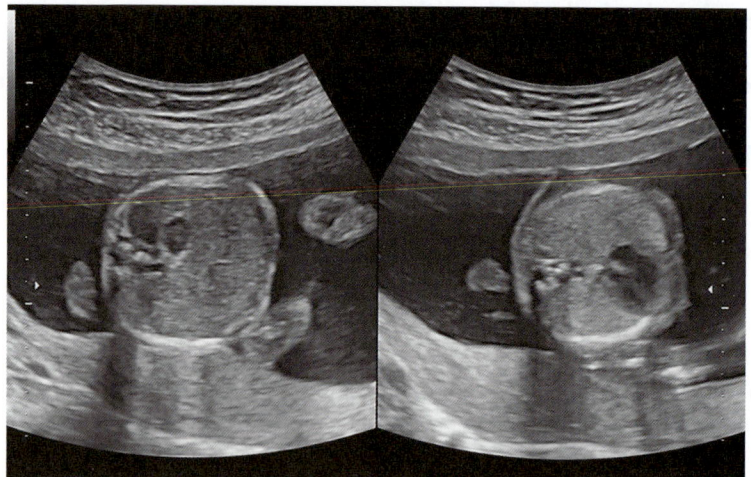

1. Identify the abnormality.
2. What are the two next important investigations?
3. Which is the main prognostic indicator in this condition?
4. Which genetic tests should be done in this case?
5. What is the recurrence risk?

Ans.

1. Heterotaxy.
2. Fetal echo and amniocentesis.
3. Cardiac defects.
4. The whole exome sequencing in addition to fetal microarray.
5. Most cases of heterotaxy are sporadic single occurrences. Approximately 10% of cases have a family history of a close relative with congenital heart disease.

OSCE 11.

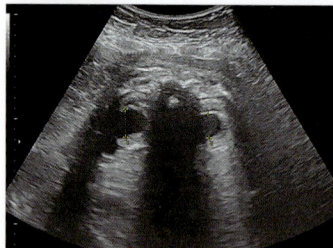 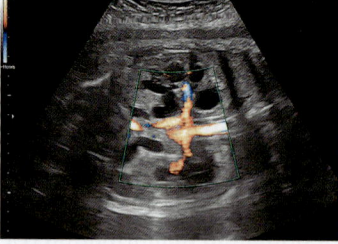 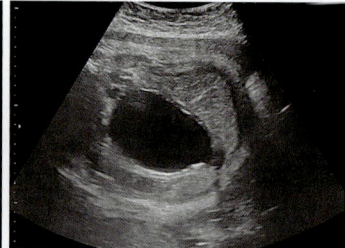

1. Identify the ultrasound findings in all three images.
2. What is the current classification system for this abnormality?
3. What is the most likely diagnosis?
4. Which is the main prognostic indicator in this condition?
5. What is the recurrence risk?

Ans.

1. Hydronephrosis, peripheral calyceal dilatation, key-hole signs.
2. Urinary tract dilatation–Antenatal (UTD–A I, II/III).
3. Posterior urethral valve (PUV).
4. Amniotic fluid index is a surrogate marker for fetal renal function. Progressive oligohydramnios is the most important poor prognostic factor.
5. Obstructive uropathies are mostly sporadic with no increased recurrence risk.

OSCE 12.

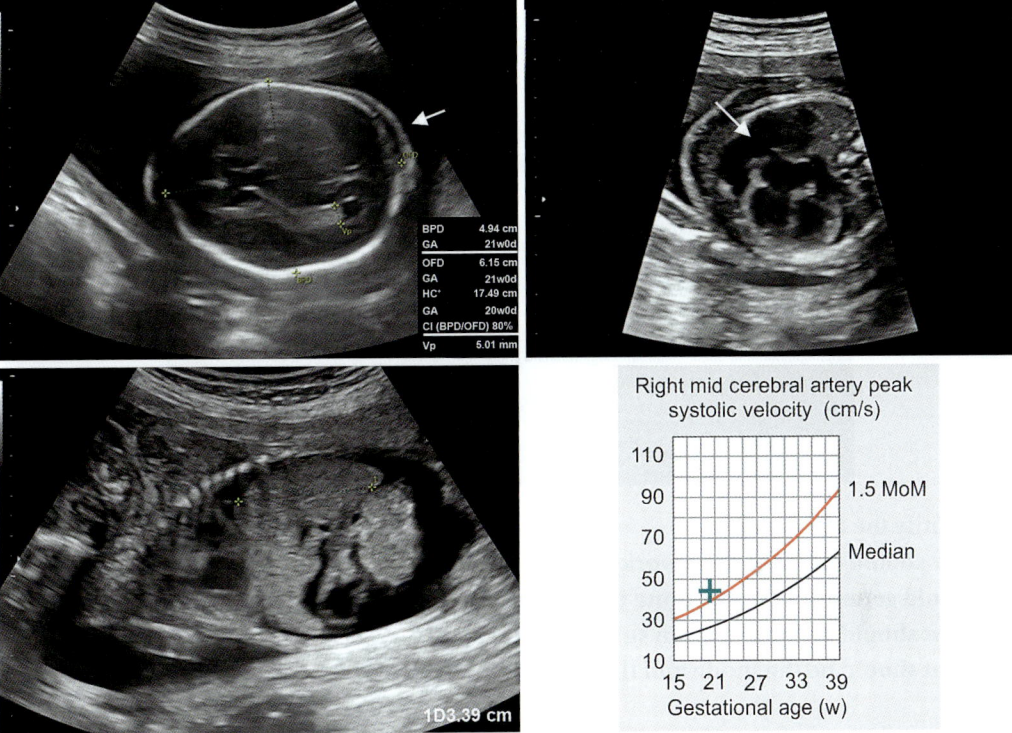

1. What does the image panel show?
2. What are the two main differential diagnoses?
3. Name two investigations, each for the mother and the fetus.
4. What is the treatment for this condition?

Ans.

1. Subcutaneous edema, pericardial effusion, ascites, and MCA PSV >1.5 MoM suggestive of fetal anemia.
2. a. Immune hydrops due to Rh incompatibility
   b. Fetal Parvovirus infection

3. *Maternal investigations:*
   a. Blood group, ICT, and atypical antibody screening
   b. Parvovirus IgM, IgG

   Fetal investigations:
   a. Fetal echocardiogram
   b. Amniocentesis and/or cordocentesis depending on maternal investigations.
4. Intrauterine transfusion with fresh O-negative, irradiated, leukodepleted blood.

OSCE 13.

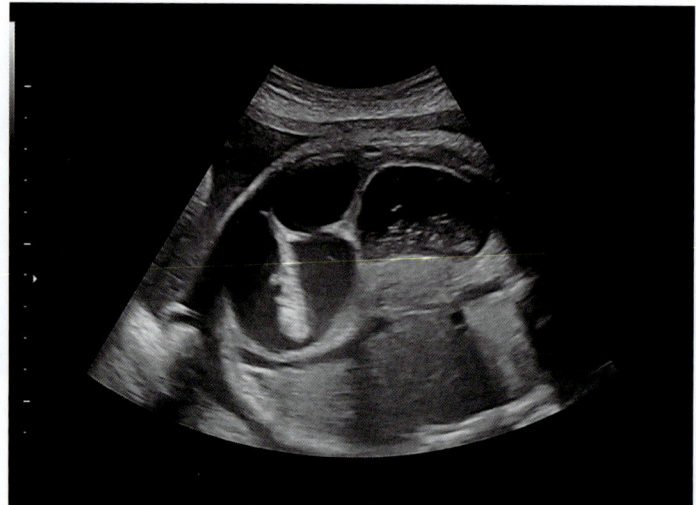

1. Identify the abnormality.
2. How should the patient be worked up?
3. Should genetic testing be done in this case?
4. What should be looked for in subsequent scans?
5. What should be the mode and timing of delivery?

Ans.

1. Bowel obstruction.
2. Detailed anomaly scan to look for associated anomalies.
3. The incidence of chromosomal abnormalities and genetic syndromes is not increased. However, there may be an association with cystic fibrosis in 10% cases and testing by amniocentesis should be offered if parents are carriers.
4. Serial USG every 2–3 weeks to look for polyhydramnios. Signs of bowel perforation and meconium peritonitis should be looked for. The association with cystic fibrosis is up to 90% when meconium peritonitis is present.
5. Delivery should be planned at term in tertiary care center with NICU and pediatric surgery facilities. Induction/cesarean should be reserved for usual obstetric indications.

Chapter 5: Congenital Malformations in Fetus

OSCE 14.

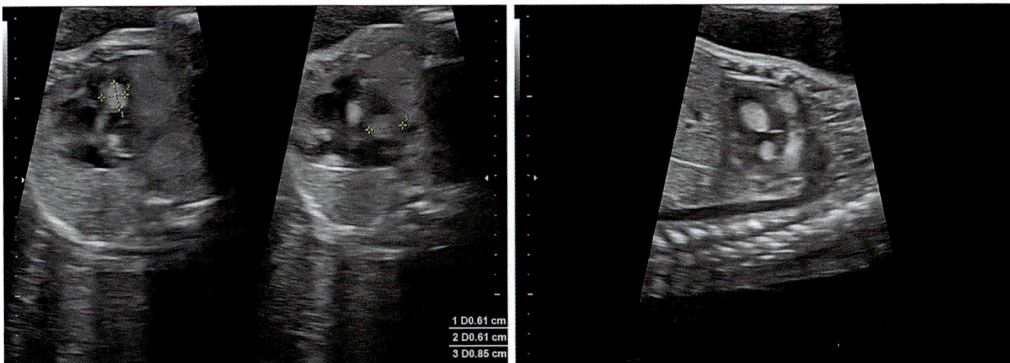

1. Identify the abnormality.
2. Which is the most common association with this finding?
3. Which is the main prognostic indicator in this condition?
4. Which genetic tests should be done in this case?
5. What is the recurrence risk?

Ans.

1. Rhabdomyomas
2. Tuberous sclerosis
3. Congestive cardiac failure leading to hydrops.
4. Genetic testing for *TSC1* and *TSC2* genes.
5. It may be sporadic or of autosomal recessive inheritance in which case both parents would be carriers of the genetic mutation.

OSCE 15.

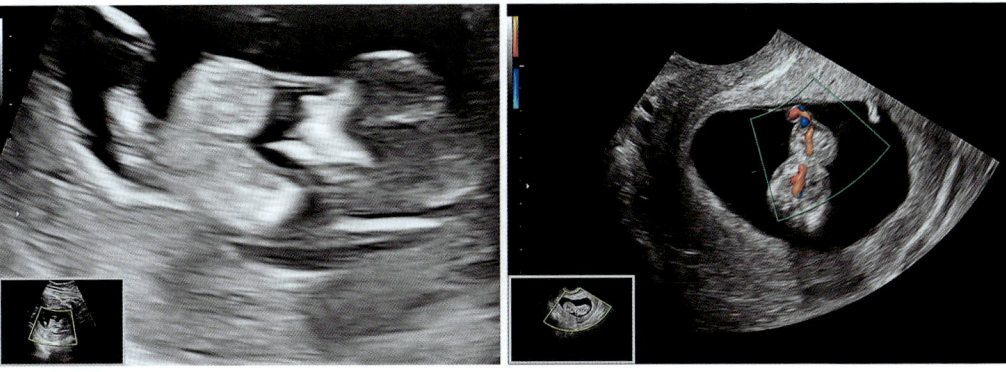

1. Identify the abnormality.
2. Name four differentials.
3. What are the main diagnostic criteria?
4. Which are the prognostic indicators in this condition?
5. Which genetic tests should be done in this case?

Ans.
1. Omphalocele
2. a. Physiological herniation (disappears by 12 weeks)
   b. Gastroschisis
   c. Cloacal exstrophy (which includes omphalocele, bladder exstrophy and external genital anomalies).
   d. Limb body wall complex
3. Cord insertion seen on the convexity of mass in the center.
4. a. Contents of the mass (if liver is not in the mass, the prognosis is excellent).
   b. Associated anomalies (mainly cardiac anomalies seen in 30–50%)
5. Amniocentesis for fetal QFPCR/FISH, microarray, and exome for single gene disorder like Beckwith-Wiedemann syndrome (chromosomal abnormalities especially trisomy 18, 13 are found in 30–50% of cases. Genetic syndromes, mainly *Beckwith-Wiedemann syndrome* found in 10% of cases).

OSCE 16. A 32-year-old Primi gravida with a monochorionic monoamniotic (MonoMono) twin pregnancy was referred at mid gestation.

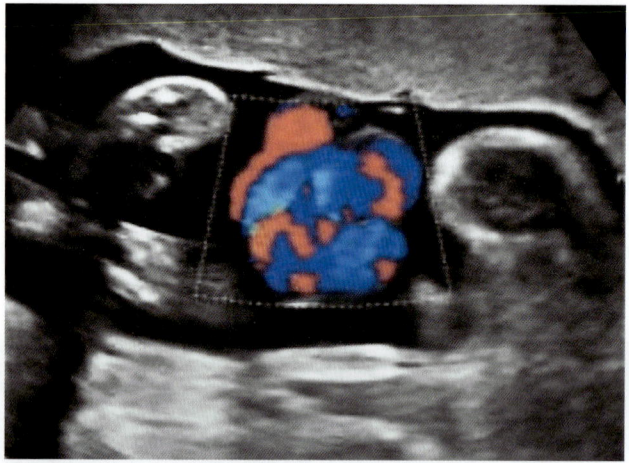

1. What does the following image of the ultrasound show?
2. How frequently should the patient be monitored?
3. Does the ultrasound finding shown above change management?
4. When and how should the delivery be planned for this patient?

Ans.
1. Cord entanglement
2. Two weekly ultrasound surveillance
3. No. MCMA twins will almost always have umbilical cord entanglement when visualized using color flow Doppler. Such a finding has not consistently been demonstrated to contribute to overall morbidity and mortality.
4. Admission at 31–32 weeks with administration of antenatal corticosteroid, delivery at 32–34 weeks by elective LSCS.

OSCE 17.

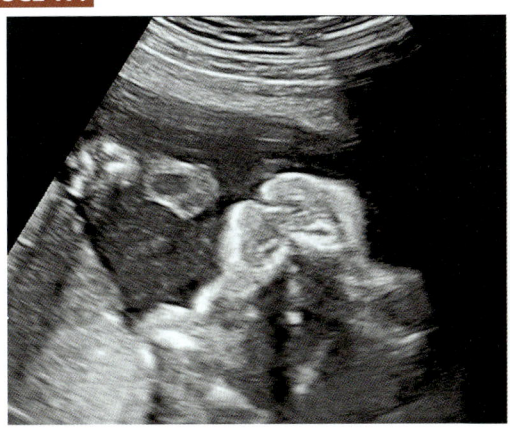
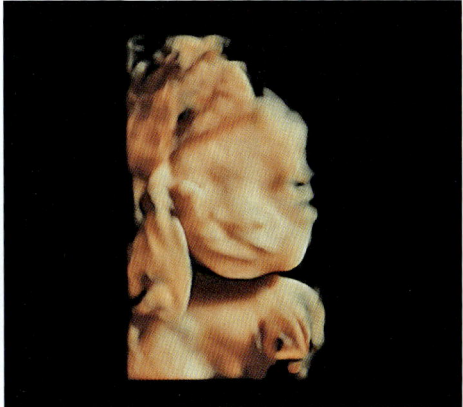

1. Identify the abnormality.
2. What are the two next important investigations?
3. Which is the main prognostic indicator in this condition?
4. Which genetic tests should be done in this case?
5. What is the recurrence risk?

Ans.

1. Unilateral cleft lip and palate.
2. Detailed anomaly scan including fetal echocardiogram and invasive testing.
3. The depth of involvement of the fetal palate
4. 70% are nonsyndromic and 30% syndromic. Amniocentesis for fetal microarray should be done.
5. a. *Isolated:* 5% if one sibling or parent is affected, and 10% if two siblings are affected.
   b. *Syndromic:* All forms of inheritance have been described, including autosomal dominant, autosomal recessive, X-linked dominant, and X-linked recessive.

OSCE 18. A 32-year-old low-risk Primi gravida referred in the third trimester with the following finding:

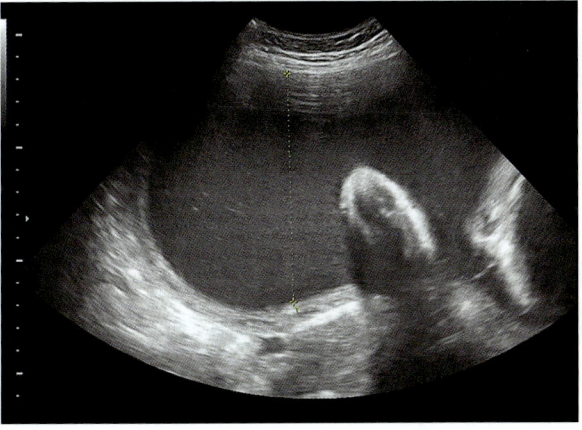
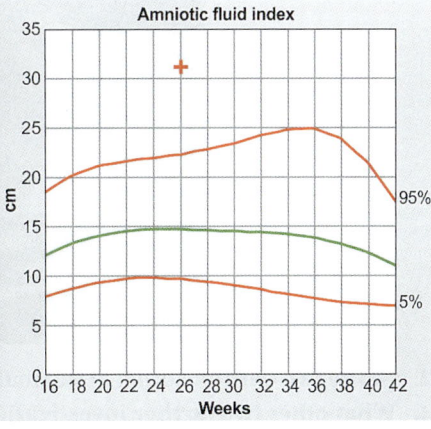

1. Identify the abnormal finding.
2. Enlist four causes.
3. Enlist four investigations
4. Detailed ultarsound showed this abnormality. Identify it.
5. Which is the most common chromosomal abnormality associated with this?

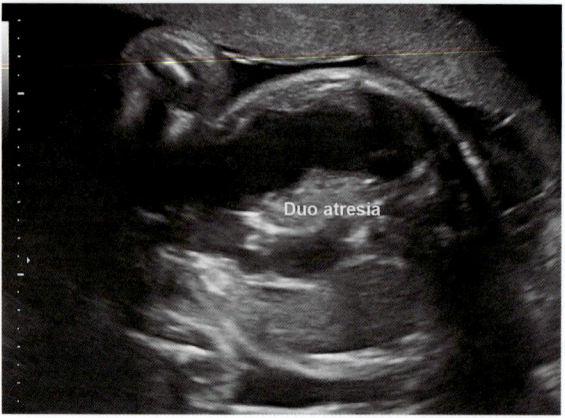

Ans.

1. Polyhydramnios, the deepest vertical pool is above the 95th centile.
2. Gestational diabetes, tracheo-esophageal fistula, Ileal atresia, Bartter syndrome.
3. Maternal OGTT, detailed fetal anomaly scan, fetal echocardiogram, amniocentesis for fetal karyotype.
4. Duodenal atresia
5. Down syndrome

OSCE 19. A 28-year-old Primigravida at 19 weeks gestation was referred for routine anomaly scan.
1. Identify the anomaly seen in this image.

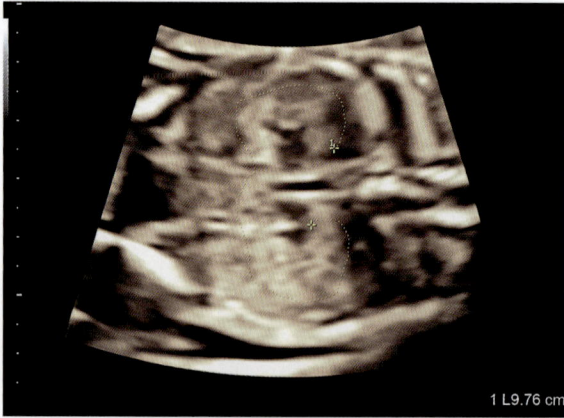

2. Name two chromosomal abnormalities associated with this anomaly.
3. What other two further investigations would you perform?

4. How would you follow up antenatally and for which common complication would you follow-up the fetus?
5. Why is postnatal follow-up advised? List two reasons.

Ans.

1. Horseshoe kidney (fusion of both the lower poles seen in front of descending aorta).
2. Turner's syndrome and Trisomy 18.
3. a. Detailed ultrasound for structural abnormalities including fetal echo
   b. Fetal MRI if additional skeletal or CNS defects are identified.
4. Ultrasound surveillance four weeks to look for development of fetal hydronephrosis.
5. Postnatal follow-up is advised because of increased risk of infections, hydronephrosis and nephrolithiasis.

OSCE 20. A 26-year-old lady Gravida 3, Para 2 with unremarkable medical history was diagnosed with the following abnormality at routine anomaly scan:

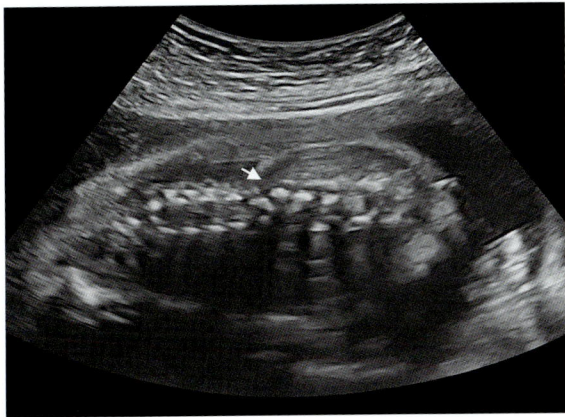

1. Identify the finding and what abnormality does it result in?
2. Name two syndromic associations of this anomaly.
3. What are the other associated structural abnormalities?
4. What are the two main prognostic indicators?
5. What is the recurrence risk and prognosis in isolated cases.

Ans.

1. Hemivertebra, it is the most common cause of congenital scoliosis and kyphoscoliosis.
2. VACTERL (Vertebral, Anorectal, Cardiac, Tracheo-Esophageal, Renal, Limb abnormalities), Jarcho-Levin syndrome, Goldenhar syndrome, and Chondrodysplasia punctata.
3. It can be associated with neural tube defects, renal anomalies, and tracheoesophageal atresia.
4. Number of vertebrae involved and associated structural abnormalities.
5. Single hemivertebra has a good prognosis with no recurrence risk. Multiple vertebrae involvement has a 5–10% recurrence risk. When part of an autosomal recessive condition, the recurrence risk is 25%. Prognosis will depend on development of kyphoscoliosis, cord tethering, and associated structural abnormalities.

CHAPTER 6

Labor

Hem Kanta Sarma

OSCE 1.

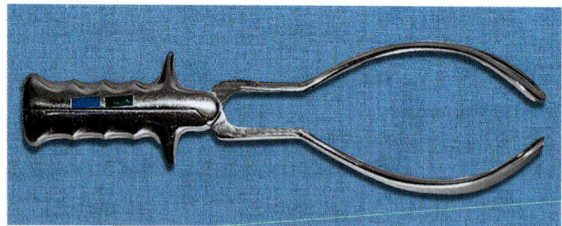

1. Write three criteria to be fulfilled before application of forceps.
2. Write two indications for use of this instrument.

Ans.

1. a. Cervix should be fully dilated
   b. Rotation should be completed
   c. Station should below 0/engaged head
2. a. Fetal compromise in second stage of labor.
   b. *Prophylactic forceps:* Medical condition like heart disease, pre-eclampsia, preterm delivery, postcesarean pregnancy, etc.

OSCE 2.

1. Write three complications associated with forceps delivery.
2. What is trial of forceps?

Ans.

1. a. Laceration of vulva, vagina and cervix and extension of episiotomy.
   b. Postpartum hemorrhage secondary to lacerations and uterine atony.
   c. Fetal injury
2. In case of borderline CPD an attempt is made with forceps in the operating room keeping everything ready for cesarean section to deliver the baby in case it fails. This is known as trial of forceps.

References

1. Oxorn-Foote Human Labor and Birth. 7th edition.
2. Seshadri L. Essentials of Obstetrics. 2nd edition.

OSCE 3.

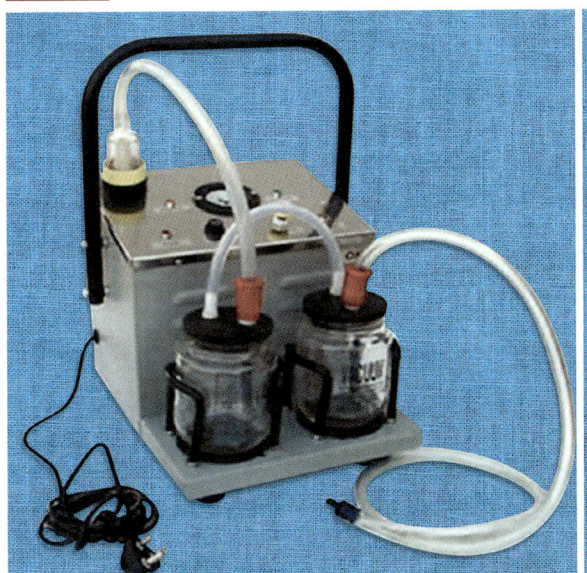
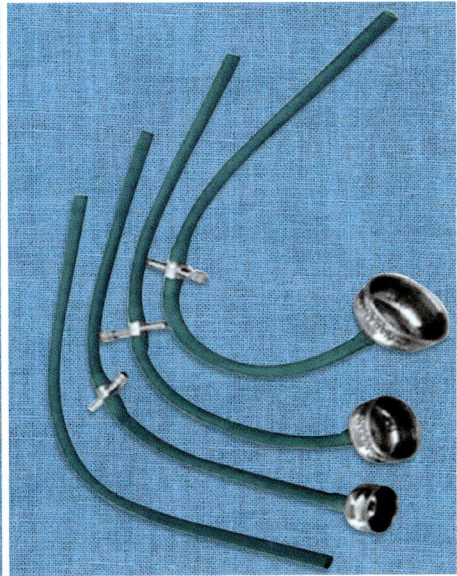

1. Define flexion point. What is the importance of flexion point?
2. What is the pressure required in ventouse delivery?
3. When to terminate the trial of ventouse delivery?

Ans.

1. Flexion point is the correct point for the placement of the ventouse cup. It is 3 cm from the posterior fontanelle and 6 cm from the anterior fontanelle such that the cup is 3 cm away from the anterior fontanelle. The cup has to be placed properly in order to promote synclitism and flexion of the fetal head, presenting the optimal diameter of fetal head to the maternal pelvis.
2. The pressure required is gradually increased at 0.2 kg/cm^2 every 2 minutes till we get 0.8 kg/cm^2 (608 mm Hg), achieved over 10 minutes
3. It is to be terminated when:
   - No descent of head with each pull
   - More than or equal to 3 pulls
   - More than 30 minutes has passes.

Reference
1. William Obstetrics. 25th edition.

OSCE 4.

1. Define postpartum hemorrhage (PPH).
2. What is the most common cause of PPH?
3. Mention three predisposing factors for atonic PPH.

Ans.

1. Cumulative blood loss greater than or equal to 1,000 mL or blood loss accompanied by signs or symptoms of hypovolemia within 24 hours after the birth process regardless of route of delivery.
2. Atonic uterus
3. a. *Overdistended uterus:* Multiple pregnancy, big baby
   b. Grand multipara
   c. Prolonged labor

OSCE 5.

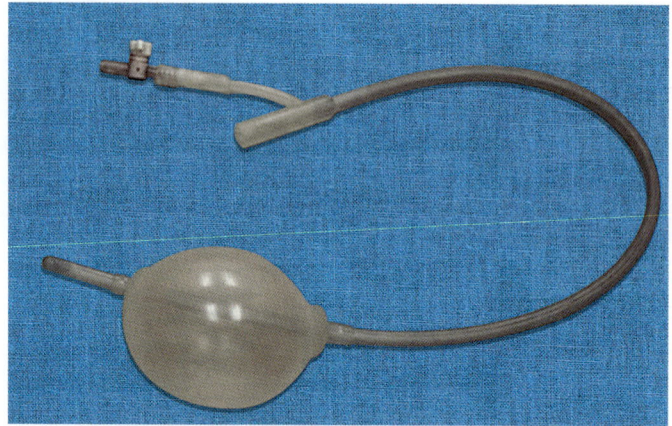

1. Identify the image and mention its use.
2. Mention the components of ATMSL.
3. Mention three drugs used in medical management of PPH.

Ans.

1. Bakri balloon. Used as a tamponade to manage postpartum hemorrhage.
2. a. Administration of uterotonics after delivery of baby
   b. Delayed cord clamping
   c. Controlled traction
3. a. Oxytocin
   b. Methylergometrine
   c. Misoprostol

Reference

1. Williams Obstetrics, ACOG guidelines.

OSCE 6.

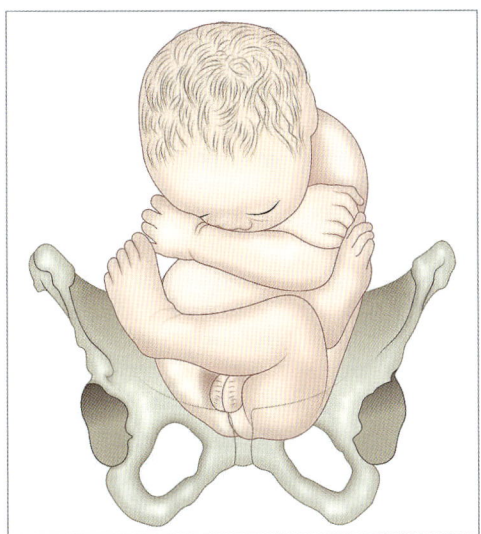

1. What is the presentation in the above image?
2. Write two contraindications for vaginal delivery.
3. At what stage episiotomy might be given?
   - Before delivery of the breech
   - Before delivery of the head
   - Before delivery of the shoulders and arm
4. Mention four complications that might happen during vaginal delivery?

Ans.

1. Breech presentation
2. a. *Large fetus:* >3800 to 4000 g
   b. Severe fetal growth restriction
   c. Oligohydramnios
   d. Incomplete breech presentation
   e. Any two
3. Before delivery of the breech
4. a. Cord prolapse
   b. Fracture or dislocation
   c. Brachial plexus injury
   d. Cervical spine dislocation or fracture
   e. Intra-abdominal organ damage
   f. Intracranial hemorrhage
   g. Birth asphyxia

OSCE 7.

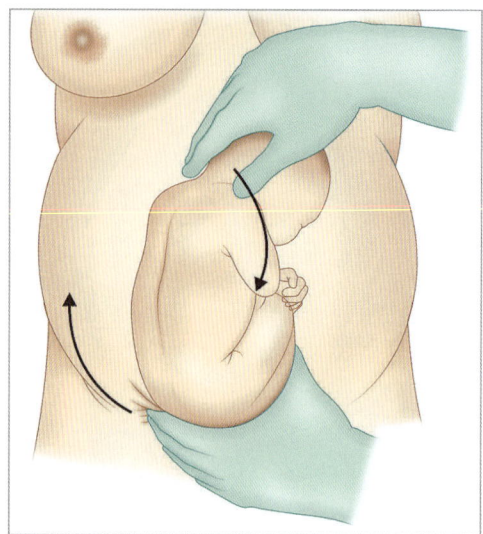

1. What is the technique called as?
2. Name two indications.
3. Name two contraindications.
4. Mention four complications that might happen during the procedure.

Ans.

1. External cephalic version
2. a. Breech presentation
   b. Transverse lie
3. a. Placenta previa
   b. If patient is in labor
   c. Oligohydramnios
   d. Fetal growth restriction
   e. Prior history of abruptio placentae
4. a. Placental abruption
   b. Preterm labor
   c. Fetal compromise
   d. Uterine rupture
   e. Amniotic fluid embolism
   f. Maternal or fetal death
   (Last three being very rare)

Chapter 6: Labor

OSCE 8. Modified WHO partogram and WHO labour care guide.

Name … Parity … Labour onset … Active labour diagnosis [Date]
Ruptured membranes [Date Time] … Risk factors

		Time	:	:	:	:	:	:	:	:	:	:	:	:	:	:	:
		Hours		1	2	3	4	5	6	7	8	9	10	11	12	1	2	3
		ALERT	←————————————Active first stage————————————→													←——Second stage——→

Supportive care	Companion	N	
	Pain relief	N	
	Oral fluid	N	
	Posture	SP	

Baby	Baseline FHR	<110, ≥160	
	FHR deceleration	L	
	Amniotic fluid	M+++, B	
	Fetal position	P, T	
	Caput	+++	
	Moulding	+++	

Woman	Pulse	<60, ≥120	
	Systolic BP	<80, ≥140	
	Diastolic BP	≥90	
	Temperature °C	<35.0, ≥37.5	
	Urine	P++, A++	

	Contractions per 10 min	≥2, >5	
	Duration of contractions	<20, >60	

Labour progress	Cervix [Plot X]	10 / 9 / 8 ≥2.5 h / 7 ≥3 h / 6 ≥5 h / 5 ≥6 h	
	Descent [Plot O]	5 / 4 / 3 / 2 / 1 / 0	

In active first stage, plot 'X' to record cervical dilatation. Alert triggered when lag time for current cervical dilatation is exceeded with no progress. In second stage, insert 'P' to indicate when pushing begins

Medication	Oxytocin (U/L, drops/min)	
	Medicine	
	IV fluids	

Shared decision-making	Assessment	
	Plan	
	Initials	

Source: https://www.who.int/publications/i/item/9789240017566

1. Identify the chart in the picture.
2. For whom should the chart be used?
3. When should plotting of this chart be started?
4. According to this chart, what is the maximum time allowed in second stage of labor?
5. According to this chart, if the cervical dilatation is at 5 cm, after how many hours it is considered as an alert.

Ans.
1. WHO labour care guide.
2. For all apparently healthy pregnant women.
3. Cervical dilatation of 5 cm or more.
4. Two hours for multigravida, 3 hours for primigravida.
5. *Alert if:* >6 hours from 5–6 cm dilatation.

OSCE 9.

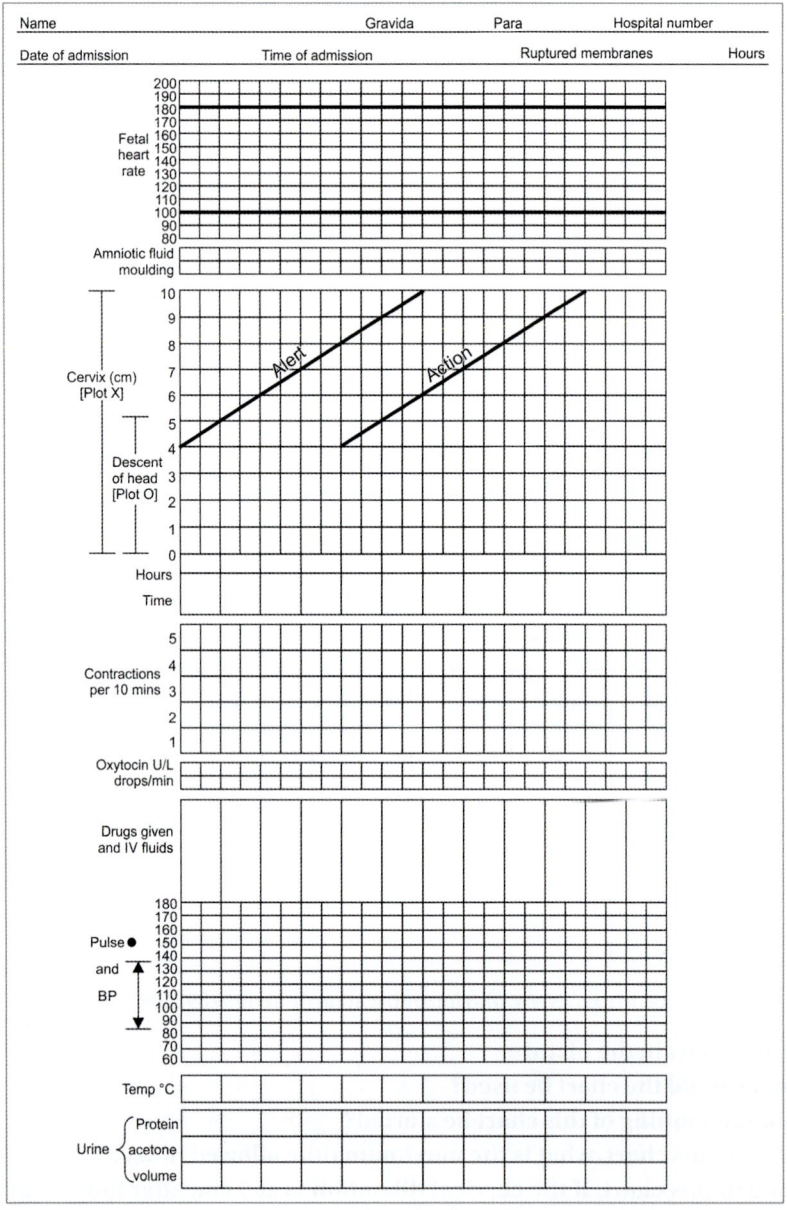

Source: https://nhm.gov.in/images/pdf/in-focus/Dakshata/Day-2/Partograph.pptx

1. Identify the chart in the picture.
2. When should plotting of this chart be started?
3. What should be the rate of dilatation of cervix according to this chart in active phase of labor?
4. What does a plot to the right of the alert line represent?
5. What is the recommended frequency of recording the fetal parameters?

Ans.

1. The modified WHO partograph
2. Cervical dilatation ≥4 cm, 2 contractions/10 minutes
3. ≥1 cm/hour
4. It represents a warning and calls for immediate intervention.
5. FHR, status of membranes and amniotic fluid-recorded every half an hour.

OSCE 10.

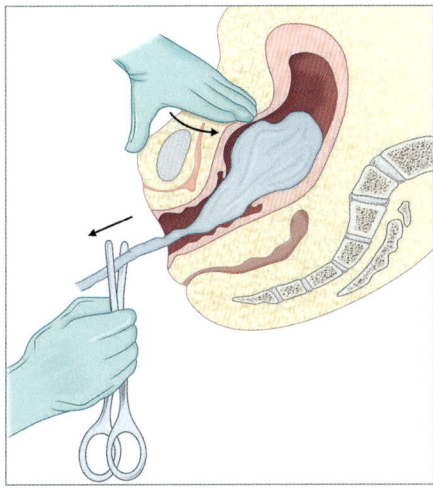

1. Identify the procedure performed in the picture.
2. State the prerequisites for the procedure.
3. State two benefits of procedure in conduct of the third stage.
4. State two complications that may occur in the improper management of the procedure.

Ans.

1. Controlled cord traction in the active management of third stage of labor.
2. a. Lengthening of the cord.
   b. Fresh gush of blood.
   c. A rise of the uterine fundus.
3. a. Shortens the third stage.
   b. Less postpartum bleeding.
4. a. Postpartum hemorrhage.
   b. Uterine inversion.

OSCE 11.

1. Mention the components of active management of third stage of labor
2. Mention the side effects of the drug when used in IV (intravenous) bolus.

Ans.

1. a. Administration of uterotonic agent.
   b. Controlled cord traction to deliver the placenta and membranes.
   c. Massaging the uterus.
   d. Oxytocin, 10 IU intramuscular either at the time of delivery of anterior shoulder or within 1 minute of the delivery of the fetus.
2. Hypotension

References

1. Munro Kerr's Operative Obstetrics. 13th edition.
2. Holland and Brews Manual of Obstetrics. 4th edition.

OSCE 12.

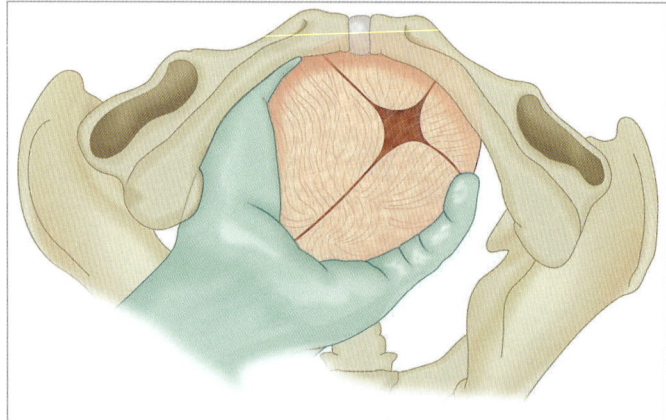

1. What is the position of fetus in the given image?
2. *Which is more common:* ROP (right occipitoposterior) or LOP (left occipitoposterior)?
3. How much rotation is needed for it to become occipitoanterior?
4. Define position of fetus in utero.

Ans.

1. ROP
2. ROP
3. 135* or 3/8th
4. Relationship of the denominator to the different quadrants of pelvis of mother.

Reference

1. Williams Obstetrics.

OSCE 13.

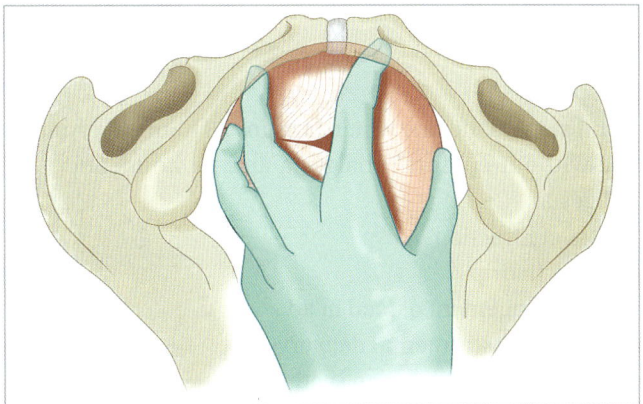

1. What is the overall most common position?
2. What is the engaging diameter in ROP position?
3. Write one maternal complication in this scenario.
4. Write three indications for C-section in OP position.

Ans.

1. LOT (left occipitotransverse)
2. Right oblique diameter
3. Extensive perinatal tear
4. Android pelvis, fetal distress, big baby

Reference
1. Williams Obstetrics

OSCE 14.

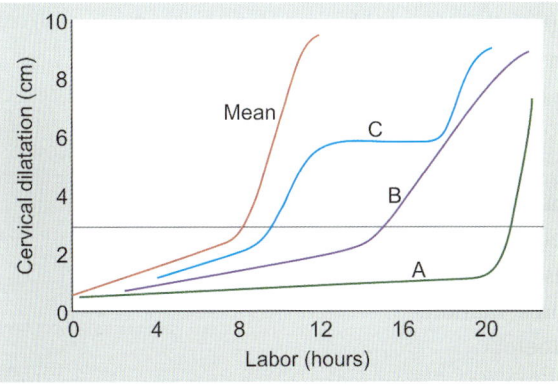

1. Identify the graphs.
2. Define prolonged second stage of labor.
3. Write management plan of prolong second stage of labor.

Ans.
1. a. Prolonged latent phase
   b. Prolonged active phase
   c. Arrested active phase
2. The prolong second stage is the one which lasts for >3 hours in primigravida and >2 hours in a multigravida without epidural analgesia and >4 hours and >3 hours respectively with epidural analgesia.
3. *Management:* Assess contractions:
   - *Inadequate:* Oxytocin drip
   - *Adequate:* Assess engagement of fetal head:
     - *Engaged:* Consider instrumental delivery.
     - *Not engaged:* Emergency cesarean section.

OSCE 15.

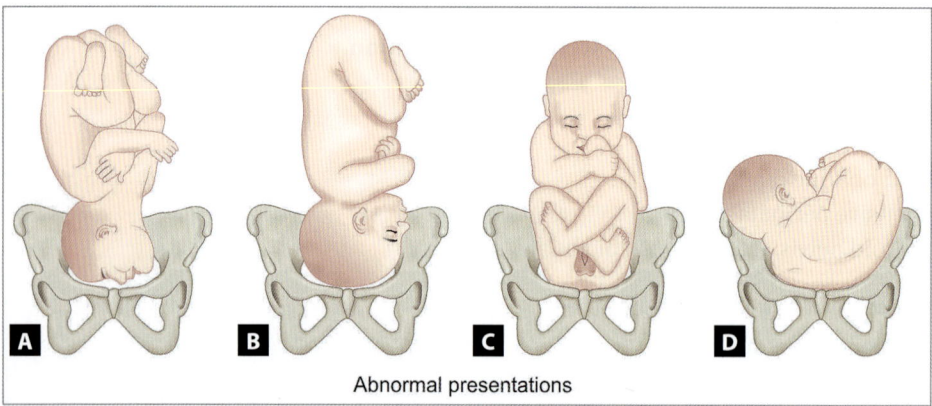

Abnormal presentations

1. Identify the abnormal presentations.
2. What is the engaging diameter for brow presentation?
3. Write mechanism of labor for persistent brow presentation.
4. What is the mode of delivery for brow presentation?

Ans.
1. a. A—Face presentation
   b. B—Brow presentation
   c. C—Breech presentation
   d. D—Shoulder presentation.
2. Mentovertical diameter.
3. The presenting diameter (mentovertical) being very large, i.e., 14 cm, there is no mechanism of labor for persistent brow presentation.
4. Cesarean delivery is done for brow presentation.

OSCE 16.
1. Write two common causes related to fault in soft tissues in case of obstructed labor.
2. Write three differentiating points between pathological Bandl's ring and physiological constriction ring.

Ans.

1. a. Cervical dystocia
   b. Uterine malformation
2. a. In pathological Bandl's ring upper uterine segment is tonically contracted with no relaxation while in case of constriction ring upper segment contract and retract with relaxation in between.
   b. Pathological retraction ring can be felt and seen abdominally and usually rises up while physiological constriction ring is not felt per abdominally and does not change its position.
   c. Uterus is normal and nontender in constriction ring whereas in Bandl's ring uterus is tense and tender.

OSCE 17.
1. Write two complications of urinary bladder due to obstructed labor.
2. Write three clinical features of obstructed labor.

Ans.

1. a. Pressure necrosis of bladder
   b. Vesicovaginal fistula.
2. a. Tonically contracted, tense and tender uterus with Bandl's ring
   b. Maternal exhaustion and sepsis
   c. Fetal anoxia which may also lead to fetal death.

OSCE 18.
1. Define induction of labor.
2. Write two indications for induction of labor.
3. Write two absolute contraindications for induction of labor.

Ans.

1. Induction of labor implies stimulation of contractions before the spontaneous onset of labor, with or without ruptured membranes.
2. Indication of induction of labor:
   a. Post-term pregnancy
   b. Gestational hypertension
3. Contraindications of induction of labor:
   a. Contracted or distorted pelvic anatomy
   b. Abnormally implanted placentas (grade II, III, IV placenta previa)

OSCE 19. A second gravida delivered a male baby 10 hours back at a peripheral center. The newborn presents with a swelling on the head.
1. Enumerate three differential diagnosis.
2. If it is following ventouse application, what is the probable diagnosis?
3. Which swelling will disappear spontaneously within 24 hours?

Ans.

1. a. Cephalohematoma
   b. Caput succedaneum
   c. Chignon
2. Chignon
3. Caput succedaneum

OSCE 20.

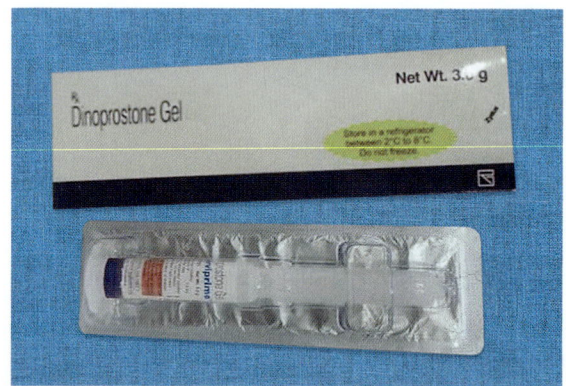

1. Identify the drug and write its use.
2. Enumerate two risks associated with the drug.
3. What are the components of Bishop Score?

Ans.

1. It is a Prostaglandin (PGE2), used for the induction of labor by causing cervical ripening.
2. *Risks:*
   a. Uterine atony
   b. Uterine rupture
3. *Components of Bishop Score:*
   - Cervical dilatation
   - Length of cervix
   - Position
   - Consistency
   - Station of the fetal head

Reference
1. Williams Obstetrics.

CHAPTER 7

Abnormal Labor

Pratik Tambe, Deepali Kale, Jyotsna S Dwivedi

OSCE 1.

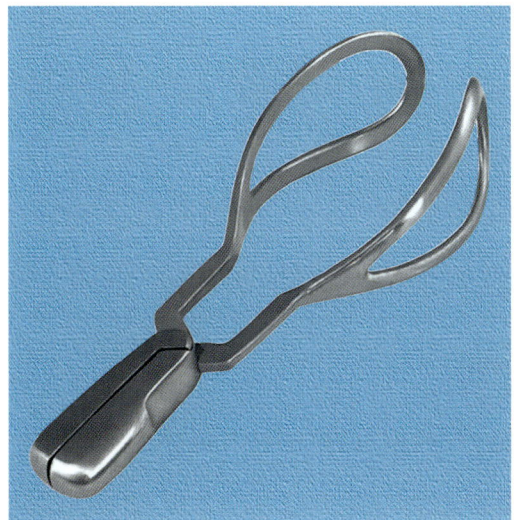

1. Identify the instrument.
2. What are the indications of using it?
3. Name the anesthetic methods used during its application.

Ans.

1. Wrigley's outlet forceps.
2. a. To deliver the fetal head when it is 3 cm below ischial spine in case of fetal distress.
   b. To cut short the second stage of labor in case of severe pre-eclampsia, cardiac disease, etc.
   c. Maternal exhaustion
   d. To deliver the floating fetal head at cesarean section.
3. a. Pudendal block
   b. Perineal and labial infiltration with 1% lignocaine.

References

1. Murphy DJ, Strachan BK, Bahl R, on behalf of the Royal College of Obstetricians Gynaecologists. Assisted Vaginal Birth. BJOG. 2020;127:e70–112.

2. O'Brien S, Siassakos D, Hinshaw K. Assisted vaginal delivery. Munro Kerr's Operative Obstetrics, 13th edition. Chapter 15. Sabaratnam Arulkumaran, Michael Robson (Eds). An Elsevier Publication.

OSCE 2.

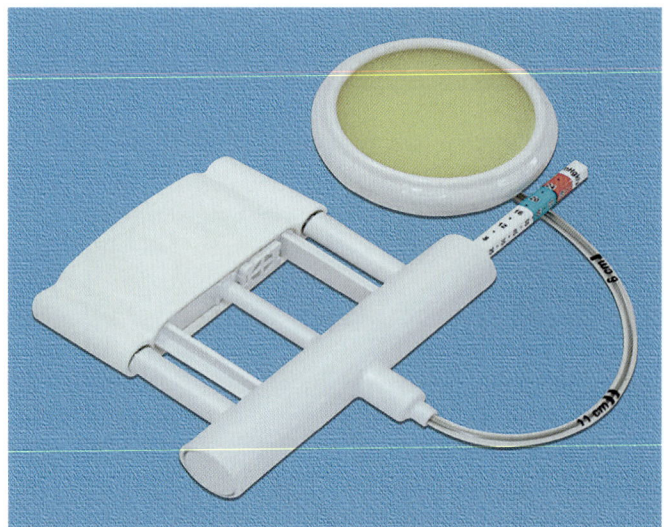

1. **Identify the instrument.**
2. **Name the parts.**
3. **Name two conditions where its application is preferred over the obstetric forceps.**

Ans.

1. The Kiwi Cup Pump
2. Parts of the Kiwi Cup are:
    - Cup
    - Suction/Traction tube
    - Traction force indicator
    - Vacuum level indicator
    - Palm pump
    - Palm pump handle
    - Button to release the suction
3. a. Occipitoposterior position
   b. Occipitotransverse position

References

1. Murphy DJ, Strachan BK, Bahl R, on behalf of the Royal College of Obstetricians Gynaecologists. Assisted Vaginal Birth. BJOG. 2020;127:e70-112.
2. Hashim N, Hussain R, Soomro N. Clinical evaluation of Kiwi omni cup: a new vacuum extraction device. 2016;41:68-71.

Chapter 7: Abnormal Labor 103

OSCE 3.

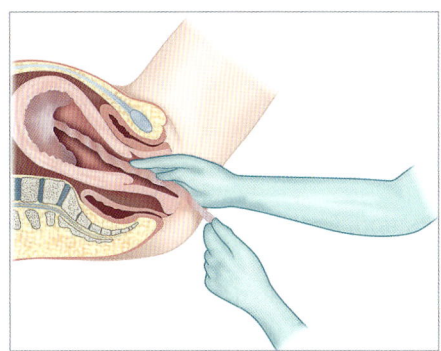

1. Name the procedure.
2. What precautions should be taken to prevent inversion of uterus?
3. When do we perform manual removal of placenta?
4. Enumerate the steps for active management of third stage of labor.

Ans.

1. Control cord traction technique of placenta removal.
2. a. Recommended to wait for signs of placental separation such as lengthening of the cord and gush of blood appearance.
   b. Traction is to be applied when the uterus is well contracted.
   c. Gentle traction should be applied on the cord and the ulnar border of left hand should be used to push the uterus.
3. When the placenta is not delivered after 30 minutes.
4. AMTSL (active management of third stage of labor) as a prophylactic intervention is composed of a package of three components:
   a. Administration of a uterotonic, oxytocin 10 units, immediately after birth of baby
   b. Controlled cord traction (CCT) to deliver the placenta
   c. Delayed cord clamping.

Reference

1. World Health Organization. WHO Recommendations For The Prevention and Treatment of Postpartum Haemorrhage, 2012. WHO: Geneva, Switzerland.

OSCE 4.

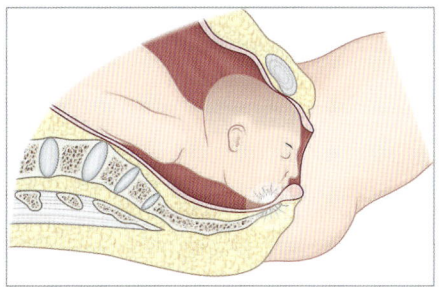

1. Identify the presentation.
2. How will you diagnose it?
3. What are the different types?

Ans.

1. Face presentation.
2. *Vaginal examination:*
   - On per vagina examination, fetal parts felt are orbital ridges, mouth, nose, and malar bones.
   - The mouth forms a triangular configuration with the malar bones whereas in case of breech presentation the anus and the ischial tuberosities are in one line.
3. a. Mento anterior face presentation.
   b. Mento posterior face presentation.

Reference

1. Murphy DJ. Normal and abnormal labor. Obstetrics by Ten Teachers, 20th edition, Chapter 12, pp. 209-10. Edited by Louis Kenny, Jenny E Mayers. CRC Press Taylor and Francis Group.

OSCE 5.

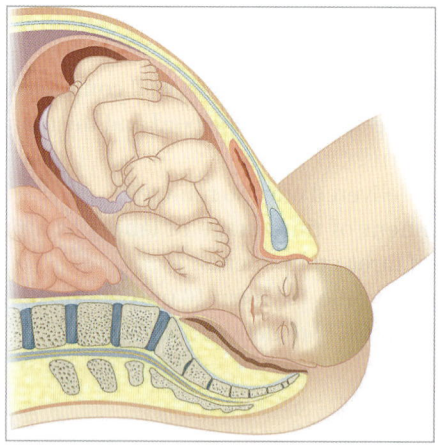

1. Identify this obstetric emergency.
2. Name the maneuvers which are carried out to complete the delivery in the above situation.
3. Most common neonatal complication.
4. Enumerate the intrapartum risk factors associated with the above condition.

Ans.

1. Shoulder dystocia
2.
   - Mc Robert's maneuver
   - Suprapubic pressure
   - Delivery of posterior arm

- Rubin's maneuver
- Woods Corkscrew maneuver
- Gaskin's knee chest/all four maneuver
- Zavanelli's maneuver
- Symphysiotomy
3. Brachial plexus impairment (Erb-Duchenne Palsy seen in >98% cases)
4. *Labor abnormalities:*
   - Prolonged first stage
   - Prolonged second stage
   - Epidural analgesia
   - Macrosomic baby
   - Operative vaginal delivery (forceps or vacuum) especially at mid-pelvic station.

Reference
1. Burd J. "Shoulder Dystocia" in Obstetrics Evidence Based Guidelines, edited by Vincenzo Berghella, CRC Press 4th edition, Chapter 27, pp. 314-18.

OSCE 6.

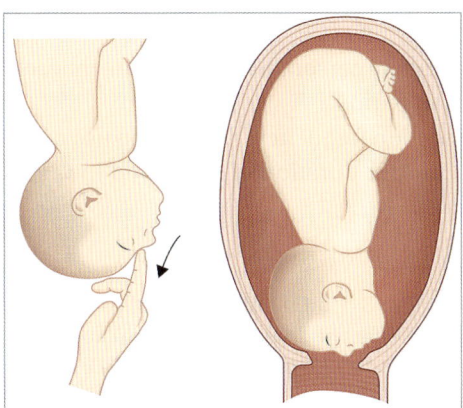

1. **Identify the presentation.**
2. **Name the attitude of the fetus in this presentation.**
3. **How will you clinically diagnose this condition?**

Ans.
1. Brow presentation
2. Deflexed (Partially extended)
3. Diagnosis is made on vaginal examination at 4–5 cm dilatation where the anterior fontanelle, frontal bones, forehead supraorbital ridges and the bridge of the nose can be palpated.

References
1. Hinshaw K. Shoulder dystocia. In: Johanson R, Cox C, Grady K, Howell C (Eds). Managing Obstetric Emergencies and Trauma: The MOET Course Manual. London: RCOG Press; 2003. pp. 165-74.

2. Gimovsky CA, Dall'Asta A, Morganelli G, Ghi T. in Obstetrics Evidence Based Guidelines, edited by Vincenzo Berghella, CRC Press 4th edition, Chapter 26, pp. 299-323.

OSCE 7.

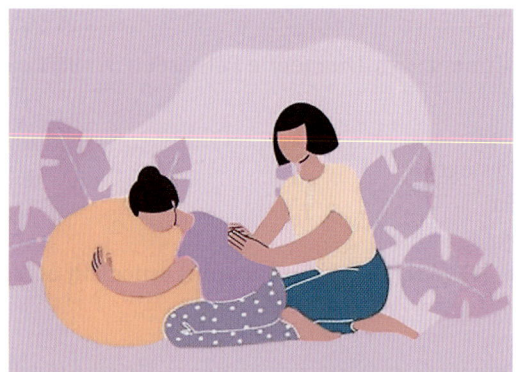

1. What is the person accompanying the laboring woman called as?
2. Enumerate the benefits of having a labor attendant during delivery.

Ans.

1. *Doula* is a continuous support person that the woman chooses for emotional support and advice during intrapartum period.
2. Reduction in cesarean section frequency, decrease in use of epidural analgesia, increased rates of breastfeeding, shorter duration of labor, and lower rates of low 5 minute Apgar score.

Reference

1. Sobczak A, Taylor L, Solomon S, Ho J, Kemper S, Phillips B, Jacobson K, Castellano C, Ring A, Castellano B, Jacobs RJ. The effect of doulas on maternal and birth outcomes: a scoping review. Cureus. 2023;15(5):e39451. doi: 10.7759/cureus.39451. PMID: 37378162; PMCID: PMC10292163.

OSCE 8.

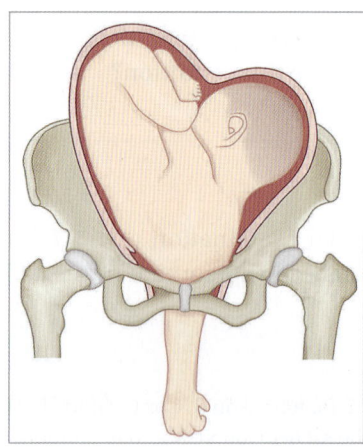

Chapter 7: Abnormal Labor

1. What is this malpresentation called?
2. What are the complications seen?
3. Mode of delivery if this malpresentation is detected in first stage of labor at 3 cm with rupture of membranes.
4. What are the predisposing factors for this malpresentation?

Ans.

1. Transverse lie
2. a. Premature rupture of membranes
   b. Cord prolapse
   c. Hand prolapse
   d. Obstructed labor
   e. Intrauterine fetal demise
   f. Uterine rupture
3. Emergency LSCS
4. a. Placenta previa
   b. Polyhydramnios
   c. Lower uterine fibroids
   d. Twin gestation
   e. Fetal anomalies

References

1. Arulkumaran S. Malpresentation, malposition, cephalopelvic disproportion and obstetric procedure. In: Edmonds DK (Ed). Dewhurst's Textbook of Obstetrics. 2006:213-26.
2. Sultana S, Rather S, Anam S, Mufti S, Qureshi A, Wani I, Wani RA. Management of term singleton transverse lie: a prospective study. Int J Sci Stud. 2018;6(4):53-6.

OSCE 9.

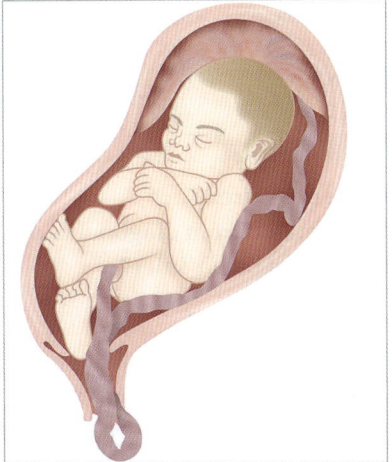

1. Identify the type of breech presentation.
2. What is the mode of delivery in this case?

3. What are the complications associated with this?
4. Name the maneuver used to deliver the extended arms.

Ans.

1. Incomplete breech with extension at one or both the hips (footling)
2. Elective LSCS if detected antenatally on imaging.
   Emergency LSCS if detected intrapartum on clinical examination.
3. Cord Prolapse
   Head Entrapment
   IUFD
4. Loveset's maneuver

References

1. Gimovsky CA, Dall'Asta A, Morganelli G, Ghi Tin Obstetrics Evidence Based Guidelines, edited by Vincenzo Berghella, CRC Press, 4th edition, Chapter 26, pp. 299-323.
2. Royal College of Obstetricians and Gynaecologists (RCOG). The Management of Breech Presentation, Guideline No. 20b December 2006; p. 1-13.

OSCE 10.

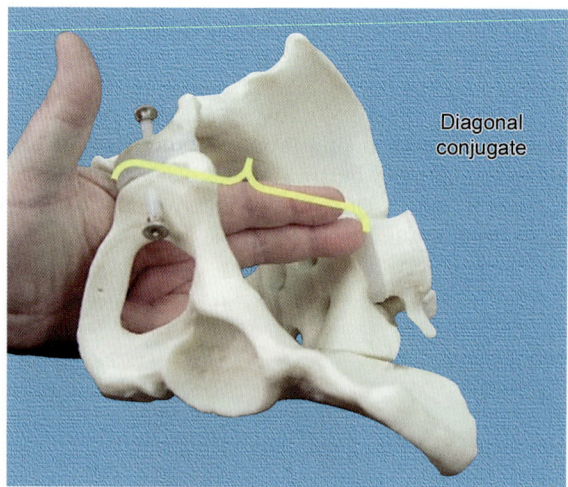

1. How is the diagonal conjugate measured?
2. How is obstetric conjugate estimated from diagonal conjugate?
3. What is the other name for plane of pelvic inlet?

Ans.

1. To measure the diagonal conjugate, a hand with palm oriented laterally extends its index finger to the promontory. The distance from the fingertip to the point at which the lowest margin of the symphysis strikes the same finger's base is the diagonal conjugate.
2. Obstetric conjugate is estimated indirectly by subtracting 1.5 to 2 cm from the diagonal conjugate.
3. The Superior Strait

Reference

1. Cunningham F, Leveno KJ, Bloom SL, Dashe JS, Hoffman BL, Casey BM, Spong CY (Eds). Williams' Obstetrics, 25th edition. McGraw Hill. 2018; Chapter 2, p. 31.

OSCE 11.

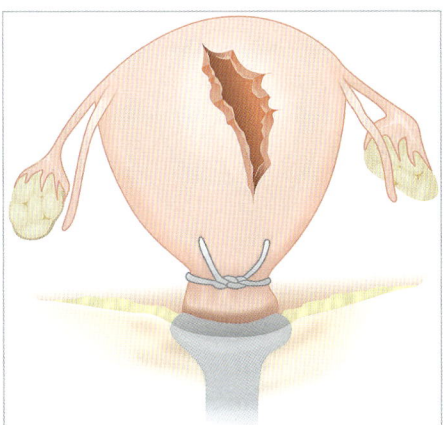

1. Identify the condition shown in this picture.
2. Mention the risk factors for the above condition in unscarred uterus.
3. What are the clinical warning signs of above?

Ans.

1. Uterine rupture
2. Risk factors for rupture of an unscarred uterus include:
   - Grand multiparity
   - Undiagnosed cephalopelvic disproportion or malpresentation
   - Oxytocin administration
   - Macrosomia
   - Placenta percreta
   - Prior uterine surgery
   - Uterine abnormalities (e.g., rudimentary horn)
3. Clinical warning signs of uterine rupture are:
   - Fetal heart rate anomalies
   - Fetal bradycardia
   - Scar pain and/or tenderness
   - Vaginal bleeding
   - Concealed bleeding (shoulder tip pain)
   - Hematuria
   - Poor progress in labor.

Reference

1. Sara Paterson-Brown, Charlotte Howell. Managing Obstetrics Emergency and Trauma, 3rd edition, pp. 365-6.

OSCE 12.

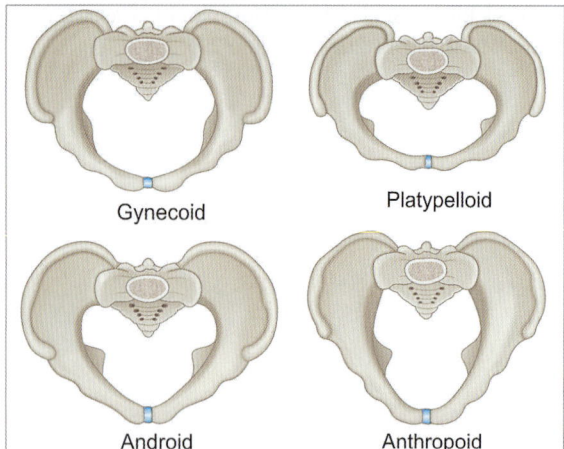

1. What is the name of this classification of types of pelvis?
2. Which type of pelvis is most favorable for normal delivery?
3. Enumerate the steps for pelvis assessment.

Ans.

1. Caldwell–Moloy classification, was given in 1933.
2. Gynecoid pelvis is most favorable for normal delivery.
3. *Pelvis assessment:*
    - After taking informed consent, the patient is made to lie down in dorsal position after emptying the bladder.
    - Assessment of pelvic inlet, mid-cavity and outlet is done.
    - Inlet is adequate if the sacral promontory is not felt.
    - If the sacral promontory is felt, then diagonal conjugate should be assessed. Sacral concavity is also examined. In a Gynecoid pelvis, the sacral concavity is well maintained. If the sacrum is flat, then the mid-cavity may be inadequate.
    - The ischial spines and sacrospinous ligaments are then examined. The mid cavity is considered adequate, if bilateral spines are not palpable simultaneously and the sacrospinous ligament accommodates three fingers.
    - To assess the outlet the subpubic angle and the intertuberous diameter are measured. The subpubic angle should accommodate three fingers and intertuberous diameter should be accommodating four knuckles.

Reference

1. Swenson PC. Anatomical variations in the female pelvis: the Caldwell-Moloy classification. Radiology. 1947;48(5):527. doi: 10.1148/48.5.527. PMID: 20240130.

OSCE 13.

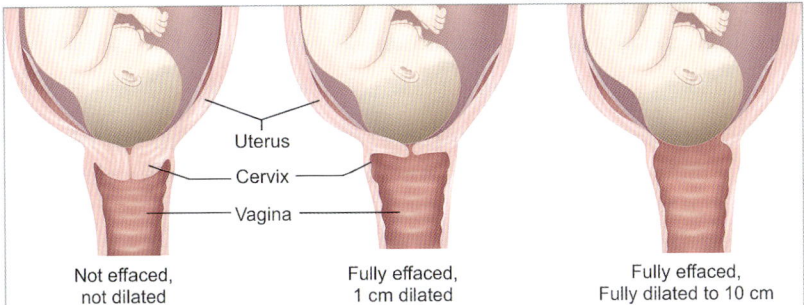

Not effaced, not dilated   Fully effaced, 1 cm dilated   Fully effaced, Fully dilated to 10 cm

1. What are the components of Bishop score?
2. What Bishop score predicts higher probability of vaginal delivery?
3. List the mechanical methods for induction/ripening of cervix.

Ans.

1. Dilation (cm), effacement (%), station, cervical consistency, position of cervix.
2. A Bishop score of >9 is usually associated with high probability of vaginal delivery.
3. Mechanical methods include the following:
   - Hygroscopic dilators (Laminaria, Lamicel, or Dilapan)
   - Balloon (Foley's catheter, double-balloon catheter)

References

1. Bishop EH. Pelvic Scoring for Elective Induction. Obstet Gynecol. 1964;24:266-8. PMID: 14199536.
2. Obstetrics Evidence Based Guidelines, 4th edition, Chapter 26, pg no 276.

OSCE 14.

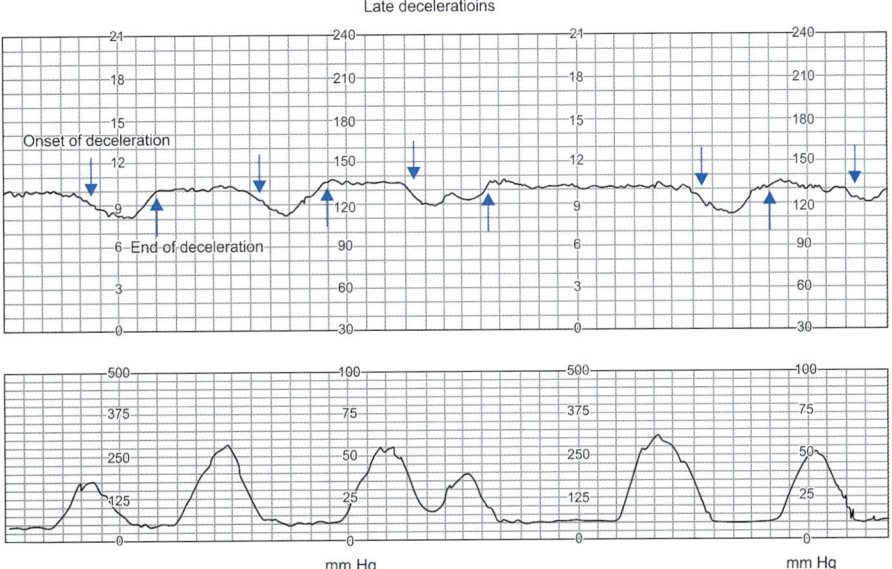

Late decelerations

1. **Enumerate the causes of late deceleration.**
2. **How do you categorize CTG traces?**
3. **Name the other fetal monitoring techniques.**

Ans.

1. Maternal and fetal conditions which can cause late decelerations are uteroplacental insufficiency, maternal dehydration, anemia, hypoxia, hypotension from epidural analgesia, uterine tachysystole and placental abruption.
2. CTG is categorized as normal, suspicious and pathological.
   It is based on whether each of the four features (i.e., contractions, baseline, variability, and decelerations) have been scored as white, amber or red.
   - Normal—no amber or red features, i.e. (all four features are white)
   - Suspicious—any 1 feature is amber
   - Pathological—any 1 feature is red or 2 or more features are amber.
3. Other tests for fetal monitoring are:
   - Digital Scalp or vibroacoustic stimulation
   - Fetal scalp blood sampling
   - Fetal electrocardiogram
   - Fetal pulse oximetry

References

1. Pillarisetty LS, Bragg BN. Late Decelerations. [Updated 2023 Jan 30]. In: StatPearls [Internet]. Treasure Island (FL): StatPearls Publishing; 2023 Jan. Available from: https://www.ncbi.nlm.nih.gov/books/NBK539820/.
2. Fetal monitoring in labor NICE guideline Published: December 2022.

Chapter 7: Abnormal Labor

OSCE 15.

Who labour care guide

Name Parity Labour onset Active labour diagnosis [Date]
Ruptured membranes [Date] Time Risk factors

		Time	:	:	:	:	:	:	:	:	:	:	:	:	:	:	:
		Hours	1	2	3	4	5	6	7	8	9	10	11	12	1	2	3
		Alert	← ────── Active first stage ────── →												← Second stage →		

Supportive care	Companion	N	
	Pain relief	N	
	Oral fluid	N	
	Posture	SP	
Baby	Baseline FHR	<110, ≥160	
	FHR deceleration	L	
	Amniotic fluid	M+++, B	
	Fetal position	P, T	
	Caput	+++	
	Moulding	+++	
Woman	Pulse	<60, ≥120	
	Systolic BP	<80, ≥140	
	Diastolic BP	≥90	
	Temperature °C	<35.0, ≥37.5	
	Urine	P++, A++	
	Contractions per 10 min	≤2, >5	
	Duration of contractions	<20, >60	

Labor progress — Cervix [plot X]: 10, 9 (≥2h), 8 (≥2.5h), 7 (≥3h), 6 (≥5h), 5 (≥6h)
Descent [plot O]: 5, 4, 3, 2, 1, 0

In active first stage, plot 'X' to record cervical dilatation. Alert triggered when lag time for current cervical dilatation is exceeded with no progress. In second stage, insert 'P' to indiate when pushing begins.

Medication: Oxytocin (U/L, drops/min); Medicine; IV fluids

Shared decision-making: Assessment; Plan; Initials

Instructions: Circle any observation meeting the criteria in the 'alert' column, alert the senior midwife or doctor and record the assessment and action taken. If, labor extends beyond 12 h, please continue on a new labor care guide.

(Y: yes; N: no; D: declined; U: unknown; SP: supine; MO: mobile; E: early; L: late; V: variable; I: intact; C: clear; M: meconium, Blood; A: anterior; P: posterior; T: transverse; P: protein; A: acetone)

1. What are the components of Labor care guide?
2. What are the points of difference in WHO modified partograph and Labor care guide?

Ans.

1. Following are the components of labor care guide: identifying information and labor characteristics at admission, supportive care, care of the baby, care of the woman, labor progress, medication, and shared decision-making.
2.

Modified partograph	Labor care guide
The active phase begins to start at cervix dilation from 4cm	The active phase begins to start at cervix dilation from 5 cm
Alert and action line fixed at 1 cm/hr	Proof-based time restrictions on cervical dilations at each centimetre
Keeps track of the intensity, frequency, and length of uterine contractions	Keeps track of span and repetition of uterine shrinking
There is no second stage	Enhanced surveillance in the second stage
No documentation of interventions for reassuring help	Companionship during labor, pain alleviation, oral fluid intake, and posture are all explicitly recorded
Besides cervical dilatation warning and action lines, there is no clear necessity to act in response to observation that differ from predictions of any labor	Requires that observation be noted, along with the provider recording the appropriate response

Reference

1. Ghulaxe Y, Tayade S, Huse S, Chavada J. Advancement in Partograph: WHO's Labor Care Guide. Cureus. 2022;14(10):e30238. doi: 10.7759/cureus.30238. PMID: 36381845; PMCID: PMC9652267.

OSCE 16.

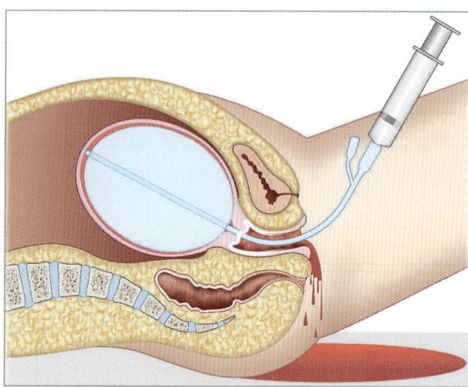

1. Explain the proposed mechanism of action of intrauterine tamponade techniques.
2. Regarding pharmacotherapy for treatment of postpartum hemorrhage, outline one first-line and two second-line agents for control of PPH.
3. Identify two purposes of continued verbal engagement with the patient during resuscitative maneuvers at this time.

Ans.

1. Application of inward-to-outward hydrostatic pressure against the uterine wall to compress endomyometrial vessels.
2. Oxytocin is the first line drug and following are the second-line drugs for control of PPH:
   - Methylergometrine
   - Carboprost
   - Misoprostol.
3. To assess her level of consciousness and to provide appropriate communication of the ongoing medical care.

Reference

1. Weeks AD, Baskett TF. Uterine and vaginal tamponade in Munro Kerr's Operative Obstetrics, edited by Sabaratnam Arulkumaran, Michael Robson, 13th edition, pp. 262-4.

OSCE 17.

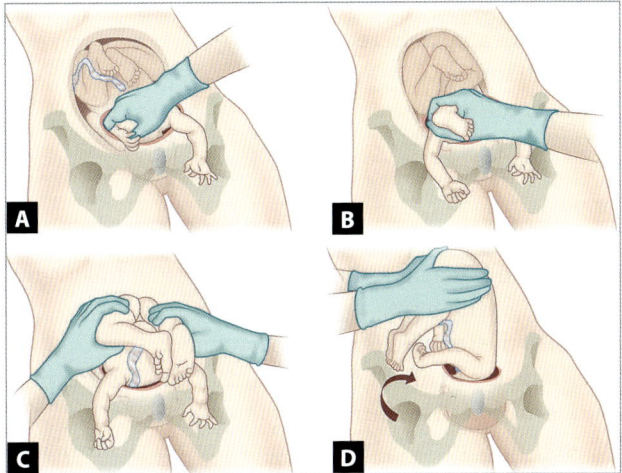

1. Identify the above technique of baby delivery.
2. What is the other name for this technique?
3. What are the complications associated with prolonged second stage?

Ans.

1. Patwardhan Technique
2. Shoulder first method or reverse breech extraction technique
3. Maternal morbidity increases due to prolonged second stage leading to increased chances of infection, postpartum sepsis, postpartum hemorrhage, long-term increased risk of obstetric fistula formation. Intraoperative there are increased chances of difficult baby delivery, extension of uterine incision, injury to uterine artery, increased blood loss, traumatic postpartum hemorrhage leading to hysterectomy and prolonged operating time. Fetal complications associated with prolonged second stage are birth asphyxia, need for NICU admission and increased chances of stillbirth.

Reference

1. Bhattacharya R, Ramesh AC. Cesarean section of an impacted fetal head at full cervical dilatation: evaluation of Patwardhan Technique. Crit Care Obst Gyne. 2020;6(4):9.

OSCE 18.

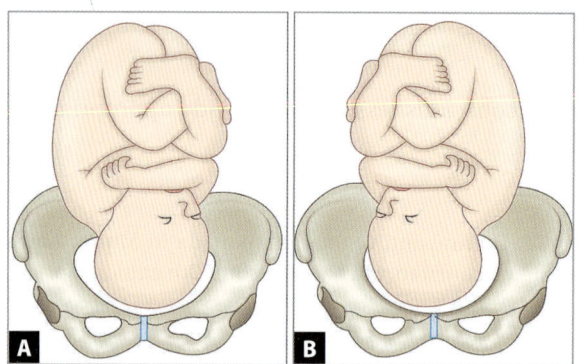

1. Identify the fetal position shown here.
2. Name the presenting diameter.
3. How is the diagnosis made?

Ans.

1. Occipitoposterior position
2. Occipitofrontal diameter measuring 11.5 cm.
3. Occipitoposterior position is diagnosed when we encounter following:
   - The head is not engaged till term.
   - The abdomen below the umbilicus appears flattened.
   - The fetal back is palpated in mother's flank and fetal limbs are present in the midline.
   - Fetal heart sounds are heard in the flank region.
   - However, the final diagnosis is made when the cervical dilatation is 4–5 cm and anterior fontanelle is palpated.

Reference

1. Othenin-Girard V, Boulvain M, Guittier MJ. Accouchement envariétéoccipito-postérieure: issues materno-fœtales et facteursprédictifs de la rotation [Occiput posterior presentation at delivery: Materno-foetal outcomes and predictive factors of rotation]. Gynecol Obstet Fertil Senol. 2018;46(2):93-8. French. doi: 10.1016/j.gofs.2017.11.006. Epub 2018 Jan 20. PMID: 29366610.

OSCE 19.

You are working as a Junior Resident, monitoring a G2P1L1 with history of gestational hypertension, well controlled on tablet labetalol 100 mg twice daily in spontaneous labor. Your on-call consultant asks you to do a CTG for this patient in latent labor. The CTG report is as below:

Chapter 7: Abnormal Labor

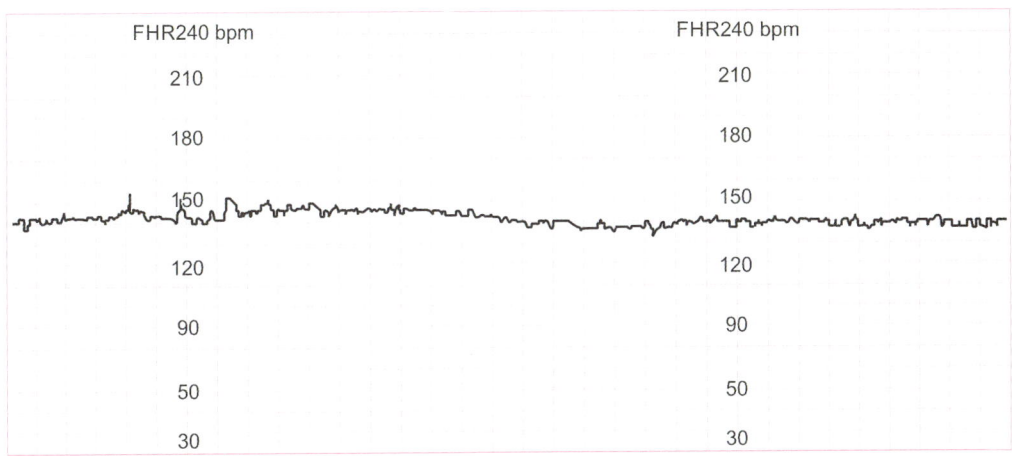

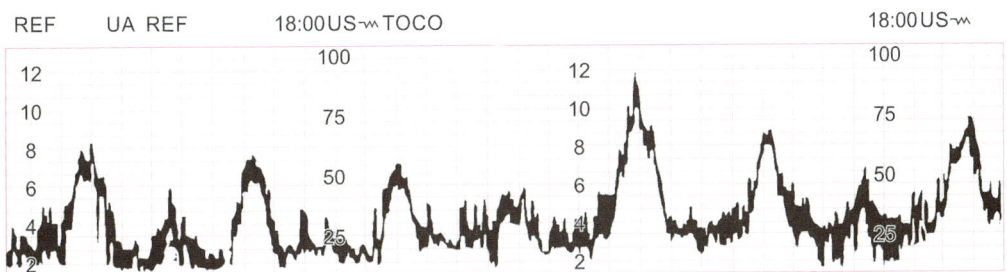

1. What is the abnormality noted?
2. What are the causes for this abnormal parameter?
3. How will you manage this patient?

Ans.

1. The abnormality noted here is reduced beat-to-beat variability.
2. Following are the causes of reduced beat-to-beat variability:
   - Fetal hypoxia/acidosis
   - Fetal sleep
   - Use of epidural analgesia
   - Use of narcotic analgesics.
3. The first step to be observed in this case is to rule out fetal sleep by repeating CTG after 1 hour.
   - If the fetal heart rate variability remains <5 bpm for >40 minutes but <90 minutes, then this is called suspicious CTG.
   - If an assessment is classified as "suspicious", a repeat assessment should be done after 30 minutes and the number of suspicious parameters must be recorded (e.g., S1 for "1 suspicious parameter").
   - Several conservative measures can be taken to clarify or improve the patterns (such as change of position, hydration).

- If the abnormality persists then fetal scalp blood sampling should be advised.
- If there is presence of acidosis on blood gas analysis, then cesarean section should be performed.

References
1. German Society of Gynecology and Obstetrics (DGGG); Maternal Fetal Medicine Study Group (AGMFM); German Society of Prenatal Medicine and Obstetrics (DGPGM); German Society of Perinatal Medicine (DGPM). S1-Guideline on the Use of CTG During Pregnancy and Labor: Long version-AWMF Registry No. 015/036. GeburtshilfeFrauenheilkd. 2014;74(8):721-32. doi: 10.1055/s-0034-1382874. PMID: 27065483; PMCID: PMC4812878.
2. Fetal monitoring in labour NICE guideline Published: December 2022.
3. Geburtshilfe Frauenheilkd. 2014;74(8):721-32. doi: 10.1055/s-0034-1382874. PMID: 27065483; PMCID: PMC4812878.

OSCE 20.

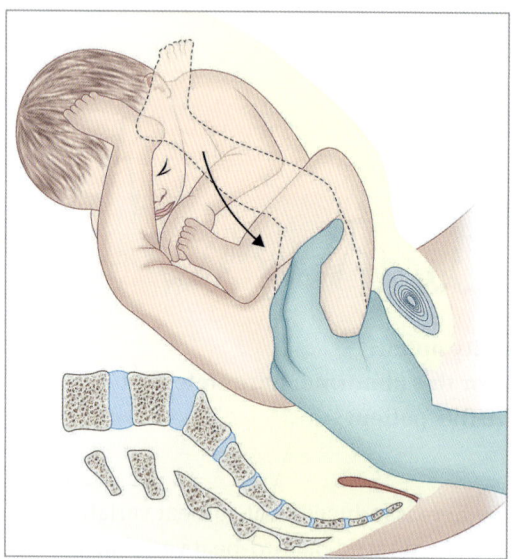

1. What is this maneuver called?
2. What is the indication to perform it?
3. Describe the method to deliver the extended arms.
4. Enumerate the methods to deliver the after coming head in breech delivery.

Ans.

1. Pinard's maneuver.
2. It is performed to deliver the extended legs.
3. Lovset's maneuver is used to deliver the extended arms:
   - The trunk of the baby is held by the pelvis and gently drawn down followed by lifting of the body to cause upward and lateral flexion.
   - The baby is then rotated 180° in one direction to deliver the posterior arm. The arm is released by sweeping the humerus across the fetal chest.

- Now the baby is rotated in the opposite direction by 180° to deliver the anterior arm. The arm is released in the similar manner as mentioned above.
- The baby is then allowed to hang down from the edge of the bed and the mother is encouraged to bear down.
- Delivery of the head is then conducted when hairline is seen.

4. Following methods are used to deliver the after coming head of breech:
   - Mauriceau-Smellie-Veit maneuver
   - Burns–Marshall technique
   - Application of obstetrics forceps (Piper's forceps, Neville Barnes forceps).

References

1. Impey LWM, Murphy DJ, Griffiths M, Penna LK. On behalf of the Royal College of Obstetricians and Gynaecologists. Management of Breech Presentation. BJOG. 2017;124:e151–77.
2. Robson MS, Calder AA, Baskett TF. Malpositions and Malpresentations. In: Munro Kerr's Operative Obstetrics. Arulkumaran S, Michael Rs, 13th edition, p. 89.

OSCE 21. You are a third-year resident doctor managing a G5P3L3MTP1 in labor. The patient's delivery is uneventful. You reassess her after 1 hour of delivery. You find her pad completely soaked and her uterine tone lost. You perform a pelvic examination and evacuate around 300 cc clots from the uterus. She has a pulse of 92 bpm and her BP is 110/68 mm Hg.

1. Identify the condition and enumerate the causes for the same.
2. What are the drugs used to control atonic postpartum hemorrhage?
3. How will you manage a case of minor PPH?
4. What should be done in case of major PPH?

Ans.

1. This is a case of postpartum hemorrhage. Following are the causes of PPH:

The four Ts	Risk factors/notes
Tone: Abnormalities of uterine contraction	
Overdistension of uterus	Polyhydramnios, multiple gestation, macrosomia
Intra-amniotic infection	Fever, prolonged rupture of membranes
Functional/anatomic distortion of uterus	Rapid labor, prolonged labor, fibroids, placenta praevia, uterine anomalies
Uterine relaxants, e.g. magnesium and nifedipine	Terbutaline, halogenated anaesthetics, glyceryl trinitrate
Bladder distension	May prevent uterine contraction
Tissue: Retained products of conception	
Retained cotyledon or succenturiate lobe	
Retained blood clots	

Contd...

Contd...

The four Ts	Risk factors/notes
Trauma: Genital tract injury	
Lacerations of the cervix, vagina or perineum	Precipitous delivery, operative delivery
Extensions, lacerations at caesarean section	Malposition, deep engagement
Uterine rupture	Previous uterine surgery
Uterine inversion	High parity with excessive cord traction
Thrombin: Abnormalities of coagulation	
Pre-existing states	
Haemophilia A	History of hereditary coagulopathies or liver disease
Idiopathic thrombocytopenic purpura	Bruising
von Willebrand's disease	
History of previous PPH	
Acquired in pregnancy	
Gestational thrombocytopenic	Bruising
Pre-eclampsia with thrombocytopenia e.g. HELLP	Elevated blood pressure
Disseminated intravascular coagulation	
a. Gestational hypertensive disorder of pregnancy with adverse conditions	Coagulopathy
b. In utero fetal demise	Fetal demise
c. Severe infection	Fever, neutrophilia/neutropenia
d. Abruption	Antepartum haemorrhage
e. Amniotic fluid embolus	Sudden collapse
Therapeutic anticoagulation	History of thromboembolic disease

2. Oxytocin 5units as IV bolus. This can be repeated once. Infusion of oxytocin containing 30–40 units can be started.

    Ergometrine 0.5 mg is administered intravenously, and this can be repeated once.
    Misoprostol 800 μg is kept per rectum.
    Inj Carboprost 0.25 mg given as IM injection. This can be repeated once in 15 minutes and a maximum of up to 8 doses can be given.

3. *PPH management for minor PPH (blood loss 500–1000 mL) without clinical shock:* The management of PPH requires a multidisciplinary approach. The anesthetist plays a crucial role in maintaining hemodynamic stability, and, if necessary, in determining and administering the most appropriate method of anesthesia (New 2016):
    - Intravenous access (one 14-gauge cannula)
    - Urgent venipuncture (20 mL) for group and screen–full blood count–coagulation screen, including fibrinogen
    - Pulse, respiratory rate and blood pressure recording every 15 minutes.
    - Commence warmed crystalloid infusion.

4. Measures for major PPH (blood loss greater than 1000 mL) and continuing to bleed or clinical shock:
   - A and B–assess airway and breathing
   - C–evaluate circulation.
   - Position the patient flat.
   - Keep the woman warm using appropriate available measures.
   - Transfuse blood as soon as possible, if clinically required.
   - Until blood is available, infuse up to 3.5 L of warmed clear fluids, initially 2 L of warmed isotonic crystalloid. Further fluid resuscitation can continue with additional isotonic crystalloid or colloid (succinylated gelatin). *Hydroxyethyl starch should not be used.*
   - The best equipment available should be used to achieve rapid warmed infusion of fluids, special blood filters should not be used, as they slow infusions.
   - *Blood transfusion:* There are no firm criteria for initiating red cell transfusion. The decision to provide blood transfusion should be based on both clinical and hematological assessment. [New 2016]
   - *Selection of red cell units for transfusion:* Major obstetric hemorrhage protocols must include the provision of emergency blood with immediate issue of group O, rhesus D (Rh-D)-negative and K-negative units, with a switch to group-specific blood as soon as feasible. [New 2016]
   - If clinically significant red cell antibodies are present, close liaison with the transfusion laboratory is essential to avoid delay in transfusion in life-threatening hemorrhage. [New 2016]

Reference

1. Mavrides E, Allard S, Chandraharan E, Collins P, Green L, Hunt BJ, Riris S, Thomson AJ, on behalf of the Royal College of Obstetricians and Gynaecologists. Prevention and management of postpartum haemorrhage. BJOG. 2016;124:e106–49.

OSCE 22.

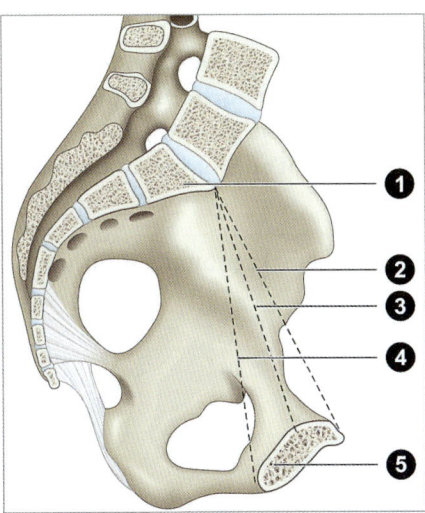

1. Name the points 1, 2, 3.
2. Is it correct to perform pelvic assessment before the onset of labor.
3. What is the best management for a woman with previous LSCS, if the length of 3 is 8 cm?

Ans.

1. (1) Sacral promontory
   (2) True conjugate
   (3) Obstetric conjugate
2. No, as the available spaces in the pelvis increase during labor due to stretching of the ligaments, decrease in fetal diameters due to complete flexion and grade 1 and grade 2 molding.
3. Perform a LSCS as the pelvic inlet is inadequate.

Reference

1. Cunningham FG, Leveno KJ, Dashe JS, Hoffman BL, Spong CY, Casey BM. Maternal Anatomy. Williams Obstetrics, edited by F Gary Cunningham, et al., 26th edn, McGraw-Hill Education, 2018, pp. 51-89.

OSCE 23.

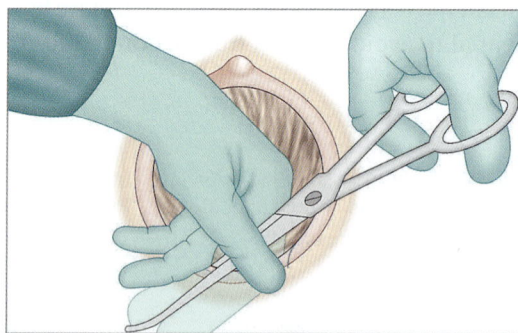

1. Mention the instruments needed for episiotomy suturing.
2. List the tissue planes that are sutured during an episiotomy.
3. How can obstetric perineal injuries be prevented?
4. What is WHO recommended rate of episiotomy in normal deliveries?

Ans.

1. Following instruments are needed for episiotomy suturing:
   - Episiotomy scissors
   - Needle holder
   - Suture
   - Surgical drape
   - Local anesthetic
   - Hemostatic forceps/tissue forceps
   - Sim's speculum

- Foley catheter
- Syringe, needles
- Scalpel/blade
- Kidney tray

2. The tissue planes that are sutured during an episiotomy include:
   - The vaginal mucosa
   - The perineal muscles
   - The perineal skin
3. In order to avoid obstetric perineal injuries, the perineum should be supported at the time of delivery by the assistant. It is said that a timely episiotomy helps to reduce perineal injuries.
4. The WHO recommends an episiotomy rate of 10% for all normal deliveries.

Reference
1. Woretaw, E., Teshome, M. &Alene, M. Episiotomy practice and associated factors among mothers who gave birth at public health facilities in Metema district, northwest Ethiopia. *Reprod Health* 18, 142 (2021). https://doi.org/10.1186/ s12978-021-01194-9

OSCE 24. You are a third-year resident attending a patient referred from primary healthcare center. The reason for referral is nonprogress of labor. On examination you find:

The patient is exhausted, dehydrated, she is in pain. Her abdominal palpation reveals the upper segment of uterus is hard and tender. The lower segment is distended and tender. The bladder is distended. On her vaginal examination the vulva is swollen, and edematous vagina is dry, hot and cervix is fully dilated with the presenting part jammed in the pelvis. There is a large caput formation.

1. What is your diagnosis?
2. How can this complication be prevented?
3. Enumerate the steps to manage this patient?

Ans.

1. The diagnosis is obstructed labor.
2. The prevention of obstructed labor can be done by:
   - Identifying antenatal high-risk factors
   - Intrapartum use of partogram or labor progress record.
3. The standard procedure for obstructed labor is cesarean section as soon as the diagnosis is made.

Prolonged or Neglected Obstructed Labor with an Intact Uterus
- *If the fetus is alive:* The woman should be prepared for expedited delivery also simultaneously attention should be paid the avoid the Sequelae of prolonged labor such as fluid electrolyte imbalance, prevention, and management of infections with broad-spectrum antibiotics and tetanus prophylaxis should be provided.
- *Method of delivery:* Emergency cesarean section should be done.

- *If the fetus is dead:* Destructive operations may be considered, particularly if the mother's condition is morbid. Resuscitation of the mother is essential before proceeding with a destructive procedure. Resuscitating the mother by correcting fluid and electrolyte imbalance, control of infection should be done.
- Anticipating PPH and keeping PPH prevention kit ready will help reduce the morbidity.

Prolonged or Neglected Obstructed Labor with a Ruptured Uterus

1. Prompt management of hypovolemia by providing adequate amount of IV fluids.
2. Laparotomy—remove fetus and placenta
3. *Secure hemostasis:* Deliver the uterus out of the abdominal incision. Assistant's hands may hold the uterus and with fingers and thumbs occlude the uterine vessels.
    - Control the bleeding edges of the uterine laceration with ring forceps.
    - Manual compression of the aorta will often enable the surgeon to identify the extent of the lacerations in the uterus.
    - Bilateral uterine artery ligation should be considered to reduce blood loss before proceeding to definitive surgery.
    - Internal iliac artery ligation may be necessary to control bleeding in the base of the broad ligament.

Before carrying out any surgical procedures on major vessels, the course of the ureter should be identified to avoid ureteric injury. The integrity of the bladder should always be carefully reviewed as there are high chances of bladder wall involvement in a lower uterine segment rupture.

Reference

1. Managing prolonged and obstructed labour: Education material for teachers of midwifery, second edition. World Health Organization, 2006. p. 51 available from: http://whqlibdoc.who.int/publications/2006/9241546662_4_eng.pdf

Chapter 7: Abnormal Labor

OSCE 25.

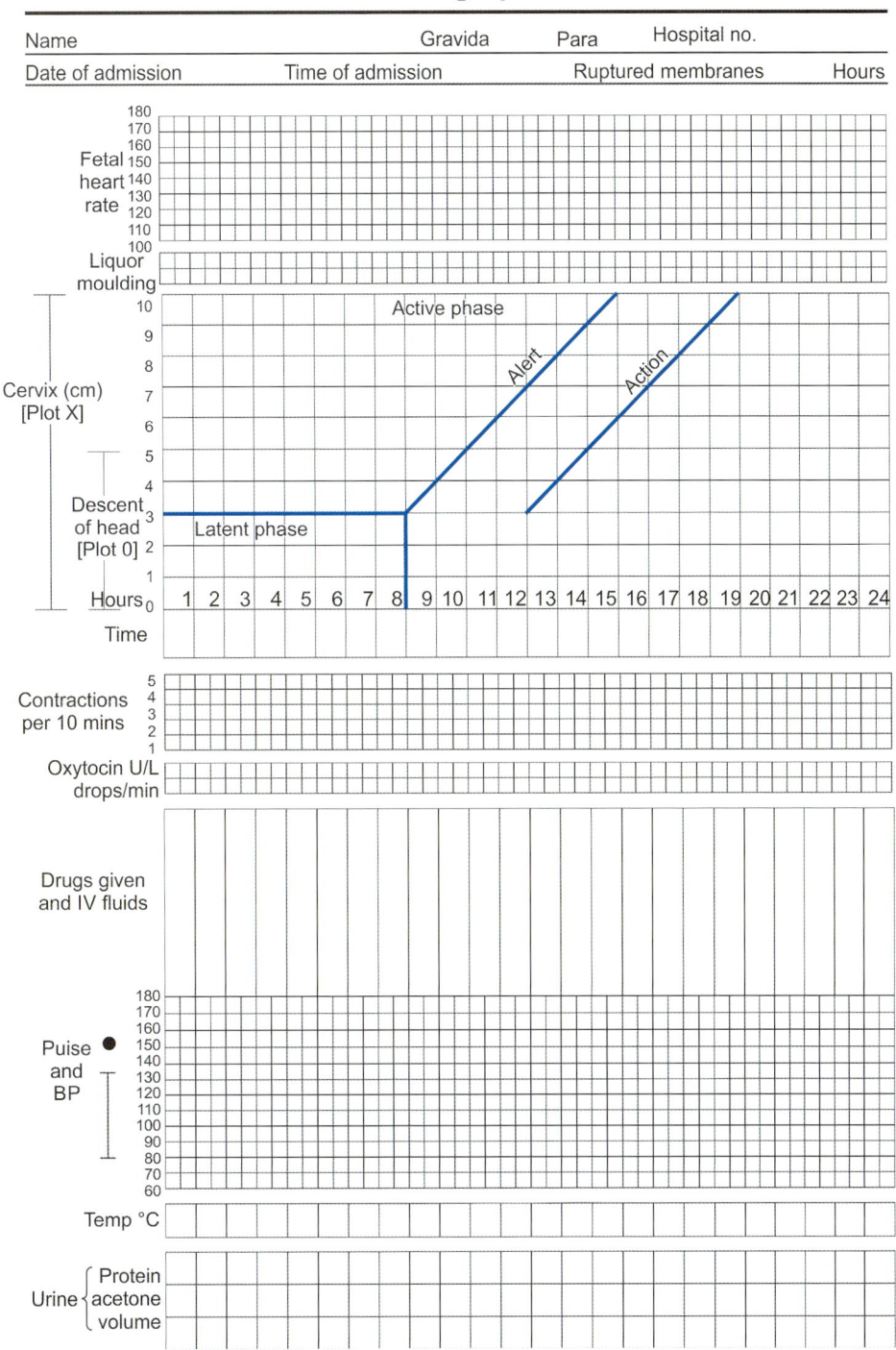

1. What are the parameters which indicate progress of labor in the partogram?
2. What are the parameters of fetal wellbeing which are monitored in partogram?
3. What are the conditions associated with tardy progress of labor?
4. What is the significance of alert and action line in partogram?

Ans.

1. Cervical dilation and descent of the fetal head.
2. Fetal heart rate, CTG findings and the color of the liquor.
3. Occipitoposterior position, brow presentation and mentoposterior face presentation.
4. The alert line goes from 4 to 10 cm and corresponds to an average dilation rate of 1 cm per hour. If the labor curve crosses to the right of this alert line, this means that the dilation is less than 1 cm per hour.

    The alert line goes from 4 to 10 cm and corresponds to an average dilation rate of 1 cm per hour. If the labor curve crosses to the right of this alert line, this means that the dilation is less than 1 cm per hour.

CHAPTER 8

Preterm Labor

Haresh U Doshi

OSCE 1.

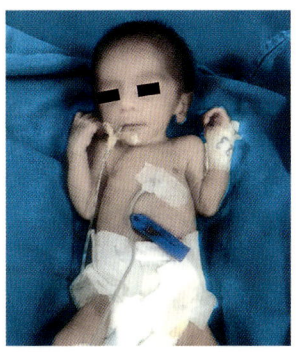

1. Enumerate the four common causes of neonatal deaths.
2. What are the four common complications in preterm newborns?
3. Write four lifestyle factors responsible for preterm labor.
4. What is the most important risk factor for preterm birth?

Ans.

1. Prematurity, IUGR, birth asphyxia, congenital anomalies, and sepsis.
2. Respiratory distress syndrome, jaundice, hypoglycemia, and hypothermia.
3. Tobacco use, smoking, alcohol, obesity, heavy physical work, and stress.
4. Past history of preterm birth.

OSCE 2.

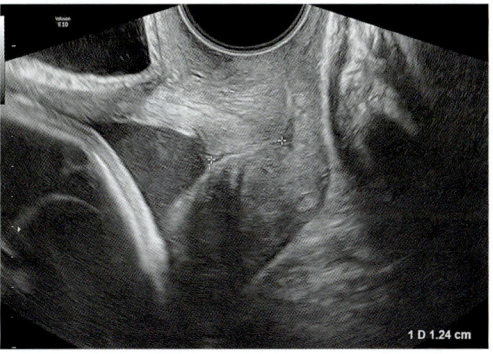

1. What is the threshold of cervical length measurement by USG for screening of preterm labor?
2. Write about the four criteria of standard technique for measuring cervical length by TVS?
3. Name four important biomarkers for screening of preterm labor?
4. For biomarkers for screening of preterm labor what is high sensitivity, specificity, positive predictive value (PPV) or negative predictive value (NPV)?

Ans.

1. 2.5 cm.
2. a. Bladder should be empty.
   b. Cervix should occupy approximately 50–75% of the image.
   c. Excessive pressure on the probe should be avoided.
   d. Three measurements should be taken. Shortest should be considered for management.
3. Fetal fibronectin, Placental alpha Macroglobulin-1(PAMG-1), Insulin-like growth factor binding protein-1 (IFGBP-1), salivary estriol
4. Negative predictive value (NPV)

OSCE 3.

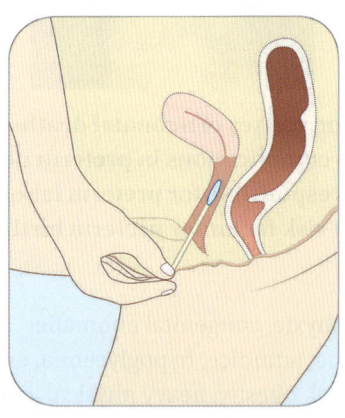

1. What is this method for screening for preterm labor?
2. At what gestational age this biomarker is normally present in cervicovaginal fluid?
3. What value is diagnostic as positive for diagnosis of preterm labor?
4. What are the reasons for the false test result?

Ans.

1. FFN (Fetal fibronectin) testing in cervicovaginal fluid by taking swab.
2. Before 16 weeks of pregnancy.
3. 50 ng/mL
4. a. Per vaginal examination prior to test
   b. Blood in the specimen
   c. PPROM, or
   d. The patient had intercourse in last 24 hours.

OSCE 4.

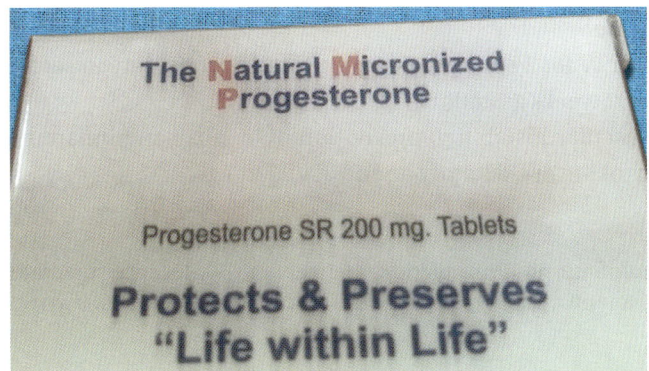

1. Which route of progesterone is most useful for prevention of preterm labor?
2. What is the dose recommended?
3. What is the latest recommendation of ACOG for intramuscular progesterone for prevention of preterm labor?
4. What is the role of progesterone in established preterm labor?

Ans.

1. Vaginal route
2. 100–400 mg by different authorities
3. USFDA withdrew approval of 17-alpha hydroxyprogesterone caproate (Makena) effective immediately for prevention of recurrent preterm labor.
4. Progesterone is not effective in established preterm labor.

OSCE 5.

1. Which are the tocolytics used for arrest of preterm labor?
2. Which tocolytic is most commonly recommended? What is the dose?
3. Tocolytics are effective up to what period of time?
4. Which two drugs are banned by FDA for use as tocolytics?

Ans.

1. Nifedipine, Betamimetics, Magnesium sulfate, Nitroglycerine, Indomethacin, Atosiban
2. Nifedipine. Initial oral dose is 20 mg followed by 10 mg every 6 hours.
3. For 3–7 days.
4. Terbutaline and Injectable progesterone 17OHPC (17-alpha-hydroxyprogesterone caproate).

OSCE 6.

1. Name the drug given to mother for neuroprotection of fetus?
2. What is the dose? How is it given?
3. It is given up to which gestational age?
4. What is the mechanism of action of the drug?

Ans.

1. Magnesium sulfate
2. It is given 1gm/hr IV for 24 hours just prior to delivery or cesarean section.
3. It is given up to 32 weeks gestational age.
4. Reduction of vascular instability, prevention of hypoxic and inflammatory damage and mitigation of cytokine or excitatory amino acid damage.

Reference

1. Magnesium sulphate neuroprotection mechanism is placental mediated by inhibition of inflammation, apoptosis and oxidative stress. ScienceDirect. https://www.sciencedirect.com › article › abs › pii

OSCE 7.

1. What are the different types of cerclage operation?
2. Which cerclage will you do in this patient?
3. What are the contraindications of this procedure?
4. Along with this procedure what other drugs will you give?

Ans.

1. There are three types of cerclage operations:
   a. History-indicated cerclage
   b. USG-indicated cerclage
   c. Rescue cerclage
2. Rescue cerclage
3. Signs of infection, active vaginal bleeding, uterine contractions, rupture of membranes.
4. Progesterone, tocolytics and antibiotics

OSCE 8.

1. G2P1L1 at 30 weeks comes with pain abdomen since 2 hours. How will you diagnose that she is in preterm labor?
2. If she is in preterm labor what 2 group of drugs will you administer?
3. For what purpose these drugs are used?
4. What is the role of maintenance therapy?

Ans.

1. The diagnosis of preterm labor generally is based on clinical criteria of regular uterine contractions accompanied by change in cervical dilation, effacement, or both.
2. Tocolytics and steroids.
3. Tocolytics are used for arresting preterm labor. Delaying labor helps the steroids to work for fetal lung maturity, and the patient can be shifted to a higher center for proper NICU care.
4. Maintenance therapy is not supported by evidence-based medicine.

Chapter 8: Preterm Labor

OSCE 9.
1. What is the drug recommended by GOI for steroid administration?
2. It is given for which gestational age and what is its dose?
3. Why steroid recommended in India is different than what is used in other countries?
4. What are the other advantages to newborns apart from preventing RDS (respiratory distress syndrome)?

Ans.
1. Dexamethasone injection
2. Dexamethasone is given IM 4 doses of 6 mg every 12 hours. It is given from 24 to 34 weeks gestation.
3. In other countries, Inj Betamethasone is recommended. The salt they use is long acting. The salt of Betamethasone available in India is short acting.
4. It prevents intraventricular hemorrhage, necrotizing enterocolitis, and PDA.

OSCE 10.
1. What is Rescue steroid?
2. When is it given and at what dose?
3. Rescue steroids are recommended for what number of times?
4. Why weekly steroids are not given now?

Ans.
1. Second course of steroids given just before delivery/cesarean is called Rescue steroid.
2. When 2 weeks or more have passed after the first course of steroids: Rescue steroid is given. It is given as a routine full course, i.e., Dexamethasone 6 mg, 12 hourly, 4 doses IM or 12 mg Betamethasone, 2 doses, 24 hours apart.
3. Only once, i.e., total 2 courses of steroids.
4. Evidence has shown that weekly steroids previously practiced resulted in fetal brain damage and fetal growth restriction apart from maternal side effects.

OSCE 11. Primi at 33 weeks of pregnancy comes with discharge per vaginum since 4 hours with no other risk factors.
1. How will you clinically confirm that it is PPROM?
2. If you cannot confirm clinically, then what test can be done for diagnosis?
3. What drugs should be administered to her?

Ans.
1. Clinically, PPROM is diagnosed by history of continuous watery discharge, sterile per speculum examination and by keeping a vulval pad for few hours to see whether it gets soaked or not.
2. Tests to confirm leaking include pH testing of vaginal discharge, microscopic examination of discharge for ferning, slide heat test, and detecting amniotic fluid protein, PAMG-1 by taking vaginal swab (Amnisure).
3. Antibiotics and steroids.

OSCE 12.
Third gravida with confirmed PPROM at 29 weeks of pregnancy is being managed conservatively.
1. How will you clinically monitor her daily?
2. What investigations should be done?
3. When should the pregnancy be terminated?
4. What are the reasons for early termination?

Ans.
1. Daily maternal evaluation is done for infection by assessing temperature, pulse, uterine tenderness, and checking for foul-smelling discharge.
2. For infection → Culture of high vaginal swab, leukocyte count, ESR, CRP.
   For fetal maturity and wellbeing → USG
3. At 37 completed weeks.
4. Indications of early termination are if chorioamnionitis develops or in case of fetal distress.

OSCE 13.
1. Enumerate four short-term common complications of preterm newborns.
2. Enumerate four long-term common complications of preterm newborns?
3. Enumerate four common interventions by neonatologists in the management of preterm newborns?
4. What are the advantages of in utero transfer?

Ans.
1. RDS, birth asphyxia, jaundice, hypoglycemia.
2. Cerebral palsy, behavioral problems, Retinopathy of prematurity, deafness.
3. Plastic wrap for extreme premature baby, surfactant administration, early CPAP and sepsis prevention bundle.
4. Possibility of immediate adequate resuscitation and less chances of infection.

OSCE 14.
1. What are the components of Kangaroo mother care (KMC) for a newborn?
2. Who can give KMC?
3. What is its role in preterm newborns?
4. Which two components are the most important in KMC?

Ans.
1. *Four components:* Kangaroo position (skin-to-skin contact), Kangaroo nutrition, Kangaroo discharge, Kangaroo support.
2. KMC can be given by a birthing parent, family member or any trained person or nurse.
3. KMC is useful in preterm newborns. It helps in proper temperature control, stabilization of cardiorespiratory system, breastfeeding and adequate sleep-in premature baby.
4. Skin-to-skin contact and exclusive breastfeeding.

OSCE 15.

1. Write any four measures for primary prevention of preterm labor?
2. Which are the clinical interventions NOT proved by evidence in preventing preterm labor?
3. GBS prophylaxis is indicated in which mothers as per ACOG guidelines?
4. Which drugs are given for GBS prophylaxis?

Ans.

1. Healthy diet provides optimum nutrition, restricting smoking, alcohol, and substance abuse.
   Avoiding stress and heavy physical work are some of the measures for primary prevention.
2. Bed rest, home uterine activity monitoring, prophylactic antibiotics in absence of PPROM and cervical pessary are not found useful by evidence for preventing preterm labor.
3. Patients with PPROM require GBS prophylaxis. As per ACOG recent guidelines, universal GBS screening is recommended between 36–38 weeks gestation and if found positive prophylactic antibiotics are indicted.
4. Penicillin and cephalosporin group of drugs are commonly used.

Reference

1. Prevention of Group B Streptococcal Early-Onset Disease in Newborns: ACOG Committee Opinion, Number 797, February 2020.

OSCE 16.

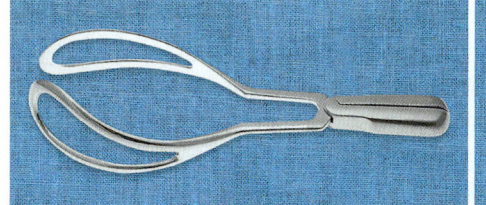 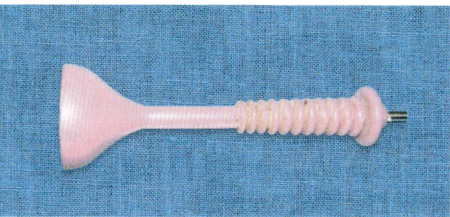

1. For instrumental vaginal delivery which instrument is used for preterm newborn? Why?
2. When should you clamp the cord in preterm delivery?
3. What is the practice of episiotomy in vaginal delivery?
4. As compared to full-term what is the difference in interpreting CTG in preterm labor?

Ans.

1. If indicated forceps is used for preterm delivery. Vacuum extraction causes intracranial hemorrhage.
2. Unless emergency resuscitation is required cord is clamped after 30 seconds up to 3 minutes.
3. Liberal episiotomy is given even if the baby is small to prevent undue compression.
4. In a very premature fetus, baseline heart rate may be more, and baseline variability and cycling may be reduced.

OSCE 17.

1. What should be the mode of delivery in idiopathic preterm labor?
2. What are the problems in doing cesarean section in preterm pregnancy?
3. If space available is less in the lower segment, what will you do to deliver the baby?
4. What anesthesia is preferred in cesarean section at preterm gestation?

Ans.

1. Cesarean section is favored in extremely preterm (<28 weeks) otherwise vaginal delivery is done if not contraindicated.
2. Lower segment is not fully formed so less space is available for delivery of fetus and malpresentation are common at preterm gestational age.
3. More curved incision, 'J' shaped incision and inverted 'T' incision can be done.
4. Spinal anesthesia is used for most preterm cesarean delivery, unless it is contraindicated by maternal disease or because of the emergency nature of the procedure, in which case general anesthesia is used.

OSCE 18.

1. What is the screening method suggested in twin pregnancy for detection of high risk for preterm labor?
2. What is the role of prophylactic vaginal progesterone in twin pregnancy?
3. What is the role of cervical pessary to prevent preterm labor in twin pregnancy?
4. What is the status of cervical cerclage in preterm labor in twins?

Ans.

1. The Society for Maternal-Fetal Medicine (SMFM) recommends that "routine cervical length screening in multiple pregnancies is not indicated",[1] while the International Society for Ultrasound in Obstetrics and Gynecology[2] states that for twin pregnancies, cervical length measurement is the preferred method of screening for preterm birth in twins.
2. Prophylactic vaginal progesterone is not recommended by evidence in twin pregnancy.
3. Cervical pessary is not proved by evidence to prevent preterm labor in twins.
4. The majority of the guidelines advise against prophylactic or USG indicated cerclage in twin pregnancy. Rescue cerclage is done when indicated.

References

1. Khalil A, Rodgers M, Baschat A, et al. ISUOG Practice Guidelines: role of ultrasound in twin pregnancy. Ultrasound Obstet Gynecol. 2016;47:247-63.
2. The Fetal Medicine Foundation. Education. Cervical assessment. Internet-based course. https://www.fetalmedicine.org/education/cervical-assessment.

OSCE 19.

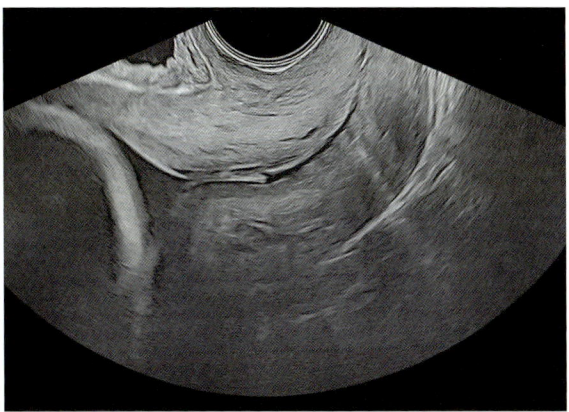

1. What cervical length has the highest sensitivity and specificity for detecting preterm labor?
2. What different shapes of cervix are considered high risk for preterm labor? Which shape is most dangerous?
3. Which is more important for screening of preterm labor. Funneling or cervical length?
4. What are the causes of false measurement of cervical length?

Ans.

1. 1.5 cm.
2. 'U', 'V', and 'Y' shapes of cervix are considered high risk for preterm labor. 'U' shape is most dangerous.
3. Cervical length.
4. Full bladder, excessive pressure by probe on the cervix, improper magnification, not having longitudinal view of cervix are the causes of false measurement of cervical length by TVS.

OSCE 20.

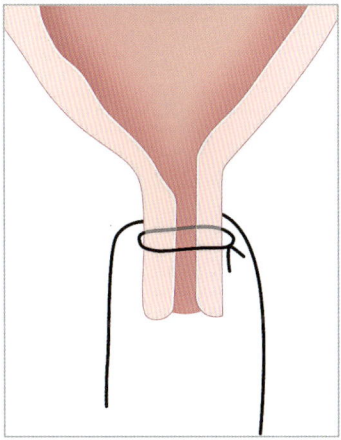

1. What are the indications of prophylactic cerclage?
2. Which are the different types for cervical cerclage?
3. Which method is commonly used for cervical cerclage? Why?
4. When is abdominal cerclage done?

Ans.

1. According to the American College of Obstetricians and Gynecologists (ACOG)[1], a history-indicated or prophylactic cerclage may be placed when there is a "history of ≥1 second-trimester pregnancy losses related to painless cervical dilation and in the absence of labor or if the woman had a prior cerclage placed due to cervical insufficiency.
2. There are 3 types of cerclages:
    a. History indicated or prophylactic cerclage
    b. USG-indicated cerclage
    c. Rescue cerclage.
3. McDonald operation is commonly used for cervical cerclage as it is easy, does not require incision on cervix or dissection, stitch removal is easy, and results are satisfactory.
4. Abdominal cerclage is performed when transvaginal cervical cerclage procedure cannot be placed or has failed previously.

Reference

1. ACOG Practice Bulletin No.142: Cerclage for the management of cervical insufficiency. Obstet Gynecol. 2014;123(2 Pt 1):372-9.

CHAPTER 9

Hyperemesis Gravidarum

Bharti Maheshwari

OSCE 1.
1. Identify the condition given in the image below:

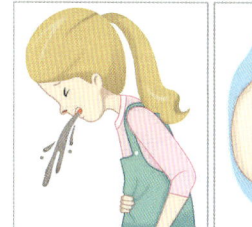
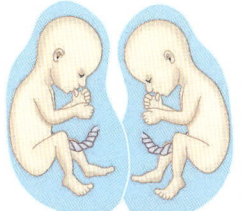
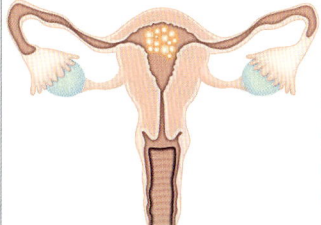
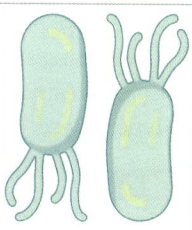

2. Enumerate four risk factors associated with the above-mentioned condition.
3. Identify the bacteria associated with the above condition.

Ans.
1. Hyperemesis gravidarum
2. Maternal obesity, multiple pregnancy, trophoblastic disease, nulliparity
3. *Helicobacter pylori*

OSCE 2.
1. Mention three diagnostic features of hyperemesis gravidarum.
2. What is the most common clinical symptom associated with hyperemesis gravidarum?

Ans.
1. Dehydration, electrolyte imbalance, more than 5% prepregnancy weight loss.
2. Vomiting

OSCE 3.
1. What percentage of pregnant women suffer from hyperemesis gravidarum?
2. Hyperemesis gravidarum is common in between which weeks of pregnancy?

Ans.
1. 0.2–3.6%
2. 8–12 weeks

OSCE 4.
1. Mention three hormones responsible for hyperemesis gravidarum.
2. Which hormone is mainly responsible for nausea in hyperemesis gravidarum?

Ans.

1. Beta-hCG, estrogen, progesterone
2. Beta hCG

OSCE 5.
1. Mention two differences between hyperemesis gravidarum and morning sickness.
2. What causes more often severe dehydration—hyperemesis gravidarum or morning sickness?

Ans.

1. a. Morning sickness is milder.
   b. Severe and persistent symptoms are present in hyperemesis gravidarum.
2. Hyperemesis gravidarum.

OSCE 6.
1. Mention two dietary modifications in hyperemesis gravidarum.
2. What should be restricted in diet of hyperemesis gravidarum?

Ans.

1. Meal high in carbohydrates and low-fat meal.
2. Alcohol, caffeine

OSCE 7.
1. Mention three essential nutritional vitamins to be replenished in diet for hyperemesis gravidarum.
2. Thiamine deficiency results in which potential maternal complication in hyperemesis gravidarum?

Ans.

1. Vitamin B_1, B_6, C
2. Wernicke's encephalopathy

OSCE 8.
1. Why is thiamine replacement essential prior to hydration therapy in the case of hyperemesis gravidarum?
2. First-line drug in treatment of hyperemesis gravidarum.
3. Role of pyridoxine in treatment of hyperemesis gravidarum.

Ans.

1. During hydration, the dextrose in the solution causes the body to metabolize thiamine, which is deficient in hyperemesis.

2. Combination of doxylamine and pyridoxine
3. Pyridoxine administration leads to correction of decreased maternal pyridoxine as decreased levels are responsible for exacerbation of physiological effects of pregnancy due to increased level of pregnancy-associated hormones.

OSCE 9.
1. What are maternal complications of hyperemesis gravidarum?
2. What are fetal complications of hyperemesis gravidarum?

Ans.

1. Hypokalemia, malnutrition, hyponatremia, Wernicke's encephalopathy, Mallory Weiss tear
2. Growth restriction, fetal death, CNS malformation

OSCE 10.
1. G1 with multiple pregnancy with excessive vomiting and nausea, not able to eat.
   O/E—signs of dehydration and ketosis.
   Mention the diagnosis.
2. Define the above condition.

Ans.

1. Hyperemesis gravidarum
2. According to ACOG, hyperemesis gravidarum is defined as a severe form of nausea and vomiting with weight loss greater than 5% of prepregnancy body weight, dehydration, and metabolic acidosis.

OSCE 11.
1. What are the differential diagnoses of hyperemesis gravidarum?
2. Identify the cause of hyperemesis by the given USG picture.

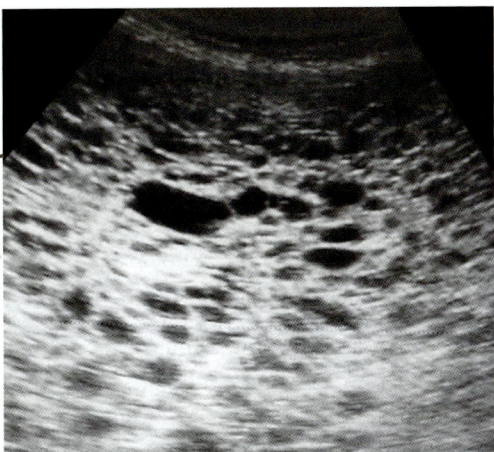

3. What is the characteristic USG appearance in this case termed as?

Ans.

1. Uremia, molar pregnancy, hepatitis, hyperthyroidism, diabetic ketoacidosis, cholecystitis
2. Hydatidiform mole
3. Snowstorm appearance

OSCE 12.
1. Identify the test.
2. What is the indication of urine Dipstick test in hyperemesis gravidarum?

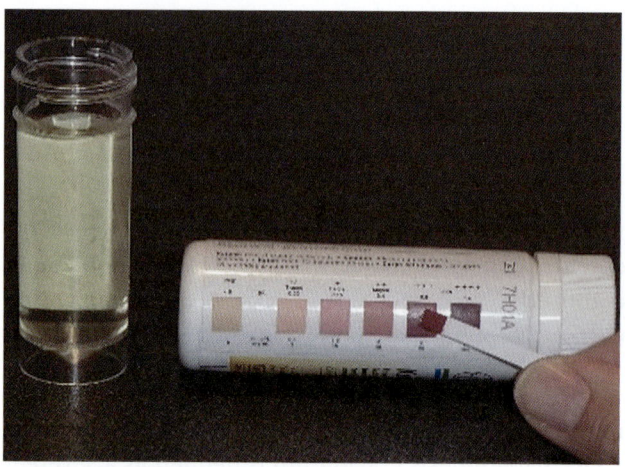

3. Name the ketone bodies found.

Ans.

1. Urine dipstick test—suggestive of positive ketone body.
2. Dehydration, intractable vomiting, signs of ketosis
3. Acetone, beta hydroxy butyrate

OSCE 13.
1. Mention four principles of management of hyperemesis gravidarum.
2. Mention two indications for hospitalization in hyperemesis gravidarum.

Ans.

1. a. To control vomiting
   b. To correct fluid and electrolyte balance
   c. To correct metabolic disturbances
   d. To prevent serious complications of severe vomiting
2. Intractable vomiting; fluid and electrolyte imbalance

OSCE 14.
1. Which foundation is associated with hyperemesis gravidarum?
2. What can be found in urine of hyperemesis gravidarum?

Ans.
1. HER foundation
2. Ketones

OSCE 15.
1. Mention five investigations for hyperemesis gravidarum.
2. Mention antiemetic drugs for hyperemesis gravidarum.

Ans.
1. Urine analysis, CBC, LFT, thyroid function test, USG scan
2. Promethazine, triflupromazine, metoclopramide

OSCE 16.
1. What do we find on physical examination of hyperemesis gravidarum?
2. How does breath of hyperemesis gravidarum patient smell?

Ans.
1. Weak, pale, and dry mucous membrane. Pulse may be elevated secondary to dehydration.
2. Ketotic breath smell

OSCE 17.
1. When is therapeutic abortion indicated in hyperemesis gravidarum?
2. What is the management of hyperemesis gravidarum?

Ans.
1. a. Intractable vomiting, not relieved on therapy.
   b. Serious maternal or fetal complications
2. a. Antiemetics
   b. Hydrocortisone
   c. Prednisolone
   d. Nutritional support—vitamin B_1, B_6, B_{12}, C

OSCE 18.
1. Name the drug banned earlier used for hyperemesis gravidarum.
2. What did the above drug cause?

Ans.
1. Thalidomide
2. Phocomelia (seal-like limbs)

OSCE 19.
1. What is the full form of a modified PUQE score?
2. Which two genes are potentially linked to hyperemesis gravidarum?

Ans.
1. Modified pregnancy unique quantification of emesis/nausea
2. *GDF15, IGFBP7*

OSCE 20.
1. What is the alternative therapy in hyperemesis gravidarum?
2. Name two antihistamines used for hyperemesis gravidarum.

Ans.
1. Acupressure therapy
2. Diphenhydramine, meclizine

CHAPTER 10

Anemia in Pregnancy

Kiran Pandey, Pavika Lal

OSCE 1. Mrs X G2P1+0 at 31 weeks 3 days was admitted with pre-eclampsia with severe features. On admission, her BP was 164/96 mm Hg which got well controlled on Labetalol 200 mg TDS and her routine investigations (CBC, LFT, KFT) were within normal limits. USG for fetal well-being was normal. After three days of admission, her general condition deteriorated. Repeat CBC showed decreasing trend of platelets and hemoglobin. LFT showed AST = 78 IU/L, ALT = 86 IU/L and bilirubin (total/direct/indirect = 2.4/0.4/2.0 mg/dL), Hb = 6.3 g/dL, platelet count = 50,000/uL, Urea = 34 mg/dL, and creatinine = 0.8 mg/dL.
1. What is the most probable diagnosis?
2. What are the other differentials for the above scenario?
3. What are the criteria for the diagnosis of the above case?

Ans.
1. *HELLP syndrome:* Hemolysis in HELLP syndrome is caused by red blood cell fragmentation that results from microvascular thrombosis, described as microangiopathic hemolytic anemia (MAHA).
2. a. *Disorders that are pregnancy specific:*
    - Pre-eclampsia with severe features
    - Eclampsia
    - Acute fatty liver disease of pregnancy
    - Disseminated intravascular coagulation (DIC)
   b. *Disorders that are pregnancy nonspecific:*
    - Congenital hemolytic anemia
    - Thalassemia
    - Sickle cell anemia
    - G-6-PD deficiency
    - Hereditary spherocytosis
    - Pyruvate kinase deficiency
    - Drug-induced hemolytic anemia
    - Transfusion-related hemolysis
3. *Tennessee classification system:* Diagnostic criteria for HELLP are—
    - Hemolysis
    - Increased LDH (>600 U/L)
    - Increased AST (>or = 70 U/L)
    - Low platelets <100×10^9/L

OSCE 2.

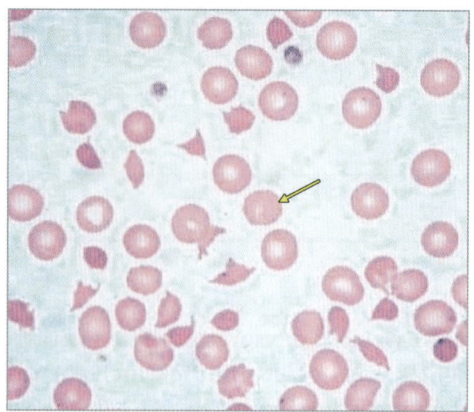

1. Identify the marked structure in the image and name the condition it denotes.
2. Enumerate the other types of cells seen in peripheral blood smear in this condition.
3. How will you manage this case?

Ans.

1. Peripheral blood smear findings are suggestive of hemolysis and the marked structure shows schistocyte.
2. Bite cells, helmet cells, spherocytes, spur cells, elliptocytes and somatotypes.
3. *Management:*
   - Assessment of the mother and fetus along with the stabilization of patient who are at a tertiary care center in HDU/ICU.
   - Transfusion of blood and blood products (PCV, FFP and platelet)
   - Antihypertensive treatment, magnesium sulfate coverage, corticosteroid coverage followed by termination of pregnancy.

OSCE 3. Mrs Y, 22-year-old, G2P1+0 at 39 weeks 4 days, was admitted for delivery of her first child on February 23, 2023. On her last visit on January 6, a routine blood examination revealed Hb 8.8 gm%, red blood cells 3,700,000 per cumm, and white blood cells 6,750 per cumm. On admission, her repeat CBC was done which demonstrated anemia, moderate thrombocytopenia, and leukopenia.

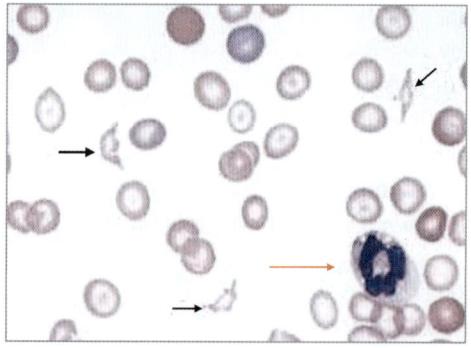

Chapter 10: Anemia in Pregnancy

1. Identify the cell marked in image and the type of anemia associated with it.
2. Name the conditions in pregnancy associated with this anemia.
3. What are the investigations done to evaluate this type of anemia?

Ans.

1. Neutrophils with more than five distinct lobes referred to as multilobed or hypersegmented seen in megaloblastic anemia.
2. Vitamin B_{12} deficiency; Folate deficiency
3. Investigations to make the diagnosis:
   - CBC including RBC indices.
   - Peripheral blood film
   - S. LDH
   - S. Homocysteine levels
   - Serum vitamin B_{12} and folate level
   - Thyroid-stimulating hormone
   - Liver function test

OSCE 4. Mrs. Y, 21-year-old, G3 P2+0 at 35 weeks was admitted for evaluation of anemia which had not responded to parenteral iron, vitamin B_{12}, and folic acid. Her Hb was 6.8 gm% and she was transfused with 2 units of PCV. She delivered at term without any complication. During her previous two pregnancies too, she had multiple packed RBC transfusion for anemia not responding to parenteral therapy.

1. What is the most probable diagnosis for the case?
2. What are the criteria for the diagnosis of refractory anemia?
3. What investigations are to be done for a case of refractory anemia?

Ans.

1. This is a case of refractory anemia which is defined as anemia which does not respond to specific treatment except for blood transfusions.
2. The criteria for the diagnosis of refractory anemia of pregnancy include:
   - The appearance of anemia during pregnancy which disappears after delivery.
   - Proved refractoriness to treatment.
   - A normal/elevated serum iron level.
   - Thrombocytopenia and granulopenia.
   - Normoblastic hypoplasia.
3. Investigations to be done in refractory anemia:
   - CBC
   - Peripheral blood smear—to exclude other types of anemias.
   - Serum Iron levels
   - Evaluation of vitamin deficiencies (Vitamin B_{12}, folate and copper)
   - Bone marrow evaluation
   - Investigations to rule out chronic systemic infection.
   - Gastrointestinal assessment

Section 1: Obstetrics

OSCE 5. Mrs X, G1P0+0 at 37 weeks was diagnosed with Thalassemia intermedia at the age of 1 year. Her parent's thalassemia status is unknown, and her three siblings have normal hemoglobin pattern. She had a history of occasional blood transfusions. Her spouse had a normal hemoglobin pattern; hence the fetus was not subjected to prenatal diagnosis of thalassemia. She delivered by emergency cesarean a live male baby of 2.6 kg with good APGAR.
1. What is thalassemia and what are its types?
2. What is its inheritance pattern?
3. What are the peripheral blood smear findings?

Ans.

1. This is a case of thalassemia, quantitative hemoglobinopathy affecting globin chain production. Its two major types are alpha- and beta-thalassemia.
2. Autosomal recessive
3. *Target cell:* Red cells with central staining with precipitated hemoglobin
   Punctate basophilia: Accumulation of ribosomes in periphery of red cell
   Howell Jolly bodies: Basophilic nuclear remnants in RBC's.

OSCE 6.
1. What should be done to differentiate between iron deficiency anemia and thalassemia?
2. Can Iron therapy be given to patients with thalassemia?
3. What points should be considered prenatally while managing a case of thalassemia intermedia/major?

Ans.

1. *Serum iron:* Decreased in IDA and normal or increased in thalassemia.
   Serum ferritin: Decreased in IDA and normal or increased in thalassemia.
2. Women with thalassemia trait only can be given oral iron therapy. Parenteral formulations should be avoided in all types of thalassemia.
3. *Prenatal counseling in thalassemia patients:*
   - Chelation therapy should be stopped, and folate supplementation should be given.
   - Prophylactic dose of penicillin therapy should be maintained especially in those who have undergone splenectomy. Pneumococcal vaccination and boosters are advised prior to pregnancy.
   - Check endocrine (TFT, blood sugar—Fasting and postprandial) and cardiac status (2D-Echo)
   - Blood transfusions are needed (usually 3 weekly) to maintain Hb above 10 gm%.
   - Prophylaxis for VTE should be counseled which is given postnatally for 6 weeks.

OSCE 7.

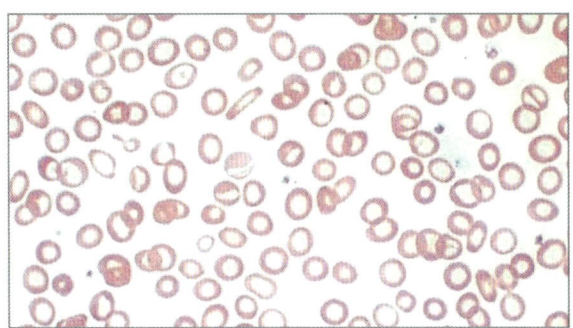

1. What does the above peripheral blood smear depict?
2. What is the most common cause for the above condition?
3. Write three other differentials for the above cause.

Ans.

1. Microcytic hypochromic anemia
2. Iron deficiency anemia
3. Sideroblastic anemia, thalassemia, and anemia of chronic diseases.

OSCE 8.
A 28 year, primigravida with easy fatigability and dyspnea has been diagnosed with iron deficiency anemia on Iron studies.
1. What is likely to be seen in CBC?
2. What is likely to be seen in peripheral blood smear (PBS)?
3. What are the findings seen in iron studies?

Ans.

1. CBC findings decreased Hb, decreased MCV, decreased MCH, decreased MCHC.
2. Microcytic hypochromic anemia
3. Serum iron—decreased, Serum Ferritin—decreased, TIBC-increased.

OSCE 9.
1. What is Pica and where is it commonly seen?
2. What is RDA of iron in normal female and during pregnancy?
3. How do we calculate iron requirement in a case of iron deficiency anemia?

Ans.

1. Pica is the consumption of nonfood items with no nutritional value like clay or ice. It is most commonly seen in iron deficiency anemia.
2. RDA in normal female 1 mg/day, RDA in pregnancy 5 mg/day
3. Iron requirement is calculated by Ganzoni formula:
   Fe requirement = 2.4 × (Target Hb–Patient Hb) × pre-pregnancy body weight + 500 mg/1,000 mg (for stores)

OSCE 10.

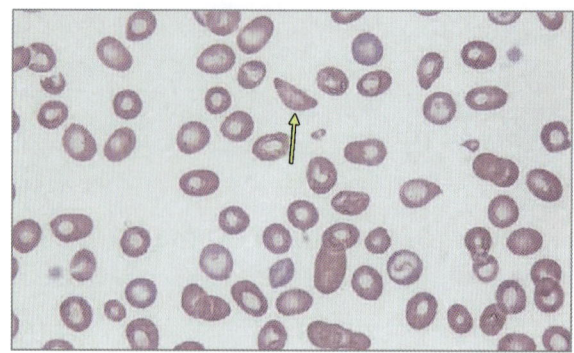

1. What does the arrowhead in PBS depict?
2. Where is this condition most commonly seen and what is the type of inheritance along with involvement of which chromosome?
3. What is the cause of sickle cell anemia?

Ans.

1. Arrowhead indicates sickle cells. Other findings are microcytic hypochromic anemia and target cells.
2. Sickle cell anemia, autosomal recessive condition with mutation in chromosome number 11 at 6th position.
3. Inherited hemoglobinopathy in the beta-globin chain, where glutamic acid is replaced by valine.

OSCE 11.

1. What investigation is done to confirm sickle cell anemia and what findings do we get?
2. What are the complications of sickle cell anemia?
3. Which is the most preferred postpartum contraceptive method advisable in patients with sickle cell anemia?

Ans.

1. High Performance Liquid Chromatography
2. Chronic pain, aseptic bone necrosis, leg ulcers, pulmonary hypertension.
3. *Depot:* Medroxy progesterone acetate injections intramuscularly 150 mg every 3 monthly as it reduces sickling and helps in reducing the incidence of veno-occlusive crisis especially in postpartum females.

OSCE 12.

1. Which drugs are contraindicated in sickle cell anemia (SCA)?
2. What vaccination is given in a patient with sickle cell anemia?
3. What does NESTROFT stand for and what is the principle behind it?

Ans.
1. Drugs like hydroxy urea are contraindicated in SCA.
2. Vaccination against capsulated organisms like *Pneumococcus*, influenza are given in SCA.
3. Naked Eye Single Tube Red Cell Osmotic Fragility Test.
   Normally, red cells put in saline solution begin to lyse at a saline concentration of 0.4–0.5% and lysis is complete at 0.32%. However, in beta-thalassemia trait, due to alteration in osmotic resistance of the affected RBCs due to volume/surface area ratio changes, lysis begins at a saline concentration between 0.4–0.35% and it may not be completed even at 0.1% solution. NESTROFT is done at a saline concentration of 0.36%.

OSCE 13.
1. What is the most common type of anemia seen during pregnancy?
2. What is the 6 × 6 × 6 policy of Anemia Mukt Bharat program.
3. What is prophylactic and therapeutic dose of IFA tablets in pregnant females?

Ans.
1. Nutritional anemia among which iron deficiency anemia is most common.
2. The 6 × 6 × 6 strategy under AMB implies six age groups, six interventions and six institutional mechanisms. The strategy focuses on ensuring supply chain, demand generation and strong monitoring using the dashboard for addressing anemia, both due to nutritional and non-nutritional causes.
3. Prophylactic 100 mg elemental Fe along with folic acid once a day for 180 days (recommended by WHO).
   Therapeutic dose 100 mg Fe+ 500 ug Folic acid Twice to thrice a day along with enhancers of iron absorption (Vitamin C).

Guidelines for management of maternal anemia
a. At 14–16 weeks of gestation

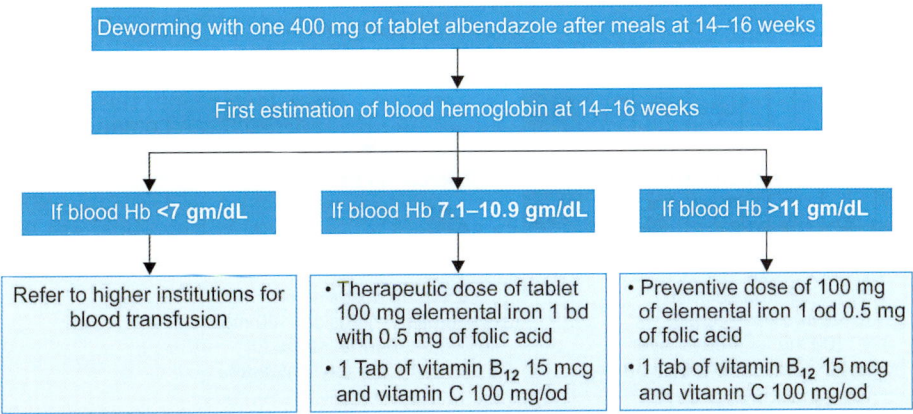

b. At 20–24 weeks of gestation

```
Second estimation of blood hemoglobin at 20–24 weeks of gestation after the consumption
of preventive/therapeutic dose of iron
```

If blood Hb <7 gm/dL	If blood Hb 7.1–8.9 gm/dL	If blood Hb 9–11 gm/dL	If blood Hb >11 gm/dL
Refer to higher institutions for blood transfusion	Injection iron sucrose infusion intravenous– 4 doses of 100 mg for 4 days over a period of 2 weeks with 2–4 days interval b/w each dose	Continue with therapeutic dose	Continue with preventive dose

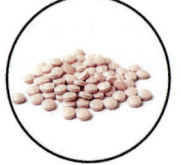
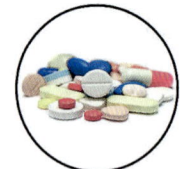

c. At 26–30 weeks of gestation

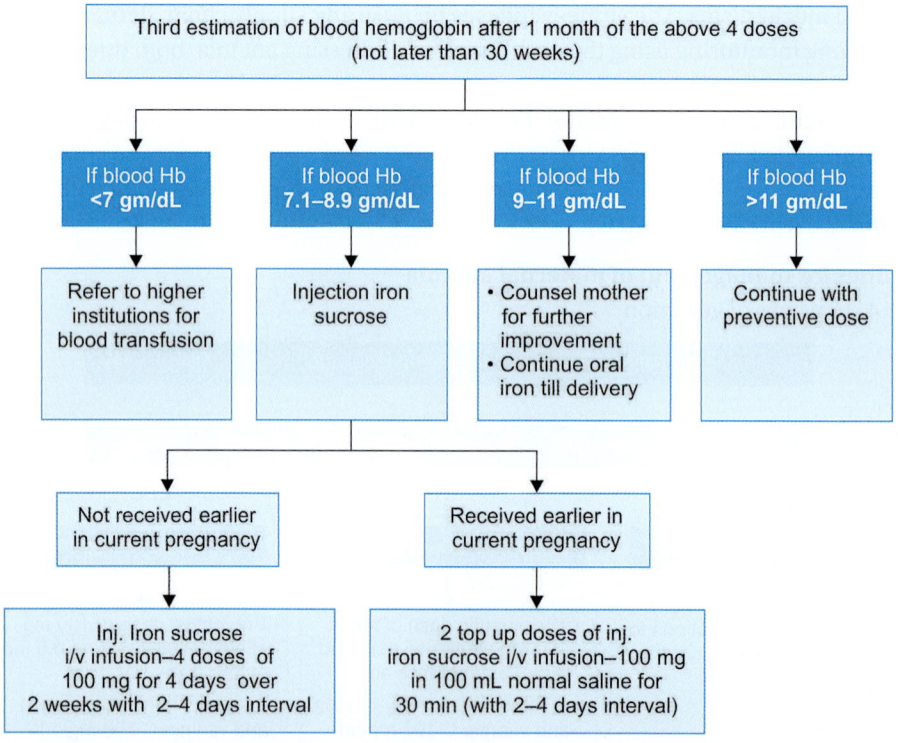

d. At 30–34 weeks of gestation

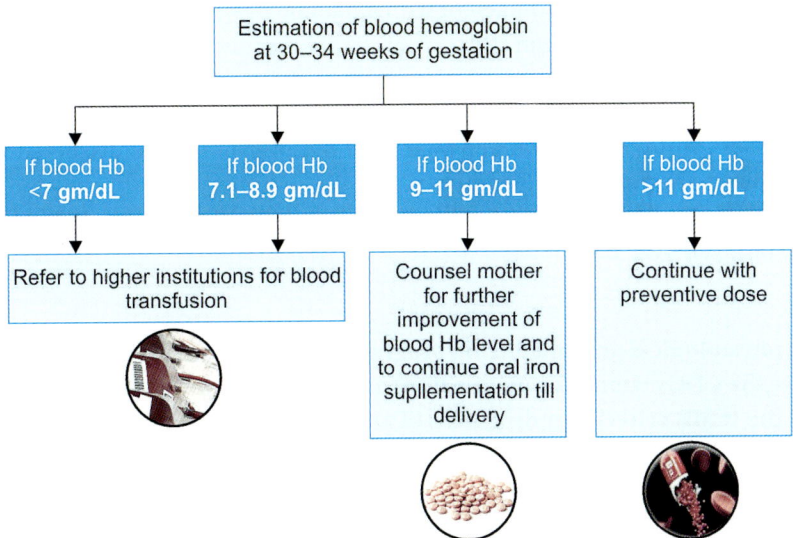

OSCE 14.
1. What are the contraindications of oral iron?
2. What are the indications of parenteral iron?
3. What are the side effects of parenteral iron?

Ans.

1. Iron therapy is contraindicated in known hypersensitivity, hemochromatosis, hemosiderosis, anemia not caused by iron deficiency.
2. Intolerance to oral iron, noncompliance, Malabsorption syndromes, history of bariatric surgery.
3. Most reactions to parenteral iron therapy occur immediately during administration of the test dose and may include dyspnea, headache, flushing, chest pain, abdominal pain, nausea, bronchospasm, fever, seizure, hypotension, urticaria and anaphylaxis.

OSCE 15.
1. What advice/counseling should be given to patients while prescribing oral iron therapy?
2. What are the various IV iron preparations available?
3. What is the minimum dilution while giving FCM and Iron sucrose respectively?

Ans.

1. a. Avoid phytates, phosphates with iron.
   b. Vitamin C enhances the absorption of iron; hence iron should be taken with citrus foods.

c. Do not take iron and calcium together.
d. Avoid taking iron empty stomach or with antacids.
2. a. 1st generation—Iron dextran (IM)
   b. 2nd generation—Iron sucrose, iron iso-maltose (IV)
   c. 3rd generation—Ferric carboxy maltose (FCM) (IV)
3. Iron sucrose—Minimal dilution (1:1), i.e., 100 mg of iron can be dissolved in 100 mL. Normal saline to be given over 30 minutes.
   FCM-Minimal dilution (2:1), i.e., 500 mg of iron can be dissolved in 250 mL of normal saline to be given over 15 minutes.

OSCE 16.
1. What is physiological anemia during pregnancy and why does it occur?
2. What are the CDC criteria for diagnosis of anemia during pregnancy?
3. What is the ICMR criteria for diagnosis of anemia during pregnancy?

Ans.

1. Physiological anemia during pregnancy is hemoglobin levels ≤11 g/dL
   It is basically dilutional and happens because plasma levels (45–50%) expansion occurs more than the red blood cells levels (20–30%).
2. CDC criteria:
   - <11 g/dL in 1st and 3rd trimester of pregnancy
   - <10.5 g/dL in 2nd trimester of pregnancy.
3. WHO criteria:
   - Mild: 9–11 g/dL
   - Moderate: 7–8.9 g/dL
   - Severe: 4–6.9 g/dL
   - Very severe: <4 g/dL

OSCE 17.
A G2P1L1 at 38 weeks presented with generalized weakness and easy fatiguability with acute onset of breathlessness in active labor?

O/E:
- PR 124/min
- Pallor +++

Investigations: Suggestive of iron deficiency anemia
- Hb 5.4%
- MCV 72 fL
- MCH 25pg
- MCHC 30%
- PBS microcytic hypochromic RBC

What precautions must be taken during these stages of labor?
1. First stage
2. Second stage
3. Third stage

Ans.
1. *First stage:*
   - Comfortable position to the mother.
   - High flow oxygen.
   - Encourage deep breathing between contractions.
   - Strict asepsis should be maintained.
2. *Second stage:*
   - Most stressful (Cardiac failure can occur)
   - A tendency for prolongation of the 2nd stage can be curtailed by forceps.
3. *Third stage:*
   - AMTSL (Active management of third stage of labor)
   - Avoid overloading of fluid-like crystalloids, etc.
   - Replenish only if hypovolemic.

OSCE 18. In the above case discussed in OSCE 17:
1. What treatment is most appropriate in the above clinical scenario?
2. What are the indications of blood transfusion in pregnancy?

Ans.
1. 1-unit packed RBCs increases Hb by 0.8–1 g/unit of 300 mL which means this patient requires 3–4 units of pRBCs to be able to reach up to 8–9 g/dL.
   Blood should be transfused slowly in a duration of 4 hours to avoid volume overload.
   It should be transfused under Lasix cover. Inj Calcium Gluconate should be administered post-transfusion as stored blood contains chelators which cause hypocalcemia.
2. *Antepartum period:*
   - POG <34 weeks:
     - Hb <5 g/dL with /without CHF
     - Hb 5–7 g/dL in presence of CHF
   - POG >34 weeks:
     - Hb <7 g/dL even without CHF
     - Severe anemia with decompensation
   - Acute hemorrhage

   Intrapartum period:
   - Hb <7 g/dL

   Postpartum period:
   - Anemia with signs of shock/acute hemorrhage/hemodynamic instability.
   - Hb <7g%

OSCE 19.
1. What are the various stages of iron deficiency anemia?
2. How does iron deficiency corelate with various parameters on iron profile?

Ans.

1. Stages of iron deficiency anemia:

	Normal	Negative iron balance	Iron-deficient erythropoiesis	Iron deficiency anemia
Iron stores				
Erythron iron				
Marrow iron stores	1–3+	0–1+	0	0
Serum ferritin (µg/L)	50–200	<20	<15	<15
TIBC (µg/dL)	300–360	>360	>380	>400
SI (µGg/dL)	50–150	NL	<50	<30
Saturation (%)	30–20	NL	<20	<10
Marrow sideroblasts (%)	40–60	NL	<10	<10
RBC protoporphyrin (µg/dL)	30–50	NL	>100	>200
RBC morphology	NL	NL	NL	Microcytic/hypochromic

2. Laboratory studies in the evolution of iron deficiency.

Measurements of marrow iron stores, serum ferritin, and total iron-binding capacity (TIBC) are sensitive to early iron-store depletion. Iron-deficient erythropoiesis is recognized from additional abnormalities in the serum iron (SI), percent transferrin saturation, pattern of marrow sideroblasts, and RBC protoporphyrin level. Patients with iron-deficiency anemia demonstrate all the same abnormalities plus hypochromic microcytic anemia. (Based on RS Hillman, CA Finch: The Red Cell Manual, 7th edn. Philadelphia, FA Davis and Co, 1996.)

OSCE 20.

1. What is autologous blood transfusion?
2. What is intraoperative cell salvage (IOCS)?
3. What are HBOCs?

Ans.

1. *Autologous blood transfusion:*
   - Pregnant patients who are at greater risk for obstetric hemorrhage are identified and blood is extracted from them and stored for preoperative autologous blood donation. It must be borne-in-mind that the patient should have a hemoglobin level of more than 11 g/dL.

- Its use is limited in pregnant patients due to risk of amniotic fluid embolism in case of Rh(D)-negative female.
- Since more than one unit of blood cannot be donated by an obstetric patient, its usefulness in severe acute hemorrhage is debatable. It may lead to anemia as well and does not completely eradicate the transfusion risk and hence is not recommended during pregnancy.

2. *Intraoperative cell salvage (IOCS) in obstetrics:* The lost blood from the patient is sucked into a reservoir, mixed with anticoagulant suction apparatus, stored in a reservoir, washed, and then transfused back. It should be performed only in centers with clinical expertise and suitable infrastructure as well as subjected to regular audit and monitoring.
3. Artificially modified hemoglobin is known as hemoglobin-based oxygen carriers. They have reached the stage of phase 2 clinical trials and are still investigational.

CHAPTER 11

Hypertensive Disorders in Pregnancy

Charmila Ayyavoo

OSCE 1.

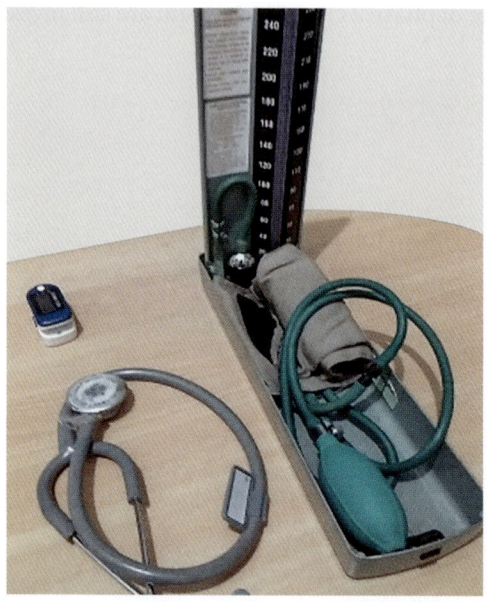

1. Identify the instrument.
2. What is the cut-off blood pressure for diagnosing HDP?
3. What is masked hypertension?
4. Write 2 main indications for home-based monitoring.

Ans.

1. BP apparatus
2. 140/90 mm Hg
3. Hypertension elevated at home and not in the clinic.
4. Chronic hypertension, masked hypertension.

Reference

1. Brown MA, Magee LA, Kenny LC, Karumanchi SA, McCarthy FP, Saito S, Hall DR, Warren CE, Adoyi G, Ishaku S. Hypertensive disorders of pregnancy: ISSHP classification, diagnosis, and management recommendations for international practice. Hypertension. 2018;72(1):24-43.

OSCE 2.

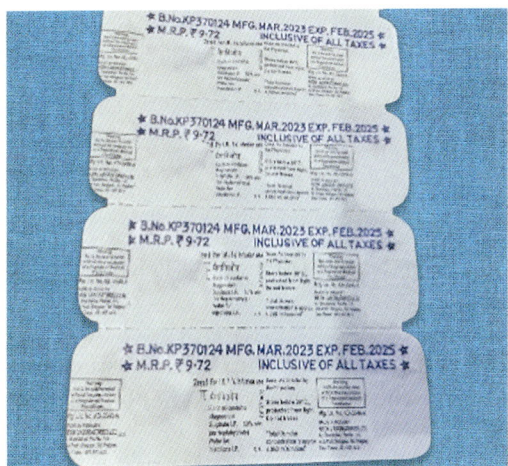

1. Enumerate two indications in pregnancy.
2. Enumerate three clinical systems to be monitored during its administration.

Ans.

1. Eclampsia, neuroprotection for preterm baby.
2. Patellar reflex, respiratory rate, urine output.

OSCE 3.

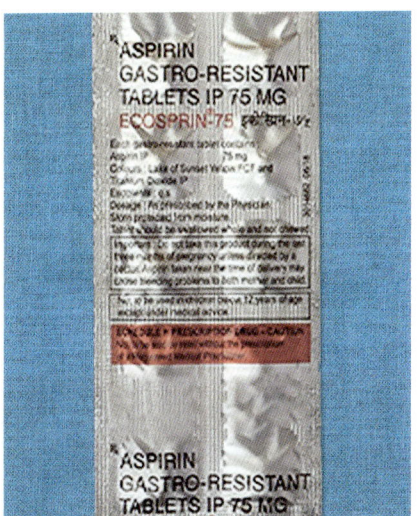

1. Enumerate one use of the above drug.
2. At what gestation should it be started?
3. When should it be stopped?
4. What is the ideal time of the day to take this drug?
5. Name the trial which studied 150 mg dose versus placebo.

Ans.

1. For prevention of pre-eclampsia.
2. Started earlier than 12 weeks.
3. Stopped 2 days before delivery.
4. Given at night.
5. ASPRE trial.

Reference

1. FOGSI-GESTOSIS-ICOG Hypertensive Disorders in Pregnancy (HDP) Good Clinical Practice Recommendations, 2019.

OSCE 4. A 19-year Primigravida, comes to the OPD at 32 weeks of pregnancy for a regular antenatal check-up. The nurse checks and says that her blood pressure is 150/100 mm Hg.
1. What will you do first?
2. What test you will do in the OPD after confirming HDP?
3. Mention two investigations to be done?
4. What is the investigation for the fetus?

Ans.

1. Keep her in bed rest and check BP after 4 hours.
2. Check for proteinuria.
3. Platelet count, peripheral smear, renal function test, liver function test.
4. Obstetric ultrasound for fetal growth restriction and doppler study.

Reference

1. Gabbe S, Niebyl JR, Simpson JL, Jauniaux ER, Driscoll DA, Berghella V, Landon MB, Galan HL, Grobman WA. Obstetrics: Normal and Problem Pregnancies: 1st South Asia Edn-E Book. Elsevier India; 2017.

OSCE 5.

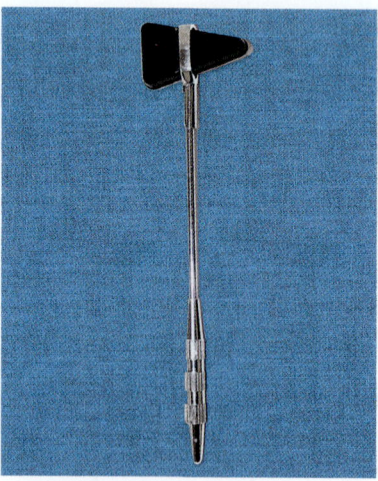

Chapter 11: Hypertensive Disorders in Pregnancy

1. Identify the instrument.
2. What is the indication for its use in HDP?
3. If knee jerk is present, what is the inference?
4. If absent knee jerk, what should be done?
5. Where should it be kept, ideally?

Ans.

1. Knee hammer.
2. Monitoring of magnesium sulphate toxicity when used in eclampsia.
3. The next dose of magnesium sulphate can be given safely.
4. Magnesium sulphate has increased to toxic levels. The next dose should be deferred.
5. A knee hammer should be a part of the eclampsia box.

OSCE 6. A 25-year Primigravida has come to OPD with a history of 34 weeks of pregnancy with upper abdominal pain. Her blood pressure is 150/100 mm Hg. The urine dipstick test shows 2+ proteinuria.
1. What are the investigations to be done for the mother?
2. What are the fetal wellbeing tests?
3. When should a coagulation profile be sent?
4. Enumerate the imminent signs and symptoms of pre-eclampsia.

Ans.

1. Renal function test, liver function test, platelet count.
2. Obstetric ultrasound, nonstress test, Doppler studies, if FGR
3. In case of thrombocytopenia
4. Altered mental status, blindness, stroke, clonus, severe headache, persistent visual scotomata, upper abdomen pain.

Reference

1. Magee LA, Brown MA, Hall DR, Gupte S, Hennessy A, Karumanchi SA, Kenny LC, McCarthy F, Myers J, Poon LC, Rana S. The 2021 International Society for the Study of Hypertension in Pregnancy classification, diagnosis and management recommendations for international practice. Pregnancy Hypertension. 2022;27:148-69.

OSCE 7.

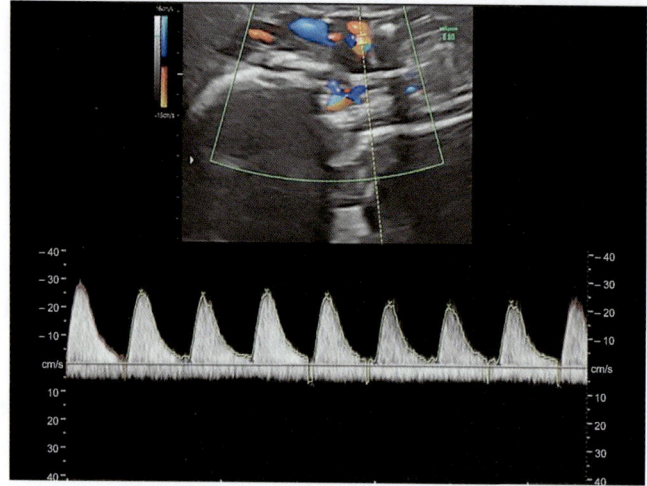

1. What is the investigation?
2. Name two indications for the above test in hypertensive disorders in pregnancy (HDP)?
3. On what changes does frequency of this test depend?
4. What are the indications of CTG testing?

Ans.

1. Umbilical artery Doppler study.
2. Pre-eclampsia or fetal growth restriction.
3. Frequency depends on the degree of umbilical artery resistance.
4. If absent or reversed flow on umbilical artery, CTG needs to be done when pregnancy prolongation is desired because of preterm status.

Reference

1. Magee LA, Brown MA, Hall DR, Gupte S, Hennessy A, Karumanchi SA, Kenny LC, McCarthy F, Myers J, Poon LC, Rana S. The 2021 International Society for the Study of Hypertension in Pregnancy: classification, diagnosis and management recommendations for international practice. Pregnancy Hypertension. 2022;27:148-69.

OSCE 8.

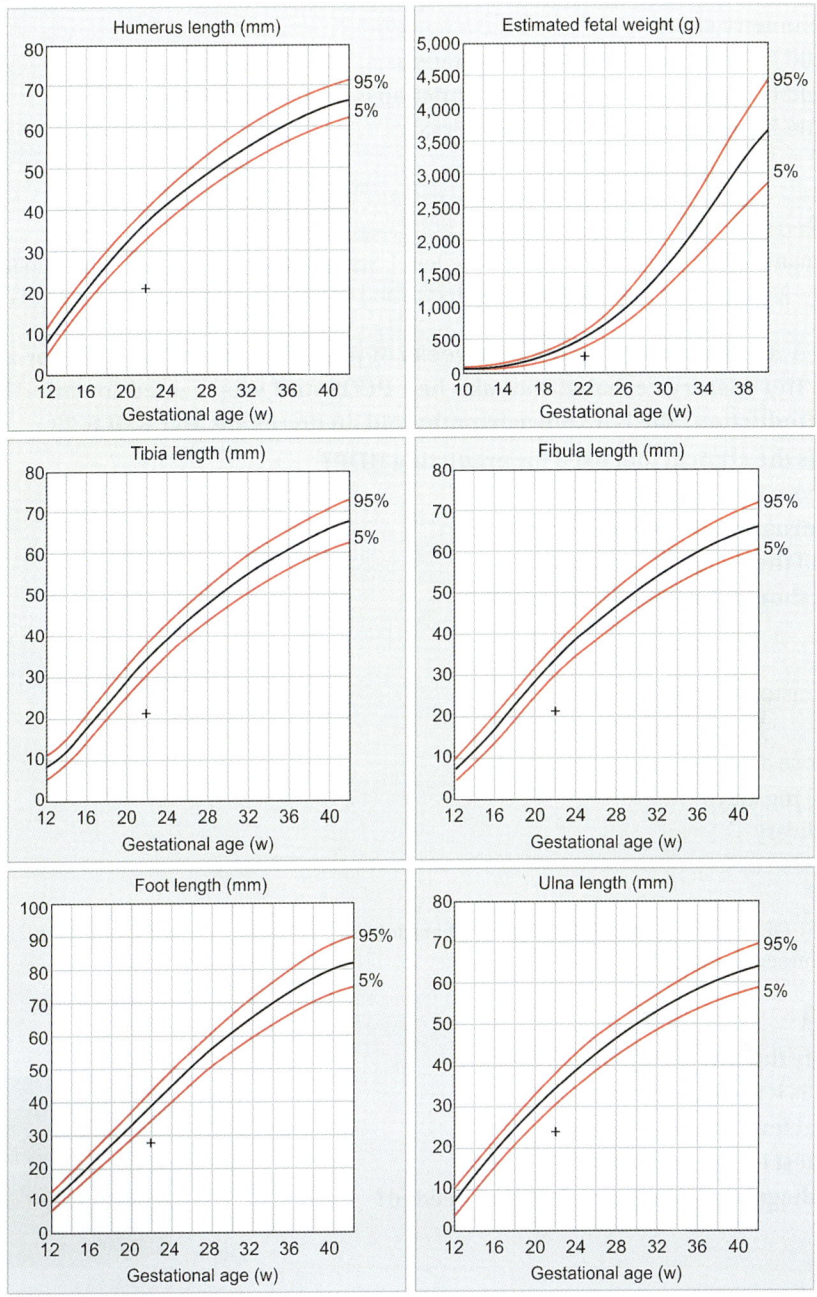

1. Name the investigation.
2. When should it be done in HDP?
3. On what basis it should be repeated?
4. How often it should be repeated?
5. Can delivery of the baby in HDP be based on fetal biometry charts?

Ans.

1. Fetal biometry chart
2. It should be done from 26 weeks of gestation.
3. It should be repeated if fetal growth restriction is diagnosed.
4. It should be repeated at 2–3 weekly intervals.
5. No

Reference

1. Lausman A, McCarthy FP, Walker M, Kingdom J. Screening, diagnosis, and management of intrauterine growth restriction. Journal of Obstetrics and Gynaecology Canada. 2012;34(1):17-28.

OSCE 9. A 30-year Primigravida at 6 weeks of pregnancy comes to OPD for antenatal checkup. Her history revealed that she had PCOS and was treated for infertility with ovulation induction. She is a known hypothyroid on thyroxine. Her BMI is 23.

1. What is the clinical tool used for predicting HDP?
2. The score for this patient is?
3. What drug should she be started on?
4. Dose of the drug?
5. When should the drug be stopped?

Ans.

1. HDP Gestosis score
2. Three
3. Low dose aspirin
4. 75–150 mg/day
5. Till delivery

Reference

1. FOGSI-GESTOSIS-ICOG Hypertensive Disorders in Pregnancy (HDP) Good Clinical Practice Recommendations, 2019.

OSCE 10.

1. Identify the test.
2. When is it measured?
3. At what level it is significant in HDP?
4. What test is more specific?
5. Once diagnosed, is repeated testing needed?

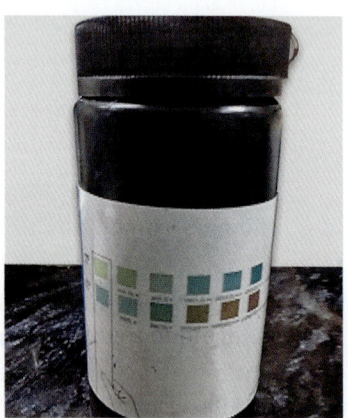

Ans.

1. Urine dipstick test
2. If there is increased blood pressure in the pregnant patient
3. ≥2+
4. Urine protein creatinine ratio
5. No need for repeat testing once proteinuria is confirmed.

Chapter 11: Hypertensive Disorders in Pregnancy

Reference
1. Magee LA, Brown MA, Hall DR, Gupte S, Hennessy A, Karumanchi SA, Kenny LC, McCarthy F, Myers J, Poon LC, Rana S. The 2021 International Society for the Study of Hypertension in Pregnancy: classification, diagnosis and management recommendations for international practice. Pregnancy hypertension. 2022;27:148-69.

OSCE 11. A 26 years Primipara is diagnosed to have severe features of pre-eclampsia at 32 weeks of gestation. She has been delivered and is in the postpartum period.
1. What is the target diastolic BP in the postpartum period?
2. BP should be monitored in the postpartum period for how many days?
3. Can NSAIDs be given for pain relief?
4. Can she breastfeed?
5. What risks should she be counselled for?

Ans.
1. 85 mm Hg
2. BP should be monitored at least once on days 3–7 postpartum.
3. If no other drug is effective for pain relief and she has no acute kidney injury, NSAIDs can be given.
4. Yes
5. She should be counseled for risks of gestational hypertension and pre-eclampsia in future pregnancies.

Reference
1. Magee LA, Brown MA, Hall DR, Gupte S, Hennessy A, Karumanchi SA, Kenny LC, McCarthy F, Myers J, Poon LC, Rana S. The 2021 International Society for the Study of Hypertension in Pregnancy: classification, diagnosis and management recommendations for international practice. Pregnancy hypertension. 2022;27:148-69.

OSCE 12. A 20-year Primipara at 32 weeks of pregnancy came with complaints of upper abdominal pain and nausea. She looked ill and on examination, her blood pressure was 150/100 mm Hg. She had 1+ proteinuria. Her blood was sent for investigations.

LABORATORY REPORT		Reference Value
Urea	: 27	10–45 mg/dL
Creatinine	: 0.6	0.5–1.4 mg/dL
LIVER FUNCTION TEST:		
Total bilirubin	: 0.3	0.2–1.2 mg/dL
Direct bilirubin	: 0.2	0.1–0.6 mg/dL
Indirect bilirubin	: 0.1	0.3–0.9 mg/dL
SGOT	: 19	Up to 37 U/L
SGPT	: 12	Up to 40 U/L
ALP	: 50	Up to 240 U/L
Total protein	: 4.8	6.0–8.0 g/dL
Albumin	: 2.5	3.5–5.0 g/dL
Globulin	: 2.3	1.5–3.5 g/dL
A/G ratio	: 1.0	0.9–1.4 g/dL

...............End of the Report ....

1. What are the tests advised to rule out severe pre-eclampsia?
2. What are the diagnostic features of HELLP syndrome?
3. What is the definitive treatment?

Ans.

1. Complete blood count, Renal function test, liver function test.
2. Hemolytic anemia, low platelet count, elevated liver enzymes.
3. Delivery of the baby.

Reference

1. Magee LA, Brown MA, Hall DR, Gupte S, Hennessy A, Karumanchi SA, Kenny LC, McCarthy F, Myers J, Poon LC, Rana S. The 2021 International Society for the Study of Hypertension in Pregnancy: classification, diagnosis and management recommendations for international practice. Pregnancy hypertension. 2022;27:148-69.

OSCE 13.

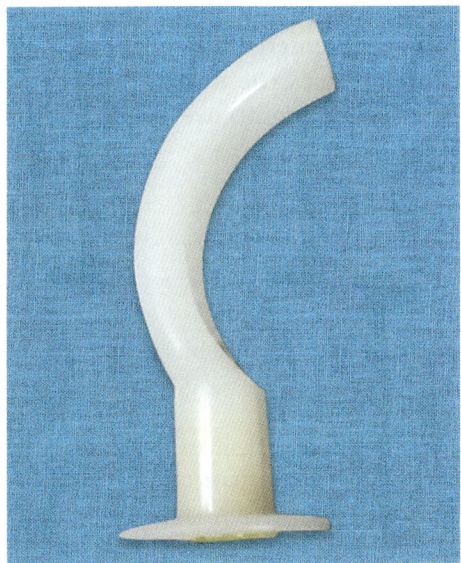

1. Identify the instrument?
2. Enumerate two indications for its use?
3. What is its benefit?
4. What else is done for the patient?

Ans.

1. Guedel airway (Mouth gag)
2. Convulsions—eclampsia, protects airway in poor GCS (Glasgow coma score) patients.
3. To prevent injuries in the mouth, protects the airway.
4. Side railbed left lateral position, injection magnesium sulphate, blood pressure monitoring and antihypertensives.

OSCE 14.

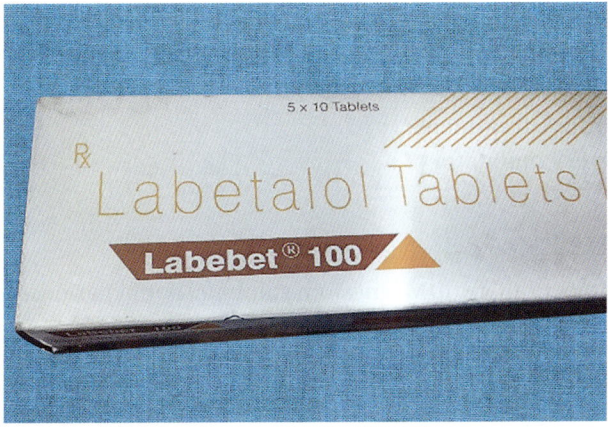

1. What is the use of the drug?
2. What is the mode of action?
3. What is the preferred route in an emergency?
4. What is the maximum dose which can be given?
5. Enumerate three contraindications for its use?

Ans.

1. Antihypertensive
2. Selective beta-1 blocker
3. Intravenous route
4. 2,400 mg/day
5. Bradycardia, congestive cardiac failure, bronchial asthma

Reference

1. Magee LA, Brown MA, Hall DR, Gupte S, Hennessy A, Karumanchi SA, Kenny LC, McCarthy F, Myers J, Poon LC, Rana S. The 2021 International Society for the Study of Hypertension in Pregnancy: classification, diagnosis and management recommendations for international practice. Pregnancy hypertension. 2022;27:148-69.

OSCE 15.

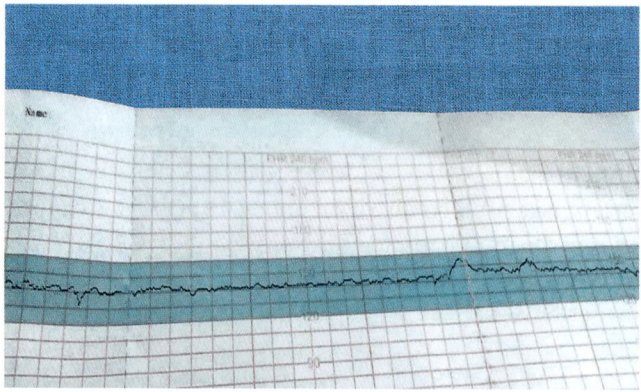

1. What is the test?
2. If it shows acute bradycardia during an eclamptic convulsion, what is the immediate treatment?
3. What is the definitive treatment?
4. Is cesarean delivery mandatory?

Ans.

1. Nonstress test
2. Resuscitation of the mother, inj. Magnesium sulphate, antihypertensives
3. Delivery of the baby
4. No

Chapter 11: Hypertensive Disorders in Pregnancy

OSCE 16. A 35-year multigravida at 37 weeks of pregnancy has come to casualty with giddiness, severe headache and reduced fetal movements. The casualty nurse checks her vital parameters, takes blood for investigations, and starts the patient on IV fluids. The patient's blood pressure is 160/110 mm Hg and she develops dyspnea after the IV fluids were started.
1. What is the complication?
2. How will you diagnose?
3. How will you avoid the complication?
4. What is the immediate treatment?
5. Any investigation to aid in the diagnosis?

Ans.
1. Pulmonary edema
2. Auscultation for basal crepitations
3. Only monitored fluid therapy in severe HDP
4. Inj. Lasix
5. Lung ultrasound

Reference
1. Magee LA, Brown MA, Hall DR, Gupte S, Hennessy A, Karumanchi SA, Kenny LC, McCarthy F, Myers J, Poon LC, Rana S. The 2021 International Society for the Study of Hypertension in Pregnancy: classification, diagnosis and management recommendations for international practice. Pregnancy hypertension. 2022;27:148-69.

OSCE 17. A second gravida with a previous normal delivery had developed severe HDP in this pregnancy. She was induced at 37 weeks and delivered vaginally. She developed PPH.
1. What uterotonic cannot be given?
2. What uterotonics can be given?
3. Dose of oxytocin for active management of third stage of labor in HDP.
4. First line treatment of PPH in HDP patients?
5. Second line uterotonic in PPH in HDP patients?

Ans.
1. Ergometrine or ergometrine with oxytocin combination.
2. Oxytocin.
3. Inj Oxytocin 10 units IM
4. Inj Oxytocin infusion.
5. Inj Carboprost or Rectal misoprostol.

Reference
1. Intrapartum care; NICE guideline [NG235] Published: 29 September 2023.

OSCE 18.

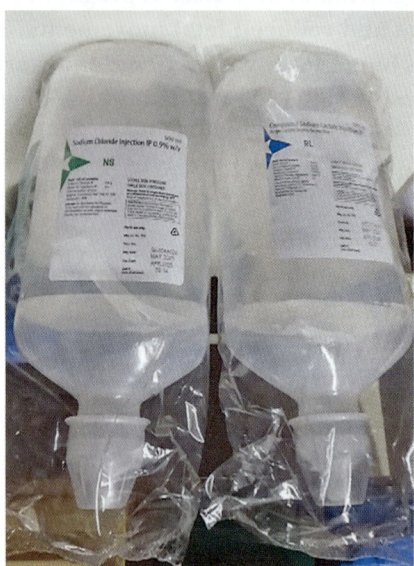

1. Which fluid should be ideally administered in a patient in labor with pre-eclampsia?
2. How much should be infused in one hour?
3. What happens if she is not given adequate hydration?
4. What happens if she is given more fluids without monitoring?
5. When should she receive preloading with fluids?

Ans.

1. Crystalloids
2. 80–100 mL/hour
3. Risk of acute kidney injury
4. Risk of pulmonary edema
5. Before hydralazine therapy.

Reference
1. Dennis AT, Castro JM. Hypertension and haemodynamics in pregnant women: is a unified theory for pre-eclampsia possible? Anaesthesia. 2014;69(11):1183-9.

OSCE 19. A 21-year Primigravida at 30 weeks pregnancy arrives with severe dyspnea of 5 hours duration. Her BP is 160/110 mm Hg, heart rate is 106 beats/minute, respiratory rate is 40/minute and labored, oxygen saturation is 90%. Her urine protein-to-creatinine ratio is 0.6. Her serum alanine transaminase is 84 IU/L and aspartate transaminase is 90 IU/L.

1. What is the most likely diagnosis?
2. What is the next immediate step?
3. What are your priority lab tests?
4. What is your management plan?

Ans.
1. Pre-eclampsia with severe features (pulmonary edema and severe hypertension).
2. Improving oxygenation is the priority.
3. Complete blood count with platelet count, renal function test.
4. Stabilize maternal status.

OSCE 20. On postpartum day 1, a 29-year primipara develops headache and blurry vision. Her blood pressure is 150/100 mm Hg and urine protein creatinine ratio is 0.5. Her neurological examination is normal.
1. What is the probable diagnosis?
2. What is the investigation needed to confirm the diagnosis?
3. Will she need antihypertensive?
4. Will mannitol help?
5. Can giving eye drops help?

Ans.
1. Posterior reversible encephalopathy syndrome (PRES)
2. MRI of the brain
3. Yes
4. Only if there is associated cerebral edema.
5. It will help if there is associated conjunctivitis.

CHAPTER 12

Heart Disease in Pregnancy

Deepa Lokwani Masand

OSCE 1. Mrs ABC, a 30-year lady presented in casualty with shortness of breath in the second trimester of pregnancy.
1. Enumerate two symptoms and two signs suggestive of cardiac disease in pregnancy.
2. Name three diagnostic modalities to confirm heart disease.

Ans.

1. Following are the diagnostic features of cardiac disease during pregnancy:
   Symptoms:
   - Progressive breathlessness (dyspnea or orthopnea)
   - Paroxysmal nocturnal dyspnea (only symptom which is diagnostic)
   - Chest pain and hemoptysis.

   Signs:
   - Cyanosis, clubbing of fingers
   - Persistent neck vein distension, thrill on palpation
   - Pathologic murmur (diastolic murmur or pansystolic >3/6 murmur)

2. *Diagnostic Evaluation:*
   - *Stress test/cardiopulmonary exercise testing (CPET)* for cause of dyspnea.
   - ECG (electrocardiography normal/Holter)
   - *Doppler transthoracic echocardiography* for the evaluation of structural, functional, and hemodynamic abnormalities during pregnancy.
   - *Echocardiography* is recommended for any pregnant patient with unexplained or new cardiovascular signs or symptoms.
   - *MRI* is a preferred imaging modality for:
     - Congenital heart conditions
     - Assessment of the aorta in patients at risk for aortic dilatation and dissection (Gadolinium contrast should be avoided during pregnancy)
   - *Cardiovascular computed tomography (CCT)* to rule out pulmonary embolism and aortic dissection.
   - *Brain natriuretic peptide (BNP) and NT-proBNP are used for the diagnostic and prognostic* differentiation of symptoms between physiological changes of pregnancy and hemodynamic deterioration.

OSCE 2. Patient XYZ, a 21-year Primigravida at 30 weeks of gestation, came with difficulty in breathing.
1. Mention whether the following hemodynamic changes in normal pregnancy are increased/decreased:

Cardiac output	
Plasma volume	
Peripheral vascular resistance	
Heart rate	

2. What are the three critical periods for cardiac failure in obstetric cases?

Ans.

1. The hemodynamic changes during pregnancy are:
   - There is a rise in cardiac output of 30–50% above baseline.
   - The plasma volume by second trimester approaches 50% above normal.
   - There is a fall in peripheral vascular resistance.
   - The heart rate increases to about 20% above baseline.

   Normal cardiovascular changes during pregnancy:
   - Variable direction of change
   - Average change in blood volume ↑ +35%
   - Plasma volume ↑ +45%
   - Red blood cell volume ↑ +20%
   - Cardiac output ↑ +40%
   - Stroke volume ↑ +30%
   - Heart rate ↑ +15%
   - Femoral venous pressure ↑ +15 mm Hg
   - Total peripheral resistance ↓ –15%
   - Mean arterial blood pressure ↓ –15 mm Hg
   - Systolic blood pressure ↓ –0 to 15 mm Hg
   - Diastolic blood pressure ↓ –10 to 20 mm Hg
   - Central venous pressure ↔ No change

2. The three critical period for cardiac failure in obstetric patients are:
   a. 29–32 weeks (as blood volume is maximum)
   b. Intrapartum (during labor)
   c. Immediately postpartum.

OSCE 3.
1. Match the grades of functional classification of heart disease in pregnancy (NYHA) with symptoms:

Class 1	Less than ordinary physical activity precipitates symptoms, patient comfortable at rest
Class 2	Discomfort with any physical activity symptoms present even at rest
Class 3	No limitations of physical activity
Class 4	Ordinary physical activity precipitates cardiovascular symptoms patient comfortable at rest

2. Enumerate two other predictors of adverse cardiac events during pregnancy?

Ans.

1. NYHA Functional classification system for cardiac disease in pregnancy.

NYHA classification system.	
Class I	No limitations of physical activity; ordinary physical activity does not precipitate cardiovascular symptoms such as dyspnea, angina, fatigue, or palpitations
Class II	Slight limitation of physical activity; ordinary physical activity precipitates cardiovascular symptoms; patients comfortable at rest
Class III	Activity limited; less than ordinary physical activity precipitates symptoms; patients comfortable at rest
Class IV	Discomfort with any physical activity; symptoms are present at rest

(NYHA: New York Heart Association)

2. Predictors of adverse cardiac events during pregnancy can be estimated by following parameters:

   N: New York Heart Association (NYHA) class >2
   O: Obstructive lesions of the left heart (Mitral valve or aortic valve area <1 cm^2)
   P: Prior cardiac event before pregnancy—Heart failure, arrhythmia, transient ischemic attack, stroke
   E: Ejection fraction <40%
   The risk of cardiac complications is 3%, 30% and 60% when none, one or more than one of these complications are present.

OSCE 4. Mrs XY, a 34-year lady with heart disease came to obstetric OPD for pregnancy counseling.

1. Name the best available risk assessment model for estimating cardiovascular risk in pregnant female with cardiac disease (congenital and acquired heart disease). How many risk categories are therein modified?
2. Enumerate three predictors used in CARPREG II and ZAHARA risk model.

Ans.

1. It is recommended to perform risk assessment in all women with cardiac diseases of childbearing age before and after conception, using the *Modified WHO classification for risk stratification of* maternal risk.

Risk category	Associated conditions
WHO 1—Risk no higher than general population	Uncomplicated, small, or mild: • Pulmonary stenosis • Ventricular septal defect • Patent ductus arteriosus • Mitral valve prolapse with no more than trivial mitral regurgitation

Contd…

Contd...

Risk category	Associated conditions
	Successfully repaired simple lesions: • Ostium secundum atrial septal defect • Ventricular septal defect • Patent ductus arteriosus • Total anomalous pulmonary venous drainage • Isolated ventricular extrasystoles and atrial ectopic beats
WHO 2—Small increase in risk of maternal mortality and morbidity	*If otherwise uncomplicated:* • Unoperated atrial septal defect • Repaired Fallot tetralogy • Most arrhythmias
WHO 2 or 3—depends on individual case	• Mild left ventricular impairment • Hypertrophic cardiomyopathy • Native or tissue valvular heart disease not considered WHO 4 • Marfan syndrome without aortic dilation • Heart transplantation
WHO 3—Significantly increased risk of maternal mortality or expert cardiac and obstetrical care required	• Mechanical valve • Systemic right ventricle—congenitally corrected transposition, simple transposition post-Mustard or -Senning repair • Post-Fontan operation • Cyanotic heart disease • Other complex congenital heart disease
WHO 4—Very high risk of maternal mortality or severe morbidity; pregnancy contra-indicated and termination discussed	• Pulmonary arterial hypertension • Severe systemic ventricular dysfunction (NYHA III-IV or LVEF <30%) • Previous peripartum cardiomyopathy with any residual impairment of left ventricular function • Severe left heart obstruction • Marfan syndrome with aorta dilated >40 mm

Modified from Thorne, 2006.

2.

The cardiac disease in pregnancy (CARPREG II) modified risk score.	
Predictor	**Points**
Prior cardiac events or arrhythmias	3
Baseline New York Heart Association functional class II or III heart failure or cyanosis	3
Mechanical valve	3
Ventricular systolic dysfunction	2
High-risk left-sided valve disease or left ventricular outflow obstruction	2
Pulmonary hypertension	2
Coronary artery disease	2

Contd...

Contd...

Predictor	Points
High-risk aortopathy	2
No prior cardiac intervention	1
Late pregnancy assessment	1

Total points	Risk
0–1	5%
2	10%
3	15%
4	22%
>4	41%

The Pregnancy in women with a congenital heart defect (ZAHARA) risk score.

Predictor	Points
History of arrhythmias	1.5
Cardiac medication before pregnancy	1.5
New York Heart Association functional class before pregnancy ≥II	0.75
left heart obstruction (peak gradient >30 mm Hg or aortic valve area <1.0 cm²)	2.5
Systemic aortic valve regurgitation (moderate or severe)	0.75
Mechanical heart prosthesis	4.25
Cyanotic heart disease (corrected or uncorrected)	1.0

Total points	Risk
0–0.5	2.9%
0.51–1.50	7.5%
1.51–2.50	17.5%
2.51–3.50	43.1%
>3.50	70.0%

OSCE 5. Mrs a 27-year Primigravida who is a known case of VSD (ventricular septal defect) presented to antenatal clinic at 7 weeks of pregnancy.
1. Name two antenatal Screening tests done for congenital heart disease in fetus.
2. Enumerate three maternal and three fetal complications in women with cardiac disease in pregnancy.

Ans.
1. a. Measurement of *nuchal fold thickness around the 12th week of pregnancy* to screen for chromosome abnormalities also screens for fetal congenital heart disease.
      For major congenital heart disease, *a 12-week ultrasound has a sensitivity and specificity of 85 and 99%, respectively.*

The incidence of congenital heart disease with normal nuchal fold thickness is about 1/1,000.

b. All women with congenital heart disease should be offered fetal echocardiography in the 19th–22nd weeks of pregnancy, with 45% of all congenital cardiac malformations identified.

2. Maternal and fetal complications of cardiac disease in pregnancy

Maternal:
- Congestive cardiac failure
- Pulmonary edema
- Pulmonary embolism
- Premature labor
- Arrythmias

Fetal:
- Increase chances of miscarriage
- Prematurity
- Fetal growth restriction
- Increase chances of fetal congenital malformations
- Fetal death.

OSCE 6. Mrs a 28-year Primigravida, known case of PAH (Pulmonary Arterial Hypertension) came to OPD after 8 weeks of pregnancy.
1. **Enumerate four indications of advising MTP in women with cardiac disease.**
2. **Mention the preferred method of MTP in such cases.**

Ans.
1. Conditions where pregnancy is contraindicated or where termination is warranted if pregnancy is diagnosed are:
   - Pulmonary arterial hypertension (Primary or Secondary)
   - Severe mitral stenosis, severe symptomatic aortic stenosis
   - Severe systemic ventricular dysfunction (LVEF <30%, NYHA III–IV)
   - Marfan syndrome with aorta dilated >45 mm.
   - Aortic dilatation >50 mm in aortic disease associated with bicuspid aortic valve.
   - Severe coarctation of aorta
   - Previous peripartum cardiomyopathy with any residual impairment
2. Surgical approach the preferred method.
   However, both medical and surgical methods are effective with similar rates of major complications.
   The greater need for unanticipated operative evacuation favors the surgical approach. High-risk patients should be managed with a multidisciplinary team.

OSCE 7. Mrs XY, a 26-year-old, married lady who is a known case of cardiac disease has come for contraceptive advice in a family planning clinic.
1. **What is the preferred choice of contraception in a female with heart disease?**

2. **Who are the candidates for permanent sterilization in females with heart disease?**

Ans.

1. Choice of contraceptive method depends on the maternal cardiac status, associated risk factors, and family completion.

   Various options available are:
   - Barrier method (safest but alone has high failure rate)
   - Combination of Progesterone only pills + Barrier method best method
   - Intrauterine contraceptive devices (LNG IUCD preferred over copper)
   - LARC (IUCD, Implants)

2. Sterilization/tubal ligation (especially with complicated cardiac disease) is advised in:
   - Women who have completed their family.
   - Women with complicated heart disease (severe pulmonary hypertension, left ventricular dysfunction, cardiomyopathy, NYHA III and NYHA IV heart failure may be considered for permanent method of contraception.)

OSCE 8.

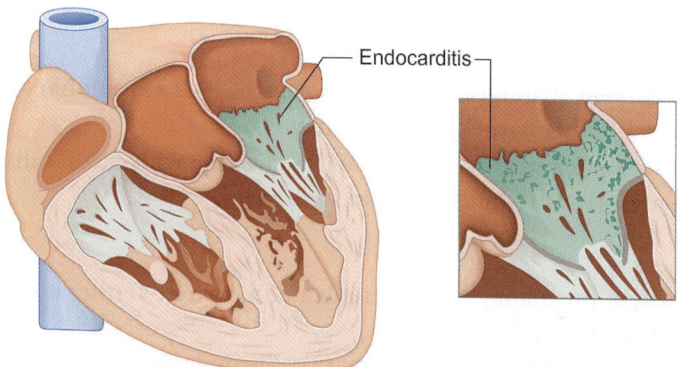

1. Identify the pathology.
2. Give two indications of using antibiotic prophylaxis for infective endocarditis (IE) in pregnancy with heart disease.
3. What is single dose antibiotic prophylaxis for IE in high risk pregnant female?

Ans.

1. Infective endocarditis (IE)
2. Routine antibiotic prophylaxis against infective endocarditis (IE) is not required for childbirth.

   It is recommended that IE prophylaxis may be given during labor in the following subgroups of patients who carry substantially high risk for mortality from IE:
   - Prosthetic cardiac valve
   - Previous IE
   - Unrepaired congenital heart disease (including palliative shunts and conduits)
   - First 6 months after completely repaired congenital heart defect with prosthetic device

- Repaired congenital heart disease with residual defects.
- Cardiac transplantation recipients who develop cardiac valvulopathy.

3. *Standard (Intravenous):* Either ampicillin 2 gm or cefazolin or ceftriaxone 1 gm

   Penicillin allergic (IV): Cefazoline or ceftriaxone 1 gm or clindamycin 600 mg

   Oral: amoxicillin 2 gm.

   If *Enterococcus* infection is of concern, intravenous vancomycin is also given.

OSCE 9. Patient XYZ, a 21 year, G2P0A1, known case of heart disease, came with pre-term labor pains at 30 weeks of gestation with Fetal growth restriction (FGR)

1. Name the safest tocolytic in pregnancy with heart disease.
2. Why are beta agonist tocolytics contraindicated in pregnant female with heart disease, enumerate two side effects?
3. Name two parameters to determine growth in FGR fetus.
4. Can we give corticosteroids for fetal lung maturity in pregnancy with heart disease?

Ans.

1. Safest tocolytic in pregnancy with heart disease is Atosiban (oxytocin antagonist).
2. Beta agonist is contraindicated in cardiac arrythmias, valvular disease and cardiac ischemia because of their *sympathomimetic* side effects such as *tachycardia, palpitation and hypotension* that can be detrimental in patients with cardiac disease.
3. Assessing fetal well-being in the context of fetal growth restriction, should be determined by *umbilical artery* and *ductus venosus* blood flow patterns in Ultrasound.

   The aim is to determine the optimal time for delivery, balancing fetal and neonatal risks.

   The chance of disability-free survival increases by 2% per day between 24 and 28 weeks, and 1% per day there after until 32 weeks.
4. Yes, Betamethasone or dexamethasone are given to enhance fetal lung maturity and can be given safely in recommended doses once without any significant adverse clinical effect on maternal cardiac disease. Maternal cardiac disease itself should not preclude steroids treatment in these patients.

OSCE 10. Mrs X, a 32-year lady, married for 10 years, G2P1+0+0+1, last childbirth 7 years ago, full-term normal vaginal delivery, known case of Rheumatic heart disease, undergone double valve replacement 6 months back, has presented in OPD with missed period and positive pregnancy test.

1. What are the choices of Anticoagulants during pregnancy, match the following:

	Weeks of gestation		Choice of anticoagulants
1.	6–12 weeks	A.	Vitamin K antagonist
2.	12–36 weeks	B.	UFH
3.	36 weeks to onset of labor	C.	LMWH
4.	Post partum	D.	LMWH/UFH

2. How do we monitor efficacy of different anticoagulants and their antidote?

Ans.

1. i (D), ii (A), iii (B), iv (C)
2.

	Anticoagulant	Monitored by	Antidote
1.	Warfarin	PT(INR)	Vit K
2.	LMWH	Anti Xa	Protamine
3.	UFH	aPTT	Protamine

OSCE 11.

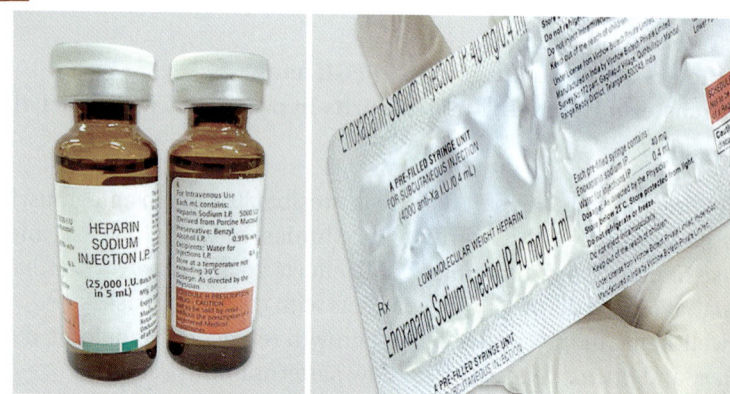

1. Identify the picture and tell three differences between LMWH and UFH.
2. Enumerate two advantages of using Warfarin during pregnancy.

Ans.

1.

Characteristics	Unfractioned heparin (UFH)	Low molecular weight heparin (LMWH)
Molecular weight	12,000–15,000 (High)	4,000–6,000 (Low)
Mechanism of action	Binds ATPIII	Binds ATPIII
Side effects	Thrombocytopenia, Osteoporosis	Lesser side effects
Half-life (hours)	1 (short)	4 (Longer)
Laboratory monitoring	APTT	Anti factor Xa
Reversal	Protamine sulfate	Protamine sulfate
Placental transfer	None	None

2. *Warfarin*
   - Low cost
   - Oral preparation
   - Better thrombolytic effect in prosthetic heart valves
   - Less side effects.

OSCE 12. Patient ABC, a 30-year Primigravida, known case of rheumatic heart disease has presented in OPD at 10 weeks of pregnancy with morning sickness.
1. What is the most common cause of RHD in developing countries like India?
2. Enumerate three common complications during pregnancy in these patients?
3. Name two characteristic clinical diagnostic signs of same?

Ans.
1. Mitral stenosis is the most common cause of cardiac disease due to rheumatic heart disease during pregnancy in India.
2. Complications associated with mitral stenosis:
   - Cardiac failure
   - Pulmonary edema
   - Atrial fibrillation
   - Thromboembolic complications
   - Severe PAH
3. Characteristic clinical diagnostic signs of mitral stenosis:
   - Diastolic thrill at cardiac apex
   - Loud S1 → HALLMARK of mitral stenosis
   - S2 → split with loud pulmonary component
   - Mitral opening snap
   - Mid diastolic murmur (rough and rumbling, low pitched)
   - Mitral stenosis with functional tricuspid regurgitation → Pansystolic murmur → ↑ with inspiration and ↓ with expiration (Carvallo's Sign)
   - Mitral stenosis with pulmonary regurgitation → Graham Steel murmur.

OSCE 13.

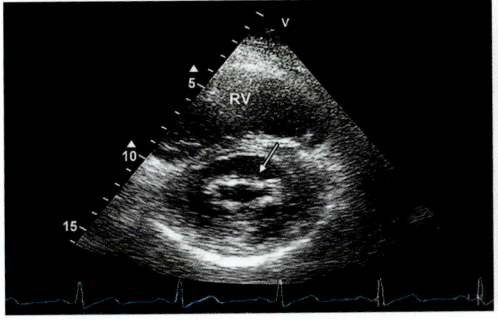
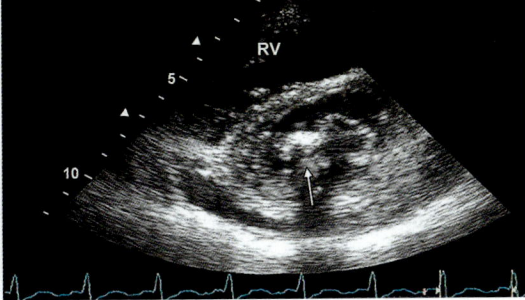

1. What is the normal mitral valve area?
2. What are the grades of severity for mitral stenosis?
3. What is the best time to operate mitral stenosis during pregnancy?
4. What is the preferred surgical procedure during pregnancy?

Ans.
1. The normal mitral valve area is 4–6 cm^2.

2. Stenosis is graded as mild MVA of >1.5 cm^2, moderate MVA of 1–1.5 cm^2 and severe MVA of <1 cm^2.
3. Second trimester (preferably 20–24 weeks of gestation) with adequate shielding of abdomen to avoid radiation risk to the fetus.
4. Percutaneous balloon mitral valvuloplasty (PBMV) is the preferred surgical procedure during pregnancy:
   - No role for prophylactic valvuloplasty in pregnancy.
   - Recommended over open mitral commissurotomy as maternal and fetal mortality is ≈35% with the latter.
   - Heavily calcified valves, severe associated regurgitation and left atrial thrombus are not suitable candidates for BMV.
   - Open heart surgery and valve replacement is indicated when valvotomy fails or valve is not suitable for valvotomy.

OSCE 14. A 35-year-old, postnatal lady gets admitted in emergency with complains of shortness of breath. She had full-term twin vaginal delivery 15 days back without any complications and was discharged from hospital in good condition. There was no significant past medical history.

On examination: Patient afebrile, BP: 130/80 mm Hg, RR: 28/min, O2: 85% on room air, bilateral basal crepitations present, ECG: Sinus tachycardia, 2D ECHO shows gross left ventricular dilatation, with poor contractility (LVEF: 35%).
1. What is clinical diagnosis and define the criteria for diagnosis.
2. Name two risk factors associated with the condition.
3. What is the role of anticoagulant in this condition?

Ans.

1. Peripartum cardiomyopathy
   Diagnostic criteria: This pregnancy-specific condition is defined as the development of cardiac failure.
   - Between the last month of pregnancy and five months postpartum
   - The absence of an identifiable cause
   - The absence of recognizable heart disease prior to the last month of pregnancy
   - Left ventricular systolic dysfunction and dilated left ventricle as per echocardiographic criteria.
2. Risk factors include:
   - Multiple pregnancy
   - Hypertension
   - Multiparity
   - Increased age
   - Afro-Caribbean race
   - Long-term tocolysis with beta-agonist.
3. Anticoagulation with LMWH is considered when the ejection fraction reaches 30–35% because of increased risk for left ventricular thrombi.

OSCE 15. Mrs ABC, a 28-year-old pregnant lady at 38 weeks of gestation, known case of heart disease is referred from peripheral center to tertiary care center for safe confinement.
1. What is the preferred mode of delivery for patients with heart disease?
2. What should be the timing of induction in these patients?
3. Mention two benefits of induction.
4. What is the best method of induction in patients with cardiac disease?

Ans.

1. Vaginal delivery is the preferred mode of delivery. Vaginal delivery is associated with less blood loss and lower risk of infection, venous thrombosis, and embolism, and should be advised for most women.
2. *Timing of delivery:* Induction of labor should be considered at 40 weeks of gestation in all women with cardiac disease. The timing of induction will depend on cardiac status, obstetric evaluation including cervical assessment, fetal well-being, and fetal lung maturity.
3. Induction of labor reduces risk of emergency cesarean section by 12% and the risk of stillbirth by 50% in women without heart disease, and the benefit is likely to be greater for women with heart disease who have higher rates of obstetric complications.
4. Labor induction:
   Mechanical methods such as a cervical ripening balloon might be preferable in patients where a drop in systemic vascular resistance would be detrimental.

   Artificial rupture of membranes and *Infusion of oxytocin* can be used safely in women with heart disease.

   Both misoprostol [25 mg, prostaglandin E1 (PGE1)] or dinoprostone [1–3 mg or slow-release formulation of 10 mg (PGE2)] through vaginal route can be used safely to induce labor in *mild cases only.*

OSCE 16.

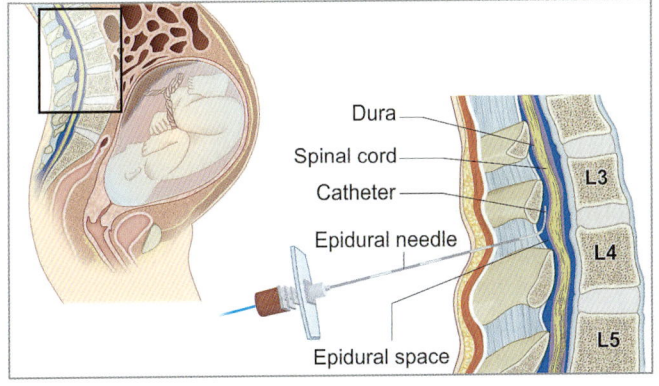

Section 1: Obstetrics

1. What is the role of analgesia in vaginal delivery of patients with heart disease?
2. What is the preferred analgesia and anesthesia for vaginal or cesarean delivery in patients with heart disease?
3. Name two conditions where General Anesthesia is preferred?

Ans.

1. Painful labor provokes catecholamine release which results in *tachycardia, hypertension and increased cardiac output* that can be detrimental for patients at risk.
   Effective labor analgesia results in greater cardiopulmonary and hemodynamic stability during labor.
2. Epidural analgesia (continuous) is preferable.
3. General anesthesia is preferred in those females with:
   - Intracardiac shunts in whom flow may be reversed.
   - Pulmonary artery hypertension
   - Aortic stenosis as ventricular output depends on adequate preload.
   Thus, in these conditions, narcotic analgesia or general anesthesia is preferred.

OSCE 17. A 23-year, primigravida at 38 weeks presented in emergency in active phase of labor. During systemic examination, diastolic murmur was present. She gave history of recurrent cold and cough with joint pains in her childhood and recently noted gradual onset of difficulty in breathing, especially on lying down.

1. Enumerate two special measures to be taken during labor.
2. Measures to prevent cardiac failure after delivery?
3. Which uterotonics should be avoided during management of third stage of labor?

Ans.

1. Team approach with an obstetrician, cardiologist, and anesthesiologist:
   - Semi recumbent position with lateral tilt of the patient
   - Intranasal O_2 if needed (5–6 L) per minute.
   - *For pain relief:* Epidural analgesia is preferred.
   - Careful monitoring of vitals (in between the contractions)
   - Cut short second stage of labor.
2. IV fluid restrictions (50–75 mL/hr)
   Diuretics (furosemide: 20–40 mg IV)
   Heart rate control in case of tachycardia with beta-blocking agents
3. Ergometrine and Prostaglandins are avoided.

OSCE 18. Mrs ABC, a 24-year Primigravida at 36 weeks of gestation is referred from a local center with shortness of breath and frothy expectorations with history of previous treatment for heart disease in childhood with the following picture of chest X-ray after abdominal shielding.

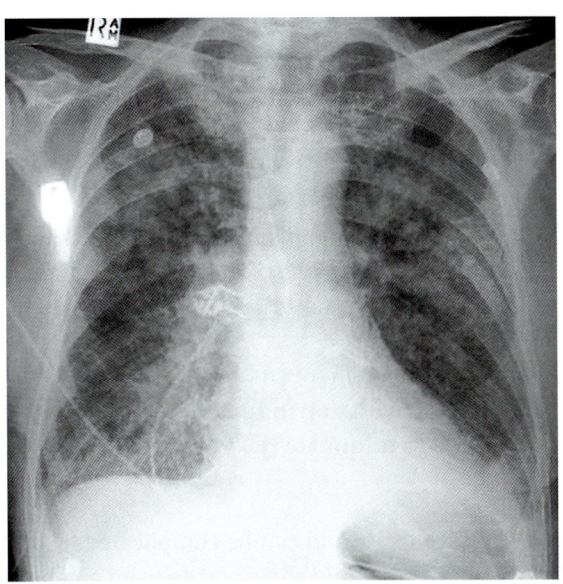

1. What are the diagnosis and precipitating causes?
2. Enumerate certain other causes of the condition.

Ans.

1. Pulmonary edema
   Precipitating factors: Cardiovascular changes during pregnancy:
   - Increase in blood volume, plasma volume, cardiac output and heart rate
   - When associated with hypertension, anemia, multiple pregnancy or intercurrent infection.
2. a. Cardiac disease
   b. Fluid overload
   c. Pre-eclampsia
   d. Pre-existing sepsis
   e. Pregnancy associated cardiac disease
   f. Administration of tocolytics

OSCE 19. A 27-year, Primigravida, known case of mitral valve replacement, on oral anticoagulant (OAC) presented in emergency room with labor pains.
1. What is the preferred mode of delivery for such patients?
2. What are four other indications of LSCS in patients with cardiac disease in pregnancy?

Ans.

1. *Cesarean section* is preferred mode of delivery if the patient is taking OAC to reduce the risk of fetal intracranial hemorrhage, even the fetus may remain anticoagulated for 10 days after discontinuation of OAC and may need to be given fresh frozen plasma as well as vitamin K.

2. Indications of LSCS in Heart Disease
   Obstetric Indications and Cardiac Indications:
   - Dilated aortic root >4 cm or aortic aneurysms
   - Acute severe congestive heart failure
   - Recent myocardial infection
   - Severe symptomatic aortic stenosis
   - Need for emergency valve replacement immediately after delivery
   - OAC administration within two weeks of delivery due to fetal risk for intracerebral hemorrhage because the fetal liver takes up to 2 weeks to metabolize warfarin.

OSCE 20. An infertile lady at 33 years, known case of RHD wants to have IVF treatment.
1. Enumerate two risks of giving ovulation induction for IVF treatment.
2. Mention three possible ways to minimize risks of assisted reproductive technique?

Ans.

1. a. Superovulation is pro-thrombotic and can be complicated by ovarian hyperstimulation syndrome (OHSS), with marked fluid shifts and an even greater risk of thrombosis.
   b. Hysteroscopy and laparoscopy can be life-threatening procedures, should be undertaken in an experienced center with appropriate support.
2. The risks can be reduced by:
   - Careful cycle monitoring
   - Using low-dose follicle-stimulating hormone in combination with a GnRH antagonist
   - Freezing all embryos
   - Only transferring a single embryo is strongly advised in women with heart disease, since conceiving a multiple pregnancy is associated with greater cardiovascular changes and more maternal and fetal complications.

REFERENCES

1. Assenza GE, et al., Management of acute cardiovascular complications in pregnancy. Eur Heart J. 2021;42(41):4224-40. doi: 10.1093/eurheartj/ehab546.
2. Nishimura RA, Otto CM, Bonow RO, et al. Thomas 2014 AHA/ACC Guideline for the Management of Patients With Valvular Heart Disease. Circulation. 2014;129:e521–e643.
3. 2018 European Society of Cardiology Guideline for the Management of CVD During Pregnancy.
4. Cardiac Disease and Pregnancy: Royal College of Obstetricians and Gynaecologists, Good Practice No. 13, June 2011.
5. Gupta A, Lokhandwala YY, Satoskar PR, et al. Ballon mitral valvotomy in pregnancy: maternal and fetal outcomes. J Am Coll Surg. 1998;187:409-15.
6. ESC Guidelines on the management of cardiovascular diseases during pregnancy: the Task Force on the Management of Cardiovascular Diseases during Pregnancy of the European Society of Cardiology (ESC). Eur Heart J. 2011;32(24):3147-97. doi: 10.1093/eurheartj/ehr218. Epub 2011 Aug 26.
7. 2018 ESC Guidelines for the management of cardiovascular diseases during pregnancy. Eur Heart J. 2018;39(34):3165-241. doi: 10.1093/eurheartj/ehy340.
8. Siu SC, Colman JM. Heart disease and pregnancy. Heart. 2001;85(6):710-5. doi: 10.1136/heart.85.6.710.

9. American College of Cardiology (citation: contraception and cardiovascular disease. Er Heart. 2015; Apr 2019 and WHO Medical Eligible Criteria for Contraceptive Usage).
10. The current UK recommendations from the National Institute for Clinical Excellence (NICE) 2008 and The British Society for Antimicrobial Chemotherapy (BSAC) 2006.
11. American College of Obstetricians and Gynecologists (2008)
12. Wilson W, Taubert KA, Gewitz M, Lockhart PB, Baddour LM, Levison M, Bolger A, et al. AHA guidelines: Prevention of Infective Endocarditis Circulation. 2007;116:1736-54.
13. ACOG Committee Opinion No. 421, November 2008, 2016: antibiotic prophylaxis for infective endocarditis. Obstet Gynecol. 2008;112(5):1193-4.
14. Cardiac Problems in Pregnancy Fourth Edition 2020 Edited by Uri Elkayam MD Department of Medicine, Division of Cardiovascular Medicine and the Department of Obstetrics and Gynecology University of Southern California Keck School of Medicine, Los Angeles, California.
15. Mehta LS, et al. Cardiovascular Considerations in Caring for Pregnant Patients: A Scientific Statement From the American Heart Association. Circulation. 2020;141:e884–e903. DOI: 10.1161/CIR.0000000000000772.
16. Arendt KW, Lindley KJ. Obstetric anesthesia management of the patient with cardiac disease. Int J Obstet Anesth. 2018, https://doi.org/10.1016/j.ijoa.2018.09.
17. AHA/ACC GUIDELINE 2018 AHA/ACC Guideline for the Management of Adults with Congenital Heart Disease A Report of the American College of Cardiology/American Heart Association Task Force on Clinical Practice Guidelines.
18. Cunningham FG, Leveno KJ, Dashe JS, Hoffman BL, Spong CY, Casey BM. Williams Obstetrics, 26th edition. Mc Graw Hill, 2023.

CHAPTER 13

Hyperglycemia in Pregnancy

Hafizur Rahman, Vandana Agarwal, Sayanti Paul

OSCE 1. Mrs SG, 25-year-old, married for 2 years is very anxious to become pregnant. She is a known diabetic for last 10 years and takes Insulin Mixtard injections twice daily. Her latest blood investigations are as follow:
FBS: 146 mg/dL
PPBS: 286 mg/dL
HbA1c: 10 gm%

1. What are the target blood sugar levels before conception?
2. What is the target HbA1c level before conception?

Ans.

1. a. Between 5 mmol/L and 7 mmol/L before breakfast (Fasting)
   b. Between 4 mmol/L and 7 mmol/L before meals at other times of the day
2. Target HbA1c before conception is below 48 mmol/mol or 6.5%.

Reference

1. Diabetes in pregnancy: management from preconception to the postnatal period, NICE guideline, 2020.

OSCE 2. A 35-year-old, G2Ab1 at 12 weeks who is known diabetic with uncontrolled sugars, comes to the OPD with the following USG report.

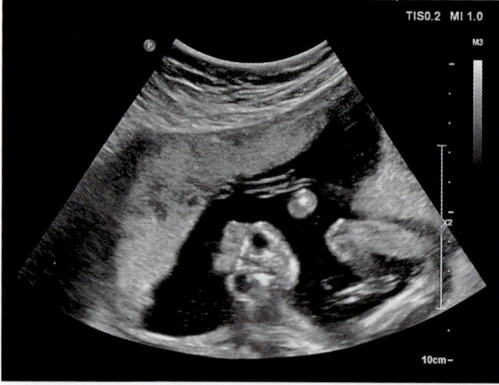

1. Identify the fetal congenital anomaly.
2. What is the characteristic ultrasound feature of this anomaly?

3. It is seen more commonly in male or female fetus?
4. Enumerate two preventive measures.

Ans.

1. Anencephaly
2. Total or partial absence of *calvarium* with absent cranial bone and/or brain and bulging orbits. A "frog eye" or "Mickey Mouse" appearance may be seen.
3. Female
4. a. Preconceptional folic acid supplementation
   b. Optimal sugar control in the preconception period as well as in early pregnancy.

OSCE 3. With respect to diabetes complicating pregnancy, answer the following questions.
1. What is the most common fetal congenital malformation associated with diabetes?
2. What is the most specific congenital malformation associated with diabetes?
3. Enumerate two malformations of the central nervous system.
4. Enumerate two malformations of the cardiovascular system.

Ans.

1. Ventricular septal defect (VSD)
2. Caudal regression, sacral agenesis
3. Malformations of the central nervous system are:
   - Open neural tube defects
   - Holoprosencephaly
   - Absent corpus callosum
   - Arnold Chiari Anomaly
   - Sacral agenesis
   - Caudal regression syndrome.
4. Malformations of the central nervous system are:
   - Transposition of great vessels
   - VSD
   - Atrial septal defect
   - Tetralogy of Fallot
   - Hypoplastic left ventricle

OSCE 4. Mrs SN, a 30-year-old primigravida at 28 weeks of pregnancy came to show 75 gm OGTT report which is as follows:
FBS: 90 mg/dL
1-hr PPBS: 190 mg/dL
2-hr PPBS: 156 mg/dL

1. What is the diagnosis?
2. Define GDM.
3. Where are the diagnostic criteria of GDM?

Ans.

1. Gestational diabetes mellitus (GDM)
2. According to WHO, gestational diabetes is a carbohydrate intolerance resulting in hyperglycemia of variable severity with onset or first recognition during pregnancy.
3. FIGO adopts the WHO criteria for diagnosis of diabetes mellitus in pregnancy.
   The diagnostic criteria used are:
   - Fasting blood sugar ≥126 mg/dL
   - 2-hour plasma glucose following 75 g oral glucose load ≥140 mg/dL
   - Random blood sugar ≥200 mg/dL in the presence of symptoms of diabetes.

   GDM is defined, if any of the values of fasting plasma glucose (FPG) ≥92 mg/dL, 1-hr PG ≥180 mg/dL, or 2-hr PG ≥153 mg/dL after 75 g glucose loading (international consensus criteria), International Association of Diabetes and Pregnancy Study Groups (IADPSG).

   Single step testing using 75 g oral glucose and measuring plasma glucose 2 hour after ingestion. The threshold plasma glucose level of ≥140 mg/dL (more than or equal to 140) is taken as cut-off for diagnosis of GDM (DIPSI).

OSCE 5. An antenatal woman at 30 weeks of gestation, detected with GDM from 20 weeks, has come to the OPD. Both MNT and OHA (oral hypoglycemic drug) have been started but her sugar levels are not controlled.
1. What do you understand by MNT?
2. What is the recommendation on calorie intake based on BM?

Ans.

1. a. MNT stands for medical nutritional therapy. It is an individualized nutrition plan developed between the woman and a registered dietician familiar with the management of GDM.
   b. The food plan should provide adequate calories to promote fetal/neonatal and maternal health, achieve glycemic goals, and promote weight gain.
   c. The DRI (Dietary Reference Intakes) for all pregnant women recommends a minimum of 175 g of carbohydrate, 71 g of protein, and 28 g of fiber.
   d. The total calorie requirement should consist of <45% carbohydrate, 30% protein and 25% fat (mainly unsaturated fats).
   e. Emphasis must be laid on monounsaturated and polyunsaturated fats while limiting saturated fats and avoiding *trans* fats.
2. Guidelines recommend calorie intake based on BMI as follows:
   - 30 kcal/kg for a BMI of 22–25
   - 24 kcal/kg for a BMI of 26–29
   - 12–15 kcal/kg for a BMI of >30

Reference

1. Kampmann U, Madsen LR, Skajaa GO, Iversen DS, Moeller N, Ovesen P. Gestational diabetes: a clinical update. World J Diabetes. 2015;6(8):1065-72.

Chapter 13: Hyperglycemia in Pregnancy

OSCE 6. A 30-year-old lady, married for 1 year and having a BMI of 32 is planning pregnancy.
1. Identify the high-risk factor in her case.
2. Enumerate two possible complications which can occur during pregnancy due to it.
3. What preconception advice should be given to her?

Ans.
1. Obesity
2. Diabetes in pregnancy, macrosomia, increased risk of cesarean, sepsis
3. *Preconception advice:*
   - Lifestyle modification—weight reduction
   - Investigation for the timely diagnosis of diabetes, hypertension, thyroid status, and their optimization.

OSCE 7.
1. Enumerate four high-risk factors for GDM.
2. Enumerate four maternal complications due to hyperglycemia in pregnancy.

Ans.
1. a. Family history of Type 2 diabetes
   b. Advanced maternal age
   c. Marked obesity
   d. History of GDM in previous pregnancy
   e. History of macrosomia
   f. Polycystic ovary syndrome (PCOS)
   g. Genetic polymorphisms
2. a. Polyhydramnios (18.8%)
   b. Infection (15.79%)
   c. Pre-eclampsia (9.9%)
   d. Prolonged labor
   e. Obstructed labor
   f. Uterine atony
   g. Postpartum hemorrhage

OSCE 8.
1. Name two imaging studies which should be performed in a pregnant lady who has overt diabetes.
2. Who should be screened for gestational diabetes?
3. How do you screen for gestational diabetes?

Ans.
1. Detailed anomaly (Level II) scan and fetal ECHO.
2. *Two approaches:*
   a. All pregnant women at first visit

b. *High-risk pregnant women:*
   - All pregnant women with factors conferring a high risk of GDM (marked obesity, previous history of GDM, glycosuria, or family history of diabetes) should be screened for GDM as soon as possible, preferably during their first antenatal visit.
   - If negative, they should be retested between 24 and 28 weeks of gestation.
   - Women who are categorized as average risk should also be screened between 24 and 28 weeks of gestation.
3. *There are two approaches for the screening of GDM:* The one-step approach and the two-step approach:
   a. In one-step approach, a diagnostic OGTT is performed without prior serum glucose screening.
   b. In two-step approach, initial screening involves glucose challenge test (GCT), which measures the plasma or serum glucose concentration after a 50 g oral glucose load. The diagnostic OGTT is performed only in women with deranged GCT (i.e. >140 mg/dL).

OSCE 9.
1. **What are the various diagnostic criteria for diabetes in pregnancy?**

Ans

1.

Criteria	Test	FBG	1-hr PG	2-hr PG	3-hr PG
WHO	75 g of OGTT	92–125 mg/dL	180 mg/dL	153–199 mg/dL	–
ACOG	100 g of OGTT	≥95	≥180	≥155	≥140
IADPSG	75 g of OGTT	≥92	≥180	≥153	–
DIPSI	75 g of OGTT	–	–	≥140	–
NICE	75 g of OGTT	≥95	–	≥140	–
ADA	75 g of OGTT	≥95	≥180	≥155	–
FIGO	75 g of OGTT	≥126	–	≥200	–

OSCE 10. A G3P2L2 at 38 weeks of gestation was induced in view of GDM with uncontrolled sugars and macrosomia. In the second stage of labor, there was difficulty in delivery of the fetal head. 'Turtle sign' was noted.

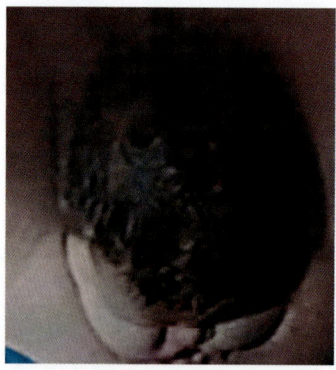

1. Identify the fetal complication.
2. Enumerate four other fetal complications which can occur in a pregnancy complicated with diabetes.

Ans.

1. Shoulder dystocia
2. Fetal complications are:
   - Shoulder dystocia, macrosomia (16–29%)
   - Neonatal hypoglycemia (18.42%)
   - Intrauterine death (15.79%)
   - Congenital malformation (5.26%)
   - Birth injuries
   - Infant respiratory distress syndrome

OSCE 11.
1. Name two oral hypoglycemic drugs (OHA) used in pregnancy.
2. What is their mechanism of action?
3. Enumerate two advantages of OHA's over insulin.

Ans.

1. Metformin (Biguanides) and Glyburide (Sulfonylurea)
2. a. Metformin acts by reducing hepatic glucose output, increasing peripheral glucose uptake in skeletal muscle and adipocytes. This leads to improved insulin sensitivity. It does not cause insulin secretion and hence does not cause hypoglycemia or weight gain.
   b. Glyburide acts primarily to enhance insulin secretion by the pancreas.
3. Advantages of OHA's over insulin are:
   - Cost-effective
   - Good patient compliance
   - No need of multiple injections as in insulin therapy and is of relevance in poor-resource setting.

OSCE 12. Answer the following with regard to blood sugar monitoring of a diabetic pregnant lady:
1. What is the target blood sugar level?
2. What is Somogyi phenomenon?
3. What is Dawn phenomenon?

Ans.

1. The ADA recommends achieving target blood sugar as follow:
   - Fasting blood sugar <95 mg/dL
   - 1-hour post mealblood sugar <140 mg/dL
   - 2-hour post mealblood sugar <120 mg/dL

2. A glucose level must be done at 2 AM to document nocturnal hypoglycemia which may occur due to excess bed-time insulin resulting in fasting hyperglycemia. This is called as Somogyi phenomenon.
3. Dawn phenomenon refers to fasting hyperglycemia without nocturnal hypoglycemia.

OSCE 13. A 30-year-old, Primigravida at 36 weeks of gestation with gestational diabetes mellitus that is well-controlled on Metformin and MNT comes to OPD to discuss regarding her delivery. She has no other co-morbidities complicating this pregnancy. Growth scan at 34 weeks showed a single, live, fetus of EFW 2.2 kg, AGA (appropriate for gestational age).
1. When should she be delivered?
2. What are the recommendations on elective cesarean in case of hyperglycemia in pregnancy?

Ans.

1. At 39 weeks:
   According to Government of India guidelines:
   - A pregnant woman with GDM with well-controlled blood sugar who has not delivered spontaneously should be induced at or after 39 weeks of pregnancy.
   - In poorly controlled blood sugar, those with risk factors like hypertensive disorder of pregnancy, previous stillbirth and other complications should be delivered earlier. The timing of delivery should be individualized by the obstetrician accordingly.
2. a. Vaginal delivery should be preferred and LSCS should be done for obstetric indications only.
   b. In case of fetal macrosomia (estimated birth weight >4 kg) consideration should be given for a primary cesarean section at 39 weeks to avoid shoulder dystocia.

Reference
1. Diagnosis and Management of GDM: Govt of India, 2018.

OSCE 14. A G3P2L2 at 37+3 weeks, with GDM on insulin and uncontrolled sugars is planned for induction of labor tomorrow.
1. What are the two important aspects to be considered regarding her sugar monitoring?
2. What is the target value of blood glucose during labor?

Ans.

1. a. Morning dose of insulin should be omitted, and fasting blood glucose is done.
   b. 2 hourly monitoring of blood sugar to be done.
   c. Intravenous infusion with normal saline to be started and regular insulin to be added according to blood sugar level.
   d. If blood glucose level is not maintained, then dextrose-insulin neutralizing drip is started. 50 units of regular insulin in 50 mL of normal saline are started.
   e. It is important to monitor vitals and fluid intake and output, urinary ketones, and blood glucose level 1–2 hourly.
2. 70–110 mg/dL.

Chapter 13: Hyperglycemia in Pregnancy

OSCE 15. A 35-year-old, G2P1L1 at 34 weeks, known diabetic, comes to the casualty with complaints of excessive vomiting, abdominal pain, and excessive thirst. On examination, she was tachypneic and had altered sensorium. Urine ketones was 3+, RBS: 320 mg/dL.
1. What is the diagnosis?
2. What are the diagnostic criteria for the above condition?
3. What is the management?

Ans.

1. Diabetic ketoacidosis (DKA)
2. Diagnosis of DKA is made when:
   - Blood sugar >250 mg/dL. It may occur at lower level also in pregnancy.
   - Ketone bodies in blood and urine.
   - Arterial pH <7.3, Serum bicarbonate level <15 mEq/L.
3. *Management includes:*
   - *Fluid replacement:* Severe dehydration may result in a large fluid deficit as much as 6–7 liters. The estimated fluid deficit must be replaced in around 12–24 hours.
   - In the first hour, one-liner of normal saline (NS) is infused followed by 300–500 mL/hour till pulse and BP returns to normal.
   - Hypokalemia generally occurs with DKA. If <4 mEq/L, 30 mEq/hr KCL must be given.
   - Insulin therapy is started as soon as possible: 0.2 U/kg IV bolus followed by 0.1 U/kg/hr in NS. Once glucose level is between 200–250 mg/dL, NS is changed to 5% dextrose.
   - Bicarbonate is required if pH falls <6.8.
   - Antibiotics to be given.
   - Periodic monitoring of pulse, BP, input and output, capillary blood glucose, urine ketones and blood arterial gases.
   - Fetal heart monitoring.
   - Treatment of cause is important.

Reference

1. Bhide A, Arulkumaran S, Damania KR, Daftary SN. Arias' Practical guide to High-risk Pregnancy and Delivery: A South Asian Perspective. Reed Elsevier India, 4th edition. 2015. p.254-66.

OSCE 16. A Primigravida who was diagnosed with GDM at 27 weeks and was on insulin therapy, thereafter, had a spontaneous vaginal delivery at 38 weeks. The delivery was uneventful. She delivered a 2.8 kg baby girl.
1. Is there any change in the insulin dose, postdelivery?
2. Enumerate two important postpartum advices that should be given to her?

Ans.

1. a. Insulin resistance decreases dramatically immediately postpartum, and insulin requirements need to be evaluated and adjusted as they are often roughly half the prepregnancy requirements for the initial few days postpartum.

b. Hence, in women-taking insulin, particular attention should be paid to hypoglycemia prevention in the setting of breastfeeding and erratic sleep and eating schedules.
2. a. Contraceptive advice should be given.
   b. All GDM women should be tested by OGTT method at 6 weeks after delivery for impaired glucose tolerance and to be linked to outpatient department for appropriate follow-up (annually if normal level) and manage (if diagnosed with high blood sugar levels).

OSCE 17.

1. What is the role of exercise in the management of gestational diabetes?
2. What is the recommended duration and frequency of these exercises?

Ans.

1. Exercises recommended in pregnancy are walking, jogging/running, aerobic dance, swimming and cycling.
2. 30 minutes of moderate intensity, aerobic exercise at least 5 days a week/minimum of 150 minutes per week (in absence of either medical or obstetric complications) is recommended.

OSCE 18.

1. A pregnant woman with overt diabetes experiences excessive weight gain. What potential maternal complication should be considered in this scenario?
2. What is the primary hormonal change that contributes to insulin resistance during pregnancy in women with overt diabetes?

Ans.

1. Risk of gestational hypertension
2. Elevated progesterone levels

OSCE 19.

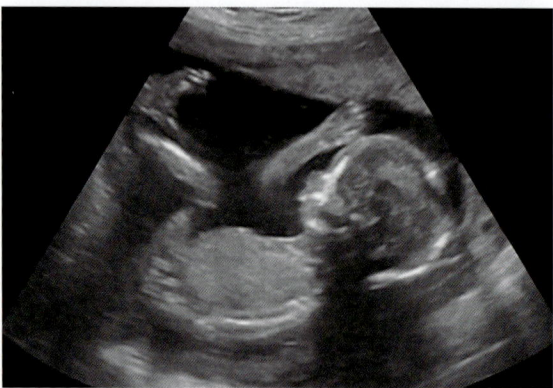

1. In the management of overt diabetes during pregnancy, which fetal parameter is particularly monitored on the ultrasound to assess the risk of macrosomia?

2. What impact can overt diabetes during pregnancy have on the mode of delivery?
3. How does overt diabetes in pregnancy affect the risk of neonatal hypoglycemia, and what measures can be taken to prevent it?

Ans.

1. Abdominal circumference
2. a. Higher risk of instrumental delivery
   b. Increased likelihood of elective cesarean section
3. Increases the risk; early and frequent breastfeeding is recommended.

OSCE 20.

1. Enumerate two long-term health implications which women with a history of gestational diabetes in pregnancy may face after childbirth.

Ans.

1. a. Increased risk of cardiovascular disease
   b. Higher risk of developing type 2 diabetes
   c. Higher risk of metabolic syndrome

CHAPTER 14

Rh-Negative Pregnancy

K Deepthi D Nair

OSCE 1. A primigravida, tests her blood group in a laboratory says its Rh-D is weak positive. She is unsure of what it means and comes to you for an opinion.
1. What are the important rhesus factor antigens?
2. What does this mean?
3. What to do next?
4. Can a woman who received Anti D, be positive in the next pregnancy in spite of receiving adequate dose?

Ans.
1. The Rhesus antigens are D, C, c E, e, G.
2. Weakened expression of D antigen is because of partial D antigen where some portions of D are missing. It is mostly due to expression of other antigens C and E.
3. Rhesus D genotyping.
4. Yes, she can, and this can be identified by antibody screening. This could be Anti-C, Anti-G antibody because of which the patient is ICT positive.

OSCE 2. A primigravida at 12 weeks of gestation comes for routine antenatal checkup. On taking her detailed history, she says she is AB –ve and her husband is B +ve. She is anxious and wants to know the risks.
1. How do you counsel this patient?
2. What test is done to know sensitization?
3. How can a primigravida be alloimmunized other than through pregnancy?
4. What are the antenatal precautions that can be taken to prevent complications?
5. What are the postnatal precautions that can be taken to prevent complications?

Ans.
1. In a Rh-negative, unless sensitized the 1st pregnancy will not be affected.
2. ICT testing
3. Maternal alloimmunization can be by:
   - Transplacental fetomaternal bleeding during any pregnancy
   - Injection with needles contaminated by RhD-positive blood.
   - Inadvertent transfusion of RhD-positive blood
   - RhD-mismatched hematopoietic stem cell transplantation.

Chapter 14: Rh-Negative Pregnancy

4. RAAPD—routine antenatal prophylaxis with anti-D Ig either with a single dose at around 28 weeks, or two-doses given at 28 and 34 weeks (RCOG guidelines).
5. Early cord clamping, monitoring of baby, identification of baby's blood group, Direct Coombs test, Anti-D if baby is Rh-positive.

OSCE 3. A G2P1L1 with previous normal delivery, Rh-negative pregnancy has come at 8 weeks gestation. Her previous baby was Rh-positive and she has taken Anti-D postnatally within 24 hours of delivery. The patient wants to know if she has any chances of complications in this pregnancy.
1. How will you test her?
2. What is the next step if the test is negative?
3. What if the test comes positive on the first visit? In that case, how do you consider follow-up?
4. What are the features that will appear in the baby in case of severe fetal anemia?

Ans.
1. Indirect Coombs test to find out if she has got antibodies against D antigen.
2. Follow-up with an ICT every visit and routine antenatal prophylaxis with Anti-D Ig should be given as single dose at 28 weeks or two doses 28 and 34 weeks.
3. If she is ICT positive, she must be followed up with titers. Monthly testing with titers is done till critical titer (1:32) is reached. If critical titer has reached, she must be checked every two weekly. Follow-up with ultrasound MCA-PSV to look for fetal anemia.
4. Fetal hydrops is seen in severe anemia when there is fluid accumulation in >2 fetal compartments like pericardial effusion, pleural effusion, ascites, and anasarca.

OSCE 4. A Rh-negative, Primigravida at 9 weeks of gestation comes to the emergency with mild bleeding per vaginum. On examination, no fresh blood was seen but her pad was partially soaked. She had no further episodes of bleeding.
1. What investigations would you like to do in particular for a Rh-negative case?
2. Her doctor has advised her to immediately report if she has bleeding PV for Anti-D, when will you give the same? Should it be given in this case?
3. Name the other conditions where Anti-D is recommended in a pregnancy of less than 12 weeks?
4. What will be the dose of Anti-D?
5. Should fetomaternal hemorrhage be tested in the above case?

Ans.
1. ICT testing to know if she is sensitized. Also, an ultrasound to see if the fetus is viable, if it is an inevitable or threatened abortion and to look for significant retrochorionic collection. If ICT is negative, then anti-D should be considered in certain conditions only.
2. In this condition as she is <12 weeks and had a single episode of bleeding which was minimal, anti-D is not recommended.

3. Anti-D Ig prophylaxis is only indicated following molar pregnancy, ectopic pregnancy, therapeutic termination of pregnancy and in cases of bleeding which is repeated, heavy or associated with abdominal pain.
4. Minimum dose 250 IU
5. Testing for fetomaternal hemorrhage (FMH) is not required.

OSCE 5. A G3P2L2, who is a Rh-negative pregnancy is tested to be ICT positive from outside and referred for further management.
1. What are the complications in the fetus and neonate when red cell antibodies are present?
2. Is karyotyping contraindicated when the woman is ICT positive?
3. When should you consider a referral to a fetal medicine specialist antenatally?
4. When should you consider a referral to a fetal medicine specialist postnatally?
5. What is the significance of Anti-K antibody?

Ans.

1. When red cell antibodies are present, there can be destruction of fetal RBCs causing severe fetal anemia and poor perinatal outcome.
2. No, when the woman is ICT positive, invasive testing is not contraindicated.
3. Antenatally when there are rising antibody levels/titers above a specific threshold (>4 IU/mL) or when the ultrasound features are suggestive of fetal anemia.
4. Postnatally refer when there is a history of unexplained severe neonatal jaundice and anemia requiring exchange transfusion, in order to exclude hemolytic disease of the fetus and newborn (HDFN).
5. Anti-K causes severe anemia secondary to erythroid suppression and immune destruction of erythroid progenitor cells, however, hyperbilirubinemia is not prominent. Here severe fetal anemia can occur even at relatively low antibody titers, so referral to fetal medicine must be considered early.

OSCE 6.

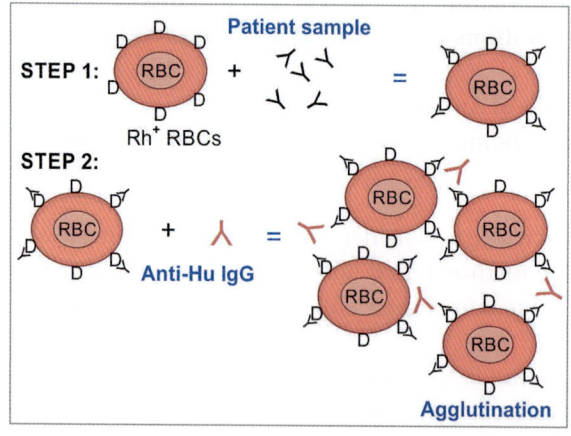

1. What is the test being done here?
2. How is it done?
3. What is Coombs reagent?
4. What is critical titer?
5. What is critical sensitizing volume?

Ans.

1. Indirect Coombs test
2. Patient's blood is taken and mixed with RBCs with known antigens. The mixture is then incubated, and Coombs reagent is added to detect agglutination of RBCs, indicating the presence of antibodies.
3. Coombs reagent is antihuman globulin. It is made by injecting human globulin into animals, which produce polyclonal antibodies specific for human immunoglobulins and human complement system factors.
4. Critical titer is clinically significant dependent on the laboratory, mostly a titer >1:16 to 1:32 is a critical titer. A value below which no case of fetal hemolysis has been reported is critical value.
5. Volume required to incite an immune response in the mother which is equivalent to 0.1 mL.

OSCE 7.

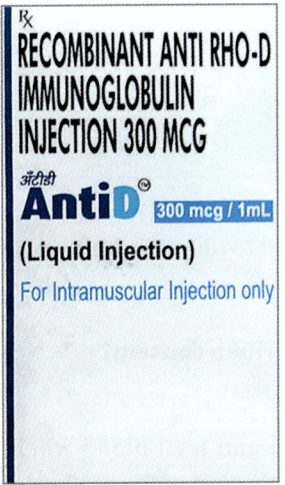

1. When is anti-D given in a pregnant woman?
2. What are the sensitizing events where we consider anti-D?
3. What dose is usually given in the third trimester or after delivery and why?
4. Where is the site of anti-D administration?

Ans.

1. In an unsensitized woman, routine antenatal prophylaxis with anti-D Ig (RAAPD) is given either with a single dose 300 μg at around 28 weeks, or two-doses given at 28 and 34 weeks

(RCOG guidelines) or it must be considered at least within 72 hours of delivery if the baby is Rh-positive.
2. Ectopic pregnancy, molar pregnancy, therapeutic termination of pregnancy and in cases of uterine bleeding where this is heavy, repeated or associated with abdominal pain, amniocentesis and chorionic villous sampling. Events after 20 weeks gestation like antepartum hemorrhage, intrauterine death, ECV (external cephalic version), abdominal trauma and in utero therapeutic interventions (shunts, surgeries).
3. 1,500 IU or 300 µg is given as it will protect from a fetomaternal hemorrhage of 30 mL fetal whole blood or 15 mL fetal RBCs and covers nearly 99.7% of the cases.
4. IM (intramuscular) only into deltoid muscle or anterolateral aspect of thigh.

OSCE 8.

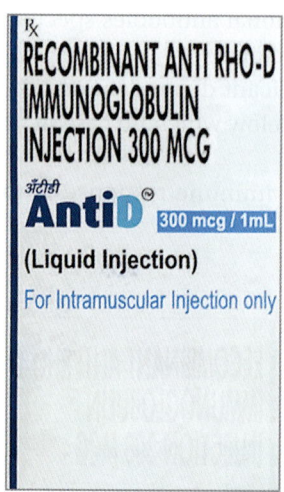

1. What is fetomaternal hemorrhage (FMH)?
2. What is the qualitative method to identify this and how is it done?
3. What is the grandmother effect?
4. How does anti-D work?
5. Does anti-D need informed written consent?

Ans.

1. Interaction between maternal and fetal blood wherein the fetal RBCs enter maternal circulation leading to the sensitization of the mother's immune system to fetal blood antigens and affects the next pregnancy.
2. Rosette test is a qualitative test that identifies whether there is Fetal D positive cells in maternal circulation. Here maternal blood is mixed with anti-D antibodies and formation of rosettes is noted which is indicative of FMH.
3. A Rh-negative female baby may be exposed to maternal Rh-positive red cells and may develop sensitization thus producing anti-D antibodies before or during her pregnancy. This is called the grandmother effect as the fetus in the current pregnancy is affected by the antibodies that were provoked by the grandmother's erythrocytes.

4. Anti-D binds on the D antigen sites on the fetal RBCs in maternal circulation and prevents their immune recognition B-lymphocytes.
5. Yes, it does as it is a blood product and has an anaphylaxis risk.

OSCE 9.

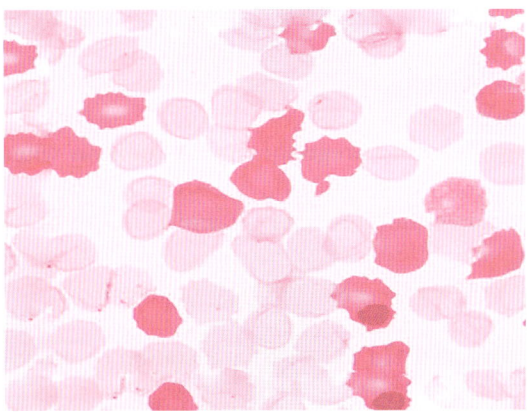

1. What is this test done here? What is its rationale?
2. What is the formula to calculate fetal blood volume?
3. How does this test help us clinically?
4. Name two conditions where this test can be inaccurate.
5. Is it recommended in India?

Ans.

1. Kleihauer-Betke or flow cytometry tests are quantitative tests that identify the amount of FMH. The rationale of this test is that fetal RBCs are more resistant to acid elution than adult RBCs. Following exposure to acid, fetal blood remains and gets stained while adult blood becomes ghost cells.
2. $FBV = \dfrac{MBV \times \text{Maternal HCT} \times \text{\% of fetal cells in KB test}}{\text{Newborn Hct}}$

   where MBV = maternal blood volume (5,000 mL approx), maternal Hct 35% and newborn Hct 50%.
3. This test can suggest whether the given dose of Anti-D will suffice or whether further doses must be given.
4. a. Maternal hemoglobinopathies in which fetal Hb may be elevated like β-thalassemia.
   b. At or near term where the fetus has a good number of Hb A (Adult Hb).
5. Quantification tests are desirable, but not mandatory as the standard dose of Anti-D 300 µg will cover nearly 99.7% of the cases.

OSCE 10. A 6-weeks, Primigravida who is Rh-negative comes with complaints of abdominal pain. On USG, there is an adnexal mass suggestive of ectopic pregnancy. Plan of management is medical with methotrexate as she is stable, and the adnexal mass is small and unruptured.

Section 1: Obstetrics

1. What investigation would you like to do specifically as she is Rh-negative?
2. Would you consider any other injection? If yes, what and suggest the dose?
3. Would your management differ if she underwent a surgical procedure instead of a medical one?
4. Is fetomaternal hemorrhage testing mandatory?

Ans.

1. Firstly, ICT should be done to know if she has been previously sensitized. If positive, no further testing is to be done.
2. If she is ICT negative, ectopic pregnancy is a condition where Anti-D of 250 IU is recommended.
3. No, for any case of ectopic the same dose of anti-D has to be given irrespective of the line of management.
4. No, for any pregnancy <12 weeks, FMH testing is not needed.

OSCE 11. An ICT negative, G2P1L1 at 36 weeks gestation comes for her regular antenatal checkup.

1. Will you consider induction and when?
2. What are the precautionary methods you would like to do in order during intrapartum and postpartum to prevent fetomaternal hemorrhage?
3. She has not been given routine antenatal prophylaxis with anti-D and wants it postpartum. When can you give it and how late can it be given?

Ans.

1. For a non-ICT negative immunized mother consider induction of labor at term, do not allow the pregnancy to go beyond date.
    - Pregnancy is not allowed to go postdate.
    - Avoid fetal blood sampling
    - Early cord clamping
    - Avoid methergine
    - Keep the cord long
    - Avoid MROP (manual removal of placenta)
2. Take cord blood sample in two tubes violet and green for: Hemoglobin, Hct, bilirubin, blood group and Rh and DCT.
3. She must be given anti-D immediately postdelivery if the baby is Rh-positive or at least within 72 hours of delivery. If not immunized or missed by chance, it can give even up to 28 days.

OSCE 12. In a case of fetal anemia where the MCA PSV is >1.5 MoM.

1. What is your line of management when the fetus is remote from term?
2. Briefly explain how it is done.
3. At what gestational age do you consider delivery when MCA PSV >1.5 MoM?
4. Other than MCA PSV, what are the signs that can tell that the baby has anemia?

Ans.

1. For a fetus that is remote from term we must consider fetal blood sampling and intra-uterine blood transfusion (IUT).
2. Cordocentesis is done under continuous ultrasound guidance with facilities for immediate analysis of the fetal blood hemoglobin and hematocrit. If Hb <2 SD for the mean gestational age or Hct <30%, then IUT is done. Crossmatched with mother's blood, O-negative, gamma-irradiated blood with a hematocrit of 75-85%. It is washed, infection free, double packed or triple packed to increase Hematocrit.
3. If the fetus has crossed 35 weeks, consider delivery.
4. Features like polyhydramnios, collection of fluid—pericardial, pleural, ascites, skin edema, cardiomegaly and features of fetal hydrops suggest fetal anemia.

OSCE 13. A primigravida who is Rh-negative and 16 weeks pregnant wants to know her baby's Rh-status and is reluctant to take any injections prior to knowing the same. She wants to know the various options available.
1. How can you identify the fetal Rh before birth?
2. How is this done?
3. When can the results be wrong?
4. What if she is ICT positive in the first pregnancy itself? How will you follow up?

Ans.

1. Noninvasive fetal genotyping using maternal blood for the following antigens—D, C, c, E, e, and K and invasive testing can be done for other antigens or when its being done for other reasons like karyotyping. These include CVS, amniocentesis or cordocentesis.
2. cffDNA—cell-free fetal DNA is used, and fetal Rh-D is identified by PCR.
3. In the case of dizygotic twins, the results may not be accurate.
4. Ideally, ICT titer estimation is done, and if more than the critical value, fetal ultrasound monitoring (MCA-PSV) for anemia is done.

OSCE 14.

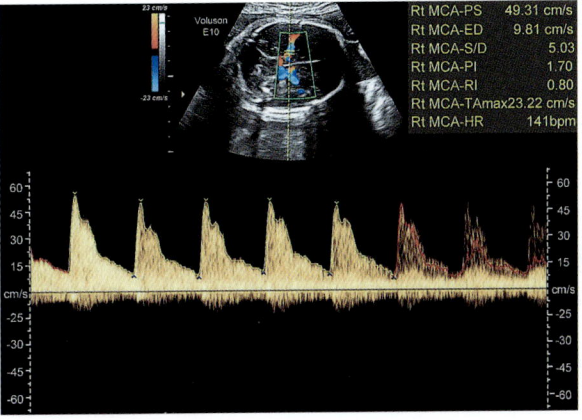

1. What is the rationale behind testing of MCA in a Rh-negative pregnancy?
2. What value is significant and what is its sensitivity?
3. Why is it considered as MoM?
4. How frequently is a normal MCA-PSV monitored?

Ans.

1. Middle cerebral artery is the artery that carries blood to the brain. In an anemic baby, the blood flow is redistributed preferentially to the brain, causing changes in the PSV and thus this is monitored. Hence, MCA is a valuable tool to detect fetal anemia.
2. Values >1.5 MoM is significant and is an indication for intervention. The sensitivity is 100% in the absence of hydrops fetalis.
3. The MCA-PSV increases as gestational age increases; hence, MoM values are taken to get the values corrected as per gestational age.
4. Normal values of MCA-PSV are monitored two weekly till it increases more than >1.5 MoM.

OSCE 15.

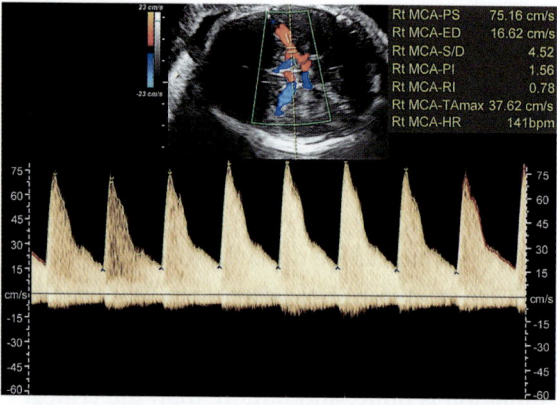

A Rh-negative G2P1L1, previous full-term normal delivery, now at 30 weeks, ICT positive and a Doppler done (image given above) showing MCA-PSV values as >1.5 MoM.
1. How will you manage this case?
2. What are the specifications for an intrauterine transfusion?
3. After intervention, how frequently should we follow-up?

Ans.

1. As the fetus is preterm and it has severe fetal anemia it can be salvaged by a procedure called intrauterine transfusion where in the fetus is given blood in-utero. Pregnancies between 24 and 34 weeks is best managed at a center by a fetal medicine specialist and must be given intrauterine transfusion under ultrasound guidance.
2. O-negative blood that is cross-matched with mother and gamma-irradiated blood with a hematocrit of 75–85%. It should be infection-free, washed, double packed or triple packed to increase hematocrit.
3. Again, the MCA-PSV is checked every 2 weekly and if >1.5 MoM, the procedure may have to be repeated.

OSCE 16.

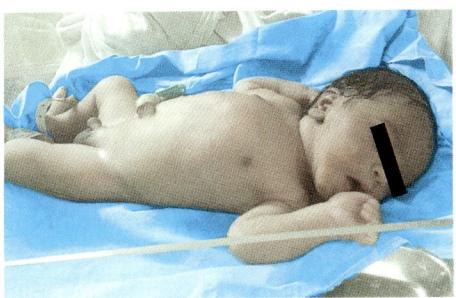

A Rh-negative unbooked mother gives birth to her second child at 37 weeks of gestation. After delivery, the neonate is admitted to the NICU with yellowish discoloration of skin.
1. What is the cause for this and the diagnosis?
2. What are the types of this condition?
3. How does it usually present?
4. What are the postnatal tests that are routinely sent for a Rh-negative pregnancy?
5. What is the relation between antibody quantification (anti-D) and this condition?

Ans.

1. This is a case of HFDN (hemolytic disease of the newborn), wherein the maternal immunoglobulin G (IgG) antibodies destroy the fetal/neonatal RBCs. This happens usually in the second pregnancy due to maternal sensitization.
2. Mild-to-moderate and hydrops fetalis
3. Mild-to-moderate presents with jaundice which is usually self-limited. It responds to phototherapy. However, rapidly rising bilirubin levels have risks like kernicterus and hemolytic anemia. Hydrops fetalis has diffuse edema, pleural and/or pericardial effusion and ascites which may require emergency exchange transfusion.
4. Blood group, Direct Coombs test, serum bilirubin, reticulocyte count.
5. Antibody quantification levels <4IU/mL is unlikely to develop HFDN and needs monitoring, 4–15 IU/mL has chance of moderate HFDN >15 IU/mL has a chance of severe HFDN.

OSCE 17.

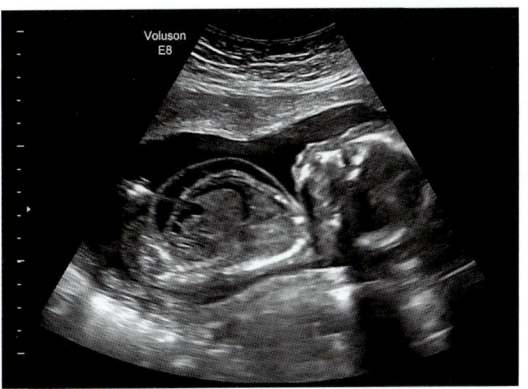

Here is a USG picture of a 32 weeks' fetus with ascites and pleural effusion seen on scan.
1. How do you define fetal hydrops?
2. What is placentomegaly?
3. What are the causes of fetal hydrops?
4. Which is more common?

Ans.
1. Fetal hydrops is defined by the presence of fluid in two or more compartments such as pleural, pericardial and ascites or one of these effusion plus anasarca.
   Sonographically, skin thickness >5 mm is fetal edema or anasarca.
2. Placentomegaly is when the placental thickness is >4 cm in the 2nd and >6 cm in the 3rd trimester. As hydrops progresses, placentomegaly, anasarca, and hydramnios follow.
3. Causes of hydrops fetalis is immune and nonimmune hydrops.
   Immune hydrops is because of transplacental passage of antibodies that destroy fetal RBCs and nonimmune hydrops is due to various causes such as aneuploidy, infections (parvovirus is the most common), cardiovascular abnormalities, other gastrointestinal, kidney-related anomalies and syndromic babies, hematological like hemoglobinopathies, TTTS in multifetal gestation, etc.
4. Nonimmune hydrops constitutes to about 90% of the cases of hydrops.

OSCE 18.

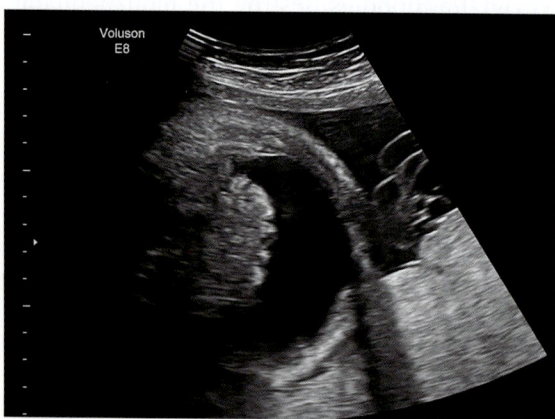

Here is a picture of a fetus who is around 26 weeks with ascites and pleural effusion.
1. What are the diagnostic tests you would do for a case of fetal hydrops?
2. What is Mirror syndrome?
3. What is the significance of isolated effusion or edema?

Ans.
1. Diagnosis for fetal hydrops is by ultrasound. To know the cause, further tests to be done are:
   - Indirect Coombs test
   - Fetal anatomical survey to look for structural anomalies like CVS (Fetal ECHO is preferred) and GIT anomalies.

- MCA PSV to detect fetal anemia.
- Amniocentesis for karyotyping and infection screening (parvovirus, toxoplasma, CMV, etc.)
- Fetomaternal hemorrhage testing with Kleihauer Betke test
- Consider tests for Inborn errors of metabolism and alpha-thalassemia.

2. Mirror syndrome is maternal edema in response to fetal hydrops where the mother mirrors the fetus.
3. Isolated effusion or edema must be strictly followed up and all the above-mentioned evaluation is to be done. It may be seen in parvovirus infection (as pericardial effusion), chylothorax (as pleural effusion), Turner's or Noonan's syndrome (as upper torso or dorsum of hands or feet).

OSCE 19. A neonate is referred to the tertiary care center with an intracranial hemorrhage and on investigation, thrombocytopenia is detected immediately following birth. The mother was a young, healthy primigravida with normal CBC, Rh-negative, low-risk and a booked case who had a full-term vaginal delivery.
1. What is the condition?
2. What is the cause of it?
3. What is the management?

Ans.
1. This is fetal and neonatal alloimmune thrombocytopenia which is the most common cause of thrombocytopenia in neonates.
2. This is due to the maternal alloimmunization to paternally inherited fetal antigens. It affects even the first pregnancy.
3. If it is diagnosed in a neonate with severe and unexplained thrombocytopenia born to a mother having normal platelet count, management is by platelet transfusion till >50,000/µL. If it is identified in the 2nd or 3rd trimester, IVIG (immunoglobulins) and steroids can be considered.

OSCE 20. A 34-year-old, Rh-negative, G2P1L1 at 11 weeks comes with a USG showing molar pregnancy. She is posted for suction evacuation.
1. Does she need anti-D?
2. What if it is a complete mole?
3. What is meant by sensibilized woman?

Ans.
1. Yes, this woman needs anti-D. It must be given to all women undergoing a surgical procedure for molar pregnancy.
2. Complete mole does not have fetal tissue and RBCs, hence, it is not theoretically necessary to give anti-D, However, it is difficult to differentiate between complete and partial mole early in pregnancy so when in doubt, it is better and safer to administer anti-D.

3. A woman who is Rh-negative and had a Rh-positive pregnancy, during postpartum has a 7–8% chance of having antibody to D-antigen which will not be detected by laboratory tests. However, when she gets pregnant again, the antibodies will rise and affect the pregnancy.

OSCE 21. Routine antenatal anti-D prophylaxis (RAAPD).
1. What is RAAPD?
2. Is it recommended in India?
3. Will ICT be positive after anti-D?
4. A pregnant lady had amniocentesis at 18 weeks and had taken anti-D, then does she need RAADP?
5. A pregnant lady had taken anti-D at 28 weeks and delivered at 32 weeks. Does she need anti-D after delivery and why?

Ans.

1. Routine antenatal prophylaxis with anti-D Ig is given either with a single dose 300 µg at around 28 weeks, or two-doses given at 28 and 34 weeks.
2. Yes, it is recommended in Indian guidelines also.
3. It may be positive, but the titers may be low 1:4 or less.
4. RAAPD is not influenced by previous doses so she must be given as usual.
5. Yes, the woman requires anti-D after delivery because the half-life of anti-D is around 24 days, so by the time she delivers the levels would not suffice the expected feto-maternal hemorrhage. If delivery occurs within 3 weeks of administration of full-dose anti-D, and if the FMH is not >15 mL of red cells, then postpartum anti-D may be omitted.
(SOGC Clinical Practice Guidelines No. 133, Sept 2003)

Images Courtesy: Shyama Devadasan, Fetal Medicine Consultant, Thrissur, Kerala, India.

CHAPTER 15

Multiple Pregnancy

Mala Srivastava

OSCE 1.
1. Enumerate three risk factors for multifetal pregnancy.
2. Why does frequency of twin pregnancy increase with age?

Ans.
1. Maternal age, parity, hereditary, infertility therapy
2. Maternal age is an important risk factor for multifetal pregnancies. Dizygotic twinning frequency rises almost fourfold between the ages of 15 and 37 years. As such, there is a paradox of declining fertility but increasing twinning rates with advancing maternal age. Another explanation for the dramatic rise in twinning with advancing maternal age may be a higher use of ART in older women. With increasing age, level of FSH increases which increases the rate of multiple follicle maturation.

Reference
1. Cunningham, Levono, Bloom, Auth H, Rouse, Sponge. Multifetal Pregnancy. Williams Obstetrics; 25th edition. p. 1339.

OSCE 2.
1. Match the following for determining chorionicity and amniocity depending on timing of zygote splitting.

Timing of cleavage	Placenta—membrane status
A. <72 hours	1. Diamniotic monochorionic
B. 4–7 days	2. Conjoint
C. 8–12 days	3. Diamniotic dichorionic
D. >13 days	4. Monoamniotic monochorionic

2. How does dizygotic twin form?

Ans.
1. A → 3
   B → 1
   C → 4
   D → 2

2. Twin fetuses usually result from fertilization of two separate ova, which yields dizygotic or fraternal twins. Less often, twins arise from single fertilized ovum that then divides to create monozygotic or identical twins.

OSCE 3.

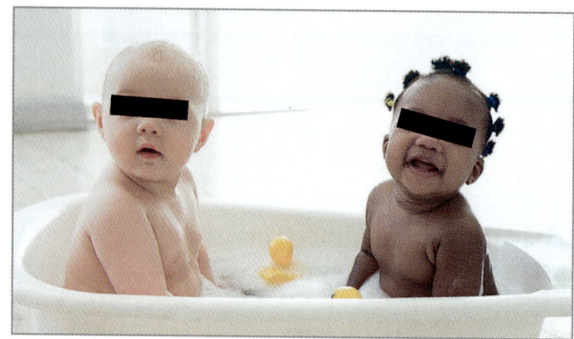

1. Name the mechanism leading to this condition in twins.
2. What is superfetation?
3. What is superfecundation?

Ans.

1. It is a consequence of superfecundation.
2. In superfetation, an interval as long as or longer than a menstrual cycle intervenes between fertilizations. Fertilization of two ova released in different menstrual cycle is superfetation. Superfetation requires ovulation and fertilization during the course of an established pregnancy, which is theoretically possible until the uterine cavity is obliterated by fusion of the decidua capsularis to the decidua parietalis.
3. Superfecundation refers to fertilization of two ova within the same menstrual cycle but not at the same coitus, nor necessarily by sperm from the same male.

Reference

1. Cunningham, Levono, Bloom, Auth H, Rouse, Sponge. Multifetal Pregnancy. Williams Obstetrics; 25th edition. p. 1338.

OSCE 4.

1. Mention five maternal physiological adaptations in twin pregnancy as compared to singleton pregnancy.

Ans.

1. a. Increase in nausea and vomiting in first trimester
   b. Greater uterine growth and weight gain
   c. Increase blood volume by 50–60% vs. 40–50% in singleton pregnancy
   d. Increased cardiac output (due to increased stroke volume) with decreased vascular resistance
   e. Increased alpha fetoprotein level, tidal volume and glomerular filtration rate.

OSCE 5.
1. What do you see in this photo?

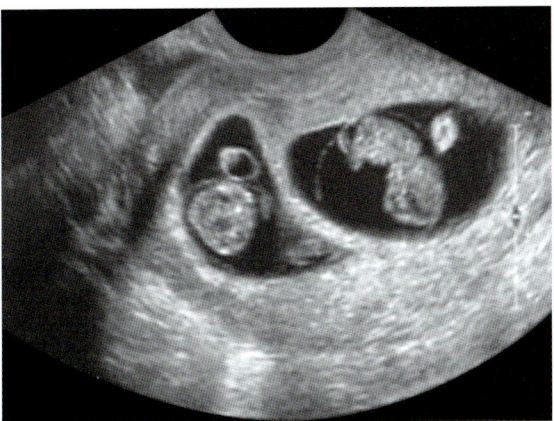

2. What type of zygosity?
3. What is the chorionicity?
4. At what weeks of gestation chorionicity is best determined?
5. Name the sign seen in this picture to determine chorionicity.

Ans.
1. It shows twin pregnancy with two gestational sacs
2. Dizogotic
3. Dichorionic
4. 11–14 weeks
5. Twin peak or delta sign or lambda sign

OSCE 6.
1. What is the chorionicity seen in this picture?

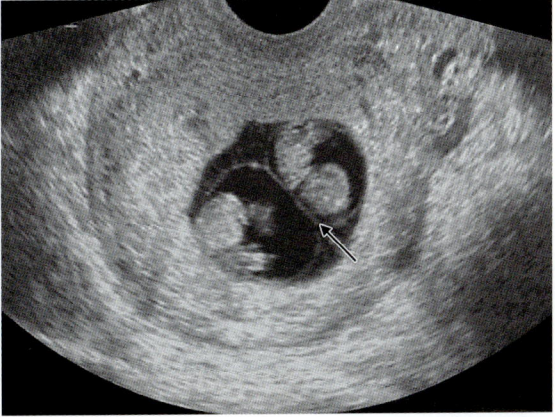

2. Mention the sign.
3. How do you determine chorionicity antenatally?

Ans.
1. Monochorionic
2. T sign
3. Determined using four features:
   a. Number of placental masses
      * *One placental mass:* Monochorionic
      * *Two distinct, separate placentas:* Dichorionic
   b. Thickness of membrane dividing sacs
      * *Dichorionicity:* Two layers of amnion and two layers of chorion and thickness >2 mm
      * *Monochorionicity:* ≤2 mm thickness
   c. Presence of intervening membrane
      * Twin peak or lambda sign or delta sign
      * Triangular projection of placental tissue extending a short distance between the layers of the dividing membrane, signifies dichorionicity
      * *T-sign:* Without apparent extension of placenta between the dividing membranes; dividing membrane thin <2 mm signifies monochorionicity, lack of a dividing membrane signals a monochorionic monoamniotic gestation.
   d. *Fetal gender:* Fetus of opposite gender signify DADC

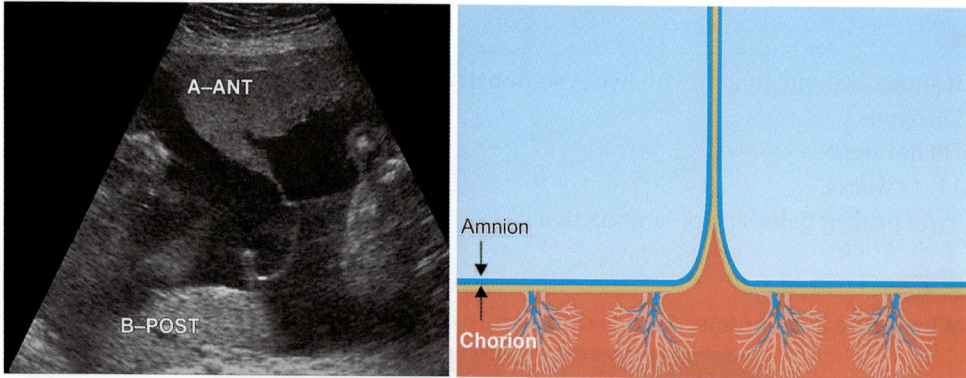

Dichorionic diamniotic.

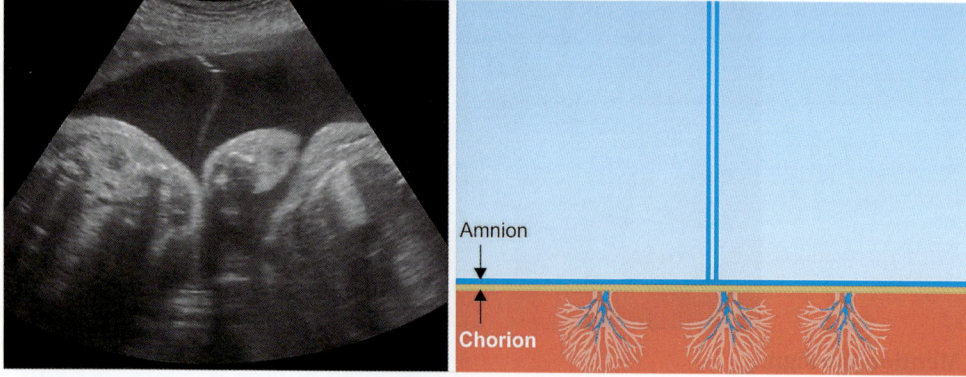

Monochorionic monoamniotic.

OSCE 7.
1. Enumerate maternal complications in twin pregnancy.
2. Enumerate four fetal complications seen in twin pregnancy.
3. What complication does the given picture depict in monoamniotic twins?

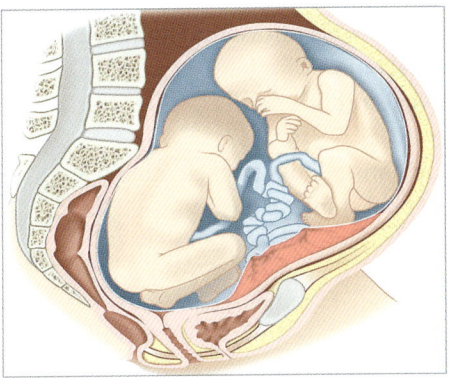

Ans.
1. a. *During pregnancy:* Spontaneous abortion, increased nausea and vomiting, antepartum hemorrhage, malpresentation, hypertension, gestational diabetes mellitus, polyhydraminos
   b. *During labor:* Early rupture of membranes, cord prolapse, preterm labor, postpartum hemorrhage
   c. *During puerperium:* Subinvolution, infection, lactational failure
2. Miscarriage, prematurity and low-birth weight (80%), discordant twin growth (20%), IUFD, vanishing twin, fetus papyraceous, fetus compressus, fetal anomalies, asphyxia and stillbirth.
3. Cord entanglement

OSCE 8.
1. What does this image show?

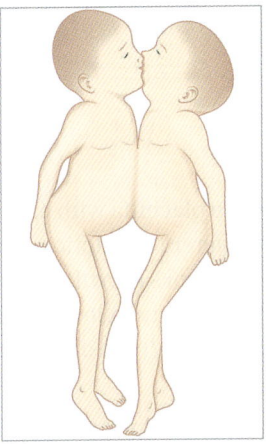

2. How is this condition diagnosed antenatally?
3. What is the mode of delivery in a term pregnancy?

Ans.

1. Conjoined twins
2. Diagnosed antenatally by following ultrasound findings:
   a. Bifid appearance of fetal pole
   b. Four vessels in umbilical cord
   c. Heads at the same level
   d. No change in fetal positions relative to each other
   e. Extended positions of fetal spine
3. Cesarean section

OSCE 9.

1. What does the picture depict?

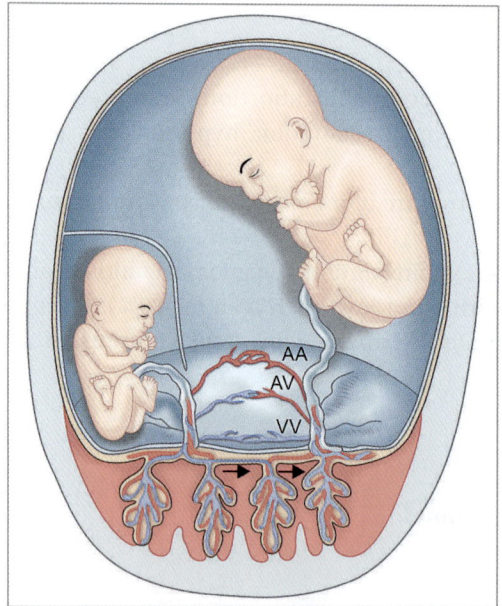

2. Name the condition.

Ans.

1. a. The given picture shows a single placenta with arterioarterial anastomosis.
   b. It is a twin pregnancy in two different amniotic cavities.
   c. In one amniotic cavity, one twin looks growth-restricted and has oligohydraminos.
   d. In another amniotic cavity, the other twin looks hydropic and has polyhydraminos.
2. Twin-twin transfusion syndrome (TTTS)/twin oligopolyhydraminos sequence (TOPS)

OSCE 10.
1. Mention two criteria for diagnosis of TTTS.
2. Name the staging of this condition.
3. Enumerate two methods for the management of this condition.

Ans.

1. Society for maternal-fetal medicine (2013).
   Two criteria:
   a. Presence of a monochorionic diamniotic pregnancy
   b. *Hydramnios:* Largest vertical pocket >8 cm in one twin and oligohydramnios <2 cm in other twin.
2. Quintero staging
3. a. Amnioreduction
   b. Laser ablation of vascular anastomoses
   c. Septostomy (Intentional creation of a communication in the dividing amniotic membrane)
   d. Selective feticide (Severe amniotic fluid and growth disturbances develop before 20 weeks)

OSCE 11.
1. Mention the condition seen in twins in the given picture.

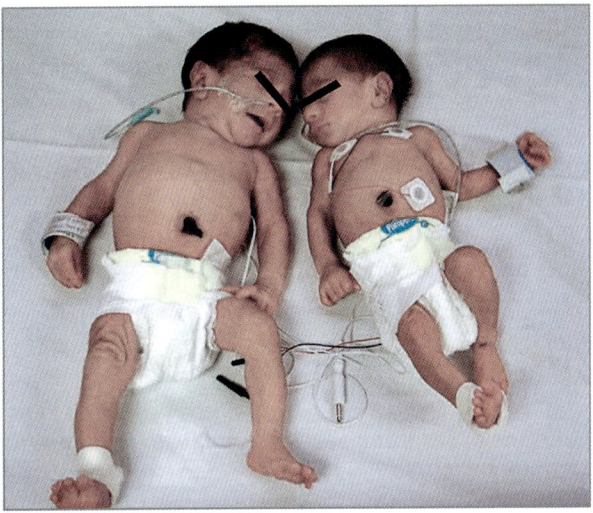

2. When do you say it to be discordant?
3. How do you calculate it?
4. What is the other parameter which can be taken into account?

Ans.

1. Discordant twin
2. When % discordancy is 20% or more

3. Percent of discordancy: $\dfrac{[\text{weight (wt) of larger twin} - \text{wt of smaller twin}] \times 100}{\text{wt of larger twin}}$
4. Abdominal circumference

OSCE 12.
1. **How frequently will you monitor the growth discordant twins with USG?**
2. **When will you terminate the pregnancy?**

Ans.

1. a. *Sonographic monitoring of twin growth:* Mainstay in management
   b. *Serial sonography:*
      - *Monochorionic twins:* 2 weekly
      - *Dichorionic twins:* 3–4 weekly
2. a. *Type I:* Normal umbilical artery Doppler, delivery by 34–36 weeks
   b. *Type II:* Intermittently absent end-diastolic flow, delivery by 34 weeks
   c. *Type III:* Persistently absent or reversed end-diastolic flow, delivery by 32 weeks

OSCE 13. Mention the weeks at which the following twins should be terminated.
1. **Uncomplicated dichorionic twins.**
2. **Uncomplicated monochorionic twins.**
3. **Uncomplicated monoamniotic twins.**
4. **Uncomplicated triplet pregnancy.**
5. **Uncomplicated >3 multiple gestation.**

Ans.

1. *Uncomplicated dichorionic twins: Delivery at around 38 weeks.* In cases of prematurity and discordant twins, timing of delivery should be based on parameters of healthy twin.
2. *Uncomplicated monochorionic twins: Delivery between 34 and $37^{6/7}$ weeks.*
3. *Monoamniotic twin: Elective delivery at 32–34 weeks recommended*
4. *Uncomplicated twin and triplet pregnancy should be planned for elective delivery at 38 weeks and 35 weeks respectively.*
5. *>3 multiple gestations: 32–34 weeks*

OSCE 14.
1. **Mention five indications of cesarean section specific to twin pregnancy.**

Ans.

1. *For twins:*
   a. Both fetuses or 1st fetus noncephalic
   b. Twins with complications (IUGR, conjoined)
   c. Monoamniotic twins
   d. Monochorionic twins with TTTS
   e. Collision of both head of at brim preventing engagement
   f. Locked twins

Obstetrics cause:
  a. Placenta previa
  b. Severe pre-eclampsia
  c. Previous cesarean section
  d. Cord prolapse of 1st baby
  e. Abnormal uterine contractions
  f. Contracted pelvis

OSCE 15. Decide the mode of delivery on the basis of presentation in cases of twin pregnancy.
1. 1st twin—cephalic; 2nd twin—cephalic
2. 1st twin—cephalic; 2nd twin—breech
3. 1st twin—breech presentation; 2nd twin—cephalic
4. Locked twins
5. Conjoined twins

Ans.

1. *Cephalic-cephalic:* Vaginal delivery preferred [*Barrett and coworkers (2013)*]
2. *Cephalic-breech:* Vaginal delivery preferred.
3. *Breech presentation of first twin:* Cesarean delivery is preferred (*ACOG* 2016)
4. *Locked twins:* Cesarean delivery preferred
5. *Conjoined twins:* Cesarean delivery preferred

OSCE 16.
1. **What does the given picture depict?**

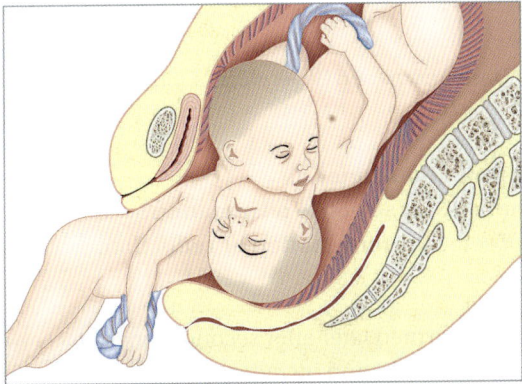

2. **Name this condition.**
3. **What is the definitive management of this condition?**

Ans.
1. First fetus is breech presentation and second is cephalic presentation. Breech of first twin has descended through birth canal and chin locked between neck and chin of second cephalic presenting co-twin.

2. Locked twin
3. Cesarean delivery preferred.

OSCE 17.
1. **Following vaginal delivery of 1st twin, cesarean delivery of 2nd twin may be required in which conditions?**

Ans.

1. Following vaginal delivery of 1st twin, cesarean delivery of 2nd twin may be required:
    a. Intrapartum fetal distress
    b. Cord prolapse
    c. Placental abruption
    d. Contracting cervix
    e. Larger (>20%) second twin with noncephalic presentation

OSCE 18.
1. **What is selective fetal reduction?**
2. **At what weeks of gestation is it performed?**
3. **Mention the three routes by which it can be performed.**

Ans.

1. In high order gestations, reduction of the fetal number to two or three to enhance survival of the remaining fetuses is called selective fetal reduction.
2. Between 10 and 13 weeks gestation.
3. Performed transcervically, transvaginally, or transabdominally. The transabdominal route is usually easiest.

Reference
1. American College of Obstetricians and Gynecologists, 2017b.

OSCE 19.
1. **When is selective termination done?**
2. **What are the prerequisites of selective termination?**
3. **Mention two risks of selective termination or reduction.**

Ans.

1. *Selective termination:* Performed later after second trimester
2. Prerequisites to selective termination include:
    a. A precise diagnosis for the anomalous fetus
    b. Absolute certainty of fetal location
3. Specific risks of selective termination or reduction are:
    a. Abortion of the remaining fetuses
    b. Abortion or retention of the wrong fetus(es)
    c. Damage without death to a fetus
    d. Preterm labor

e. Discordant or growth-restricted fetuses
f. Maternal complications; potential infection, hemorrhage, or disseminated intravascular coagulopathy because of retained products of conception.

OSCE 20. A 27-year-old lady with twin pregnancy presented in labor. On examination, os was 8 cm dilated, 80% effaced, head station: +2. Pelvis was adequate.
1. What will be your preferred mode of delivery?
2. Following the delivery of 1st twin, you found that the 2nd twin has transverse lie. What maneuver can be done in order to deliver it vaginally?
3. If there is cord prolapse of second twin, what mode of delivery is preferred?
4. Following delivery of 1st twin, enlist 2 parameters which needs to be assessed in second twin.

Ans.
1. Vaginal delivery
2. External cephalic version or internal podalic version
3. Cesarean delivery
4. Following delivery of 1st twin presenting part of second twin, its size and its relationship to the birth canal should be quickly and carefully ascertained by combined abdominal, vaginal and at times real-time ultrasound.

CHAPTER 16: Liver Disease in Pregnancy

Sarita Bhalerao, Latika Chawla, Ashwin Shetty, Kausha Shah

OSCE 1.

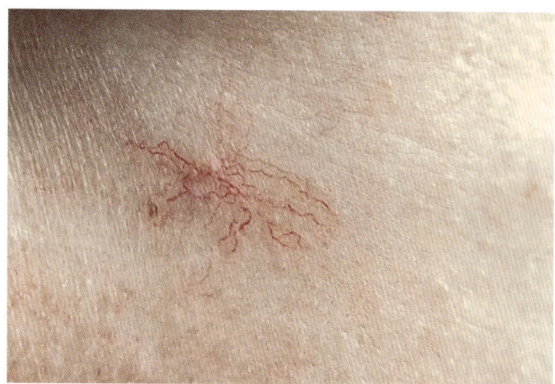

1. Name two skin findings in liver disease which can be seen in normal pregnancy.
2. Which liver biochemical test increases markedly in normal pregnancy?
3. Which liver biochemical test is increased in hyperemesis gravidarum?

Ans.

1. Spider angiomata and palmar erythema
2. Serum alkaline phosphatase
3. ALT and AST

OSCE 2.
A 28-year-old, primigravida comes with severe itchiness in palms and soles of feet. She is 33 weeks pregnant.
1. Which lab tests would you ask for?
2. What is the most likely diagnosis?
3. What are the possible triggers?
4. Which drug is used as first-line treatment, and in what dose?

Ans.

1. SGOT, SGPT, and bile acids.
2. Cholestasis of pregnancy
3. Genetic susceptibility and geographic variability
4. Ursodeoxycholic acid 10–20 mg/kg/day

Chapter 16: Liver Disease in Pregnancy

OSCE 3. A 25-year-old, primigravida comes to the emergency room at 36 weeks complaining of headache. Her BP is found to be 180/90 mm Hg and urine albumin 3+. Her blood tests show SGOT 325, SGPT 200, and platelets 80,000.
1. What is the most likely diagnosis?
2. What are the maternal risks?
3. What are the fetal risks?
4. How should this patient be managed?

Ans.
1. HELLP syndrome
2. Eclampsia, DIC
3. IUFD
4. Stabilize condition and expedite delivery.

OSCE 4. A 35-year-old primigravida, Asian, presented to OPD with severe itching at 32 weeks of gestation. However, there is no history of allergies/drug reaction. BP is normal.
1. What is the most probable diagnosis?
2. Which is the single definitive blood test that confirms IHCP?
3. Based on clinical features and laboratory parameters, how can IHCP be classified?
4. In singleton pregnancies, total bile acid conc. above what level has positive association with increased chances of IUFD?
5. In a case of pruritus in pregnancy to establish diagnosis of IHCP raised levels of this marker is the only one that can predict increased risk of stillbirth.

Ans.
1. Intrahepatic cholestasis of pregnancy (IHCP)
2. Raised total bile acid concentration
3. a. *Mild ICP:* Itching + raised peak bile acid = 19–39 μmol/L
   b. *Moderate ICP:* Itching + raised peak bile acid = 40–99 μmol/L
   c. *Severe ICP:* Itching + raised peak bile acid = more than 100 μmol/L
4. 100 μmol/L
5. Bile acid concentration alone.

OSCE 5. A 34-year-old lady with moderate IHCP came in labor at 37 weeks of gestation.
1. What investigations have not had a positive relation and are not required to be done in case of IHCP?
2. What postnatal follow-up should be taken? When should it be done?
3. In patients of IHCP what are the additional maternal risks?
4. Enumerate 2 perinatal risks in IHCP?

Ans.
1. LFT, hepatitis C, coagulation screen.
2. Repeat S. bile acids after 4 weeks postdelivery.

3. a. Increased risk of pre-eclampsia 12%
   b. Increased risk of gestational diabetes 13%
4. Chances of meconium-stained amniotic fluid and chances of stillbirth

OSCE 6. A 32-year-old primipara with 30 weeks MCDA twin pregnancy walks into your OPD complaining of reduced fetal movements since a few hours. She has had 3–4 episodes of vomiting and looks visibly agitated. On examination, she is icteric, and her BP is 160/100 mm Hg.
1. What is your diagnosis based on this clinical picture?
2. What is the most important therapeutic intervention for this patient?
3. Which liver function test helps differentiate between HELLP and AFLP?

Ans.
1. AFLP
2. Urgent delivery
3. PT and aPTT, low blood sugar

OSCE 7. Below are the LFTs of a 38-year-old multipara with 26 weeks singleton pregnancy admitted in your ward for management of uncontrolled pregnancy-induced hypertension. She is currently on maximum dosage of oral labetalol. You have added a second antihypertensive (nifedipine) hoping to control the blood pressure. She has been complaining of severe epigastric pain since morning. BP is 150/90 mm Hg, urine protein on dipstick is 3+. She had pre-eclampsia in her previous pregnancy and had to be delivered at 32 weeks.

LFTs 2 pm: Total bilirubin 0.6 mg/dL, direct bilirubin 0.1 mg/dL, ALT 100 IU/L, AST 120 IU/L, albumin 1 g/dL, LDH 512 IU/L.
1. What is your diagnosis?
2. Enumerate four risk factors for developing this condition.
3. What is the risk of maternal mortality in this condition?

Ans.
1. HELLP
2. Previous HELLP, pre-eclampsia, advance maternal age, multiple pregnancy
3. <1%

OSCE 8. Primi who reports to you at 9 weeks pregnancy with a viable pregnancy on scan and routine booking blood test showing *HbsAg positive*.
1. What are the implications for her pregnancy?
2. What are the implications for the baby?
3. What would you advise for delivery and breastfeeding?
4. If she also showed positivity for HBeAg what additional implications will be there for her pregnancy?

Ans.

1. a. Immunological changes during pregnancy and the postpartum period have been associated with hepatitis flares. Pregnant women who are HBsAg positive should have further testing to measure baseline HBeAg, hepatitis B e antibody (anti-HBe), HBV DNA, and aminotransferase levels. Those who have a high HBV DNA (>106 copies/mL), elevated aminotransferase levels, and/or a positive HBeAg should be referred to a hepatologist to see if early initiation of antiviral medications is needed.
   b. Women with cirrhosis are at significant risk for perinatal complications and poor maternal and fetal outcome.
   c. Antiviral therapy is recommended for patients with a persistently elevated ALT >2 times the upper limit of normal and an elevated HBV DNA (HBV DNA >20,000 international units/mL in HBeAg-positive patients or HBV DNA ≥2,000 international units/mL in HBeAg-negative patients to reduce the risk of mother-to-child transmission.
      Tenofovir disoproxil fumarate (TDF) is antiviral therapy used.
      Women with cirrhosis fetal risks are intrauterine growth restriction, intrauterine infection, premature delivery, and intrauterine fetal demise.

2. a. The risk of mother-to-child transmission of hepatitis B virus (HBV) from hepatitis B surface antigen (HBsAg)-positive mothers to their infants has been reported to be as high as 90% without the use of active and passive immunization
   b. Transmission can occur in utero, at birth, or after birth
      The risk of HBV transmission is significantly reduced with the introduction of universal maternal HBV screening, hepatitis B vaccination of all newborns, and the use of prophylactic hepatitis B immune globulin (HBIG) and the first dose of hepatitis B vaccine at birth for infants of HBsAg-positive mothers. It is important that the infant complete the hepatitis B vaccine series.
   c. Transmission was significantly associated with having a mother who was hepatitis B e antigen (HBeAg) positive, had a HBV viral load >2,000 international units/mL, or was <25 years old; transmission was also associated with receiving <3 doses of the hepatitis B vaccine series.
   d. Maternal serum HBV DNA levels correlate with the risk of transmission. Vertical transmission of hepatitis B occurs in 9–39% of infants of highly viremic mothers despite postnatal vaccination.

3. a. Cesarean delivery is not routinely recommended for carrier mothers for the sole purpose of reducing HBV transmission.
   b. Breastfeeding and transmission—transmission of HBV through breastfeeding is unlikely, particularly in infants who received HBIG and hepatitis B vaccine at birth.
   c. Mothers with chronic hepatitis B who are breastfeeding should also exercise care to prevent bleeding from cracked nipples. HBsAg-positive mothers should not participate in donating breast milk.

4. a. The most important risk factors for mother-to-child transmission, despite proper administration of prophylaxis (HBIG and first dose of hepatitis B vaccine given within 12 hours of birth and completion of hepatitis B vaccine series), appear to be a positive HBeAg and/or a high HBV DNA level in the mother.
   b. Children born to HBeAg-positive mothers remain at risk for HBV infection, even if they receive hepatitis B vaccination and HBIG.
   c. According to the World Health Organization (WHO), HBeAg may be used as an indicator for antiviral prophylaxis when testing for HBV DNA is not available

OSCE 9. Primi with a known *hepatitis C infection* gets pregnant and reports to you at 10 weeks following a dating scan showing viable intrauterine gestation.
1. How would you investigate her further?
2. What are implications for her pregnancy and the baby?
3. How would you advise on delivery and lactation?

Ans.

1. a. Most women chronically infected with HCV will have an uneventful pregnancy without worsening of liver disease or other adverse effects on the mother or fetus.
   b. Transmission of HCV from the mother to the newborn can occur, with estimated rates of transmission between 3 and 10%. Vertical transmission refers to viral transmission from the mother to the infant during pregnancy, at the time of delivery, or during the first 28 days after birth.
   c. Women with cirrhosis are at significant risk for perinatal complications and poor maternal and fetal outcomes. The management of cirrhosis in a pregnant woman does not differ from that of nonpregnant patients. Variceal screening with endoscopy is still recommended and is safe during pregnancy. Active variceal bleeding should be managed the same way with banding.
2. a. Women with cirrhosis fetal risks are intrauterine growth restriction, intrauterine infection, premature delivery, and intrauterine fetal demise.
   b. The safety and efficacy of direct-acting antiviral agents during pregnancy and in neonates have not yet been assessed, and these agents should not be used.
3. a. The mode of delivery does not appear to be associated with the risk of vertical transmission of HCV. Invasive obstetric procedures, such as scalp electrode monitoring of the fetus during delivery, may increase the risk of HCV transmission. Avoiding prolonged rupture of membranes >6 hours in HCV-infected women is recommended.
   b. If mother has a coinfection with HIV-cesarean delivery may decrease the risk of HCV transmission. This is minimized if mother is on antiretroviral therapy for HIV.
   c. The available evidence suggests that breastfeeding by an HCV-infected mother does not appreciably increase the risk of transmitting HCV to her offspring.
   d. Women should abstain from breastfeeding if their nipples are cracked or bleeding.

OSCE 10. A 34-year-old primipara is admitted in the ICU for management of HELLP syndrome. She is 28 weeks pregnant. Answer the following as true/false with respect

to antenatal corticosteroid (CS) therapy in patients with HELLP syndrome awaiting delivery.
1. Delivery should be planned 24 hours after the last dose.
2. It has been shown to be effective in severe pre-eclampsia but it seems to be less beneficial in the HELLP syndrome.
3. Along with fetal lung maturation benefits, CS reduces maternal mortality in women with HELLP.
4. Multiple doses are not recommended.

Ans.
1. T
2. T
3. F
4. T

CHAPTER 17

HIV in Pregnancy

Sheela Mane, Radhika MS

OSCE 1.

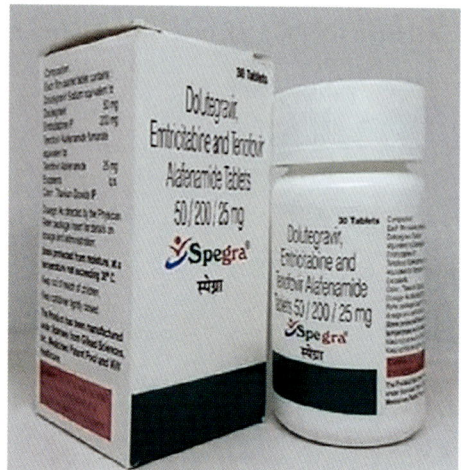

1. Expand HAART.
2. What are the principles of HAART?
3. What is the classification of HAART?
4. Enumerate two side effects of Abacavir.
5. What is the normal regimen followed in pregnancy?

Ans.

1. Highly active antiretroviral therapy
2. Principles of antiretroviral therapy:
   - Medication adherence is critical to maintain viral suppression and minimize emergence of viral resistance.
   - Avoid monotherapy to prevent emergence of resistance and drug failure.
   - Three or more antiretroviral agents are more effective than two agents.
   - First regimen provides best chance for complete viral suppression and immunologic recovery.
   - Never add a single agent to a failing regimen.
   - Resistance to one drug is likely to alert resistance to another drug in the same class (Resistance testing).

3. Classification of HAART.
    - Non-nucleoside reverse transcriptase inhibitors (NNRTIs)
    - Nucleoside reverse transcriptase inhibitors (NRTIs)
    - Protease inhibitors (PIs)
    - Integrase inhibitors
4. Side effects of abacavir:
    a. Hypersensitivity in HLA B5701 carriers.
    b. Hyperlactatemia
    c. Lactic acidosis
5. Normal regimen followed in pregnancy to start ART as soon as diagnosed and not wait for CD4 counts.
    - Tenofovir
    - Lamivudine
    - Efavirenz

OSCE 2.

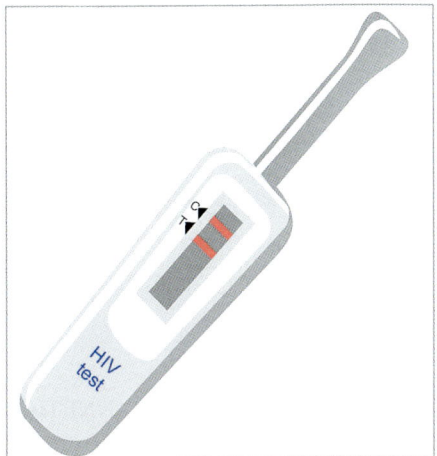

1. Name the test.
2. What is the principle of this test?
3. What is the screening of HIV in routine antenatal care?
4. What is opt-in and opt-out approach?
5. Enumerate CD4 count testing principles in a retropositive pregnant woman.

Ans.

1. ELISA
2. *Principle of the above test:* ELISA is also known as a solid-phase enzyme immunoassay that is used to detect the presence of a specific protein (antigen or antibody) in blood samples. The basic principle of ELISA is to use an enzyme to detect the binding of antigen (Ag) or antibody (Ab).
3. Voluntary counseling and testing center (VCTC) at the antenatal clinic to all pregnant women with an 'opt-out' approach is offered.

4. a. *Opt-in HIV testing:* Requires health provider to provide counseling and a separate written informed consent, which patients must sign before being permitted to have an HIV test.
   b. *Opt-out HIV testing:* Patients are informed either orally or via general medical consent that HIV testing will be included as part of the routine blood tests. Patients can decline the HIV test (opt-out). Assent is inferred unless the patient declines testing.
5. CD4 counts testing principles in retropositive ANC.
   - In women conceiving on ART there should be a minimum of one CD4 cell count at baseline and one at delivery.
   - Who commence CART in pregnancy, a CD4 cell count should be performed as per routine initiation of cART with the addition of a CD4 count at delivery even if starting at CD4 >350 cells/mm.
   - HIV viral load should be performed 2–4 weeks after commencing cART, at least once every trimester, at 36 weeks and at delivery.
   - Liver function tests (LFTs) should be performed as per routine initiation of cART and then with each routine blood test.

OSCE 3.

1. What is the ATT (Antituberculosis treatment) regimen in a retropositive pregnant woman?
2. What is the drug interaction of ATT with ART?
3. What is the management of TB with HIV in pregnancy?

Ans.

1. First-line drugs:
   - Isoniazid
   - Rifampicin
   - Ethambutol
   - Pyrazinamide
2. All non-nucleoside reverse transcriptase inhibitors (NNRTIs) are metabolized in the liver by CYP3A isoenzymes.
   - Efavirenz (EFV) and nevirapine (NVP) also are substrates of CYP2B6 enzymes, and etravirine (ETR) is a substrate of CYP2C9 and CYP2C19 enzymes.
   - Co-administration with drugs that induce or inhibit these enzymes can alter NNRTI drug concentrations, resulting in virologic failure or adverse effects.
   - All NNRTIs (except Rilpivirine [RPV]) induce or inhibit CYP isoenzymes.
   - EFV acts as a mixed inducer and inhibitor, but, similarly to NVP, it primarily induces CYP3A and 2B6 enzymes.
3. For persons with HIV who are not already on ART, treatment for HIV should be initiated during treatment for TB disease, rather than at the end, to improve outcomes among TB patients co-infected with HIV.
   - Antiretroviral therapy should ideally be initiated within the first 2 weeks of TB treatment for patients with CD4 cell counts <50/mm^3 and by 8–12 weeks of TB treatment initiation for patients with CD4 cell counts ≥50/mm^3.
   - An important exception is HIV-infected patients with TB meningitis, in whom antiretroviral therapy should not be initiated in the first 8 weeks of antituberculosis therapy.

Chapter 17: HIV in Pregnancy

OSCE 4.
1. What are the do's and dont's of intrapartum management in a HIV positive pregnant woman?
2. What are the principles of augmentation?
3. What is cord clamping principle?

Ans.

1. Elective cesarean delivery reduces the risk of vertical transmission by about 50%.
   - Avoidance of breastfeeding, HAART therapy and appropriate mode of delivery has reduced MTCT rates from 25–30% to <1%. Baby may be bathed immediately.
   - Planned cesarean delivery is recommended (RCOG-2019) at 39 weeks for women taking HAART who have plasma viral load >50 copies/mL measured at 36 weeks.
2. Amniotomy and oxytocin augmentation for vaginal delivery should be avoided whenever possible.
   - Invasive procedures that might result in break in the skin or mucous membrane of the infants (procedures like attachment of scalp electrode and determination of scalp blood pH) are contraindicated.
   - Instrumentation (ventouse) is avoided.
3. Delayed cord clamping is safe and reduces neonatal anemia.
   - Intrapartum IV ZDV is not advised for women receiving ART regimens with HIV RNA copies <50/mL near delivery.
   - Perioperative or peripartum broad spectrum antibiotics should be given as per hospital protocol.

OSCE 5.
1. What is the principle of testing and prophylaxis of a newborn of a HIV positive mother?
2. Enumerate two adverse birth outcomes in a HIV positive woman.
3. What are the principles of breastfeeding in them?
4. What is the protocol for weaning?

Ans.

1. *Neonatal care:* Antiretroviral therapy (ART) should be given to all neonates regardless of breastfeeding within 4 hours of birth. A confirmatory HIV antibody test is done at 18 months. Once this test is negative, the child is declared to be free of HIV.
2. Preterm birth, low birthweight, stillbirth/intrauterine fetal death (IUFD), baseline risk of mother-to-child transmission (MTCT) of 20–25%
3. a. *Infant feeding:* Women living with HIV may feed their babies with formula milk (high income settings).
   b. Woman on CART who chooses to breastfeed is allowed to do so. She is informed about the low risk of transmission of HIV through breastfeeding.
   c. The woman and her infant need monthly review for HIV RNA viral load testing during and for 2 months after stopping breastfeeding.
   d. Maternal cART helps to minimize HIV transmission through breast milk and also protects the women. WHO recommends exclusive breastfeeding.

Breastfeeding considerations:
- Arrange for free formula as breastfeeding is contraindicated for the infant's health (jurisdictional variations exist).
- Beware of possible psychological repercussions to the patient for whom lactation is contraindicated; provide support services.
- Consideration for cabergoline to suppress lactation (BHIVA-2020)
- Off-label use for HIV-positive women
- Inform the patient about the earlier return of ovulation in absence of breastfeeding

4. The baby has to be weaned at 6 months abruptly and no mixed feeds to be done since mixed feeds will cause intestinal injury causing higher risk for viral entry through mucosa.

OSCE 6.
1. When should postexposure prophylaxis (PEP) be initiated?
2. What is the regimen and duration of PEP?
3. Enumerate the drugs used in PEP.

Ans.

1. Postexposure prophylaxis should be initiated within 72 hours of suspected exposure
2. Triple therapy for 4 weeks reduces the risk of seroconversion by more than 80%
3. Zidovudine 200 mg TID + Lamivudine 150 mg BID + Indinavir 800 mg TID

OSCE 7.
1. What are the current care recommendations contributing to decreased MTCT (mother to child transmission) of HIV?
2. What are the important postpartum issues to be discussed with a retropositive mother?

Ans.

1. a. Provide continued psychosocial support services, either within the medical system or available community resources.
   b. Screening for, and treatment of postpartum depression
   c. May administer MMR vaccine, if indicated for rubella nonimmunity, given the patient's CD4 count is >200 cells/mm (otherwise, exercise caution with live-viral vaccinations among HIV-positive individuals)
   d. Counsel the patient on preexposure prophylaxis for her partner if they are serodiscordant and if her HIV viral load is not suppressed.
2. a. Arrange for routine postpartum obstetrical follow-up
   b. Arrange Papanicolaou cervical cytology screening (particularly important for women living with HIV)
   c. Encourage adherence with long-term follow-up with primary care provider and virologist.
   d. Support completion of neonatal postexposure prophylaxis and pediatric care follow-up
   e. Recommend future preconceptional counseling

Chapter 17: HIV in Pregnancy

OSCE 8.
1. Enumerate two important points to be considered in prenatal care?
2. How is the disease progression assessed?
3. How is laboratory monitoring of a HIV positive pregnant woman done?

Ans.

1. Voluntary Counseling and Testing Center (VCTC) at the Antenatal Clinic (ANC) to all pregnant women with an opt-out approach is offered.
   In seropositive cases the following additional tests should be done:
   - Test for other STDs such as hepatitis B and C viruses, syphilis, *Chlamydia*, herpes and rubella, serological testing for cytomegalovirus and toxoplasmosis.
   - Timely diagnosis of tuberculosis and any fungal opportunistic infections.
   - Husband should be offered serological testing for HIV.
   - Counseling with education to the patient is done about the impact of HIV infection on pregnancy; perinatal transmissions, side effects of medications and mode of delivery. Pregnancy does not affect the progression of HIV disease.
   - Advise for vaccination (pneumococcal, hepatitis, Tdap and influenza) given.
2. Progression of the disease is assessed by CD4 T-lymphocyte counts and HIV RNA (viral load).
   - Assessment is done at every 3–4 months interval. A patient with low viral load (<3000 copies/mL) and high CD4 count (>750 cells/mm) has nearly a zero probability of progressing to AIDS within 3 years.
   - Women with CD4 count (≤350 cells/mm^3) or HIV RNA level ≥50,000 copies/mm^3 should be initiated with HAART (WHO)
3. HIV care needs a Multidisciplinary Team (MDT).
   - *Laboratory monitoring:* HIV resistance testing to be done before the start of treatment. Women on combined antiretroviral therapy (cART), viral load should be estimated 2–4 weeks after start of cART, once in each trimester, at 36 weeks and at delivery.
   - *Laboratory monitoring:* (a) CD4 cell count, (b) Viral load (HIV RNA-PCR), (c) HIV genotype, (d) HIV resistance testing, (e) complete blood count (CBC), platelet count, LFI, serum urea, creatinine, electrolytes, amylase and G6PD.

OSCE 9.
1. Enumerate two important points to be considered during contraceptive counseling of a HIV positive patient.
2. What are the methods of contraception which can be used in them?

Ans.

1. Contraceptive particularities for a HIV patient with CD4 count >200 cells/mm are:
   - Dual contraception is ideal; stress importance of condoms with HIV infection.
   - Avoid use of diaphragms or nonoxyl-9 spermicides.
   - No restrictions for use of combined hormonal contraceptives, however, potential drug-drug interactions between hormonal contraceptives and antiretroviral therapy may lead to failed contraception; individualized assessment is required.
   - Intrauterine contraceptive device (IUCD) is an option to be considered.

2. Barrier methods of contraception (condom or female condom) is effective in preventing transmission of the virus:
   - COCs (combined oral contraceptive pills) are avoided as drug interactions with ARV (antiretroviral drugs) affect their efficacy and safety.
   - IUCD (Copper IUCD and LNG-IUS) are safe and effective.
   - Implants and injectables can be safely used.
   - However, condom use should be continued regardless of the use of other method of contraception. The disease could be prevented predominantly by health education and by practice of safer sex.

OSCE 10.

1. What are the recommendations when an urgent invasive fetal procedure is required in a HIV infected patient who is not yet on treatment and has detectable viral load?
2. Enumerate the general interventions for a patient where combined ART appears to fail in viral suppression despite resistance analysis.
3. Write about the health maintenance of a HIV positive pregnant woman.

Ans.

1. Treatment recommendations:
   - Single-dose oral nevirapine 200 mg should be given 2–4 hours prior to the invasive prenatal procedure.
   - Commence an integrase-inhibitor containing combined antiretroviral therapy regimen (i.e., Raltegravir).
   - Achieves rapid viral load reduction
2. Procedural advice:
   - Avoid transplacental needle entry
   - Single entry technique
   - Review treatment adherence, exploring potential confounders or drug interactions with concomitant medications.
   - Consider therapeutic drug monitoring, if available
   - Consider intensifying/optimizing treatment regimen with input from virologist.
3. Vaccinate for HAV, influenza, pneumococcus, and pertussis (patient is immune to HBV); ensure receipt of COVID-19 vaccination:
   - Repeat third-trimester screening for syphilis, gonorrhea, and chlamydia (e.g., at 28–34 weeks' gestation)
   - Ensure access to psychosocial support services especially given a new diagnosis of HIV (Encourage and support treatment adherence)
   - Access to evaluation of domestic violence and perinatal mental health
   - Recommend delivery in a tertiary center or facility with access to pediatric care
   - Prepare the patient that breastfeeding is not recommended among women with HIV in resource-rich nations, irrespective of an undetectable viral load
   - Continued evaluation for onset of opportunistic infections.

CHAPTER 18

Fetal Growth Restriction

Pushpa Junghare

OSCE 1. A 35-year Primi with PIH came for her 4th visit to ANC OPD at 32 weeks of gestation. There was no maternal weight gain for the last 3 weeks. Symphysiofundal height (SFH) was 28 cm.
1. What do you suspect?
2. Name the investigation done for diagnosis.
3. When will you repeat fetal biometry?

Ans.
1. FGR (Fetal growth restriction)
2. Ultrasonography with Doppler imaging.
3. Fetal biometry is performed every 3 weekly.

OSCE 2.

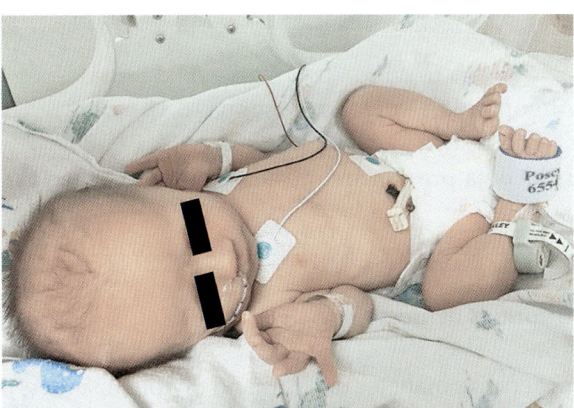

1. How do you define FGR fetus?
2. Which type of FGR this baby is having?
3. What are the types of FGR and what is the frequency of the 2 types?

Ans.
1. Fetus which fails to reach its normal growth potential with ultrasound estimated weight (EFW)/Abdominal circumference (AC) <3rd percentile is termed as FGR.

2. Asymmetrical FGR.
3. a. Asymmetric or late onset FGR, seen in 70% of cases.
   b. Symmetric FGR or early onset FGR, seen in 30% of cases.

Reference
1. Gordijn SJ, Beune, et al (2016). Consensus definition of fetal growth restriction: a Delphi procedure. Ultrasound Obstet Gynecol. 48:333-39. https://doi.org/10.1002/uog.15884

OSCE 3. The following diagram shows various factors causing fetal growth restriction.
1. Identify factor 1 and enumerate the causes under it which may lead to FGR.
2. Identify factor 2 and enumerate the causes under it which may lead to FGR.
3. Identify factor 3 and enumerate the causes under it which may lead to FGR.
4. Identify factor 4 and enumerate the causes under it which may lead to FGR.

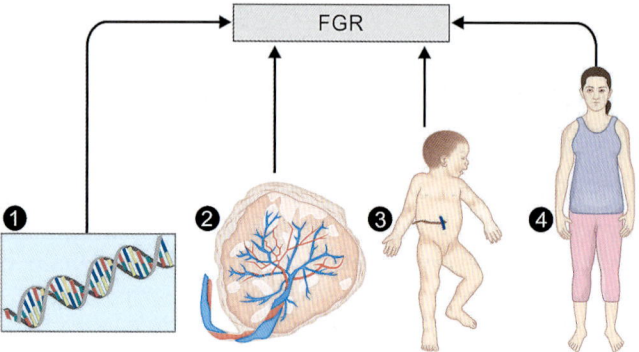

Ans.
1. *Genetic causes:* Aneuploidies such as Trisomy 13,18 and 21, Turner syndrome and chromosomal aberrations such as deletions.
2. *Placental factors:* Placenta previa, circumvallate placenta, chorioangioma and multiple placental infarcts.
3. *Fetal causes:* Multiple pregnancies, congenital diaphragmatic hernia, and omphalocele.
4. *Maternal causes:*
   - Hypertensive disorders of pregnancy
   - Chronic infections
   - Endocrine disorders like diabetes mellitus and thyroid disorders
   - Anemia
   - COPD, valvular heart disease, chronic renal diseases and APLA syndrome
   - Congenital abnormalities of uterus.

OSCE 4.

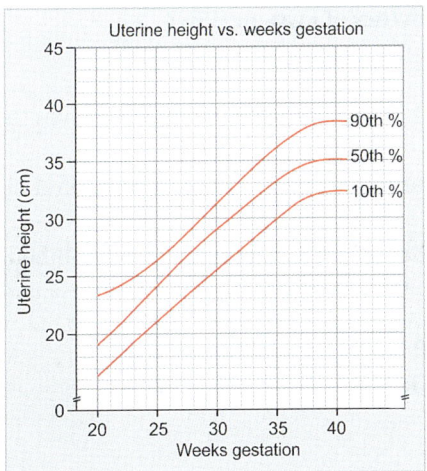

1. What does the graph represent?
2. What is Ponderal Index (PI)? What is the normal range?
3. How is PI calculated?
4. How is it affected in growth restriction?

Ans.

1. Gravidogram
2. Ponderal index determines how thin or fat a fetus is. Normal values range from 2.32 and 2.85.
3. It is calculated by the formula: $\dfrac{\text{Estimated fetal weight in gm} \times 100}{\text{Fetal length in cm}^3}$
4. Ponderal index <2 diagnoses an FGR baby.
   a. PI is normal in symmetric FGR/Early onset FGR
   b. PI is low in Asymmetric FGR/Late onset FGR

OSCE 5.

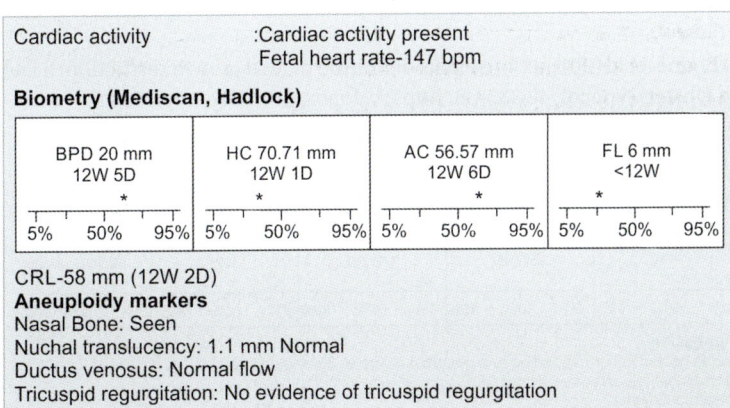

1. What is the most accurate parameter that should be measured to determine gestational age on ultrasound?

2. In the above picture, what are the parameters used for fetal growth estimation?
3. What are accurate predictors of FGR on USG?

Ans.

1. Crown rump length (CRL) measured at 8 to 13 weeks gives the most accurate gestational age.
2. Biparietal diameter, head circumference and abdominal circumference are the parameters of fetal growth.
3. Estimated fetal weight or abdominal circumference combined with Doppler studies.

OSCE 6.

1. Name the 2 types of FGR based on gestational age?
2. Define the 2 types of FGR.

Ans.

1. Early onset FGR (<32 weeks of gestation) and late onset FGR (>32 weeks gestation) in absence of congenital anomalies.
2. *Early FGR is defined as:*
   AC/EFW <3rd centile or UA (umbilical artery)-AEDF
   Or
   a. AC/EFW <10th centile *combined with*
   b. UtA-PI (Uterine artery-pulsatile index) >95th centile *and/or*
   c. UA-PI (Umbilical artery-pulsatile index) >95th centile

   Late FGR is defined as:
   AC/EFW <3rd centile
   Or
   At least two out of three of the following:
   a. AC/EFW <10th centile
   b. AC/EFW crossing centiles >2 quartiles on growth centiles
   c. CPR <5th centile or UA-PI >95th centile.

Reference

1. Gordijn SJ, Beune, et al (2016). Consensus definition of fetal growth restriction: a Delphi procedure. Ultrasound Obstet Gynecol. 48:333-39. https://doi.org/10.1002/uog.15884

OSCE 7.

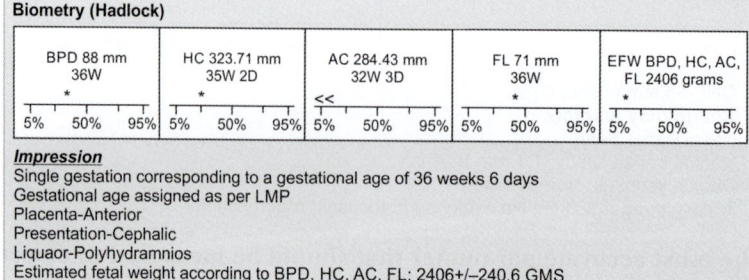

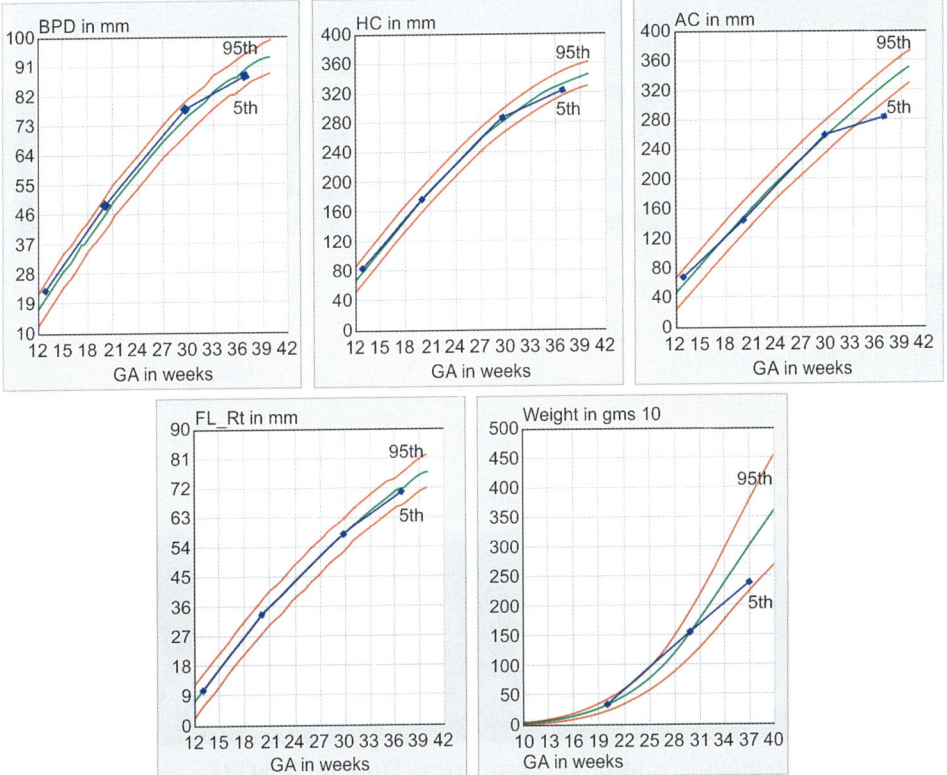

1. **What is the diagnosis?**
2. **What is the other terminology used for this diagnosis?**
3. **Enumerate the complications of FGR?**

Ans.

1. Asymmetrical FGR
2. Late onset FGR
3. Complications of FGR:
   - Perinatal asphyxia
   - Intraventricular Hemorrhage
   - Meconium Aspiration
   - Respiratory Distress syndrome
   - Hypothermia
   - Hypoglycemia
   - Necrotizing Enterocolitis

OSCE 8. The following picture shows Doppler images of umbilical arteries.
1. Identify image A.
2. Identify image B.
3. Identify image C.
4. Identify image D.

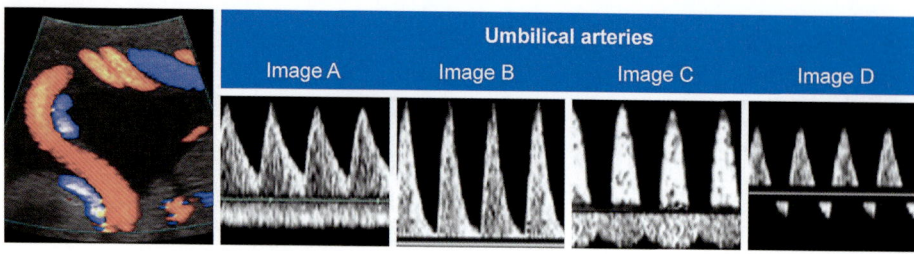

Ans.
1. Normal umbilical artery Doppler.
2. Raised Pulsatile index (PI).
3. Absent end diastolic flow (AEDF).
4. Reversal in end diastolic flow (REDF).

OSCE 9. With regard to middle cerebral artery (MCA).

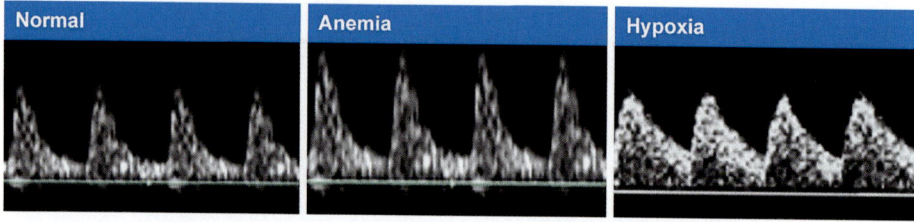

1. What are the changes in middle cerebral artery Doppler in FGR?
2. What does it indicate?
3. What is cerebro placental ratio (CPR)?
4. What is the significance of CPR?

Ans.
1. The pulsatile index (PI) is reduced in MCA in FGR.
2. It indicates brain sparing effect. It is a surrogate marker of fetal hypoxia.
3. Cerebro placental ratio is the ratio of MCA PI/Umbilical artery PI.
4. It is the most sensitive marker of redistribution of blood in fetal hypoxia.
   CPR less than 1 is the earliest sign of cerebral hypoxia and is a very important marker in late onset FGR.

OSCE 10. The following diagram shows Doppler image of ductus venosus.

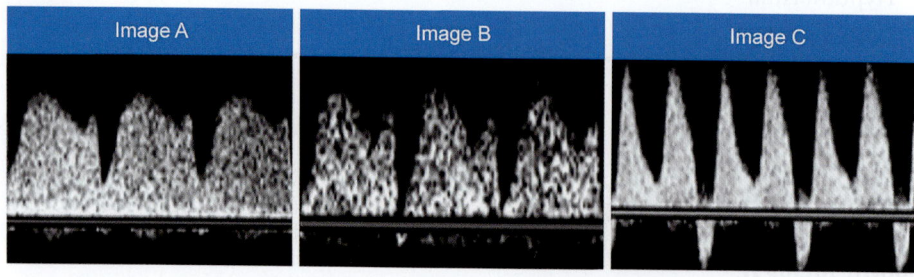

1. Identify image A.
2. Identify image B.
3. Identify image C.

Ans.

1. Normal ductus venosus Doppler.
2. Absent a-wave.
3. Reversal of a-wave.

OSCE 11.

1. What is the significance of ductus venuses (DV) Doppler in FGR?
2. What does pulsatile DV indicate?
3. What are other USG indications for early termination of pregnancy?

Ans.

1. DV waveform becomes abnormal in advanced stages of fetal compromise: first there is absence of a wave and then reversal of a wave.
2. Pulsatile DV is a gross abnormality and is an indication to deliver the fetus irrespective of gestational age.
3. a. Abnormal Biophysical score.
   b. Oligohydramnios.
   c. Poor or no growth of fetus over a week.

OSCE 12.

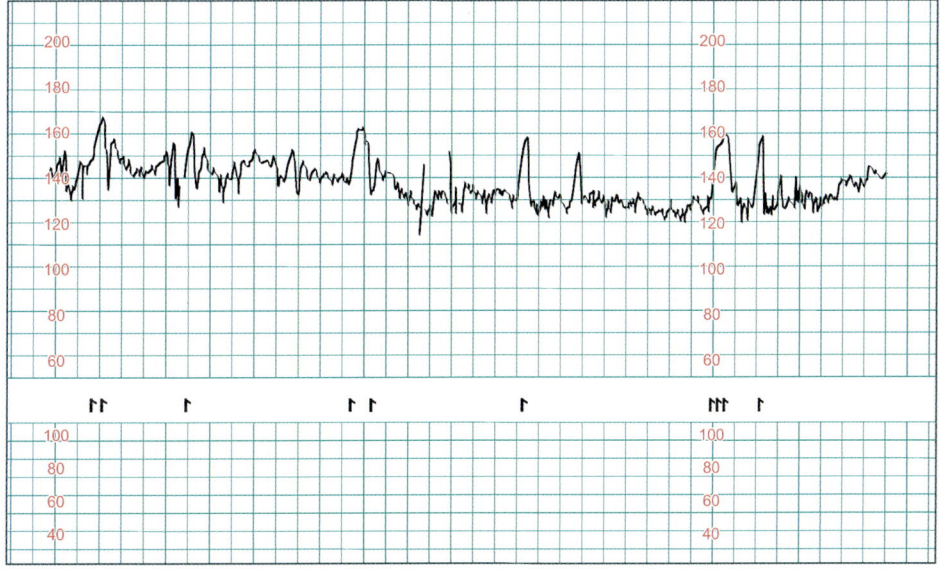

1. Name four methods for fetal surveillance in FGR?
2. How often should NST be repeated if it is reactive?
3. What are the various types of decelerations on CTG?

Ans.
1. Methods for fetal surveillance in FGR are:
   a. DFMC (daily fetal movement count) by the patient.
   b. Clinical examination/Gravidogram
   c. Modified Biophysical profile on ultrasonography
   d. NST (Nonstress test)
2. NST should be repeated every 72 hours
3. Early, Late and Variable deceleration.

OSCE 13. Primigravida at 37 weeks of gestation with PIH (pregnancy induced hypertension) came with the following USG report:

Fetal Biometry:
- *BPD:* **8.71 cm-35 w 1 d**
- *HC:* **30.93 cm-34 w 4 d**
- *AC:* **29.55 cm-33 w 4 d**
- *FL:* **6.94 cm-35 w 4 d**

Average maturity by USG is *34 w 6 d. EFW-2454 gm*

Fetal muscle tone: **No movement in 30 minutes**

Fetal body movements: **Two in 30 minutes**

Fetal breathing movements: **None**

AFI- 6 cm

NST was reactive:
1. What is her Biophysical Profile Score?
2. What does her USG biometry indicate?
3. What further investigation should be advised?

Ans.
1. 4
2. FGR
3. Obstetric color Doppler study.

OSCE 14. A Primigravida at 35 weeks comes with USG report showing AC (abdominal circumference) corresponding to 2nd centile and Umbilical artery PI (Pulsatile Index) >95th centile.
1. What is the diagnosis?
2. At what gestation should she be delivered?
3. What would be the mode of delivery?

Ans.
1. FGR Stage 1
2. 37 weeks

3. Vaginal delivery by labor induction according to Bishop's score. A caesarean section would have to be done in case of other obstetric reasons like malpresentation/placenta previa etc.

Reference
1. Lees CC, Stampalija, et al (2020). ISUOG Practice Guidelines: diagnosis and management of small-for-gestational-age fetus and fetal growth restriction. Ultrasound Obstet Gynecol. 56:298-312. https://doi.org/10.1002/uog.22134

OSCE 15. A Primigravida at 32 weeks comes with USG report showing AEDF in the umbilical artery.
1. What is the diagnosis?
2. How frequently should Doppler be monitored in her case?
3. At what gestation should she be delivered if Doppler on further monitoring does not worsen?
4. What would be the mode of delivery?

Ans.
1. FGR stage 2
2. Biweekly
3. 34 weeks
4. Labor induction depending on Bishop's score should be done. However, the risk of emergent caesarean section at labor induction exceeds 50%, therefore, elective caesarean section remains a reasonable option.

Reference
1. Lees CC, Stampalija, et al. (2020), ISUOG Practice Guidelines: diagnosis and management of small-for-gestational-age fetus and fetal growth restriction. Ultrasound Obstet Gynecol. 56:298-312. https://doi.org/10.1002/uog.22134

OSCE 16. A G2P1L1 with previous vaginal delivery presents at 30 weeks with USG report showing REDF in the umbilical artery.
1. What is the diagnosis?
2. How frequently should Doppler be monitored in her case?
3. Within what time duration should she be delivered?
4. What would be the mode of delivery?

Ans.
1. FGR stage 3
2. Monitoring every 24–48 hours until delivery is recommended.
3. Within 48 hours.
4. Caesarean section.

Reference
1. Lees CC, Stampalija, et al. (2020). ISUOG Practice Guidelines: diagnosis and management of small-for-gestational-age fetus and fetal growth restriction. Ultrasound Obstet Gynecol. 56:298-312. https://doi.org/10.1002/uog.22134

Section 1: Obstetrics

OSCE 17. A Primigravida presents at 29 weeks with USG report showing EFW at 2nd centile along with abnormal ductus venosus Doppler.
1. What is the diagnosis?
2. What is the management?
3. What would be the mode of delivery?

Ans.

1. FGR Stage 4
2. Steroid prophylaxis and Magnesium sulphate for neuroprotection along with termination of pregnancy.
3. Caesarean section.

Reference
1. Lees CC, Stampalija, et al. (2020), ISUOG Practice Guidelines: diagnosis and management of small-for-gestational-age fetus and fetal growth restriction. Ultrasound Obstet Gynecol. 56:298-312. https://doi.org/10.1002/uog.22134

OSCE 18.
1. What additional drug should be administered in case of delivery of fetus before 34 weeks?
2. What are the advantages of administering this drug?
3. Name one maternal condition in which additional precaution and monitoring is required while administering the above drug.

Ans.

1. Steroid prophylaxis by Betamethasone/dexamethasone.
2. Steroid prophylaxis helps in fetal lung maturity, prevention of RDS (respiratory distress syndrome) and necrotizing enterocolitis.
3. Diabetes complicating pregnancy since steroid can cause hyperglycemia.

OSCE 19. A 36 year, Primigravida with IVF conception presents at 32 weeks of gestation with BP of 160/110 mm Hg. The height of uterus is 28 weeks.
1. What is the diagnosis?
2. What investigations will you carry out?
3. What medications will you give her?
4. How will you manage this patient?
5. What are indications for caesarean in patients with FGR?

Ans.

1. Hypertensive disorder of pregnancy with FGR
2. a. PIH profile
   b. Fundoscopy
   c. Biophysical profile with fetal biometry and Doppler study

3. Antihypertensive drugs, Magnesium sulphate for neuroprotection and steroids.
4. Termination of pregnancy apart from management of hypertension.
5. Indications for caesarean section:
   - Obstetrical indications
   - Foetal hypoxia
   - Severe oligohydramnios
   - Breech presentation.

OSCE 20.

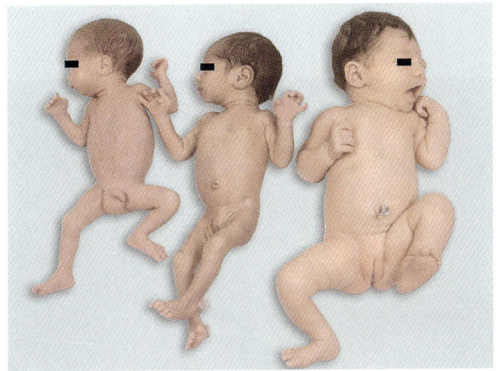

1. What is the problem with the first two babies?
2. What parameters should be assessed after delivery?
3. What are the indications for admission to NICU?
4. What are the long-term complications of FGR?

Ans.

1. FGR babies
2. Parameters to be assessed after delivery:
   - Weight
   - Height
   - Head circumference
   - Congenital abnormalities to be ruled out.
   - Assessment of physical and neuromuscular maturity
3. Indications for NICU admission are:
   - Prematurity
   - Birth weight less than 1.8 kg
   - Complications like RDS, meconium aspiration.
4. The potential long-term complications of FGR are:
   - Cerebral palsy
   - Behavioral and Learning problems
   - Altered postnatal growth
   - Metabolic syndrome

CHAPTER 19

Antepartum Hemorrhage

Jaya Chawla

OSCE 1.

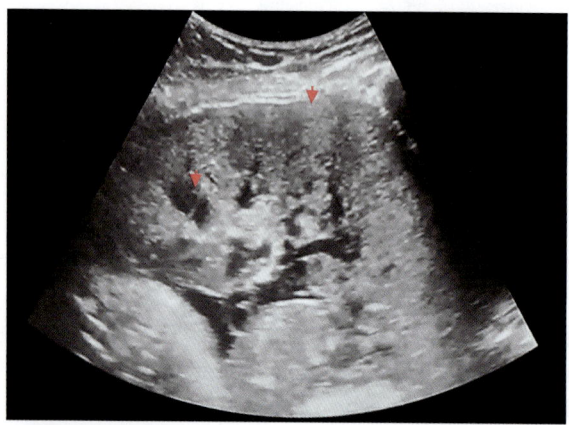

1. What is the provisional diagnosis?
2. Name three 2D gray scale features that support your diagnosis.
3. How can you confirm this diagnosis in a posteriorly situated placenta?

Ans.

1. Placenta accreta spectrum
2. Multiple vascular lacunae within placenta, loss of retroplacental hypoechoic zone and reduction in retroplacental myometrial thickness to <1 mm.
   Others:
   a. Bladder wall interruption—loss or interruption of the bright bladder wall (the hyperechoic band or 'line 'between the uterine serosa and the bladder lumen).
   b. Placental bulge deviation of the uterine serosa away from the expected plane, caused by an abnormal bulge of placental tissue into a neighboring organ, typically bladder.
   c. Exophytic mass—placental tissue seen breaking through the uterine serosa and extending beyond it. Most often seen inside a filled urinary bladder.
3. Magnetic resonance imaging (MRI)

Reference

1. Placenta Accreta Spectrum, Obstetric Care Consensus Number 7, December 2018.

OSCE 2.

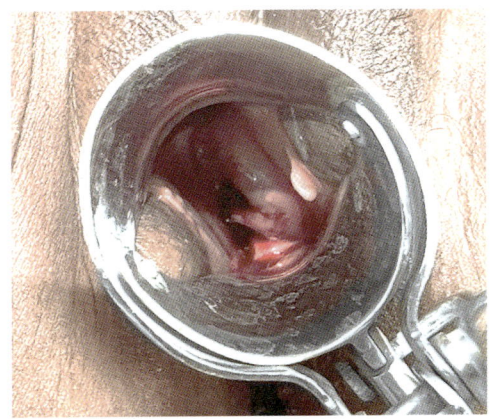

A 32-year-old lady, G2+1+0+1 prior cesarean birth, presents to the outpatient department at 27 weeks with complaints of bleeding per vaginum 48 hours ago. Her per speculum picture is as above. Her blood group is O negative and her husband's is O positive. Her indirect Coomb's test is negative at 26 weeks.
1. What medication should be offered to reduce the risk of isoimmunization and in what dose?
2. Enumerate the routes of administration of this medication.

Ans.

1. Anti-D immunoglobulin; 1,500 IU or 300 µg
2. Intramuscular and intravenous

Reference

1. Visser GHA, Thommesen T, Di Renzo GC, Nassar AH, Spitalnik SL. FIGO/ICM guidelines for preventing Rhesus disease: A call to action. 2021;152(2):144-7.

OSCE 3.

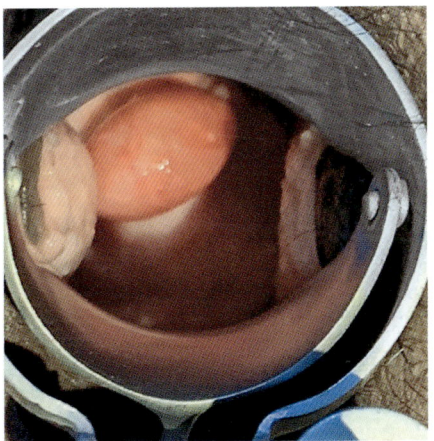

Section 1: Obstetrics

A 33-year-old lady presents to the gyne outpatient department at 26 weeks gestation with complaints of bleeding per vaginum following intercourse two days back. She is a second gravida with prior one normal vaginal birth 3 years back. There is no associated abdominal pain or leaking. She has no comorbidities. The uterus is relaxed and nontender. Fetal heart sounds—152 beats per minute. Speculum examination is as shown above.

1. What is the most likely cause of bleeding in this case?
2. What test shall be most appropriate to confirm the diagnosis?
3. Cervical cancer screening is mandatory during pregnancy as per Indian guidelines. True/false?
4. Name the most appropriate test for cervical cancer screening as per currently available evidence.

Ans.

1. Cervical polyp
2. Histopathology
3. False
4. Pap smear

Reference

1. Zagorianakou N, Mitrogiannis I, Konis K, Makrydimas S, Mitrogiannis L, Makrydimas, G. The HPV-DNA Test in Pregnancy: A Review of the Literature. Cureus. 2023;15(5):e38619.

OSCE 4. A 37-year-old, G2P1L1 at 34 weeks and 2 days gestation presented with severe pain abdomen since last night. Her last pregnancy details included the birth of a baby weighing 1.8 kg at 38 weeks with history of bleeding per vaginum after which the labor had been augmented. She had also been on antihypertensives in her last pregnancy. At present pulse = 130 per minute; BP = 130/60 mm Hg; uterus is 36 weeks, tetanic contraction on palpation.

Test Name	Result	Unit	Biological ref. Interval
Prothrombin time			
Patient's time	20.7	In seconds	
Control time	12.8	In seconds	
I.N.R	1.70		1.0–1.3
Activated partial thromboplastin time #(APTT)			
Patient's time	55.0	In seconds	
Control time	28.5	In seconds	
Reference Rnage: 24–40 seconds			

Her coagulation profile report is attached above:

1. What classification is used to assess the severity of the condition described above?
2. What is the class of disease as assessed from above findings, as per the classification?

3. What blood product should be transfused to correct hypofibrinogenemia?
4. One unit of the blood product of choice raises the fibrinogen levels by .... mg/dL.

Ans.

1. Page's classification
2. Class 4
3. Cryoprecipitate
4. 10

References

1. Page EW, King EB, Merrill JA. Abruptio placentae, dangers of delay in delivery. Obstet Gynecol. 1954;3:385-93.
2. Escobar MF, Nassar AH, Theron G, et al. FIGO recommendations on the management of postpartum hemorrhage 2022. Int J Gynecol Obstet. 2022;157(Suppl 1): 3-50.

OSCE 5.

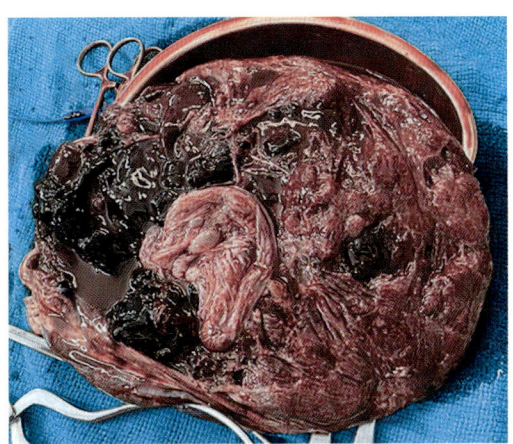

The case in previous question is optimized and labor augmented. She delivers a stillborn baby with retroplacental hemorrhage as shown in the picture above. During the course of her optimization, she is found to be rhesus negative, nonisoimmunized pregnancy. Her husband is O positive.

1. What would be the most appropriate time for administration of anti-D injection in the case?
2. What percentage of cases develop DIC after retained intrauterine dead fetus?
3. What is the test used to quantify the dose of anti-D required for prophylaxis of alloimmunization?
4. Antenatal ultrasound has good sensitivity and specificity for diagnosis of placental abruption. True/false?

Ans.

1. As soon as intrauterine fetal death (IUFD) is confirmed.
2. 10% at 4 weeks

3. Kleihauer Betke test
4. False

Reference
1. Antepartum Hemorrhage Green–top Guideline No. 63 November 2011.

OSCE 6. A 26-year-old, primigravida reports to obstetric triage with 36 weeks pregnancy and profuse bleeding per vaginum that she has noticed since morning as she got up from bed. There have been episodes of spotting per vaginum earlier at 32 and 34 weeks as well. The emergency ultrasound performed suggests placenta covering the os. She is in shock.
1. What will be the mode of termination of this pregnancy?
2. She has lost three liters of blood during surgery. What is the ratio in which blood products should be replaced?
3. How is massive transfusion protocol defined?
4. What are the percentage chances of her developing a placenta accreta in the next pregnancy after this one prior cesarean section if she develops placenta previa again?

Ans.
1. Emergency cesarean section
2. 1:1:1 for PRBC:Platelets:FFP
3. Requirements of ≥4 PRBC units (some articles considered ≥10 PRBC within 24 hours), replacement of total blood volume within 24 hours, or replacement of 50% of blood volume within 3 hours.
4. 3%

Reference
1. Escobar MF, Nassar AH, Theron G, et al. FIGO recommendations on the management of postpartum hemorrhage 2022. Int J Gynecol Obstet. 2022;157(Suppl 1): 3–50. doi:10.1002/ijgo.14116

OSCE 7. A 32-year-old G2P1L1with prior cesarean section is undergoing trial of labor at 39 weeks gestation. She has been augmented with injection Oxytocin in the active phase of labor. She has been fully dilated for one hour with head station at +2 station. The resident on duty reports a sudden prolonged deceleration of >5 minutes and seeks consultant opinion. Upon examination, the consultant finds a tonically contracted uterus and the head station to be 0. Also, the gloved finger is smeared with blood.
1. What is your provisional diagnosis?
2. Match the following risks of trial of labor after prior cesarean section with their corresponding percentage occurrence:
    a. Surgical injury   1. 0.71%
    b. Blood transfusion   2. 0.3–1.3%
    c. Uterine rupture   3. 0.66%

Ans.
1. Rupture uterus
2. a-2, b-3, c-1

References

1. Birth After Previous Caesarean Birth Green-top Guideline No. 45 October 2015.
2. ACOG Practice bulletin no. 115: Vaginal birth after previous cesarean delivery. Obstet Gynecol. 2010;116(2 Pt 1):450-63.
3. Ayres-de-Campos D, Spong CY, Chandraharan E. FIGO consensus guidelines on intrapartum fetal monitoring: Cardiotocography. Int. J Obstet Gynaecol. 2015;131(1): 13-24. https://doi.org/10.1016/j.ijgo.2015.06.020.

OSCE 8. A 36-year-old, primigravida presents to obstetric triage at 32 weeks singleton gestation with complaints of bleeding per vaginum since last evening. She has soaked three pads since last evening. She is hemodynamically stable. USG reveals a placenta covering the os. The resident doctor on duty seeks consultant review to administer steroids for fetal lung maturity and also tocolysis until the cover is completed.

1. Tocolysis is always indicated in a case of antepartum hemorrhage when presenting preterm: True/False?
2. Nifedipine is the drug of choice when tocolysis is indicated in antepartum hemorrhage: True/False?
3. Name two contraindications to tocolysis in antepartum hemorrhage.

Ans.

1. False
2. False
3. Hemodynamic instability/Placental abruption

Reference

1. Antepartum Hemorrhage Green-top Guideline No. 63 November 2011.

OSCE 9. A 34-year-old primigravida is undergoing induction of labor for uncontrolled pre-eclampsia with severe features. The growth scan suggests an appropriately grown fetus with adequate liquor and admission test is normal. Per abdomen, the fundal height corresponds to 32–34 weeks gestation with engaged head. The resident doctor on duty performs an artificial rupture of membranes at 4 centimeters dilatation. The gloved finger is smeared with small amount of blood. The post ARM cardiotocography trace shows a prolonged deceleration of >5 minutes.

1. What is the most likely provisional diagnosis?
2. What category cesarean is indicated in a sudden prolonged deceleration?
3. What are two most common causes of prolonged sudden deceleration?
4. What are two most common conditions associated with vasa previa?

Ans.

1. Vasa Previa
2. Category 1 cesarean
3. Rupture uterus, severe abruptio placentae, cord prolapse
4. Velamentous insertion of cord and succenturiate lobe or bilobed placenta, IVF, placenta previa or low-lying placenta in the second trimester, and multiple gestation.

References

1. Jauniaux ERM, Alfirevic Z, Bhide AG, Burton GJ, Collins SL, Silver R on behalf of the Royal College of Obstetricians and Gynaecologists. Vasa praevia: diagnosis and management. Green-top Guideline No. 27b. BJOG 2018.
2. Society of Maternal-Fetal (SMFM) Publications Committee, Sinkey RG, Odibo AO, Dashe JS. #37: Diagnosis and management of vasa previa. Am J Obstet Gynecol. 2015;213:615-9.
3. Ayres-de-Campos D, Spong CY, Chandraharan E. FIGO consensus guidelines on intrapartum fetal monitoring: Cardiotocography. Int J Gynaecol Obstet. 2015; 131(1):13-24.

OSCE 10. Please refer to the picture below and answer the following questions:

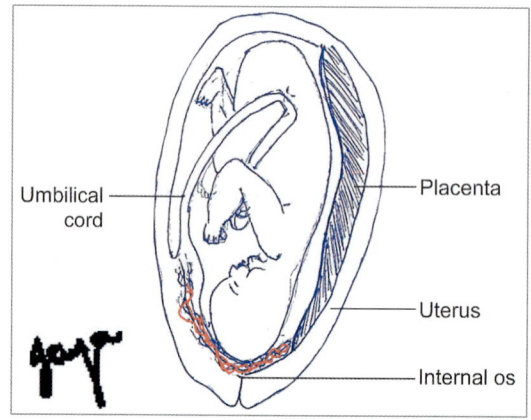

1. Give a provisional diagnosis.
2. Give one differential diagnosis of this condition.
3. Give one cardiotocographic abnormality associated with this condition.
4. When should elective birth be planned for women diagnosed with vasa previa?

Ans.

1. Vasa previa
2. Cord presentation
3. Sinusoidal pattern or prolonged deceleration
4. Between 34 and 37 weeks

Reference

1. Society of Maternal-Fetal (SMFM) Publications Committee, Sinkey RG, Odibo AO, Dashe JS. #37: Diagnosis and management of vasa previa. Am J Obstet Gynecol. 2015;213:615-9.

OSCE 11. A 31-year-old G5P1L1A3 lady was admitted for change over from warfarin to unfractionated heparin (UFH) at 36 weeks. She has a history of both mitral as well as aortic valve replacement with mechanical valve prosthesis when she was 10 years of age. She was also on aspirin (150 mg OD) prophylaxis as she had tested positive for lupus anticoagulant on two occasions 16 weeks apart as part of her investigations for recurrent pregnancy loss.

During switch over day 3, she had received 7 mg tablet warfarin, and 10,000 units twice a day of subcutaneous UFH. She developed per vaginum bleed.

1. What would be the preferred mode of birth in this case?
2. What can be done to optimize her coagulation status prior to initiating termination of pregnancy?
3. How soon can the anticoagulation be initiated postpartum if hemostasis is ensured, in case of (i) vaginal birth (ii) cesarean section.

Ans.

1. Cesarean section
2. Fresh-frozen plasma/four-factor prothrombin concentrate
3. (i) 4–6 hours (ii) 6–12 hours

Reference

1. Regitz-Zagrosek V, Roos-Hesselink JW, Bauersachs J, Blomström-Lundqvist C, Cífková R, ESC Scientific Document Group, et al. 2018 ESC Guidelines for the management of cardiovascular diseases during pregnancy. Eur Heart J. 2018;39(34):3165-241. doi: 10.1093/eurheartj/ehy340

OSCE 12. A 34-year-old, G4P3L3 patient was referred from a peripheral hospital as a case of diamniotic dichorionic twin gestation with 24 weeks amenorrhea with intrauterine demise of both twins, profuse vaginal bleeding since 2 hours and shortness of breath. She had history of fever since three days. PR = 120/minute; BP = 130/80 mm Hg; Temp: 99°C; respiratory and cardiovascular systems NAD; Hb: 7.4 g/dL; platelet count: 54,000/cu mm; PT/aPTT within normal limits. USG revealed twin intrauterine demise both 24 weeks, with large retroplacental collection. NS1 antigen positive.

1. What are the four WHO criteria for dengue hemorrhagic fever?
2. Name two specific blood tests for diagnosis of dengue.
3. Enumerate warning signs of dengue fever.

Ans.

1. a. Ongoing fever or recent history of fever that lasts 2–7 days.
   b. Hemorrhagic manifestations
   c. Platelet count <100,000/cu mm
   d. Any evidence of increased vascular permeability.

Reference

1. World Health Organization. Dengue and Dengue Haemorrhagic Fever. Fact sheet 117, 2009.

2. (i) Dengue NS1 antigen and (ii) dengue IgM antibody are used for the diagnosis of dengue during the acute phase of infection.
3. The warning signs are as follow:
   a. Severe abdominal pain
   b. Persistent vomiting
   c. Mucosal bleed
   d. Clinical fluid accumulation
   e. Lethargy, restlessness

Reference
1. Dengue: Guidelines for Diagnosis, Treatment, Prevention and Control: New Edition. Geneva: World Health Organization; 2009. 4, Laboratory Diagnosis and Diagnostic Tests. Available from: https://www.ncbi.nlm.nih.gov/books/NBK143156/

OSCE 13. In case of placenta accreta spectrum disorders, state whether following practices are supported by currently available evidence:
1. Bilateral internal iliac artery ligation is of proven benefit. True/false?
2. Balloon occlusion is advocated irrespective of the degree of hemorrhage. True/False?
3. Tranexamic acid if available should be administered immediately prior to cesarean birth. True/False?
4. Subtotal hysterectomy has been proven to reduce the incidence of urinary tract injury. True/false.

Ans.
1. False
2. False
3. True
4. False

Reference
1. Allen L, Jauniaux E, Hobson S, Papillon-Smith J, Belfort MA. FIGO consensus guidelines on placenta accreta spectrum disorders: Nonconservative surgical management. Int J Gynecol Obstet. 2018;140:281-90.

OSCE 14. State true/false:
1. Triple P procedure is a method of nonconservative management of placenta accreta spectrum.
2. Enumerate the three steps involved in triple P procedure.

Ans.
1. False
2. a. Perioperative ultrasound localization of the upper edge of placenta
   b. Preoperative placement of intra-arterial balloon catheters (anterior division of the internal iliac arteries)
   c. Large myometrial excision and uterine repair without any attempt to remove the placenta

Reference
1. Sentilhes L, Kayem G, Chandraharan E, Palacios-Jaraquemada J, Jauniaux E. FIGO consensus guidelines on placenta accreta spectrum disorders: Conservative management,. Int J Gynecol Obstet. 2018;140:291-8.

OSCE 15.

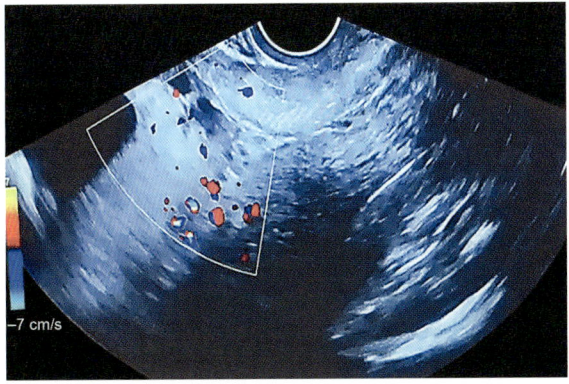

Above is a transvaginal scan of a pregnant lady with a placental pathology.
1. Identify the condition in the above image.
2. Name three high risk factors that are associated with this condition.

Ans.

1. Placenta previa
2. Prior cesarean, smoking, ART.

Reference

1. Placenta Praevia and Placenta Accreta: Diagnosis and Management Green-top Guideline No.27a September 2018.

OSCE 16. What percentage of women with placenta previa are likely to develop placenta accreta after:

1. Two cesarean sections
2. Three cesarean sections
3. Four cesarean sections
4. Five cesarean sections

Ans.

1. 11%
2. 40%
3. 61%
4. 67%

Reference

1. Placenta Accreta spectrum Obstetric care Consensus, Number 7, December 2018.

OSCE 17. With respect to placenta previa, please answer the following questions:

1. Beyond what period of gestation is the term *'Low Lying Placenta'* used for placental localization?

2. What should be the distance of lower placental margin from internal os for the placenta to be called low-lying at the mid trimester anomaly scan?
3. At what period of gestation should a follow-up scan be offered to confirm or refute a persistently low-lying placenta initially diagnosed at mid trimester anomaly scan?
4. What is the recommended approach/route of ultrasound to confirm a low-lying placenta in the third trimester?

Ans.

1. 16 weeks
2. 2 cm
3. 32 weeks
4. Transvaginal scan

Reference

1. Jauniaux ERM, Alfirevic Z, Bhide AG, Belfort MA, Burton GJ, Collins SL, Dornan S, Jurkovic D, Kayem G, Kingdom J, Silver R, Sentilhes L on behalf of the Royal College of Obstetricians and Gynaecologists. Placenta Praevia and Placenta Accreta: Diagnosis and Management. Green-top Guideline No. 27a. BJOG. 2018.

OSCE 18.

1. Name two conditions that must be fulfilled for conservative management of placenta previa to be offered.
2. Write any two components of the McAfee regime for placenta previa.

Ans.

1. Pregnancy less than 37 weeks, patient hemodynamically stable.
2. McAfee Regime
   Conservative management of placenta praevia:
   - Hospitalization at 32 weeks until 38 weeks/delivery.
   - Bed rest along with strict pad chart monitoring.
   - Monitor vital signs.
   - Ultrasound monitoring for placenta localization is done every 2 weeks to look for placenta migration, possible prior to 34 weeks.
   - Fetal monitoring by CTG and biophysical profile.
   - Daily fetal movement count chart.
   - 2 doses of dexamethasone, 12 mg administered IM 12 hours apart to enhance lung maturity and prevent interventricular hemorrhage in preterm babies.
   - Ensure availability of 2 units grouped and cross matched blood
   - Round the clock availability of cesarean section.

OSCE 19.

1. Name four conditions when McAfee's regime should be discontinued.
2. Enumerate two maternal complications due to placenta previa.
3. Enumerate two fetal complications due to placenta previa.

Ans.

1. a. When pregnancy has reached 38 weeks or more
   b. When there is premature rupture of membrane (PROM)
   c. Antepartum fetal distress
   d. Congenital anomaly
   e. Intrauterine fetal death (IUFD)
   f. When a patient goes in labor
2. Maternal complications which can occur due to placenta previa are:
   a. Antepartum hemorrhage
   b. Malpresentation
   c. Postpartum hemorrhage
   d. Increased risk of puerperal sepsis
3. Fetal complications which can occur due to placenta previa are:
   a. FGR
   b. Premature delivery
   c. Fetal distress due to hypoxia
   d. Intrauterine fetal demise

Reference

1. Jauniaux ERM, Alfirevic Z, et al on behalf of the Royal College of Obstetricians and Gynaecologists. Placenta Praevia and Placenta Accreta: Diagnosis and Management. Green-top Guideline No. 27a. BJOG. 2018.

OSCE 20.

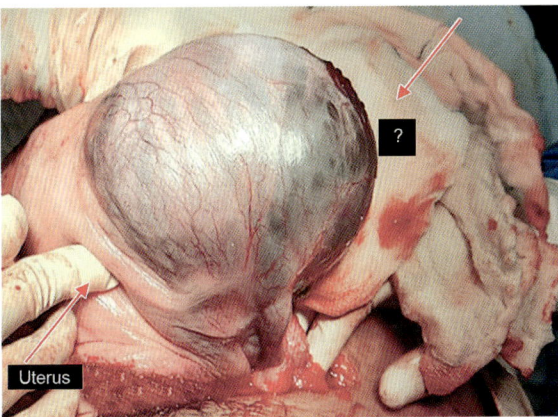

1. Identify the complication.
2. Name two most common high risk factors associated with this complication.
3. What would be the appropriate gestational age to terminate this pregnancy in case the diagnosis is certain?
4. What would be the instances where the pregnancy would be terminated earlier than the usual gestation. Give two such conditions.

Ans.

1. Placenta percreta
2. Placenta previa and previous cesarean birth, other uterine surgery including repeated curettage.
3. 34+0 to 35+6 weeks gestation
4. Persistent bleeding/rupture of membranes/uncontrolled maternal comorbid conditions/intra uterine demise/malformed fetus

References

1. RCOG Green-top Guideline No. 126, 2018.
2. Placenta Accreta spectrum Obstetric care Consensus, Number 7, December 2018.

CHAPTER 20

Pregnancy beyond Expected Date of Delivery

Indu Lata

OSCE 1.

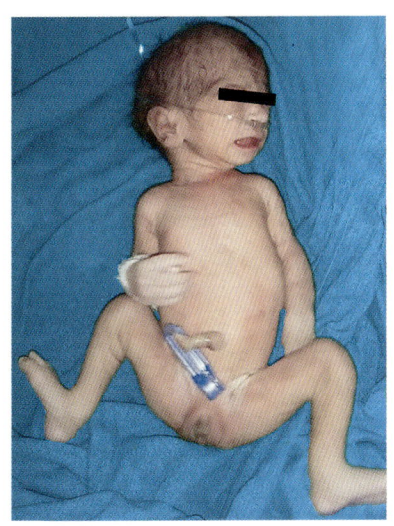

1. Identify the newborn appearance?
2. What is the name of this condition?
3. What is found decreased in these newborns?
4. Name two physical features lacking in these babies just after birth?
5. Name the immediate risk to these newborns?

Ans.

1. Old man appearance
2. Postmaturity or dysmaturity syndrome
3. Subcutaneous fat
4. Lanugo and vernix
5. Meconium aspiration due to increased incidence of meconium-stained liquor.

Reference

1. Gabbe's Obstetrics, 8th edition, Chapter 29, Late and Postterm pregnancy.

OSCE 2.

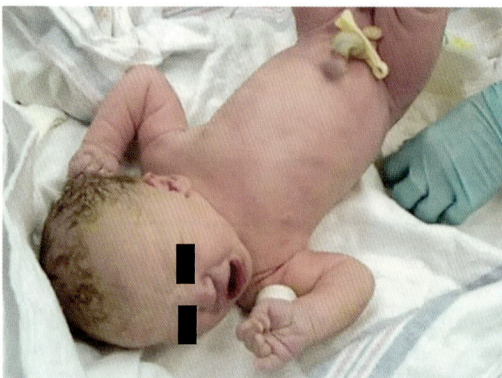 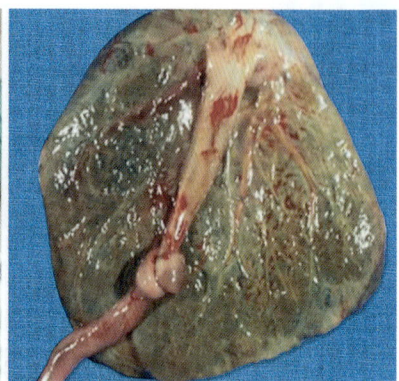

1. What is seen in these pictures?
2. At what gestation there is significant risk of meconium-stained liquor?
3. What could be the finding on nonstress test?
4. Name one immediate serious neonatal condition?
5. Name one serious neonatal complication?

Ans.

1. Meconium-stained fetus and placenta
2. In post-term pregnancy
3. Late decelerations
4. Meconium aspiration
5. Chemical pneumonitis.

Reference

1. Gabbe's Obstetrics, 8th edition, Chapter 29, Late and Postterm pregnancy.

OSCE 3.

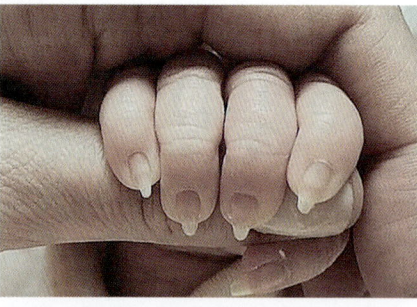 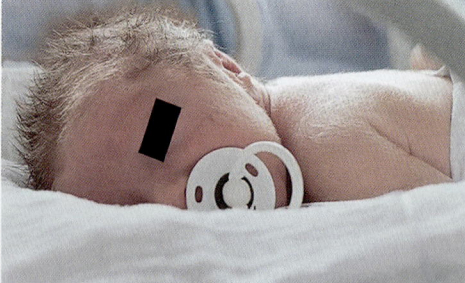

1. What do these pictures show?
2. What is this syndrome known as?
3. Name the condition in which it is seen.
4. Write two other features seen in this condition.
5. Name the significant risk in this condition.

Ans.

1. Long finger nails and abundant hair of baby
2. Postmaturity syndrome
3. Post-term pregnancy
4. Decreased subcutaneous fat and lack of lanugo and vernix.
5. Meconium-stained liquor.

Reference
1. Gabbe's Obstetrics, 8th edition, Chapter 29, Late and Postterm pregnancy.

OSCE 4. A Primigravida patient come to hospital after 10 days of her expected date of delivery for consultation. She is anxious that she still does not have any pain in abdomen.
1. What is condition known as?
2. What is her gestational age?
3. What are three most commonly used methods to determine the expected date of delivery?

Ans.

1. Late term pregnancy
2. 41 weeks 3 days
3. a. Last menstrual period
   b. Timing of intercourse or embryo transfer
   c. Early ultrasound assessment.

Reference
1. Gabbe's Obstetrics, 8th edition, Chapter 29, Late and Postterm pregnancy.

OSCE 5.

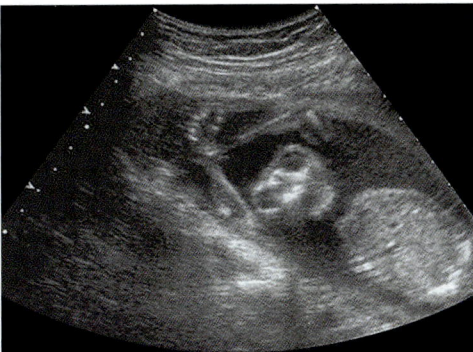
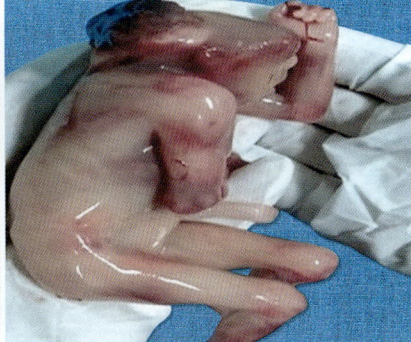

1. What is this fetal anomaly?
2. Which maternal condition is commonly associated with it?
3. How it is responsible for prolonged gestation?
4. How early can we detect this anomaly on ultrasound?
5. What is a specific sign of this anomaly on ultrasound?

Ans.

1. Anencephaly
2. Late and post-term pregnancy
3. Dysfunction of HPA Axis
4. 11 weeks
5. Frog eye sign

Reference

1. Gabbe's Obstetrics, 8th edition, Chapter 29, Late and Postterm pregnancy.

OSCE 6. A primigravida patient presents with body mass index of 33 present with complain of no labor pains even after 2 weeks of her expected date of delivery.
1. What is this condition?
2. What are her risk factors?
3. What is the probable cause for it?
4. What are 2 methods of fetal surveillance?
5. What is management?

Ans.

1. Post-term pregnancy
2. Primigravida and obesity
3. Low levels of circulating Cortisol
4. Nonstress test and modified biophysical profile.
5. Induction of labor if no obstetrical contraindications.

Reference

1. Gabbe's Obstetrics, 8th Edition, Chapter 29, Late and Postterm pregnancy.

OSCE 7.

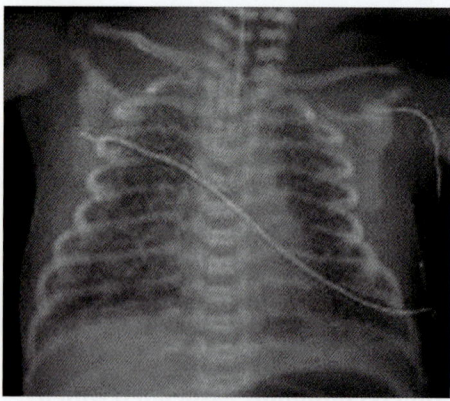

A primigravida obese patient delivers a male baby after 2 weeks of her expected date of delivery. The liquor was meconium stained. Baby was admitted in Neonatal intensive care unit Investigation done.

1. What is probable cause of meconium-stained liquor?
2. What is probable cause of Neonatal intensive care admission?
3. What this fetal X-ray shows?
4. What is cause of this fetal lung X-ray abnormality?
5. What are risk factors in this patient?

Ans.

1. Post-term pregnancy
2. Respiratory distress of neonate
3. Aspiration pneumonitis
4. Meconium aspiration
5. Primigravida, obesity and male baby.

Reference

1. Gabbe's Obstetrics, 8th edition, Chapter 29, Late and Postterm Pregnancy.

OSCE 8. A Primigravida patient with 41 weeks 4 days pregnancy with Amniotic fluid index of 5 cm on obstetric ultrasound. On nonstress test there is prolonged deceleration.
1. What is this maternal condition called?
2. Name the ultrasound abnormality seen at this gestation.
3. Name the two most common risks to the baby in this condition?
4. What is the cause of late deceleration?

Ans.

1. Late term pregnancy or pregnancy beyond expected date of delivery.
2. Oligohydramnios
3. Meconium passage and Birth asphyxia
4. Cord compression

Reference

1. Gabbe's Obstetrics, 8th edition, Chapter 29, Late and Postterm pregnancy.

OSCE 9.

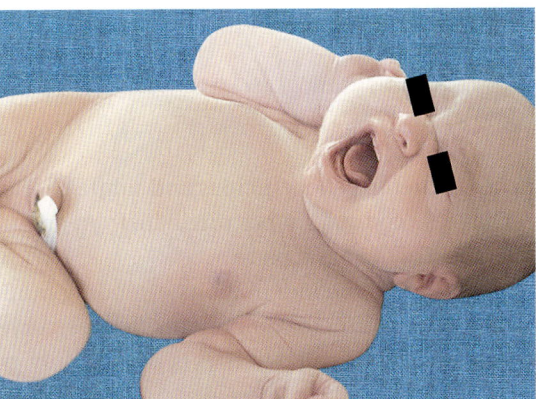

Section 1: Obstetrics

A primigravida with 41 weeks 6 days gestation presented with labor pains and delivers male baby.
1. Name the condition of the newborn seen in the picture?
2. What is the definition of this neonate condition?
3. Name two common maternal conditions where such neonates are born.

Ans.

1. Macrosomia/Large for gestational age
2. When the fetal weight is more than 95th percentile for that gestational age.
3. Maternal diabetes and post-term pregnancy.

Reference

1. Williams Obstetrics, 25th edition, Chapter 43, Postterm pregnancy.

OSCE 10.

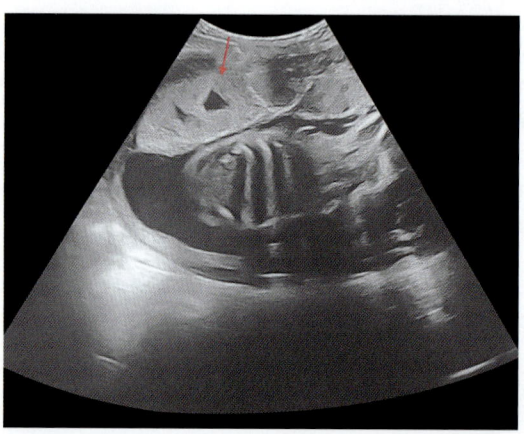

A G2P0010 with 41 weeks pregnancy with Hypothyroidism come for antenatal visit. Her ultrasound and Biophysical profile were done. On ultrasound:
1. Name the marked structure?
2. Write the grading of placenta seen on ultrasound?
3. What is placental apoptosis?

Ans.

1. Mature placenta
2. Grading of placenta
   - *Grade I:* Placenta has scattered echogenicities and subtle chorionic plate undulations.
   - *Grade II:* Large, echogenic comma shapes originate from an indented chorionic plate, but their curve falls short of the basal plate.
   - *Grade III:* Placenta has echogenic indentations extending from the chorionic plate to the basal plate, which create discrete components that resemble cotyledons.
3. Placental apoptosis is programmed cell death. It is significantly greater at 41 to 42 completed weeks compared with that at 36 to 39 weeks.

Reference
1. Williams Obstetrics, 25th edition, Chapter 6 and 43, Placenta & Postterm pregnancy.

OSCE 11.

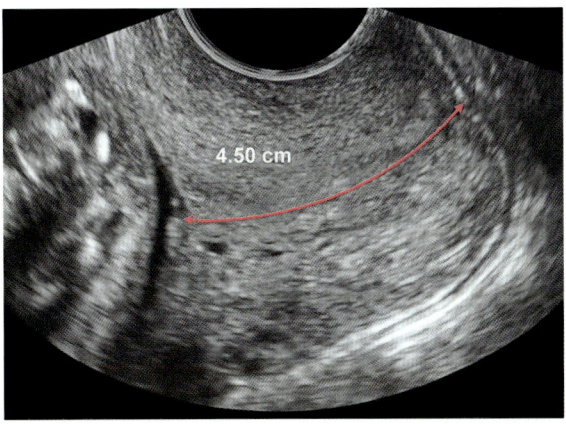

A second gravida with previous one abortion presented at 40 weeks 5 days. Her ultrasound at 32 weeks gestation had this finding.
1. Name the structure?
2. Mention how its length is associated with probable gestational age for delivery.
3. Name the two routes to measure it on ultrasound.
4. Write the prerequisites for these two routes.

Ans.

1. Cervix
2. In nulliparas, those whose cervical length at mid-pregnancy is longer are twice as likely to deliver after 42 weeks.
3. Two routes to measure cervical length are:
   a. Transabdominal route
   b. Transvaginal route
4. For Transabdominal route Urinary bladder should be filled whereas for Transvaginal route urinary bladder should be empty.

Reference
1. Williams Obstetrics, 25th edition, Chapter 43, Postterm pregnancy.

OSCE 12.

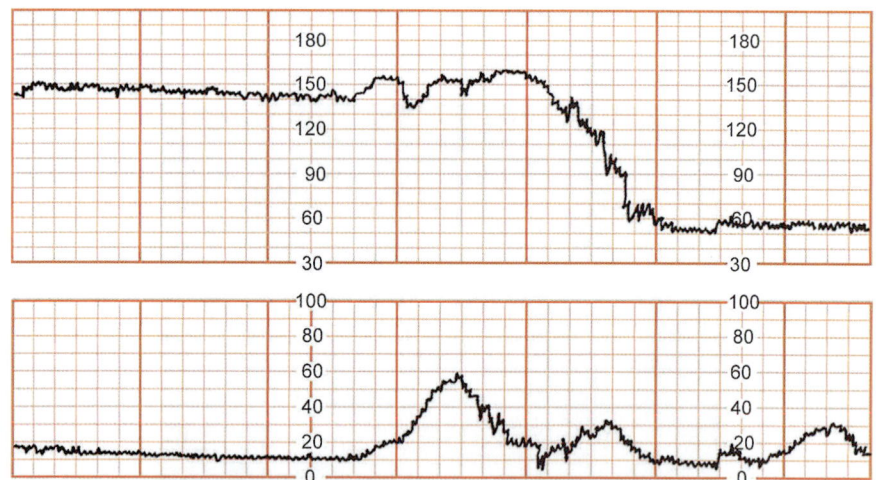

1. Name the method of fetal surveillance.
2. What is depicted in upper part of test?
3. What is depicted in lower part of graph?
4. What is the interpretation of this test?
5. Write the cause of this type of test in post-term pregnancy.

Ans.

1. Cardiotocography
2. Fetal heart rate tracing
3. Uterine contractions
4. Prolonged fetal heart deceleration
5. Post-term pregnancy with oligohydramnios.

Reference

1. Williams Obstetrics, 25th edition, Chapter 43, Postterm pregnancy.

OSCE 13.

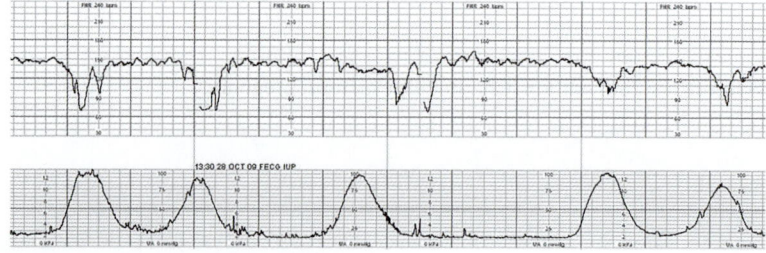

1. Name the method of fetal surveillance.
2. What is depicted in upper part of test?
3. What is depicted in lower part of graph?

4. What is the interpretation of this test?
5. Write the cause of this type of test in post-term pregnancy.

Ans.
1. Cardiotocography
2. Fetal heart rate tracing
3. Uterine contractions
4. Prolonged fetal heart deceleration.
5. Post-term pregnancy with oligohydramnios with cord compressions.

Reference
1. Williams Obstetrics, 25th edition, Chapter 43, postterm pregnancy.

OSCE 14.

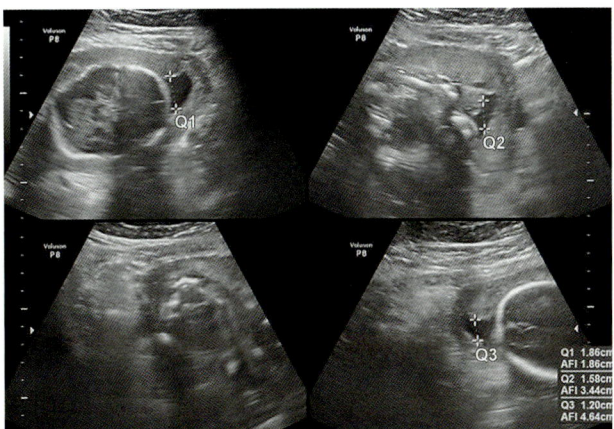

Primigravida at 41 weeks 5 days pregnancy with hypothyroidism presented for ultrasound in view of decreased fetal movements. On ultrasound her Amniotic fluid index was below normal limit.
1. Write the name of above maternal condition.
2. What happens to amniotic fluid in above maternal condition?
3. What is being measured in above ultrasound image?
4. What is oligohydramnios?
5. Amniotic fluid index is measured in how many quadrants?

Ans.
1. Pregnancy beyond expected date of delivery
2. Reduction in Amniotic fluid/Oligohydramnios
3. Amniotic fluid index
4. When Amniotic fluid index is less than 5 cm
5. Four quadrants.

Reference
1. Williams Obstetrics, 25th edition, Chapter 43, postterm pregnancy.

OSCE 15. A pregnant patient Gravida 2 with previous one abortion presents with 42 weeks pregnancy in Antenatal Outdoor clinic. She was admitted for safe confinement. After pelvic assessment induction of labor planned.

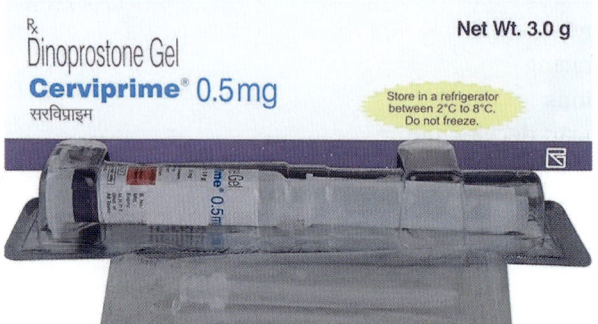

1. Name the method of induction of labor.
2. What type of Prostaglandin analogue is it?
3. When is this method used in post term pregnancy?
4. Name two obstetrical complications that can occur on using it.

Ans.

1. Pharmacological method for induction of labor
2. Prostaglandin E2
3. Induction of labor is used when cervix is not favourable or a Bishop score <6
4. a. Uterine Tachysystole
   b. Uterine Hyperstimulation.

Reference

1. Gabbe's Obstetrics, 8th edition, Chapter 29, Late and Postterm pregnancy.

OSCE 16. A pregnant patient Gravida 3 with previous two abortion presents with 42 weeks pregnancy in Antenatal Outdoor clinic. She was admitted for termination of pregnancy. After pelvic assessment induction of labor was planned with this agent.

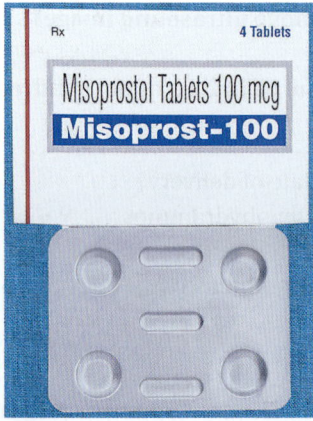

Chapter 20: Pregnancy beyond Expected Date of Delivery **267**

1. Name the method of induction of labor.
2. What type of Prostaglandin analogue is this?
3. When is this method used in post-term pregnancy?
4. Name two obstetrical complications that can occur on using it?

Ans.

1. Pharmacological method for induction of labor
2. Prostaglandin E1
3. Induction of labor is used when cervix is not favourable or a Bishop score <6
4. a. Uterine Tachysystole
   b. Uterine Hyperstimulation.

Reference

1. Gabbe's Obstetrics, 8th edition, Chapter 29, Late and Postterm pregnancy.

OSCE 17. A primigravida patient with 41 weeks uncomplicated pregnancy presented for antenatal checkup. She was advised fetal surveillance.
1. Name two methods for fetal surveillance.
2. Name the components of modified biophysical profile.

Ans.

1. Fetal kick count, Nonstress test (NSTs), Contraction stress test (CSTs), biophysical profile
2. Nonstress test and Amniotic fluid index

Reference

1. Gabbe's Obstetrics, 8th edition, Chapter 29, Late and Postterm pregnancy.

OSCE 18. A Gravida 2 previous one abortion (G2P0010) pregnant patient with 41 weeks uncomplicated pregnancy presented for antenatal checkup. She was advised fetal surveillance.
1. Name the types of biophysical profile used for fetal surveillance.
2. Name the components of biophysical profile.
3. Name the components of modified biophysical profile.
4. What is the time to start and frequency of fetal surveillance by ACOG Recommendation?

Ans.

1. Two types of biophysical profile–complete and modified biophysical profile.
2. Fetal breathing, fetal body movement, fetal tone, amniotic fluid on ultrasound and Nonstress test
3. Nonstress test and Amniotic fluid index
4. At 41weeks or beyond at least once a week.

Reference

1. Williams Obstetrics, 25th edition, Chapter 43, postterm pregnancy.

Section 1: Obstetrics

OSCE 19. Second gravida with previous one male child (G2P1001) with 42 weeks 2 days with history of post-term pregnancy in last pregnancy comes in obstetric emergency with labor pains.
1. Write the name of this condition.
2. Write four common maternal complications.
3. Write four common perinatal adverse outcomes.

Ans.
1. Post-term pregnancy
2. Fetal Macrosomia, Oligohydramnios, Pre-eclampsia, and caesarean delivery.
3. Stillbirth, Postmaturity syndrome, meconium aspiration and Neonatal Intensive care unit admission.

Reference
1. Williams Obstetrics, 25th edition, Chapter 43, postterm pregnancy.

OSCE 20. Primigravida pregnant patient with BMI of 30 whose expected date of delivery (EDD) was 1st of October 2023. Today 7 days have passed after EDD. She attended antenatal outdoor for further advice.
1. Name the condition.
2. Write the two steps in her management if pregnancy is uncomplicated.
3. What would be her management plan if pregnancy is complicated with pre-eclampsia or oligohydramnios?
4. What would be the management plan if she attends hospital after two weeks of her EDD?

Ans.
1. Pregnancy beyond expected date of delivery (EDD)
2. If uncomplicated pregnancy, then—
    a. Pregnancy continuation with fetal surveillance.
    b. It should be followed by labor induction if she crosses 42 weeks.
3. If complicated pregnancy, then labor induction
4. After 42 weeks straightway labor induction.

Reference
1. Williams Obstetrics, 25th edition, Chapter 43, postterm pregnancy.

CHAPTER 21

Postpartum Hemorrhage

Ruby Bhatia, Sanjum Yasmin Malik, Vidushi Tewari, Vanisha Anand, Darryl Gibson Edwin

OSCE 1. A 35-year, G3P2L2 admitted in labor room in active phase of labor at 39-week POG and has an uncomplicated spontaneous vaginal delivery. She is 30 min postpartum and has excessive vaginal bleeding and feels dizzy. On general physical examination, BP 90/60 mm Hg, Pulse rate 122/minute, Respiratory rate 20/minute, SPO_2 96%, chest and CVS examination is normal. On per abdominal examination, uterus is flabby and on pelvic examination, about 200 cc of clots removed from vagina with fresh bleed.

1. What is your diagnosis in this case?
2. What are the criteria for diagnosing postpartum hemorrhage?
3. What are the types of postpartum hemorrhage?
4. Enumerate four causes of postpartum hemorrhage.
5. What should you do to immediately manage a case of atonic PPH?
6. What is the medical management for atonic PPH?
7. Any other drug apart from above-mentioned drugs for management of atonic PPH.
8. Name the first line agent used for treatment of atonic PPH.
9. Which drugs are used only for treatment of PPH and not for prevention?
10. Enumerate four conditions in which methylergometrine is contraindicated.

Ans.

1. Atonic postpartum hemorrhage.
2. a. PPH is defined as blood loss from the genital tract, exceeding 500 mL within 24 hours of vaginal delivery and 1,000 mL during a cesarean section.
   b. Blood loss >500 mL within 24 hours after birth and severe PPH is blood loss >1,000 mL within the same time frame. (WHO 2017)
   c. Cumulative blood loss >1,000 mL or blood loss accompanied by signs or symptoms of hypovolemia within 24 hours after birth process regardless of route of delivery. (ACOG 2019)
   d. Minor PPH includes 500–1000 mL and major PPH includes >1,000 mL of blood loss after delivery. (RCOG 2016)
3. a. *Primary hemorrhage (within 24 hours of delivery):*
   - Atonic
   - Traumatic
   b. Secondary/Late hemorrhage (>24 hours to 12 weeks after delivery)

4. a. Tone – uterine tone. Incidence is 70%
   b. Trauma – laceration, rupture, tears – 10%
   c. Tissue – retained tissue, blood clots, or placenta accreta spectrum (PAS) – 20%
   d. Thrombin – coagulopathy <1%
5. a. To alert obstetric and anesthetic seniors (Call for help).
   b. Restore and maintain intravascular volume by crystalloids and colloids by two wide bore cannulas (16G cannula).
   c. Maintain adequate oxygenation (O_2, by face mask at 10–15 L/min).
   d. To send blood for ABO and Rh-typing, crossmatch and to arrange blood and blood products and to catheterize the patient for continuous I/O monitoring.
   e. Massage the uterus to stimulate uterine contractions.
   f. Start oxytocin 40 units in 1 liter of NS at the rate of 60 drops/min.
6. The first line management in stepwise manner till bleeding is controlled:
   - Uterine massage
   - Oxytocin 40 units in 1 liter of NS, IV at the rate 60 drops per minute
   - INJ Methylergometrine 0.2 mg IM, can be repeated at 2–4 hours intervals up to a max of 4–5 doses.
   - INJ Carboprost (PGF2-alpha) 250 µg IM can be repeated at intervals of 15–90 minutes up to maximum of 8 doses.
   - Misoprostol (PGE1 analog) 600–1,000 µg per rectally (ACOG 2019); 800 µg per rectally (FIGO 2017)
   - Tranexamic acid 1gm IV slowly over 10 min, given within 3 hours of PPH. (ACOG 2019)
   - Bimanual uterine compression
   - Aortic compression (Both these are temporary measures for management of PPH)
7. Syntometrine (0.5 µg of methylergometrine + 5 units of oxytocin)
8. Oxytocin
9. a. Carboprost
   b. Tranexamic acid
10. a. Severe anemia
    b. Heart diseases
    c. Pre-eclampsia/eclampsia
    d. Rh-incompatibility
    e. After delivery of 1st twin
    f. Not to be used in HIV patients on protease inhibitors as it causes Hypertension.

References
1. *(For Questions 2–5, 7, 9, 10)* Cunningham FG. Causes of obstetrical hemorrhage. In: Cunningham FG, Leveno KJ, Hoffman BL, et al (Eds). Williams Obstetrics. 26th edition. New York: Graw Hill; 2022;42:731-48.
2. *(For Question 4)* Arias F. Postpartum hemorrhage. In: Bhide AG, Arulkumaran S, Damania K, Daftary SN (Eds). Practical Guide to High-risk Pregnancy and Delivery: a south Asian Perspective, 5th edition. Elsevier Health Sciences; 2019;23:359-69.
3. *(For Questions 6, 8)* World Health Organization (WHO) recommendations: Uterotonics for the prevention of postpartum hemorrhage. Geneva, WHO 2018.

Chapter 21: Postpartum Hemorrhage

OSCE 2. A 38-year, G5P4L4 admitted in labor room at 40 weeks period of gestation with polyhydramnios, delivers a live baby of 4 kg. Half an hour later after delivery, there is increased vaginal bleeding with clots. On general physical examinations, BP 90/50 mm Hg; pulse rate 124/minute, respiratory rate-24/minute, SpO_2 94% on room air, chest and CVS examination is normal. On per abdominal examination, uterus is not palpable, and on pelvic examination, excessive bleeding with clots is present.

1. Name the most common cause of PPH.
2. What is active management of the third stage of labor?
3. What are the methods used for placental separation?
4. What is the main goal of AMTSL?
5. Define" Golden first hour".
6. Define the "Rule of 30".
7. What is the major concern regarding postpartum hemorrhage?
8. What are the risk factors in the above-mentioned case?
9. Mention the other risk factors for postpartum hemorrhage.
10. How will you prevent postpartum hemorrhage?

Ans.

1. Uterine atony
2. a. Administer uterotonic agent (oxytocin 10 units IM) within 1 minute of delivery of baby
   b. Delayed cord clamping (1–3 minutes)
   c. Deliver placenta by controlled cord traction-optional (Modified Brandt–Andrew's technique)
   d. Intermittent assessment of uterine tone
3. a. *Schultze method:* In this method, placenta separates from center, blood from placental site pours into the membrane sac, does not escape externally, until the extrusion of placenta.
   b. *Duncan method:* The placenta separates from periphery and blood collects between the membranes and the uterine walls and escapes from vagina.
4. The goal of AMTSL is to:
   - Decrease blood loss
   - Prevent PPH
   - Reduce maternal morbidity and mortality.
5. The "golden first hour" is the time at which resuscitation must begin to achieve maximum survival, before metabolic acidosis sets in.
6. When a woman loses 30% of her blood volume, her systolic BP is likely to fall by 30 mm Hg, heart rate to increase by 30/minute, respiratory rate is likely to be increased by 30/minute, and hematocrit is likely to drop by 30% and her urine output is likely to fall by <30 mL/hr. If one or more of these features develop, it indicates moderate shock.
7. Obstetric hemorrhage is the major direct cause of maternal morbidity and mortality in India and other developing countries.

8. a. Grand multipara
   b. Macrosomia
   c. Polyhydramnios
9. a. *Obstetrical factors:* Obesity, previous history of PPH, sepsis, pre-eclampsia, eclampsia, anemia
   b. *Injuries to the birth canal:* Episiotomy, instrumental delivery, uterine rupture, cesarean delivery, obstructed labor, breech extraction, tachysystole, high parity
   c. *Uterine atony:* Uterine overdistention, large fetus, multiple pregnancies, polyhydramnios, retained clots, rapid labor, prolonged labor, chorioamnionitis
   d. *Abnormal placentation* (Placenta Previa, Placenta Accreta Spectrum, Abruptio placenta)
   e. *Coagulation defects:* Sepsis, HELLP syndrome, AFLP, IUFD (intrauterine fetal demise), anticoagulation treatment
   f. *Vulnerable patients:* Chronic renal insufficiency
10. a. *Antenatal preventive measures:*
    - Correction of anemia
    - Placental localization by USG in case of prior cesarean delivery
    b. *Intrapartum preventive measures:*
    - Institutional delivery
    - Active management of third stage of labor
    - Sensitization of resident doctors and skilled birth attendants regarding the mode of delivery and to attempt fetal head delivery in shortest possible fetal head diameter.

References

1. *(For Questions 1, 3, 4, 8–10)* Cunningham FG. Causes of obstetrical hemorrhage. In: Cunningham FG, Leveno KJ, Hoffman BL, et al. (Eds). Williams Obstetrics, 26th edition. New York: Graw Hill; 2022:42:731-48.
2. *(For Question 2)* World Health Organization: WHO recommendations for the prevention and treatment of postpartum hemorrhage. Geneva, WHO 2012.
3. *(For Questions 5–7)* Arias F. Postpartum hemorrhage. In: Bhide AG, Arulkumaran S, Damania K, Daftary SN (Eds). Practical Guide to High-risk Pregnancy and Delivery: a south Asian Perspective, 5th edition. Elsevier Health Sciences; 2019;23:359-69.

OSCE 3.

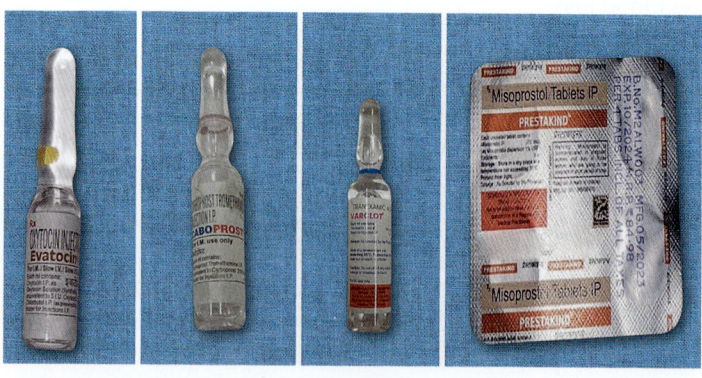

1. Define PPH bundle approach.
2. What is the aim of this approach?
3. Name the three components of PPH bundle care.
4. Which interventions are used for PPH prevention in bundle approach?
5. What is 'First Response PPH Bundle'?
6. What is 'Response to Refractory PPH Bundle'?
7. Define refractory PPH.
8. How is aortic compression done?
9. What are the criteria to use 'Response to Refractory PPH Bundle'?
10. Define acronym "MOTIVate".

Ans.

1. Small sets of evidence-based interventions for a defined patient population and care setting that, when implemented together in case of PPH, result in significantly better outcome.
2. a. To increase uptake and compliance to recommended interventions.
   b. To reduce rate of PPH-related morbidity and mortality.
3. a. Prevention and recognition of PPH
   b. First response to PPH
   c. Response to refractory PPH
4. a. Uterotonics
   b. Controlled cord traction
   c. Uterine tone assessment
5. a. Uterotonics drugs
   b. Isotonic crystalloids
   c. Tranexamic acid and
   d. Uterine massage
6. Uterotonics, tranexamic acid, compressive measures (aortic compression, bimanual uterine compression), intrauterine balloon tamponade, nonpneumatic antishock garment.
7. Defined as threatening postpartum hemorrhage that is unresponsive to conservative treatment and inevitably require surgical intervention.
8. Aortic compression is done manually or with the help of resuscitative endovascular balloon occlusion of aorta (REBOA)
9. 'Response to Refractory PPH Bundle' is intended to treat critically ill women who continues to bleed despite first response measures.
10. "MOTIVate" means Massage, Oxytocic, Tranexamic acid and IV fluids.

References

1. Resar R, et al. Using care bundles to improve health care quality. IHI Innovation series white paper. Cambridge, MA: Institute for Healthcare Improvement; 2012)
2. *(For Questions 3–7, 9, 10)* Althabe, et al. Postpartum hemorrhage care bundles to improve adherence to guidelines: a WHO technical consultation. Int J Gynecol Obstet. 2019;148:290-99.

3. *(For Question 8)* Cunningham FG. Management of obstetrical hemorrhage. In: Cunningham FG, Leveno KJ, Hoffman BL, et al (Eds). Williams Obstetrics, 26th edition. New York: Graw Hill; 2022; 44:770-82.

OSCE 4.

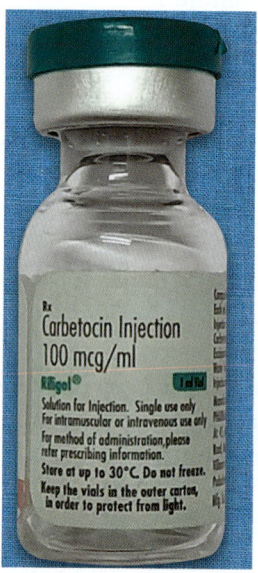

1. Identify this.
2. Where do you use this drug?
3. Mechanism of action of Carbetocin.
4. Dose of Carbetocin.
5. Can Carbetocin be used for management of PPH?
6. What is the half-life of Carbetocin?
7. What is the advantage of Carbetocin over Oxytocin?
8. Benefits of oxytocin over carbetocin.
9. What are the other drugs used for prophylaxis of PPH?
10. Why is oxytocin not given as IV Bolus dose?

Ans.

1. Carbetocin
2. Carbetocin is used for the prevention of PPH.
3. Carbetocin is a synthetic oxytocin analog, stimulates the myometrium of fundus to contract rhythmically, which constricts the spiral arteries and decreases blood flow through uterus.
4. 100 μg IV slowly or IM, single dose.
5. No, it is used only for prevention of PPH.
6. 40 minutes.
7. a. Carbetocin is heat stable and does not need cold chain transport and storage. Therefore, it is convenient to be stored at room temperature in low-income countries.

b. Half-life of Carbetocin is 40 minutes which is longer than Oxytocin and duration of action is 24 hours after an IM injection, thus avoiding the side effects of IV injection.
8. a. Low cost of Oxytocin
   b. Oxytocin can be repeated while Carbetocin is only for single use.
   c. Oxytocin can be used for prevention as well as for management of PPH, while Carbetocin is used only for prevention of PPH.
9. *Oxytocin, if not available:*
   - Methyl ergometrine
   - Misoprostol
10. Oxytocin is never given as an undiluted bolus dose because severe hypotension or cardiac arrythmias can develop.

References

1. *(For Questions 2–5)* Cunningham FG. Vaginal delivery. In: Cunningham FG. Leveno KJ, Hoffman BL, et al (Eds). Williams Obstetrics, 26th edition. New York: Graw Hill; 2022;27:497-17.
2. *(For Question 3)* Arias F. Postpartum hemorrhage. In: Bhide AG, Arulkumaran S, Damania K, Daftary SN (Eds). Practical Guide to High-Risk Pregnancy and Delivery: A south Asian Perspective, 5th edition. Elsevier Health Sciences. 2019;23:359-69.
3. *(For Questions 4–8)* Jin et al. Carbetocin versus oxytocin for prevention of postpartum hemorrhage after vaginal delivery: A meta-analysis. Medicine. 2019;98:47.
4. *(For Questions 9, 10)* Cunningham FG. Causes of obstetrical hemorrhage. In: Cunningham FG. Leveno KJ, Hoffman BL, et al (Eds). Williams Obstetrics, 26th edition. New York: Graw Hill; 2022;42:731-48.

OSCE 5. A 30-year, G4P3L3 admitted in labor room in active phase of labor at 39 weeks 4 days period of gestation and has a spontaneous vaginal delivery. On assessment after 15 minutes, BP 90/62 mm Hg, Pulse rate 130/minute, Respiratory rate 22/minute, SPO$_2$ 95%, chest and CVS examination is normal. On per abdomen examination, uterus is flabby and on pelvic examination, excessive bleeding with clots is present and there is no evidence of any birth canal injury. A diagnosis of atonic PPH is made. First line management with all uterotonics done but patient still has profuse bleeding.

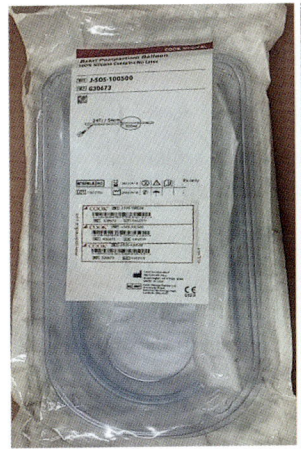
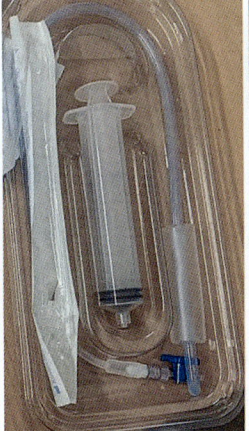
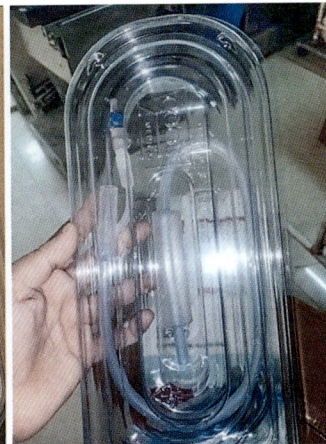

1. What is the diagnosis?
2. Identify the above picture?
3. What is the next second line procedure used in PPH, when medical management fails?
4. What is the capacity of Bakri balloon?
5. What are the other devices used for tamponade?
6. Mechanism of action of balloon tamponade?
7. Balloon tamponade is recommended in which type of PPH?
8. What are the prerequisites before using Balloon tamponade?
9. Which temporary measure is recently not used to treat PPH?
10. What is the most common complication of balloon tamponade?

Ans.

1. Atonic postpartum hemorrhage intractable to first-line medical management.
2. Intrauterine Bakri balloon
3. Intrauterine balloon tamponade
4. A total of 300–500 mL of normal saline.
5. a. Foley's catheter 24–30 F
   b. Condom catheter
   c. Sengstaken-Blakemore catheter
6. Balloon tamponade compresses the open venous sinuses and reduces bleeding.
7. It is used in the treatment of PPH, due to uterine atony which does not respond to standard first line medical management.
8. a. When first line treatment protocol of primary PPH implemented (including use of uterotonics, IV fluids) and all other causes of PPH (retained tissue, trauma) are reasonably excluded.
   b. Immediate access to surgical intervention and blood products is possible if needed.
   c. Maternal condition can be regularly monitored for prompt identification of any signs of deterioration.
9. Uterine packing.
10. Postpartum endometritis.

References

1. *(For Questions 3, 6)* Arias F. Postpartum hemorrhage. In: Bhide AG, Arulkumaran S, Damania K, Daftary SN (Eds). Practical Guide to High-risk Pregnancy and Delivery: a south Asian Perspective, 5th edition. Elsevier Health Sciences. 2019;23:359-69.
2. *(For Questions 4, 5, 10)* Cunningham FG. Causes of obstetrical hemorrhage. In: Cunningham FG, Leveno KJ, Hoffman BL, et al (Eds). Williams Obstetrics, 26th edition. New York: Graw Hill; 2022;42:731-48.
3. *(For Questions 7, 8)* World Health Organization: WHO Recommendation for using IBT to treat postpartum hemorrhage. Geneva, WHO, 2022.
4. *(For Question 9)* World Health Organization: WHO recommendations: Uterotonics for the prevention of postpartum hemorrhage. Geneva, WHO 2018.

Chapter 21: Postpartum Hemorrhage

OSCE 6.

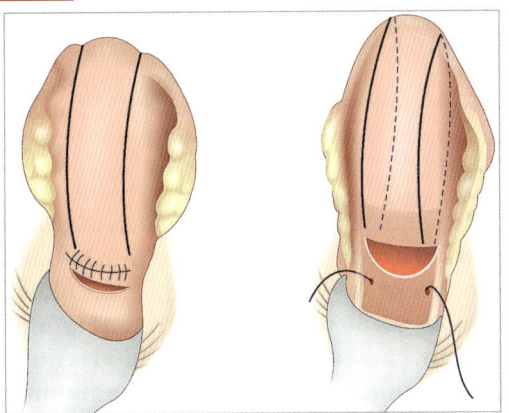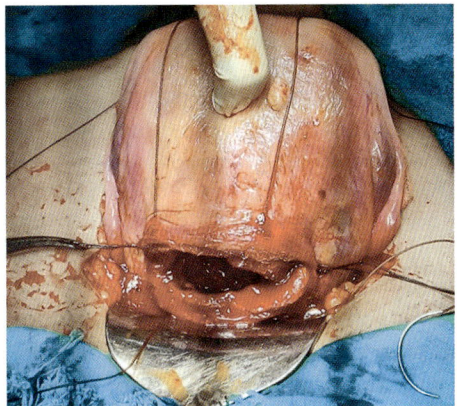

1. Identify the procedure?
2. Name the compression suture used in this technique.
3. Name the most common uterine compression suture.
4. Which suture is most commonly used for this technique?
5. Name the other Uterine compression sutures.
6. What are the indications of uterine compression sutures?
7. What are the criteria for applying uterine compression sutures?
8. Mechanism of action of uterine compression suture.
9. How effective are compression sutures?
10. What are the complications of uterine compression sutures?

Ans.

1. Uterine compression suture (Hemostatic suture), as second line modality for management of atonic PPH.
2. B-Lynch suture.
3. B-Lynch suture.
4. Chromic catgut no. 2.
5. a. Hayman suture (Multiple vertical suture)
   b. Cho square suture
   c. Gun Shella suture
6. a. Atonic PPH
   b. DIC-associated bleeding, along with blood transfusion
7. a. When medical management fail to control atonic PPH
   b. When the patient is hemodynamically stable.
8. The main aim of compression suture is to stop bleeding from placental site by opposing anterior and posterior uterine wall together.
9. The effectiveness of compression sutures is approximately 60–75%.
10. a. Uterine Ischemic necrosis with peritonitis
    b. Uterine wall defect
    c. Uterine synechiae (Rarely)

References

1. *(For Questions 2–4, 6, 10)* Cunningham FG. Causes of obstetrical hemorrhage. In: Cunningham FG, Leveno KJ, Hoffman BL, et al (Eds). Williams Obstetrics, 26th edition. New York: Graw Hill; 2022;42:731-48.
2. *(For Questions 5, 7–9)* Arias F. Postpartum hemorrhage. In: Bhide AG, Arulkumaran S, Damania K, Daftary SN (Eds). Practical Guide to High-risk Pregnancy and Delivery: a south Asian Perspective, 5th edition. Elsevier Health Sciences. 2019;23:359-69.

OSCE 7. A 22-year, primigravida presented in spontaneous labor at 38 weeks of gestation with heart disease with a good size baby. Patient has a term vaginal delivery with RMLE with outlet forceps. After expulsion of placenta, there is excessive bright red bleeding with constant trickle. On general examination, BP 90/60 mm Hg, Pulse rate 120/minute, respiratory rate 18/minute, SPO_2 96% on room air, chest and CVS examination is normal. On per abdomen examination, uterus is well retracted and on pelvic examination, excessive bleeding is present. Per speculum examination, is as seen in below picture:

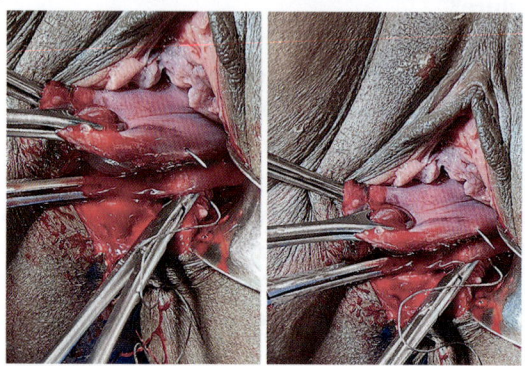

1. What is your diagnosis?
2. Identify the above picture.
3. Enumerate four causes of traumatic postpartum hemorrhage.
4. What is the most common cause of traumatic postpartum hemorrhage?
5. Enumerate four risk factors for traumatic postpartum hemorrhage?
6. What is the most common location of cervical tear?
7. Which artery supplies the cervix?
8. How many sponge-holding forceps are required to stitch cervical tear?
9. How will you repair cervical tear?
10. Enumerate two complications of cervical tear in subsequent pregnancies?

Ans.

1. Traumatic postpartum hemorrhage
2. Cervical tear
3. a. Vulvovaginal lacerations
   b. Cervical tear
   c. Perineal tear
   d. Uterine rupture
   e. Puerperal hematomas.

4. Cervical tear.
5. *Risk factors:*
   - High parity
   - Instrumental delivery
   - Breech extraction
   - Obstructed labor
   - Macrosomia
   - Shoulder dystocia
   - Previously scared uterus
   - Cesarean delivery
   - Tachy-systole
   - Intrauterine manipulation.
6. 3'o clock >9'o clock.
7. Descending cervical branch of uterine artery at 3 and 9 o'clock position.
8. Minimum three sponge-holding forceps.
9. Cervical Tear is repaired by using chromic catgut 2-0 or polyglactin. The first suture is placed in tissue above the angle of cervix and subsequently either interrupted or continuous locking sutures are serially placed towards the edges.
10. a. Recurrent lacerations
    b. Cervical incompetence
    c. Preterm labor
    d. Cesarean delivery

References

1. *(For Questions 3, 5–10)* Cunningham FG. Causes of obstetrical hemorrhage. In: Cunningham FG, Leveno KJ, Hoffman BL, et al (Eds). Williams Obstetrics, 26th edition. New York: Graw Hill; 2022;42:731-48.
2. *(For Question 4)* Arias F. Postpartum hemorrhage. In: Bhide AG, Arulkumaran S, Damania K, Daftary SN (Eds). Practical Guide to High-risk Pregnancy and Delivery: a south Asian Perspective, 5th edition. Elsevier Health Sciences. 2019;23:359-69.

OSCE 8.

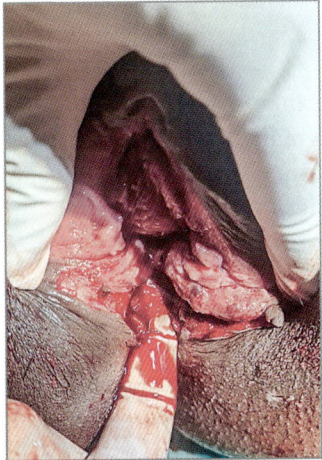

1. See the above picture to make the diagnosis.
2. What is the classification of perineal tear?
3. Define OASIS (Obstetric Anal Sphincter Injuries).
4. Enumerate 4 risk factors of perineal tear.
5. How to prevent perineal tear?
6. What is modified Ritgen's maneuver?
7. Name the techniques used to repair third degree perineal tear.
8. Overlapping technique is used for which perineal tear repair?
9. What postoperative care should be done after repair of perineal tear?
10. Enumerate four complications after Perineal tear repair.

Ans.

1. Perineal tear (Grade 3b)
2. *Grade of perineal tear:*
   - Grade I—involving vaginal epithelium and perineal skin
   - Grade II—tear of perineal muscles
   - Grade III—involvement of anal sphincter:
     a. <50% involvement of external anal sphincter thickness
     b. >50 % involvement of external anal sphincter thickness
     c. Internal anal sphincter is involved.
   - Grade IV—tear in anal epithelium or rectal mucosa.
3. 3rd degree and 4th degree tears are referred to as OASIS.
4. a. Nulliparity
   b. Persistent occipitoposterior position
   c. Macrosomia
   d. Shoulder dystocia
   e. Instrumental delivery
   f. Tachysystole
   g. Rapid labor/Precipitate labor
   h. Previous history of perineal tear
   i. Breech extraction.
5. a. Perineal massage
   b. Warm compresses on perineum
   c. Follow modified Ritgen's maneuver
6. Manually supporting the perineum with right hand and deflex the head of fetus with left hand to avoid perineal injuries.
7. a. End-to-end anastomosis (most common)
   b. Overlapping technique.
8. This method is used only in type 3C lacerations, those with complete external anal sphincter rupture.
9. a. Single shot of second generation cephalosporins at the time of repair is considered.
   b. Warm Sitz bath and Icepacks to reduce swelling and allay discomfort.
   c. Pain relief using NSAIDs.

    d. Stool softeners for a week
    e. Avoid pregnancy for at least six months.
10. a. Infections
    b. Breakdown of repair
    c. Pain
    d. Scarring
    e. Dyspareunia
    f. Fistula formation
    g. Endometriosis of scar (rarely).

References
1. *(For Questions 2,3,9)* Arias F. Postpartum hemorrhage. In: Bhide AG, Arulkumaran S, Damania K, Daftary SN (Eds). Practical Guide to High-risk Pregnancy and Delivery: a south Asian Perspective, 5th edition. Elsevier Health Sciences. 2019;22:345-58.
2. *(For Questions 4,7–9)* Cunningham FG. Causes of obstetrical hemorrhage. In: Cunningham FG, Leveno KJ, Hoffman BL, et al (Eds). Williams Obstetrics, 26th edition. New York: Graw Hill; 2022; 27:497-17.
3. *(For Questions 5, 6)* World Health Organization: WHO recommendations: Uterotonics for the prevention of postpartum hemorrhage. Geneva, WHO 2018.

OSCE 9.

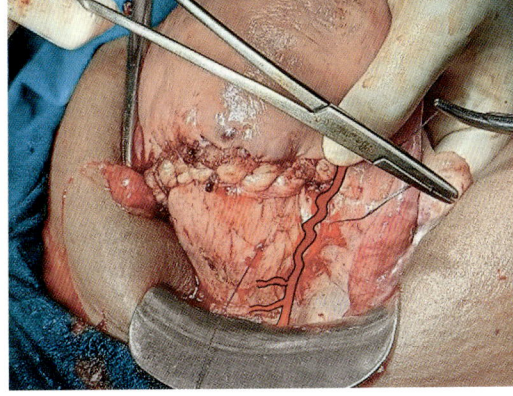
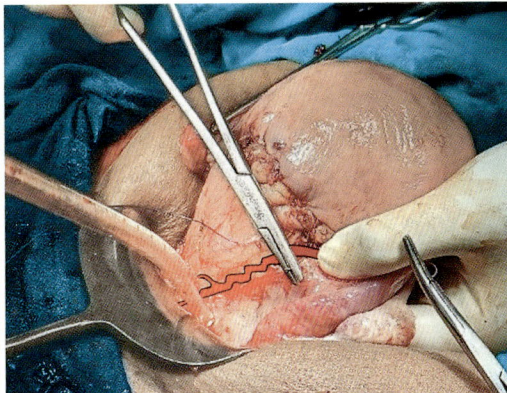

1. Name of the procedure.
2. What is the name of the technique used for uterine artery ligation?
3. What is the origin of uterine artery?
4. What are the indications of uterine artery ligation?
5. Name the most common indication for uterine artery ligation.
6. Name the structure which is most likely to be injured during uterine artery ligation.
7. What is the relationship of uterine artery to ureter?
8. Name the branches of uterine artery.
9. What are the indications of Uterine artery embolization?
10. Enumerate four complications of uterine artery embolization?

Ans.

1. Left-sided uterine artery ligation
2. O'Leary technique
3. From anterior division of internal iliac artery
4. a. Uterine atony
   b. Abnormal placentation
   c. Hysterotomy incision laceration
5. Uterine artery ligation is mainly done for PPH, when first line management and Intrauterine balloon tamponade fails to control bleeding.
6. Ureter
7. From its origin, the uterine artery crosses medially to the lateral side of uterus and after that it crosses over the ureter approximately 2 cm lateral to the cervix.
8. a. Sampson artery (Round ligament)
   b. Ovarian and tubal branches (ovary and fallopian tubes)
   c. Vaginal and descending cervical branches (upper vagina and lower cervix)
   d. Fundal branch (fundus)
   e. Arcuate, radial, spiral and basal arteries supplying uterus.
9. Uterine artery embolization should be considered when there is:
   - Persistent bleeding in the women who is hemodynamically stable, when primary measures have failed.
   - Uterine AV malformation.
10. a. Endometritis
    b. Intrauterine synechia
    c. Migration of embolus
    d. Bladder wall necrosis
    e. Uterine necrosis
    f. Vaginal fistula (rarely)

References

1. *(For Questions 2–6)* Cunningham FG. Management of obstetrical hemorrhage. In: Cunningham FG, Leveno KJ, Hoffman BL, et al (Eds). Williams Obstetrics, 26th edition. New York: Graw Hill; 2022; 44:770-82.
2. *(For Questions 7, 8)* Cunningham FG. Maternal Anatomy. In: Cunningham FG, Leveno KJ, Hoffman BL, et al (Eds). Williams Obstetrics, 26th edition. New York: Graw Hill; 2022;2:12-29.
3. *(For Questions 9, 10)* Arias F. Postpartum hemorrhage. In: Bhide AG, Arulkumaran S, Damania K, Daftary SN (Eds). Practical Guide to High-risk Pregnancy and Delivery: a south Asian Perspective, 5th edition. Elsevier Health Sciences. 2019;23:359-69.

OSCE 10.

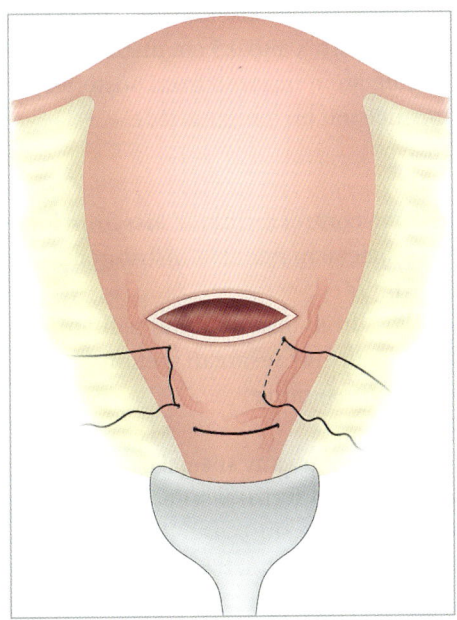

1. Identify this procedure?
2. Who discovered this stitch?
3. Which suture is used for this stitch?
4. Where do you use Ashok Anand stitch?
5. What is the objective behind using this stitch?
6. How Ashok Anand stitch can control blood loss?
7. What is the technique of applying this stitch?
8. Name the advantages of this stitch.
9. Name the limitations of this stitch.
10. What is its benefit over uterine artery embolization?

Ans.

1. Ashok Anand stitch.
2. This stitch was discovered by Dr Ashok Anand, professor in OBS and GYNAE department, Grant Medical College and Sir JJ Groups of Hospital, Mumbai, in 2007.
3. Polyglactin 910 number 1.
4. Ashok Anand stitch is used to control blood loss in case of placenta previa as well as in morbidly adherent placenta during cesarean section.
5. a. To reduce blood loss and the need for blood transfusion.
   b. To reduce complications in case of placenta previa as well as in morbidly adherent placenta during cesarean section.
6. It de-vascularizes the lower segment of uterus by bilaterally occluding the collaterals supplying the lower part of uterus. As these are end arteries, their occlusion leads to hemostasis in the lower segment.

7. Polyglactin number 1 is mounted on straight needle (number 18) after ligation of bilateral uterine arteries. The needle is inserted into the cervix, from anterior to posterior, 1 cm above the level of lateral fornix and 0.5 cm medial from lateral cervical musculature. The same suture and needle are reinserted from posterior to anterior 0.5 cm, below the lower edge of the uterine incision on the same side.
8. a. Simple and less invasive
   b. Cost effective
   c. Rapid effective method to control the blood loss from lower uterine segment.
   d. It does not require any special material or instrument.
   e. Does not affect the fertility.
9. It only controls the blood loss from lower uterine segment in case of placenta previa and morbidly adherent placenta during caesarean section.
10. a. It is simple and nontime consuming
    b. Cost effective
    c. Easy to take and does not require any special expertise.
    d. Can be done in the setting where there is lack of facilities and interventional radiologist at the time of delivery.

Reference

1. Anand AR et al. Reducing intraoperative lower segment blood loss in placenta previa with Ashok Anand stitch. Int J Reprod Contracept Obstet Gynecol. 2013 J; 2OSce.

OSCE 11.

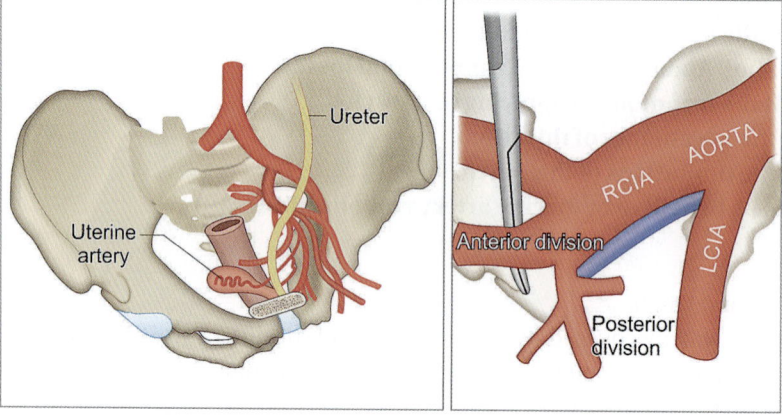

1. Identify the procedure?
2. What is the site for internal iliac artery ligation?
3. What is the principle of ligating anterior division of internal iliac artery?
4. What are the steps of Stepwise Devascularization?
5. Which artery provides maximum blood supply to the pelvis?
6. Name the branches of anterior division of Internal iliac artery?
7. Name the branches of posterior division?
8. What are the indications of Internal Iliac artery ligation?

9. Relation of Internal Iliac artery to the ureter.
10. What are the complications which occur after angiographic embolization of Internal Iliac artery?

Ans.

1. Ligation of anterior division of Internal iliac artery.
2. Ligation of internal iliac artery is 3–5 cm distal to the common iliac artery bifurcation and after the origin of posterior division of internal iliac artery.
3. Ligation reduces the pulse pressure by 85% in arteries distal to the ligation.
4. a. Unilateral uterine artery ligation
   b. Bilateral uterine artery ligation
   c. Low uterine vessel ligation
   d. Unilateral ovarian vessel ligation
   e. Bilateral ovarian vessel ligation
   f. Anterior division of internal iliac artery ligation.
5. Branches of internal iliac artery.
6. a. Inferior gluteal artery
   b. Internal pudendal artery
   c. Middle rectal artery
   d. Vaginal artery
   e. Uterine artery
   f. Obturator artery
   g. Umbilical artery and its continuation as superior vesical artery.
7. a. Superior gluteal artery
   b. Lateral sacral artery
   c. Iliolumbar arteries.
8. a. Uncontrolled bleeding due to placenta previa.
   b. PPH intractable to first and second-line management.
9. As Ureter enter pelvis, it crosses over the bifurcation of Common Iliac Artery, and after descending into pelvis, it lies medial to Internal Iliac artery and anterolateral to Uterosacral Ligament.
10. a. Perforation of Internal Iliac artery
    b. Occlusion of External Iliac artery leading to Ischemia of lower limbs.
    c. Paraplegia.

References

1. *(For Questions 2, 3, 8)* Cunningham FG. Causes of obstetrical hemorrhage. In: Cunningham FG, Leveno KJ, Hoffman BL, et al (Eds). Williams Obstetrics, 26th edition. New York: Graw Hill; 2022; 44:770-82)
2. *(For Questions 4, 10)* Arias F. Postpartum hemorrhage. In: Bhide AG, Arulkumaran S, Damania K, Daftary SN (Eds). Practical Guide to High-Risk Pregnancy and Delivery: A south Asian Perspective, 5th edition. Elsevier Health Sciences. 2019:23:359-69.
3. *(For Questions 5–7, 9)* Cunningham FG. Maternal Anatomy. In: Cunningham FG, Leveno KJ, Hoffman BL, et al (Eds). Williams Obstetrics, 26th edition. New York: Graw Hill; 2022:2:12-29.

OSCE 12.

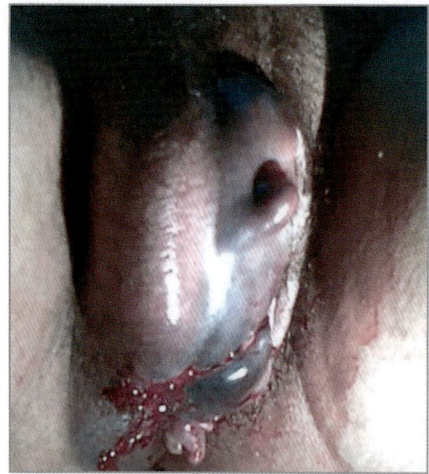

1. Identify the above picture.
2. Most common site of pelvic hematoma.
3. Define the anatomic classification of puerperal hematomas.
4. How are vulval hematomas formed?
5. Enumerate four risk factors for puerperal hematomas.
6. Paravaginal hematoma occurs due to injury of which artery?
7. How will you diagnose hematoma?
8. What are the indications for surgical management of hematoma?
9. Which puerperal hematomas are also managed by embolization?
10. How will you manage hematoma?

Ans.

1. Vulval hematoma.
2. Vulval hematoma.
3. a. Vulvar
   b. Vulvovaginal
   c. Paravaginal
   d. Retroperitoneal hematomas.
4. Vulval hematoma occurs due to injury of vestibular bulb or the branches of pudendal artery (inferior rectal, perineal and clitoris branches).
5. a. Vaginal or perineal lacerations
   b. Episiotomy
   c. Operative vaginal delivery.
6. Descending branch of uterine artery.
7. *Symptoms:*
   - Severe pelvic pain or pelvic pressure
   - Urinary retention/inability to pass urine
   - Signs of hypovolemia.

Signs: On local examination, tense, tender, bluish fluctuant swelling encroaches the vaginal lumen and causes overlying skin ecchymotic with locally raised temperature.

8. a. Patient is hemodynamically unstable or in shock
   b. Falling hematocrit
   c. Size of hematoma is increasing.
   d. Excruciating pain (It indicates that hematoma extended to muscles).
9. Supralevator or retroperitoneal hematoma, if surgical attempts of hemostasis have failed or if hematoma is difficult to access surgically.
10. a. Stabilize the patient with crystalloids, colloids, blood, and blood products with resuscitative measures.
    b. Drain hematoma and ligate bleeding points, then obliterate the cavity of hematoma with absorbable sutures.
    c. Infralevator hematomas are evacuated by vaginal approach, while Supralevator hematomas need laparotomy or angiographic embolization.

Reference

1. *(For Questions 2–10)* Cunningham FG. Causes of obstetrical hemorrhage. In: Cunningham FG, Leveno KJ, Hoffman BL, et al (Eds). Williams Obstetrics, 26th edition. New York: Graw Hill; 2022:42:731-48.

OSCE 13. A 27-year, primigravida presented to labor room in active phase of labor at 39 weeks 3 days period of gestation. The patient has spontaneous vaginal delivery following which there was torrential bleeding P/V. On general physical examination, BP 80/52 mm Hg, pulse rate 130/minute, respiratory rate 24/minute, SpO$_2$ 92%, chest and CVS examination is normal. On per abdomen examination, uterine fundus is not palpable. On pelvic examination, a round boggy congested hyperemic mass is noted in the vagina with smooth surface with profuse bleeding.

1. What is your diagnosis?
2. Define uterine inversion.
3. What is the most common cause of shock immediately after delivery?
4. What is the cause of shock after uterine inversion?
5. What are the degrees of uterine inversion?
6. Enumerate four risk factors for uterine inversion.
7. What is the most common cause of uterine inversion in developing countries?
8. Define first line management of uterine inversion.
9. What is O'Sullivan hydrostatic method?
10. Name the surgical methods used to treat uterine inversion.

Ans.

1. Uterine inversion.
2. Uterine inversion occurs when the uterine fundus collapses into the endometrial cavity, turning the uterus partially or completely inside out.
3. Uterine inversion.
4. Neurogenic shock due to stretching of para-sympathetic nerves.

5. a. *1st degree (incomplete inversion):* Fundus within the endometrial cavity
   b. *2nd degree (complete inversion):* Fundus protrudes through the cervical os.
   c. *3rd degree (prolapsed inversion):* Fundus protrudes to or beyond the introitus.
   d. *4th degree (total inversion):* Both the uterus and vagina are inverted.
6. Risk factors:
   - Cord traction applied before placental separation
   - Atonic uterus
   - Excessive fundal pressure
   - Placental implantation at the fundus
   - Abnormally adherent placenta
   - Short cord
   - Uterine wall weakening at implantation site
   - Uterine tumor
7. Mismanaged third stage of labor.
8. a. Immediate assistance is summoned, including obstetrical and anesthesia personnel.
   b. Resuscitate with crystalloids, colloids, blood and blood products.
   c. Manual replacement of uterus (Johnson's maneuver) using cupping technique. If placenta is still attached to uterus, first manually replace the uterus, then placenta is manually removed.
   d. Once uterus is reverted to its normal configuration, oxytocin and other uterotonics agents are given for atony, after that Balloon tamponade may be used to maintain repositioned uterus.
9. This method involves infusing 2–3 L of warm saline into vagina under pressure. The resulting distention of vagina pushes the fundus upward to its normal position by hydrostatic pressure.
10. a. *Abdominal:* Huntington procedure and Haultain procedure
    b. *Vaginal:* Kustner and Spinelli procedure.

References
1. *(For Figures 2,4,9)* Macones G. In: Puerperal uterine inversion. Berghella V (Ed). Up-to-date. Waltham, MA: Wolters Kluwer Health, 2019)
2. *(For Figures 3, 5–10)* Cunningham FG. Causes of obstetrical hemorrhage. In: Cunningham FG, Leveno KJ, Hoffman BL, et al (Eds). Williams Obstetrics, 26th edition. New York: Graw Hill; 2022:42:731-48.

OSCE 14. A 29-year, P1L1 readmitted in labor room, 2 weeks postdelivery due to excessive vaginal bleeding. Patient reported that the bleeding began on the 10th day after delivery and increased in severity subsequently. Patient had a spontaneous vaginal delivery with right mediolateral episiotomy (RMLE), 2 weeks back, however doctor at the time of delivery fails to examine the placenta due to busy labor room. On general physical examination, BP 90/60 mm Hg, pulse rate 110/minute, respiratory rate 20/minute, SPO_2 96%, Chest and CVS examination is normal. On per abdomen examination, uterus is well retracted and on per vaginal examination, bleeding is present.

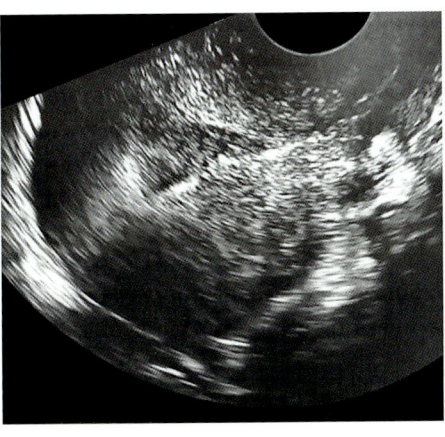 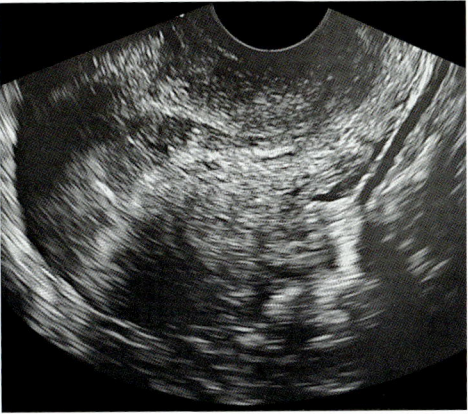

1. Identify the above picture.
2. What is your diagnosis?
3. Define secondary/late postpartum hemorrhage.
4. Enumerate four causes of secondary postpartum hemorrhage.
5. Enumerate four risk factors of secondary postpartum hemorrhage.
6. What are the clinical features of endometritis?
7. How will you clinically diagnose the subinvolution of uterus?
8. Can you differentiate subinvolution of uterus from retained products of conception sonographically, If yes, then how?
9. How will you manage a case of secondary postpartum hemorrhage?
10. What are the indications of surgical management (curettage) in case of secondary PPH?

Ans.

1. Vascularized retained products of conception.
2. Secondary postpartum hemorrhage with retained placental products.
3. Secondary postpartum hemorrhage is defined as significant uterine bleeding occurring between 24 hours and 12 weeks postpartum.
4. a. Retained products of conception
   b. Subinvolution of placental bed
   c. Infection (endometritis)
   d. AV malformation
   e. Pseudoaneurysm of uterine artery or vaginal artery
   f. Dehiscence of cesarean scar
   g. Infected polyp or submucosal fibroid
   h. Bleeding diathesis.
5. a. Placental abnormalities
   b. Prolonged labor
   c. Chorioamnionitis
   d. Manual removal of placenta
   e. History of secondary postpartum hemorrhage in previous pregnancy.

6. *Clinical features of endometritis:* Fever, tachycardia, uterine tenderness, malodorous discharge, excessive bleeding.
7. a. *Symptoms:* Excessive/irregular bleeding, prolonged Lochia.
   b. *Signs:* On bimanual examination, uterus is soft and larger than usual size.
8. a. *RPOCs:* Thickened endometrium or endometrial mass and increase vascularity in the area.
   b. *Subinvolution:* Enlarged uterus with tubular hypoechoic areas in the myometrium.
9. a. Stabilize/resuscitate the patient with crystalloids and blood products
   b. Determine and treat the cause of bleeding
   c. Uterotonic agents in case of subinvolution of uterus
   d. Antibiotics if uterine infection is present (endometritis)
   e. Surgical procedures (suction and curettage), when medical management fails or vascularized retained placental products are identified sonographically
10. a. Vascularized placental retained products are seen in uterine cavity sonographically
    b. If excessive bleeding is present.
    c. Bleeding recurs after medical management.

References

1. *(For Question 3)* American College of Obstetricians and Gynecologists: postpartum hemorrhage. Practice Bulletin No.183, October 2017d.
2. *(For Questions 4, 5, 8–10)* Cunningham FG. The Puerperium. In: Cunningham FG, Leveno KJ, Hoffman BL, et al (Eds). Williams Obstetrics, 26th edition. New York: Graw Hill; 2022;36:634-48.
3. *(For Questions 6, 7)* Cunningham FG. Puerperal Infection. In: Cunningham FG, Leveno KJ, Hoffman BL, et al (Eds). Williams Obstetrics, 26th edition. New York: Graw Hill; 2022;37:649-63.

OSCE 15. A 36-year, primigravida with term pregnancy with obstructed labor admitted in labor room as a referral from CHC. On admission, BP 80/40 mm Hg, pulse rate 136/minute, respiratory rate 24/minute, SPO_2 92%, chest and CVS examination is normal. On per abdominal examination, uterine contour could not be assessed, fetal parts are felt superficially, and fetal heart rate is absent. On per vaginal examination, dry hot vagina, fully dilated cervix, with molding and caput is present. USG confirmed IUFD.

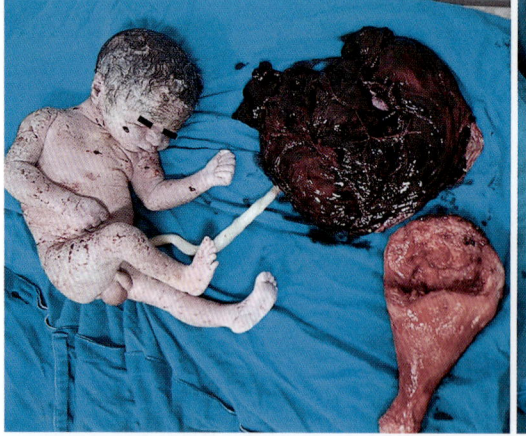
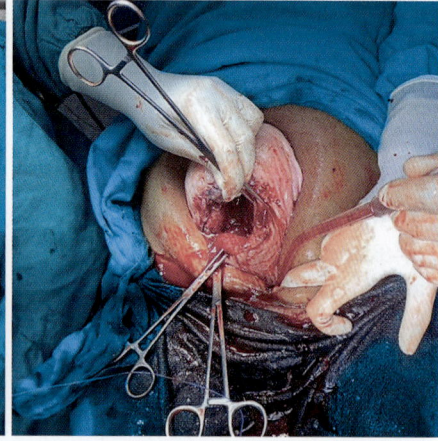

1. What is your diagnosis?
2. What is uterine rupture?
3. What are the types of uterine rupture?
4. Enumerate causes of uterine rupture.
5. What is the most common cause of uterine rupture in developing countries?
6. Enumerate two risk factors for rupture in our case.
7. Enumerate four clinical manifestations of uterine rupture.
8. What is the most significant sign of uterine rupture?
9. Enumerate four complications of uterine rupture.
10. How will you manage a case of uterine rupture?

Ans.

1. Rupture uterus.
2. Uterine rupture is complete disruption of all uterine layers, including the serosa, leading to changes in maternal and fetal status.
3. a. *Primary:* Rupture occurring in a previously intact and unscarred uterus
   b. *Secondary:* Rupture associated with a preexisting incision, anomaly or injury of myometrium (scarred uterus)
4. *Causes of uterine rupture:*
   a. *Surgery involving myometrium:* Cesarean delivery or hysterotomy, previously repaired uterine rupture, myomectomy, operative hysteroscopy, trauma.
   b. *Congenital:* Pregnancy in rudimentary uterine horn, defective connective tissue disorders
   c. *Uterine abnormality in current pregnancy:* Uterine overdistention (polyhydramnios, multifetal pregnancy), external version, persistent intense contractions, labor stimulation by oxytocin, difficult instrumental delivery, breech extraction, difficult manual removal of placenta, placenta accreta spectrum, gestational trophoblastic neoplasia.
5. Obstructed labor and scarred uterus.
6. a. Obstructed labor
   b. Advanced maternal age
7. a. Abdominal pain
   b. Abnormal fetal heart rate
   c. Cessation of contractions
   d. Loss of uterine contour and tone
   e. Hemodynamic instability
   f. Vaginal bleeding
   g. Hematuria
   h. Loss of station of presenting part
8. Nonreassuring fetal heart pattern with variable deceleration that may evolve into late decelerations and bradycardia followed by absent fetal heart rate.
9. *Maternal complications:*
   - Shock

- Hemorrhage
- Extension of uterine tear to broad ligament, cervix, and bladder
- Need for blood transfusion
- Need for laparotomy and peripartum hysterectomy

Fetal complications:
- Fetal—hypoxia and fetal death.

10. a. Resuscitation of patient with crystalloids and blood products
    b. Exploratory laparotomy with uterine defect repair in 2–3 layers with bilateral tubectomy
    c. If uterine repair is not possible, peripartum hysterectomy is done depending upon the extent of uterine damage, desire for future pregnancy, and hemodynamic instability.

Reference

1. *(For Questions 2-5, 7-10)* Cunningham FG. Causes of obstetrical hemorrhage. In: Cunningham FG, Leveno KJ, Hoffman BL, et al (Eds). Williams Obstetrics, 26th edition. New York: Graw Hill; 2022; 42:731-48.

OSCE 16.

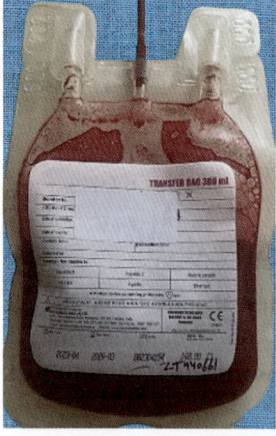
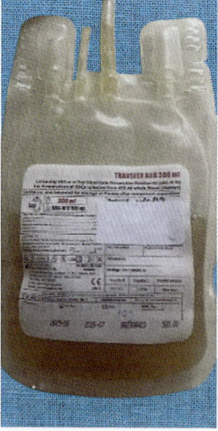
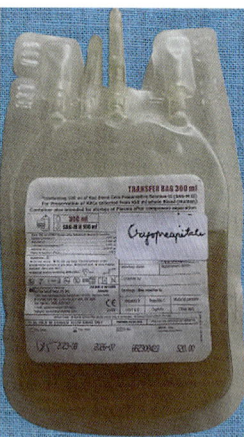
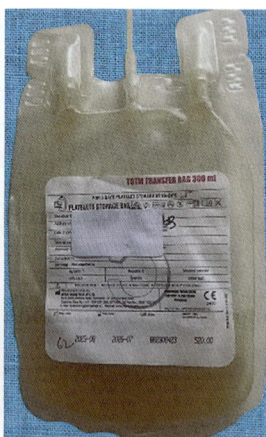

1. What are the blood products commonly transfused in obstetric hemorrhage?
2. Define massive transfusion.
3. What is shock index?
4. What is the triad of massive blood transfusion protocol?
5. Define 1:1:1 transfusion protocol.
6. Name the indications of massive transfusion.
7. What are the standard coagulation parameters, need to be maintained on massive hemorrhage?
8. Enumerate four complications of massive blood transfusion.
9. What is the significance of massive blood transfusion protocol?
10. What is the protocol of blood transfusion?

Ans.

1. Whole blood, Packed red blood cells, Fresh frozen plasma, Cryoprecipitate, Platelets.
2. Defined as transfusion of 10 units of packed red blood cells within a 24-hour period.
3. It refers to heart rate/systolic blood pressure. Normal value is 0.5–0.7. If SI increases by 0.9 to 1.1, intensive resuscitation and blood transfusion may be required in 80% of cases.
4. a. Acidosis
   b. Hypothermia
   c. Coagulopathy
5. It describes the unit ratio of packed red blood cells to plasma to platelets.
6. Acute blood loss and hemodynamic instability due to:
   - Obstetric catastrophe
   - Surgeries
   - Trauma
   - GI bleed
7. *Standards:*
   - Hemoglobin >8 g/dL
   - Platelet count >75 x 10^9
   - Fibrinogen >1.0 g/L
   - Prothrombin <1.5 mean control
   - APTT <1.5 × mean control
8. *Complications:*
   - Metabolic alkalosis
   - Electrolyte imbalance (hypocalcemia, hypothermia, hyperthermia, hyperkalemia)
   - Transfusion related acute liver injury
   - Transfusion associated circulatory overload
   - Bacterial and viral infections from contaminated blood products
   - Transfusion of incompatible blood may result in acute hemolysis, acute kidney injury and death.
9. They provide rapid blood product delivery for immediate resuscitation and avoid dilutional coagulopathy and hypoxic injury.
10. In case of active hemorrhage:
    - Two units of PRBC are given and if bleeding continues, two more units of PRBC and two units of FFP are transfused.
    - Platelets are transfused if PC is less than 50000/mcL.
    - Cryoprecipitate is transfused if fibrinogen level is less than 150 mg/dL.
    - Prolonged PT or APTT is an indication for replacement of FFP.

References

1. *(For Questions 1, 8, 9)* Cunningham FG. Management of obstetrical hemorrhage. In: Cunningham FG, Leveno KJ, Hoffman BL, et al (Eds). Williams Obstetrics, 26th edition. New York: Graw Hill; 2022; 44:770-82.

2. *(For Questions 2–7)* Arias F. Postpartum hemorrhage. In: Bhide AG, Arulkumaran S, Damania K, Daftary SN (Eds). Practical Guide to High-risk Pregnancy and Delivery: A south Asian Perspective, 5th edition. Elsevier Health Sciences. 2019;23:359-69.

OSCE 17.

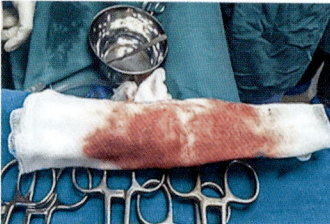
Soiled asnitary towel 30 mL

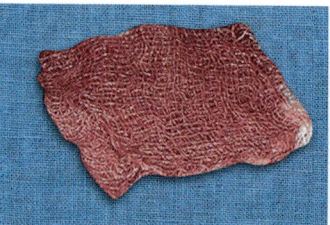
Small soaked gauze piece 10 cm x 10 cm

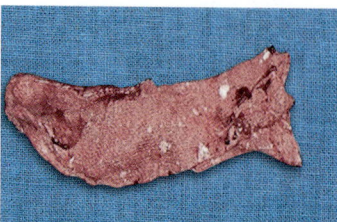
Soiled sanitary towel 60 mL

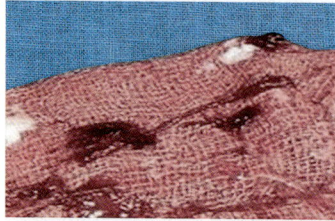
Incontinence Pad 250 mL

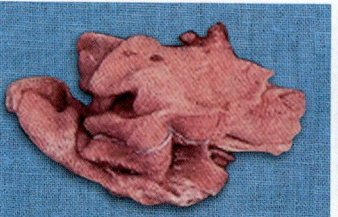
Large soaked swab 40 cm x 40 cm 350 mL

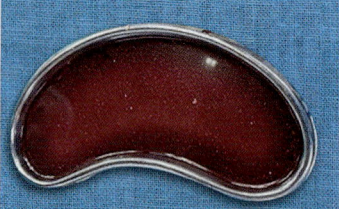
Full kidney tray 500 mL

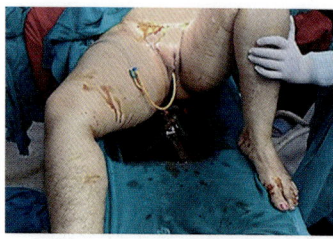
PPH on bed only 1000 mL

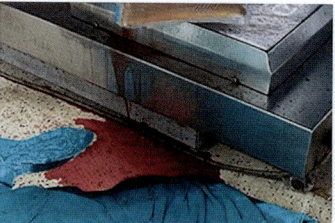
100 cm floor spill 1500 mL

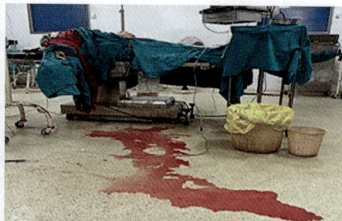
PPH spilling to the foor 2000 mL

1. Name the various methods used for estimation of blood loss?
2. Which method is most commonly used to assess severe blood loss?
3. What does the above image depict?
4. What is the advantage of visual assessment of blood loss?
5. Name the limitation of qualitative method (visual assessment of blood loss).
6. What are the initial steps to prevent blood loss?
7. What is a risk assessment tool kit?
8. What are the benefits of risk assessment tools?
9. Mention about urgency grid based on obstetric shock index.
10. Define modified shock index.

Ans.

1. a. *Qualitative methods:* Visual assessment of blood loss

b. *Quantitative methods:*
   - Gravimetric analysis
   - Colorimetric analysis
2. Quantitative methods are commonly used to identify severe hemorrhage, as they are more accurate.
3. It is a pictorial reference guide to help in visual estimation of blood loss in obstetric hemorrhage.
4. Accurate visual assessment leads to:
   - Quick and easy recognition of severe blood loss
   - Reduce the need of blood transfusion
5. This method has been shown to underestimate the actual blood loss by 33–50%, when volume is high and overestimate it when volume is low.
6. Initial management steps: *The HAEMOSTASIS Algorithm*
   General medical management
   - H: Ask for Help (Multidisciplinary approach, Senior Obstetrician, Anesthetists, OT staff, Hematologists, Blood bank, ICU)
   - A: Assess (vital parameters, blood loss) and resuscitate
   - E: Establish etiology, Ensure availability of blood
   - M: Massage the uterus
   - O: Oxytocic

   Specific surgical management
   - S: Shift to operating theater, bimanual compression, antishock garment, especially if transfer is required
   - T: Tissue and Trauma exclude and proceed to tamponade balloon, uterine packing
   - A: Apply compression sutures
   - S: Systematic pelvic devascularization (uterine, ovarian, internal iliac)
   - I: Interventional radiology, uterine artery embolization
   - S: Subtotal or total abdominal hysterectomy
7. *California Quality Improvement Tool Kit*

Low risk	Medium risk	High risk
• Singleton pregnancy • Fewer than four previous deliveries • No previous uterine surgery • No history of PPH	• Prior uterine surgery • More than four previous deliveries • Multiple gestation • Large fibroids • Chorioamnionitis • Magnesium sulphate or prolonged oxytocin infusion	• Morbidly adherent placenta • Hematocrit <30% • Bleeding at admission • Bleeding diathesis/coagulation defect • History of PPH • Tachycardia, hypotension

8. a. These are readily available.
   b. Identify 60–85% of patients who will experience a significant obstetric hemorrhage
   c. Reduce maternal morbidity and mortality.

9. *Urgency grid based on obstetric score index*

Loss of blood volume/% Blood Volume	Blood Pressure Systolic (SBP)	Symptoms and signs	Obstetric shock Index	Degree of shock/urgency
500–1,000 mL 10–15%	Normal SBP	Palpitation, mild tachycardia, dizziness	<1	Compensated Grade 4
1,000–1500 mL 15–30%	• Slight fall in SBP (SBP = 80–100 mm Hg) • A rise in diastolic blood pressure leading to increased pulse pressure	Weakness, marked tachycardia, sweating	>1	Mild Grade 3
1,500–2,000 mL 30–40%	Moderate fall in SBP (70–80 mm Hg)	Restlessness, marked tachycardia, pallor, oliguria	>1.5	Moderate Grade 2
>2,000 mL >40%	Marked fall in SBP (50–70 mm Hg)	Collapse, Air Hunger, Anuria	>2	Severe Grade 1

10. Modified Shock Index = HR/MAP.
    - Normal (0.7–1.3)
    - If value >1.3, it indicates increase in ICU admissions and mortality.

References

1. *(For Questions 1, 4)* Cunningham FG. Management of obstetrical hemorrhage. In: Cunningham FG, Leveno KJ, Hoffman BL, et al (Eds). Williams Obstetrics, 26th edition. New York: Graw Hill; 2022: 44:770-82.
2. *(For Question 2)* American College of Obstetricians and Gynaecologists: Quantitative blood loss in obstetric haemorrhage. Committee Opinion No. 794, November, 2019b.
3. *(For Questions 5–9)* Arias F. Postpartum hemorrhage. In: Bhide AG, Arulkumaran S, Damania K, Daftary SN (Eds). Practical Guide to High-risk Pregnancy and Delivery: a south Asian Perspective, 5th edition. Elsevier Health Sciences. 2019;23:359-69.

OSCE 18.

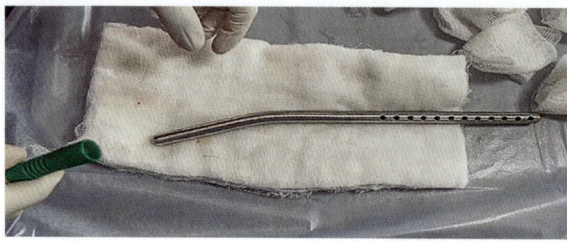

1. Name the device.
2. What is the use of this device?
3. What is the principle of this device?
4. What is the pressure used in the device?

5. What are the dimensions of this device?
6. What is this device made of?
7. Enumerate four advantages of this device.
8. What are the limitations of this device?
9. What is the estimated cost for this device?
10. What is the success rate of this device currently?

Ans.

1. Panicker's vacuum suction hemostatic device.
2. This is a negative intrauterine pressure suction device (NIPSD) used for:
   - Atonic PPH
   - Abnormal uterine bleeding
3. This device creates negative pressure within the uterine cavity, resulting in cessation of bleeding from the uterus. The device is inserted into the uterine cavity and connected to suction apparatus to create a negative pressure of 650 mm Hg, which ultimately creates soft cervical tissue to get sucked into small holes of cervical portion of cannula and becomes adherent. Further application of negative pressure results in constriction, contraction and firm retraction of uterus which stops atonic bleeding.
4. This device creates negative pressure, up to 650 mm Hg and is maintained for 15 minutes.
5. This device is made of stainless steel or plastic.
6. It is 25 cm long with a diameter of 12 mm, with multiple holes of 4 mm diameter over the distal end of the cannula.
7. a. It is a safe and simple technique for treating PPH in low-resourced and primary care settings.
   b. Can be used in patients allergic to drugs.
   c. Can be used in asthma, severe anemia, and cardiac diseases (where some uterotonic are contraindicated)
   d. Reusable
   e. Anesthesia is not required for the usage of this device.
8. a. It is effective only in managing uterine sources of bleeding.
   b. Cost-effective
   c. All Obstetric care unit-staff and paramedical personal needs to be trained to use it.
9. Approximate cost of this device in India is ₹ 4,500–7,000.
10. Success rate is 94–98% with Panicker's vacuum suction device for treating PPH.

Reference

1. Panicker TN. Panicker's vacuum suction haemostatic device for treating post-partum haemorrhage. J Obstet Gynaecol India. 2017;67(2):150-51.

OSCE 19.

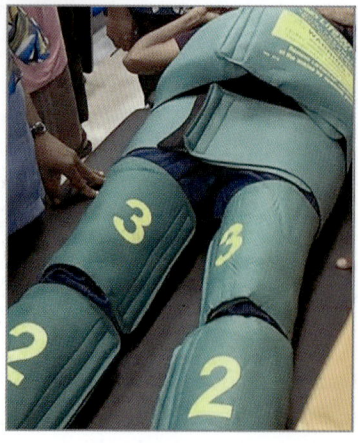
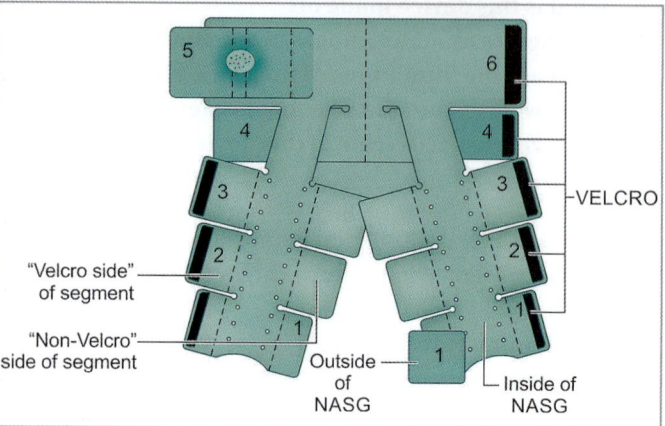

1. Name the above device.
2. What is NASG made of?
3. What is the principle of NASG?
4. What are the advantages of this device?
5. How many times can this device be reused?
6. How can you apply this device?
7. What are the criteria for removal of this device?
8. Enumerate two contraindications of NASG.
9. What is the success rate of this device?
10. What are the limitations of this device?

Ans.

1. This device is known as NASG (Nonpneumatic antishock garment).
2. NASG is made of Neoprene and Velcro with a small foam to provide uterine compression.
3. NASG is an innovative First Aid device, that is designed to provide external pressure to the lower segment of body, thereby increasing circulation in the vital organs of upper body and thus serves the purpose to reverse hypovolemic shock, when all other methods have failed to stop the bleeding or while waiting for definitive treatment.
4. a. This device provides time for transportation, blood transfusion or surgery in under-resourced and overcrowded settings.
   b. It is lightweight and reusable.
   c. It can keep a woman with PPH alive for 48 hours.
5. NASG is reusable up to 72–144 times.
6. a. *Criteria for NASG usage:* Any postpartum or pregnant woman with profuse hemorrhage showing signs of shock/hemorrhage instability, at the primary healthcare centers or cases requiring referral to higher centers: EBL 500 mL, SBP <100 mm Hg, pulse >100 bpm; at high-level facilities: EBL >1,000, SBP <90 mm Hg, pulse >110 bpm.
   b. Patient is made to lie on open NASG.

c. Make sure that NASG is placed properly, so that the top of the NASG segment lies at patient's lowest rib, and the pressure ball lies over umbilicus.
   d. Tightly close each segment pair, beginning at the ankle, first segments, and then ending with fifth and sixth segments directly over the umbilicus.
   e. The NASG is also adjustable for short women: fold back the ankle segment into the number two segment and close it on the ankle.
   f. To check whether the NASG is tight enough or not, place one or two fingers under the top layer of NASG segment, pull back the fabric, and let it go. The tightly closed segment will sound like snapping of fingers.
   g. After placing it, make sure that the woman is breathing normally.
   h. Watch for dyspnea and decreased urine output as potential signs of the NASG being too tight. If anyone of these two occurs, slightly loosen the NASG fifth or sixth abdominal segments.
7. a. Women is not bleeding more than 25–50 mL of blood/hour.
   b. SBP should be >100 mm Hg and pulse rate should be <100 bpm for at least 2 hours.
   c. Hb level should be >7gm/dL or hematocrit ≥20%
8. There are no absolute contraindications to NASG use. Relative contraindications are:
   - Severe CHF
   - Pre-existing MS
   - Trauma to chest or head, where redistribution of blood to injured area with NASG placement raises possibility of increased hemorrhage.
9. NASG showed survival rate of approximately 96% following its use.
10. a. Relatively high cost and low availability
    b. Training of staff is required.
    c. Nonavailability in all PHC and CHC centers
    d. Low awareness regarding NASG use.

References

1. *(For Questions 1–4, 6–8, 10)* FIGO Safe Motherhood and Newborn Health Committee, Non-pneumatic Anti-shock Garment to Stabilize Women with Hypovolemic Shock Secondary to Obstetric Hemorrhage. International Journal of Gynecology and Obstetrics, Elsevier, Amsterdam, November 2015.
2. *(For Questions 5, 9)* Unicef.org; Non-pneumatic Anti-Shock garment: product profile. UNICEF supply division, October 2020.

OSCE 20. A 29-year, P3L3 delivered at CHC few hours back, referred with shock and intractable vaginal bleeding. Patient received in labor room, on inotropic support with bleeding from cannula and catheter site. On general physical examination, BP 80/50 mm Hg, pulse rate 132/ minute, respiratory rate 24/minute, SPO$_2$ 92%, chest and CVS examination is normal. On per abdominal examination, uterus is flabby and on pelvic examination, fresh bleed along with clots is present and trauma has been ruled out. Despite all 1st and 2nd line modalities of treatment, patients still have extensive vaginal bleeding. Hematological investigation revealed: Hb 5.2 g/dL, platelet count 32,000/mcL, fibrinogen level 90 mg/dL, deranged LFTs and prolonged APTT and PT.

1. What is the most probable cause of extensive bleeding in this case?
2. Define DIC.
3. What is the incidence of DIC in PPH?
4. Enumerate four obstetrical causes of DIC.
5. What is the most common cause of severe consumptive coagulopathy in obstetrics?
6. Enumerate four clinical manifestations of consumptive coagulopathy.
7. What is ISTH scoring system and what are its parameters?
8. How will you diagnose DIC on the basis of laboratory findings?
9. How do you differentiate between consumptive coagulopathy and dilutional coagulopathy?
10. How will you manage a case of DIC?

Ans.

1. The most probable cause of extensive bleeding in this case is disseminated intravascular coagulation (DIC) syndrome.
2. Disseminated intravascular coagulation (DIC) is an acquired syndrome characterized by the intravascular activation of coagulation cascade leading to deposition of fibrin and formation of microvascular thrombi in small blood vessels throughout the body, leading to multiple organ dysfunction.
3. Incidence of DIC varies from 0.03 to 0.35%.
4. *Obstetrical causes of DIC:*
    - Placental abruption
    - Postpartum hemorrhage
    - Pre-eclampsia/eclampsia/HELLP syndrome
    - Acute fatty liver of pregnancy
    - *Pregnancy-related sepsis:* Septic abortion, severe chorioamnionitis, and postpartum endometritis
    - Prolonged retention of dead fetus
5. Placental abruption
6. *Symptoms:*
    - Severe vaginal bleeding
    - Persistent bleeding from venipuncture sites or mucosa of bladder
    - Spontaneous bleeding from gums, nose, or GI Tract
    - Purpura or petechiae at pressure sites

   Signs:
    - Systemic:
        ◆ Tachycardia
        ◆ Hypotension
        ◆ Weak peripheral pulses
        ◆ Altered mental status
        ◆ Cool extremities
    - *Organ dysfunction:*
        ◆ Acute kidney injury
        ◆ Hepatic dysfunction

- Acute lung injury
- Neurological dysfunction

7. ISTH (International Society on Thrombosis and Haemostasis) scoring system is used for diagnosis of overt DIC in pregnant females. Parameters of ISTH scoring system are:
    - Platelet Count
    - Prothrombin time/INR
    - Fibrinogen levels

    A value of ≥5 indicates overt DIC.

8. *Major findings in DIC:*
    - Platelet count—mildly to moderately reduced
    - Prolonged APTT and PT
    - Deranged clot retraction time (CRT)
    - Hypofibrinogenemia—serum fibrinogen levels <150 mg/dL
    - Increased D-dimer
    - Abnormal liver function test—suggest acute liver injury
    - Deranged renal function test—suggest acute kidney injury

9. Dilutional coagulopathy is differentiated from consumptive coagulopathy on the basis of peripheral blood smear reports.
    - *Dilutional coagulopathy:* There is no evidence of microangiopathy (Schistocytes) on peripheral blood smear.
    - *Consumptive coagulopathy:* There is evidence of microangiopathy (Schistocytes) on peripheral blood smear.

10. a. Early and accurate recognition of DIC is the hallmark of success in the treatment of this dire complication.
    b. It is an acute obstetrical emergency requiring a multidisciplinary approach. A team effort of obstetricians, anesthesiologists, hematologists, physicians, nursing, and paramedical staff in all maternity units.
    c. Resuscitation aims to achieve euvolemia, optimal tissue oxygen delivery, and correction of acidosis by appropriate fluid therapy (crystalloids and colloids) and blood transfusion (packed red blood cells, plasma, and platelets) by 1:1:1 transfusion protocol. FFP remains the treatment of choice in coagulation failure associated with PPH along with supportive care.
    d. Identify and treat the underlying condition and the triggering event leading to coagulation failure.
    e. Regular clinical and laboratory surveillance should be done until the patient is stabilized.

Reference

1. Cunningham FG. Management of obstetrical hemorrhage. In: Cunningham FG, Leveno KJ, Hoffman BL, et al (Eds). Williams Obstetrics, 26th edition. New York: Graw Hill; 2022;44:770-82.

Images Courtesy: Department of Obstetrics and Gynecology, MMIMSR, Ambala, Haryana, India.

CHAPTER 22

Obstetric Critical Care

Jyotsna Suri, Suchandana Dasgupta

OSCE 1.

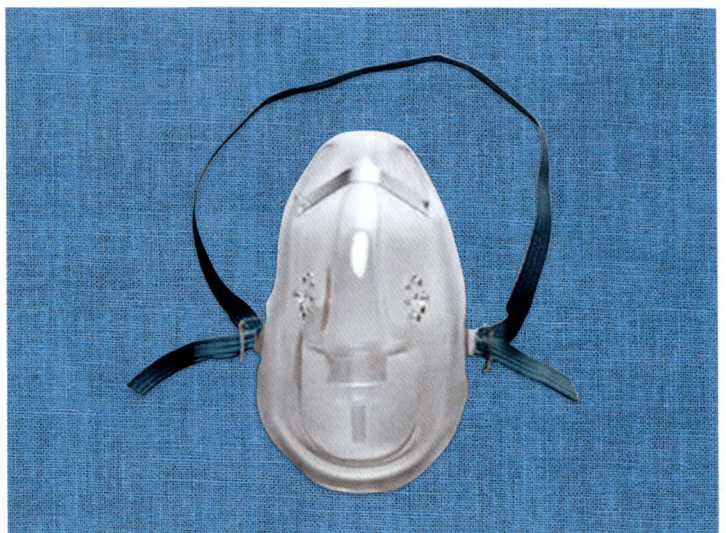

1. Identify this device.
2. Define FiO_2.
3. What is the FiO_2 in room air?
4. What is the minimum flow rate for this device?
5. What is the maximum FiO_2 which can be delivered by this device?

Ans.
1. This is a simple face mask
2. FiO_2 is the fraction of inspired oxygen.
3. FiO_2 in room air is 0.21.
4. The minimum flow rate of oxygen with face mask is 5 L/min.
5. The maximum FiO_2 with face mask is 0.60.

Reference
1. Critical Care PROMPT CiPP Cambridge University Press, 2019.

OSCE 2.

Blood gas values			
↓pH	7.027		[7.350–7.450]
↓pCO$_3$	34.2	mm Hg	[35.0–45.0]
↓pO$_3$	59.7	mm Hg	[53.0–108]
Temperature corrected values			
pH(T)	7.027		
pCO$_3$(T)	34.2	mm Hg	
pO$_3$(T)	59.7	mm Hg	
Acid base status			
cHCO$_3$-(P)c	8.5	mmol/L	
cHCO$_3$-(Pst)c	8.9	mmol/L	
cBased(B)c	−20.2	mmol/L	
cBased(Ecf)c	−20.1	mmol/L	
Cximetry values			
↓ctHb	5.8	g/dL	[12.0–16.0]
↓sO$_3$	83.5	%	[95.0–99.0]
FMetHb	1.0	%	
FO$_2$Hb	81.7	%	
FCOHb	1.1	%	
FHHb	16.2	%	
Electrolyte values			
cNa$^+$	136	mmol/L	[135–145]
?↑ck$^+$	5.1	mmol/L	[4.3–4.5]
↓cCa^{3+}	0.79	mmol/L	[1.15–1.29]
↑ cCl$^-$	120	mmol/L	[98–106]
Metabolite values			
↑cGlu	135	mg/dL	[70–105]
↑cLac	9.5	mmol/L	[0.5–1.5]

1. Identify the primary acid-base disorder from this ABG strip.
2. What is the Winter's formula?
3. Is the compensation adequate in this case?
4. How do you calculate the anion gap?
5. What is the anion gap in this case?

Ans.

1. Primary disorder is metabolic acidemia
2. Winter's formula is used to calculate the compensation in metabolic acidosis. It is calculated as: PCO$_2$ = 1.5 [HCO$_3^-$] + 8 ± 2
3. In this case, the predicted PCO$_2$ is 1.5 (8.5) + 8 ± 2 = 18.75 – 22.75. However, since the PCO$_2$ is 34.2, the compensation is not adequate (there is respiratory acidosis along with metabolic acidosis)
4. Anion gap is = Na$^+$ − (Cl$^-$ + HCO$_3^-$)
5. Anion gap in this case is 7.5

Reference

1. Suri J, Gandhi A, Mittal P, Arora M. Practical Approach to Critical Care in Obstetrics. 2018, 1st edition.

OSCE 3.

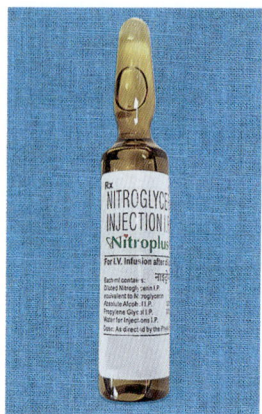

1. What is the main indication of NTG in obstetrics?
2. What is the mechanism of action?
3. What is the dose in which NTG is administered?
4. Name any two side effects of this drug.

Ans.

1. Main indication is hypertension with pulmonary edema.
2. The mechanism of action is vasodilatation (decreases preload) and arteriolar dilatation (decreases afterload).
3. The dose starts from 5 microgram/min and maximum dose is 100 microgram/min.
4. Headache, flushing, methemoglobinemia, nausea and vomiting.

Reference

1. Regitz-Zagrosek V, Lundqvist CB, Borghi C, et al. ESC guidelines on the management of cardiovascular diseases during pregnancy: The Task Force on the Management of Cardiovascular Diseases during Pregnancy of the European Society of Cardiology.

OSCE 4.

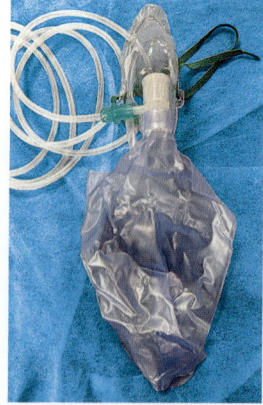

1. Identify this device.
2. At what oxygen flow rate does it work?
3. How much FiO_2 is administered by this device?
4. What is the most important precaution while using this device?
5. What are the disadvantages of this device?

Ans.

1. This is a nonrebreathing mask for administering oxygen therapy.
2. It is used at an oxygen flow rate of 10–15 liter/min.
3. This device can achieve a FiO_2 of 0.8–0.9.
4. The main precaution while using this device is that reservoir bag must be inflated throughout the entire respiratory cycle (at least two-third full) to ensure adequate CO_2 clearance and highest possible FiO_2.
5. The main disadvantage of this device is risk of absorption atelectasis and oxygen toxicity.

Reference
1. Critical Care PROMPT CiPP Cambridge University Press, 2019.

OSCE 5.

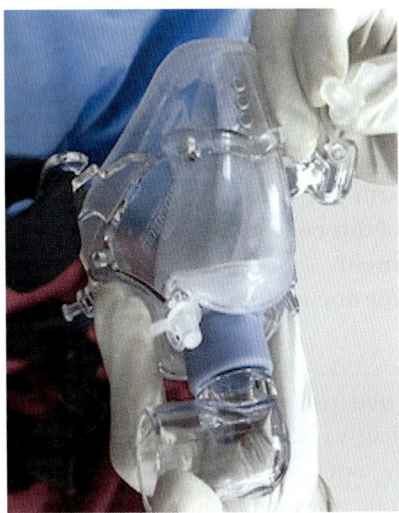

1. Identify this device.
2. What is the main advantage of NIV over invasive ventilation?
3. What is the indication of NIV in obstetrics?
4. What is the most important contraindication for use of this device?
5. Name complications of this device.

Ans.

1. This is a noninvasive ventilation mask also called the CPAP mask.

2. The main advantage of this is that it avoids endotracheal intubation. In pregnancy there is 4-fold increase in difficult intubation and 8-fold increase in failed intubation. Other advantages are:
   a. Preservation of speech and swallowing
   b. Maintenance of upper airway protective mechanisms—glottic barrier maintained—no pooling of secretions—lesser nosocomial pneumonia
3. The main indications of NIV in obstetrics are—respiratory failure due to:
   a. Pulmonary edema—noncardiogenic
   b. Pulmonary edema—cardiogenic
   c. ARDS
   d. Pneumonia
   e. COPD
   f. Asthma
4. The most important contraindication is a poor mental status (GCS) with inability to protect airway. Others are—cardiorespiratory collapse, hemoptysis, GI bleed, status eclampticus and facial injury.
5. The main complications are facial and nasal pressure sores/injury and gastric distention.

References
1. Critical Care PROMPT CiPP, Cambridge University Press 2019.
2. Irwin and Rippes Intensive Care Medicine, 8th edition.

OSCE 6. A 25-year-old primigravida at 35 weeks is brought in the emergency with history of convulsions. She is not responding to verbal commands. Her BP is 160/108 mm Hg.
1. How will you address the safety of the patient?
2. What initial assessment will you do?
3. What is the likely cause of this condition?
4. List the immediate treatment.
5. What are the key points for documentation in the case records?

Ans.
1. Patient to be nursed in bed/trolley with side rails and in lateral position to prevent aspiration, oropharyngeal airway to prevent tongue bite and maintain airway.
2. Pulse, BP, respiratory rate, SpO_2, GCS, pallor, icterus, any sign of injury, temperature. Lungs will be auscultated, obstetric examination including FHS and urine output (after inserting indwelling catheter).
3. Most important differential is eclampsia; other important diagnosis to be ruled out is CVA due to severe hypertension and pre-existing seizure disorder.
4. Immediate treatment consists of:
   a. *Preventing further seizure:* Magnesium sulfate is drug of choice
   b. *Treating hypertension:* IV Labetalol is the preferred antihypertensive
   c. *Supportive care:* Oxygen therapy, IV fluids
   d. *Definitive treatment:* Consists of termination of pregnancy

5. Key points for documentation are the history, examination findings, investigations sent, treatment advised, plan for delivery and communication with the relatives of the patient.

Reference
1. Critical Care PROMPT CiPP, Cambridge University Press 2019.

OSCE 7.

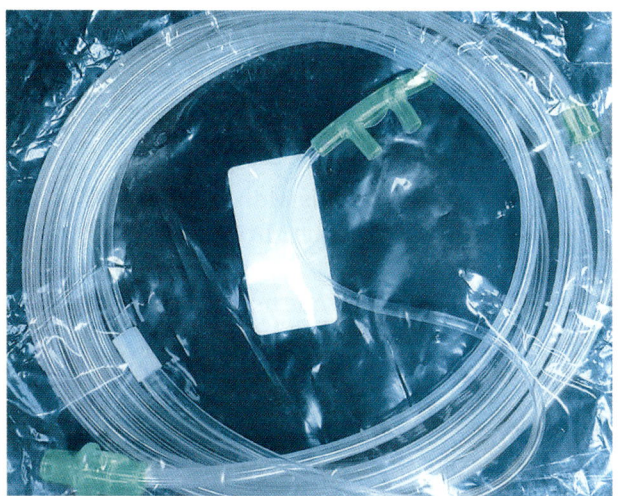

1. What is this device?
2. What is the maximum flow rate and FiO_2 that can be delivered by this device?
3. Name two pulmonary effects of oxygen toxicity.

Ans.

1. This is an oxygen nasal cannula/nasal prongs.
2. Maximum flow rate is 6 L/min and maximum FiO_2 that can be delivered is up to 0.44.
3. Pulmonary effects of oxygen toxicity are:
    a. Hypoventilation
    b. Absorption atelectasis
    c. Pulmonary vasodilatation
    d. Decreased mucociliary clearance
    e. Bronchopulmonary dysplasia

Reference
1. Critical Care PROMPT CiPP, Cambridge University Press 2019.

OSCE 8.

A 22-year-old P0L0A1 with postabortal day 10 (history of MTP pill intake) referred to emergency with history of fever since last 7 days, and bleeding per vaginum on and off since last 5 days with foul smelling discharge. On examination, GCS—15/15, PR— 128/min, BP—82/44 mm Hg, RR—28/min, SpO_2—96% (room air), pallor present. Per abdomen

examination normal, per vaginal examination reveals bulky uterus with cervical motion tenderness, B/L adnexa tender and gloved finger stained with blood and foul-smelling discharge.
1. What is the likely diagnosis?
2. What is septic shock?
3. Within how much time of recognition of sepsis should antibiotic be administered for best outcome?
4. What is the fluid of choice in septic shock?
5. How much fluid should be administered?

Ans.

1. Septic abortion in shock
2. Septic shock is defined as presence of sepsis with:
   a. Vasopressor requirement to maintain the MAP of >65 mm Hg
   b. Serum lactate level >2 mmol/L
3. Antibiotic should be administered within one hour of recognition of sepsis.
4. Crystalloids (RL) is the fluid of choice in septic shock.
5. In the initial resuscitation from sepsis induced hypoperfusion at least 30 mL/kg crystalloid should be given within 3 hours

Reference
1. Surviving Sepsis Campaign Guidelines 2021.

OSCE 9.

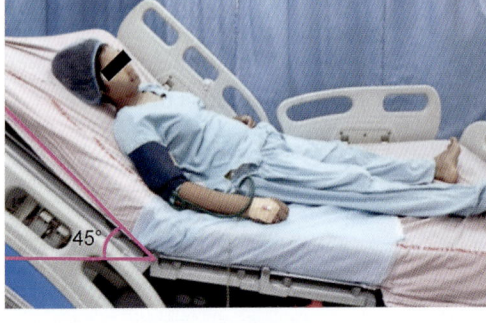 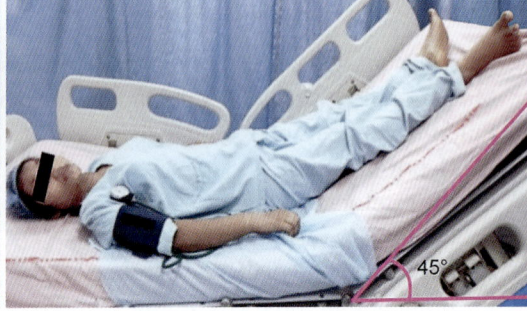

1. What is this test called?
2. What is this used for?
3. How do you interpret it at the bedside?
4. What are the two types of tests to assess fluid responsiveness?
5. Name another bedside noninvasive test used for the same purpose.

Ans.

1. The test is called passive leg raising test (PLR).
2. This test is a dynamic test used for assessing the fluid responsiveness.

3. Baseline pulse pressure is taken (SBP-DBP) when patient's head end is raised at 45°. Patient's legs are then passively raised at 45° for around 1–3 minutes and pulse pressure is repeated. If pulse pressure has increased by 9% from baseline the patient is fluid responsive and further fluid boluses can be given if patient is still hypotensive.
4. Fluid responsiveness is assessed by static tests and dynamic tests.
5. Another test used for the same purpose is inferior vena cava collapsibility test.

References
1. Surviving Sepsis Campaign 2021.
2. Practical Approach to Critical Care in Obstetrics 2018, 1st edition.

OSCE 10.

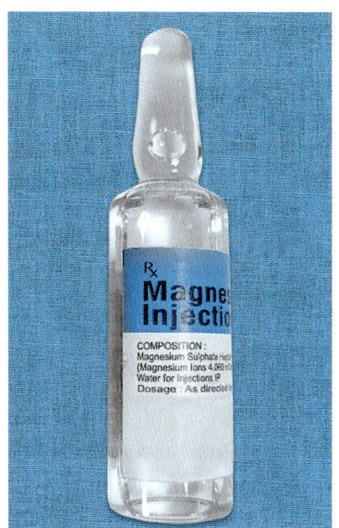

1. What is this drug?
2. Name two important uses in obstetrics.
3. Name two contraindications of using this drug.
4. What is the antidote?
5. Name one indication of Zuspan regime.

Ans.
1. This is magnesium sulfate.
2. It is used in seizure prophylaxis in hypertension and neuroprotection in preterm baby (<32 weeks).
3. The contraindications are myasthenia gravis and renal failure.
4. The antidote is 10 mL, 10% calcium gluconate.
5. HELLP syndrome with platelet count less than 50,000 cumm

Reference
1. William Obstetrics 26th edition.

OSCE 11.

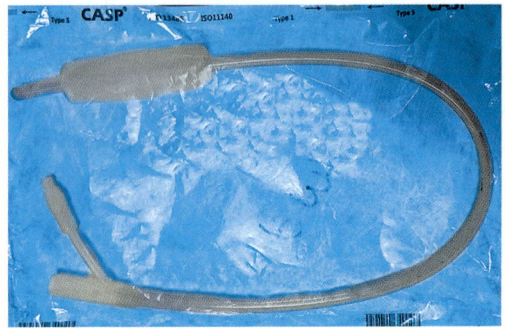

1. What is this device?
2. When is this used?
3. How much fluid to be instilled in this?
4. Name any other alternative device used for the same purpose.
5. What is the next step if this method fails during managing postpartum hemorrhage?

Ans.

1. This is Bakri balloon.
2. This is used as tamponade when medical methods for managing postpartum hemorrhage fails.
3. 500–550 mL fluid is to be instilled.
4. Other methods of tamponade are using condom catheter, Chhattisgarh balloon, Rosch balloon, Sengstaken-Blakemore balloon.
5. The next step is to proceed for surgical management or uterine artery embolization (if patient hemodynamically stable) when available.

Reference

1. William's Obstetrics, 25th edition.

OSCE 12.

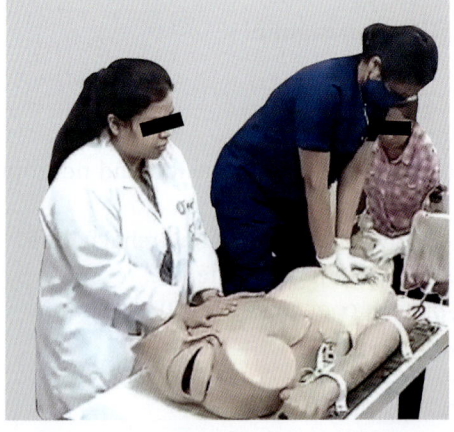

A primigravida at 38 weeks found pulseless, BP not recordable just after entering the emergency room.
1. What should be done next?
2. Name the maneuver which is done differently while resuscitating pregnant women.
3. If CPR is ongoing for 3 minutes and the pregnant lady is still pulseless what should be the next step?
4. Where should a perimortem cesarean delivery be done?
5. Should perimortem cesarean delivery be done if the fetus is an IUFD?

Ans.
1. Initiate code blue and start CPR immediately.
2. Left uterine displacement (LUD) to reduce the pressure of the gravid uterus on the inferior vena cava, which will make the compressions more effective.
3. The next step should be resuscitative hysterotomy or perimortem cesarean section.
4. It should be done at the place where CPR is being given.
5. It is done even if there is an IUFD as it is a resuscitative procedure for the mother.

Reference
1. American Heart Association Guidelines for CPR 2020.

OSCE 13.

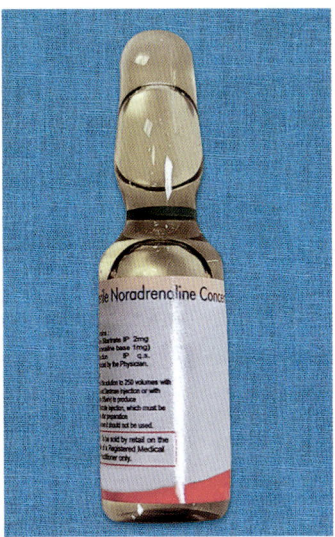

1. What is this drug?
2. What is the mechanism of action and what is its use?
3. What is the target mean arterial pressure (MAP) while using this drug?
4. In what doses is it used in septic shock?

Ans.
1. This is noradrenaline for IV infusion.

2. This is vasopressor, works on alpha and beta receptors, helps in increasing the systemic vascular resistance. Thus, it is used in most types of shock.
3. The target MAP is >65 mm Hg.
4. Its dose in septic shock is 0.05–1.5 mcg/kg/min.

References
1. Surviving Sepsis Campaign Guidelines, 2021.
2. Practical Approach to Critical Care in Obstetrics, 2018, 1st edition.

OSCE 14.

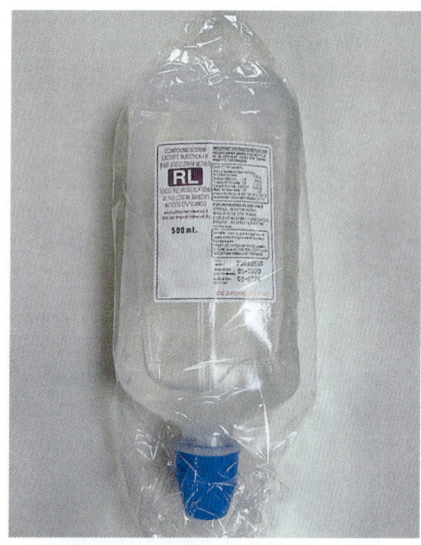

1. What type of fluid is this?
2. What is the sodium content in this fluid?
3. In which condition it is relatively contraindicated?
4. Why should we not administer it in the same IV line as blood?
5. Does this fluid cause metabolic acidosis?

Ans.
1. This is a crystalloid.
2. The sodium content is 130 mmol/L.
3. It is relatively contraindicated in patients with hyperkalemia.
4. RL if administered in the same IV line with blood causes chelation of blood because of calcium in the RL.
5. This fluid does not cause metabolic acidosis as the lactate is metabolized to bicarbonate in the liver.

Reference
1. Suri J, et al. Practical Approach to Critical Care in Obstetrics, 2018, 1st edition.

OSCE 15.

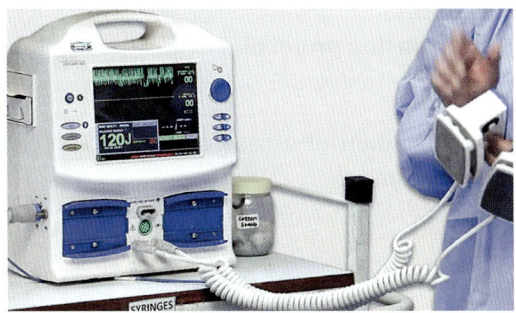

1. What is this device?
2. What is the indication to give shock during CPR?
3. What are the contraindications of its use?
4. How many Joules of energy is recommended in pregnant women?
5. Name any additional precaution that has to be taken in pregnant women.

Ans.

1. This is defibrillator.
2. Defibrillation is to be used if ECG waveform shows ventricular fibrillation or ventricular tachycardia in a patient having cardiac arrest.
3. It should not be used in:
   a. Asystole
   b. Supraventricular tachycardia
4. The amount of shock to be given in a biphasic defibrillator is 120–200 Joules which is same as in nonpregnant.
5. Attachment of any maternal monitors and fetal electrodes are to be disconnected prior to giving shock.

Reference

1. American Heart Association CPR Guidelines, 2020.

OSCE 16.

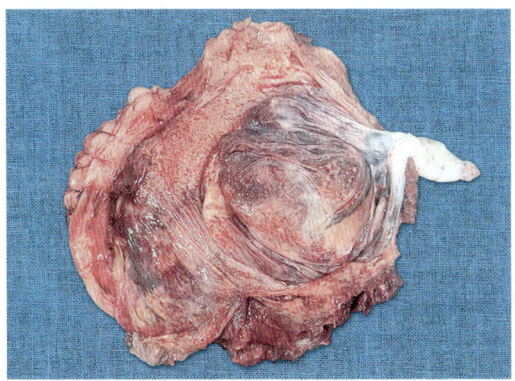

1. What is this condition? What are the types?
2. What is "triple P" procedure?
3. Define massive blood transfusion protocol.

Ans.

1. This is a hysterectomy specimen of a case of placenta accreta spectrum/morbidly adherent placenta. The types are:
   a. Placenta accreta
   b. Placenta increta
   c. Placenta percreta
2. "Triple P" procedure, which is a conservative procedure to avoid hysterectomy, involves
   a. Perioperative localization of the upper placental edge
   b. Pelvic devascularization
   c. Placental nonseparation with myometrial excision followed by the repair of the myometrial defect.
3. Massive blood transfusion is defined as:
   a. Replacement of 10 units of red cells in 24 hours or
   b. 3 units of red blood cells over one hour or
   c. Any four blood components in 30 minutes or
   d. Replacement of more than one blood volume in 24 hours

Reference

1. William Obstetrics 26th edition.

OSCE 17.

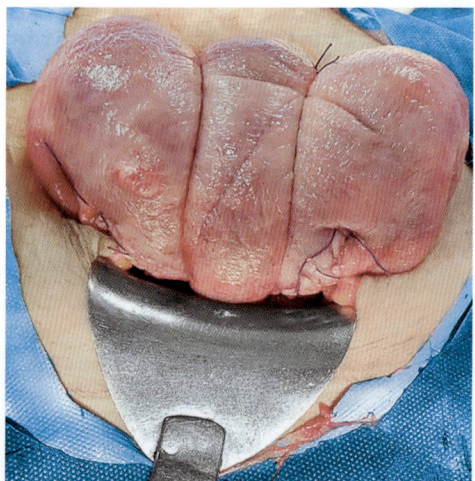

1. Identify this.
2. Name two more similar kinds of sutures.
3. What is the site of internal iliac artery ligation? Which branch of internal iliac artery is ligated during management of PPH?

Ans.
1. This is a compression suture for management of atonic PPH—Hayman's suture.
2. Two other compression sutures are:
   a. B-Lynch suture
   b. Cho square suture
3. Internal iliac artery is ligated 3–5 cm distal from the point of its division. The anterior branch of internal iliac artery is ligated.

Reference
1. William's Obstetrics, 25th edition.

OSCE 18.

A 23-year-old, primigravida presented in the emergency with complaints of shortness of breath and palpitation. Her SpO_2 on room air is 91%, PR 108/min, BP 104/62 mm Hg, RR 40/min. She had history of high grade fever 3 days back along with cough and expectoration. ABG done and the PF ratio was 180. She was admitted in the OBS-CCU and bedside ECHO was normal. Her chest X-ray is shown below.

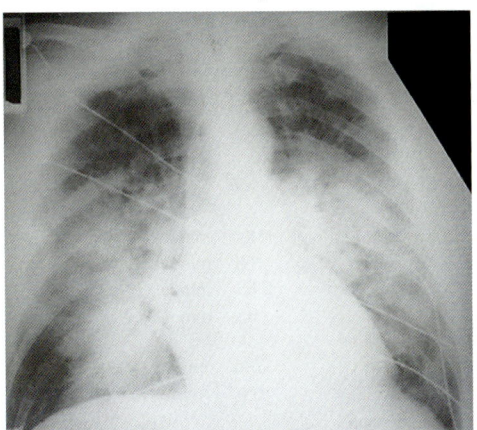

1. What is the diagnosis?
2. What are the criteria used for defining this condition?
3. What is the normal pH, target PaO_2 and $PaCO_2$ in pregnant female?

Ans.
1. This is a case of acute respiratory distress syndrome (ARDS).
2. The criteria used for diagnosis in ARDS is Berlin's criteria.
3. The normal pH in pregnancy is 7.40–7.46, target PaO_2 is 95–105 mm Hg and PCO_2 is 28–35 mm Hg in a pregnant woman.

References
1. Suri J, et al. Practical Approach to Critical Care in Obstetrics, 2018, 1st edition.
2. Pandya ST, Krishna SJ. Acute respiratory distress syndrome in pregnancy. Indian J Crit Care Med. 2021;25(Suppl 3):S241-S247.

OSCE 19.

A 35-year-old primigravida presented at 31 weeks of gestation with altered mentation, cold clammy extremity, dehydrated tongue and sweet smell in breath. PR 110/min, BP 100/56 (MAP 62 mm Hg), SpO_2 80% (room air), RR 26/min. She had leaking per vagina since 1 week, she is a known case of diabetes who was being treated with insulin and in the referral center she received injection betamethasone. She was intubated and admitted to the ICU. Her ABG at an FiO_2 of 1 is shown below:

Blood gas values			
↓ pH	7.053		[7.350–7.450]
pCO_2	38.5	mm Hg	[35.0–45.0]
↑pO_2	191	mm Hg	[83.0–108]
Temperature corrected values			
pH(T)	7.053		
pCO_2(T)	38.5	mm Hg	
pO_2(T)	191	mm Hg	
Acid base status			
$cHCO_3^-$(P)c	10.2	mmol/L	
$cHCO_3^-$(P.st)c	10.3	mmol/L	
cBase(B)c	–18.8	mmol/L	
cBase(Ecf)c	–18.1	mmol/L	
Cximetry values			
↓ctHb	8.5	g/dL	[12.0–16.0]
sO_2	95.6	%	[95.0–99.0]
FMetHb	1.8	%	
FO2Hb	94.0	%	
FCOHb	–0.1	%	
FHHb	4.3	%	
Electrolyte values			
↓cNa^+	121	mmol/L	[135–145]
↓cK^+	3.8	mmol/L	[4.3–4.5]
↓cCa^{2+}	0.63	mmol/L	[1.15–1.29]
↓cCl^-	93	mmol/L	[98–106]
Metabolite values			
↑cGlu	298	mg/dL	[70–105]
cLac	0.9	mg/dL	[0.5–1.5]
Calculated values			
Anion Gap c	17.6	mmol/L	
AnionGap K^+c	21.4	mmol/L	
$ctCO_2$(P)c	25.6	1/0%	

1. What is the likely diagnosis?
2. What are the main components of treatment of this condition?
3. What is the indication for giving bicarbonate in this patient? Is it indicated in this case?

Ans.

1. The diagnosis is diabetic ketoacidosis.
2. The main three component of treatment are:
    a. Resuscitation for correction of fluid loss with intravenous fluids (NS initially)
    b. Correction of hyperglycemia with IV plain insulin
    c. Correction of electrolyte disturbances, particularly potassium loss
3. Injection sodium bicarbonate has to be given only if the pH is <7.0. In this case it is not indicated.

Reference

1. ACOG guideline on pregestational diabetes mellitus 2018.

OSCE 20.

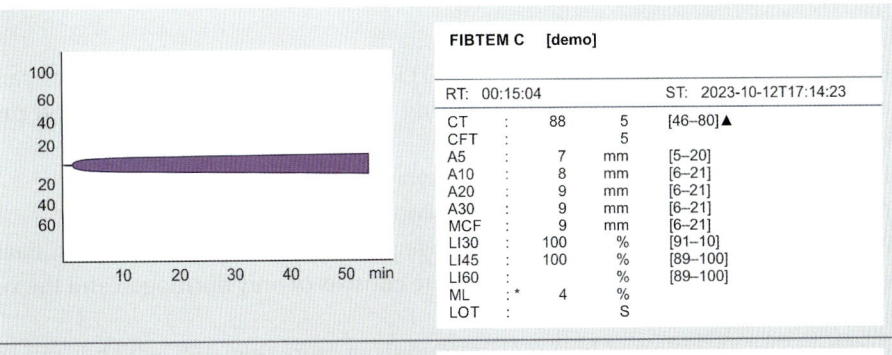

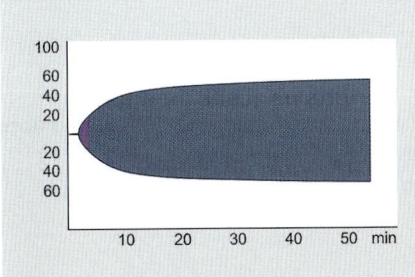

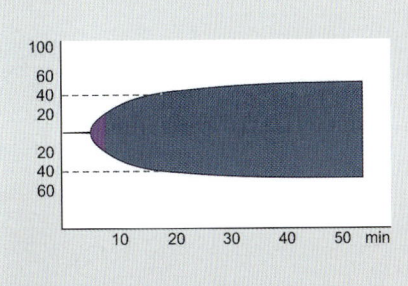

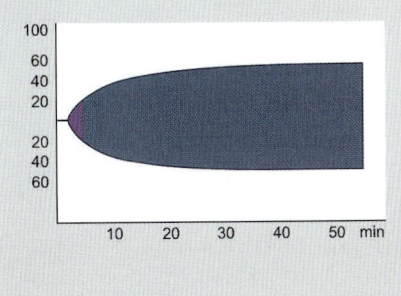

FIBTEM C [demo]

RT: 00:15:04   ST: 2023-10-12T17:14:23

CT	:	88	5	[46–80]▲
CFT	:		5	
A5	:	7	mm	[5–20]
A10	:	8	mm	[6–21]
A20	:	9	mm	[6–21]
A30	:	9	mm	[6–21]
MCF	:	9	mm	[6–21]
LI30	:	100	%	[91–10]
LI45	:	100	%	[89–100]
LI60	:		%	[89–100]
ML	:*	4	%	
LOT	:		S	

EXTEM C [demo]

RT: 00:34:24   ST: 2023-10-12T17:14:28

CT	:	93	5	[50–80]▲
CFT	:	132	5	[46–149]
A5	:	33	mm	[32–52]
A10	:	43	mm	[43–63]
A20	:	51	mm	[52–70]▼
A30	:	53	mm	[54–72]▼
MCF	:	55	mm	[55–72]
LI30	:	100	%	
LI45	:	100	%	[98–100]
LI60	:		%	[94–100]
ML	:*	0	%	
LOT	:		S	

INTEM C [demo]

RT: 00:53:55   ST: 2023-10-12T17:14:58

CT	:	322	5	[161–204]▲
CFT	:	161	5	[63–130]▲
A5	:	29	mm	[33–52]▼
A10	:	39	mm	[43–62]▼
A20	:	47	mm	[50–68]▼
A30	:	50	mm	[51–69]▼
MCF	:*	52	mm	[51–69]
LI30	:	100	%	[98–100]
LI45	:	100	%	[92–100]
LI60	:		%	[87–100]
ML	:*	0	%	
LOT	:		S	

APTEM C [demo]

RT: 00:52:56   ST: 2023-10-12T17:15:57

CT	:	103	5	[41–80]▲
CFT	:	150	5	[62–184]
A5	:	30	mm	[28–50]
A10	:	40	mm	[39–61]
A20	:	48	mm	[48–68]
A30	:	51	mm	[51–71]
MCF	:	52	mm	[52–71]
LI30	:	100	%	
LI45	:	100	%	[98–100]
LI60	:		%	[93–100]
ML	:*	0	%	
LOT	:		S	

Section 1: Obstetrics

1. What is this test?
2. What does INTEM reflect?
3. What does FIBTEM reflect?
4. What is the difference between FFP and cryoprecipitate?
5. Does the above graph show any evidence of hyperfibrinolysis?

Ans.

1. This is rotational thromboelastometry (ROTEM) report which is a point of care test to diagnose/assess coagulopathy in bleeding patient and guide in the blood product transfusion
2. INTEM reflects the intrinsic coagulation pathway
3. FIBTEM reflects the fibrinogen levels in the blood
4. FFP is fresh frozen plasma which has fibrinogen and other coagulation factors. Each unit has a volume of 50–70 mL. The cryoprecipitate consists of only fibrinogen and the volume of each unit is only 15–20 mL
5. Hyperfibrinolysis is reflected by a maximum lysis of more than 15% which is not seen in this case

References

1. Mallaiah S, Barclay P, Harrod I, et al. Introduction of an algorithm for ROTEM-guided fibrinogen concentrate administration in major obstetric haemorrhage. Anaesthesia. 2015;70:166.
2. Irwin & Rippes Intensive Care Medicine, 8th edition.
3. ROTEM Interpretation, NHS, 2021.

CHAPTER 23

Maternal and Neonatal Health Programs

Aruna Nigam, Zeba Khanam

OSCE 1. The National Health Mission was launched by the Ministry of Health and Family Welfare, Government of India in 2005 to strengthen healthcare delivery system in the country. It aims to ensure comprehensive, accessible, affordable, and quality health care to all citizens (Universal Health Coverage), especially poor people and those living in remote and rural areas.
1. Enumerate four major initiatives under the NHM.
2. What is the new name proposed for NHM?

Ans.

1. Major initiatives under NHM include:[1]
    (1) Accredited Social Health Workers (ASHAs) as facilitators, mobilizers, and providers of community health care; *Certification of ASHA* by the National Institute of Open Schooling (NIOS).
    (2) *Rogi Kalyaan Samiti/Patient Welfare Committee/Hospital Management Society:* A registered society whose trustees manage hospital affairs and ensure provision of better facilities to patients. They are funded by the government.
    (3) *United Grants to Subcentres*
    (4) *Village Health Sanitation and Nutrition Committee (VHSNC):* Community empowerment and participation at grassroot level to address environmental and social issues.
    (5) Enhancing health human resource, training of MBBS in Emergency Obstetric Care (*EmOC*), Life Saving Anesthesia Skills (*LSAS*), and laparoscopic surgeries, colocation of AYUSH services at public health facilities, capacity building of nursing staffs and ANMs.
    (6) *Janani Suraksha Yojna (JSY):* Cast incentivizing scheme for increasing rates of institutional deliveries to reduce maternal and neonatal deaths.
    (7) *Janani Sishu Suraksha Karayakaram (JSSK):* Free and cashless delivery and care to sick infant up to one year of age for pregnant women and infants assessing public healthcare systems.
    (8) *Facility-based newborn care:* Establishment of Newborn Care Corners (NBCCs) at delivery points/DPs, Special Newborn Care Units (SNCUs) at district hospital/medical colleges, and Newborn Stabilisation Units (NBSUs) are First Referral Units (FRUs).

(9) *National Mobile Medical Units (NMMUs) Service*
(10) *National Ambulance Service:* Dial 108 is an emergency response system against critically ill patients, or patients of trauma or accidents; Dial 102 is a basic patient transport system, including for pregnant women and children.
(11) Mainstreaming of *AYUSH*
(12) *Mother to Child Tracking System (MCTS) and Mother to Child Tracking Facilitation Centre (MCTFC):* MCTS captures information on and tract all pregnant women and children up to the age of 5 so that receive full maternal and child healthcare services; the MCTFC is operationalized by the National Institute of Health and Family Welfare (NIHFW) through helpdesk agents to validate data entered in MCTS and to guide the beneficiaries and service providers with updated information on mother and childcare services through phone calls and interactive voice response system (IVRS), to collect feedback on the services provided from the beneficiaries, and to raise awareness about the public mother and child-related health programmes.
(13) *India Newborn Action Plan (INAP):* Targeted strategy to increase the rate of decline in preventable neonatal death and stillbirths with the goal of achieving single digit neonatal mortality rate and stillbirth rate by 2030. It is implemented within the RMNCH+A framework.
(14) *Intensified Diarrhoea Control Fortnight (IDCF):* Aims to prevent deaths due to childhood diarrhea.
(15) *Rashtriya Bal Swasthya Karyakaram (RBSK):* It aims to screening and early intervention through early detection and treatment of 4 Ds in children, namely Defects at birth, Diseases, Deficiencies, and Developmental delays including Disabilities.
(16) *Rashtriya Kishor Swasthya Karyakaram (RKSK):* It aims to target adolescent boys and groups in their own spaces through peer-led interventions at community levels while focusing on reproductive, sexual, and other aspects of life (life skills, nutrition, injuries, violence, gender-based violence, noncommunicable diseases, and substance abuse).
(17) *MCH (Maternal and Child Health) wings:* 100/50/50 bedded MCH wings are being built in public healthcare facilities with high bed occupancy to meet increased demand.
(18) *Free Drugs and Free Diagnostic Service* to all patients attending public healthcare facilities.
(19) *National Iron Plus Initiative (NIPI)* and *Intensified NIPI-Anemia Mukt Bharat*
(20) *Reproductive, Maternal, Newborn, Child, and Adolescent Health services (RMNCH+A):* It is a continuum of care approach to improve health of women across all stages of life cycle (newborn, child, adolescent, reproductive, pregnancy and lactational stages) by strengthening linkages between community and facility-based health services and between various levels of healthcare system.[2]
(21) Establishment of *Delivery Points (DPs):* Health facilities with high demand for service and performance are identified as delivery points with the objective of providing comprehensive RMNCH+A services at these facilities.
(22) Achieving *Universal Health Coverage (UHC)* by 2030.

(23) Single and comprehensive *Quality Assurance* approach under the National Quality Assurance Standards (NQAS).
(24) *MusQan initiative:* This initiative ensures quality child-friendly services in public health facilities within the existing National Quality Standards Framework (NQAS) to reduce preventable morbidity and mortality in children of 0–12 years of age group.

2. The new name proposed by the central government for the National Health Mission is Pradhan Mantri Samagra Swasthya Mission.

OSCE 2. District medical officers and other providers of labor room of the Southeast district were subjected to a clinical update cum skills training that was focused on intrapartum and immediate postpartum care. The training was mentored by master trainers at a high load Community Health Centre (CHC) and was aimed at strengthening competencies of the providers.

1. What is this initiative called?
2. In which year did the Government of India launch this initiative?
3. Mention four pause points in the initiative?
4. Where should such training of providers ensue?
5. What do you understand by a high delivery load facility?

Ans.

1. This initiative is called DAKSHTA initiative.
2. It was launched by the Ministry of Health and Family Welfare Government of India in 2015. It is based on the WHO derived Safe Childbirth Checklist.[3]
3. The four pause points include: At the time of admission; just before pushing or at cesarean section; within 1 hour of delivery; at the time of the discharge.
4. The place should have a high delivery load and can be a district hospital or a community health centre (CHC), etc.
5. A high delivery load facility is the one which records a delivery per month of 50 or more.

OSCE 3. The Janani Shishu Suraksha Karyakaram (JSSK) was launched in June 2011 to improve access to maternal and child health care in India.

1. What is the goal of this programme?
2. Who are the beneficiaries?
3. What are the entitlements in the JSSK for the pregnant woman delivering at a public healthcare facility?

Ans.

1. The goal of this programme is to provide an absolutely free, out-of-pocket expense delivery (including cesarean section) and care of the newborn.[1]
2. The JSSK covers all pregnant women and infants up to the age of one year who are assessing public healthcare system.
3. Entitlements for the woman are free drugs, free consumables, free diagnostics, free blood, and free diet for up to 3 days in case of a vaginal delivery and for up to 7 days in case

of cesarean delivery. It also includes transportation of the woman between healthcare facility, between facilities, from home to a facility and vice versa. The same applies for the infant up to one year of age.

OSCE 4. SUMAN initiative was launched under the flagship of RMNCH+A framework.
1. It was launched under the flagship of?
2. What does SUMAN stand for?
3. What is the aim of this initiative?
4. Enumerate two services guaranteed to the beneficiary under this initiative?

Ans.

1. RMNCH+A framework.
2. SUMAN stands for Surakshit Martitivya Aashwasan.[2]
3. *Aim:* To provide assured, dignified, respectful and quality health care at zero cost and zero tolerance for denial of services for every pregnant woman and newborn visiting a public healthcare system in order to end all preventable maternal and neonatal deaths and morbidities and provide a positive birthing experience.
4. The services that are guaranteed are:
    - Zero tolerance to any negligence
    - Integration of existing initiatives such as JSY, JSSK, PMSMA, LaQshya, FRUs, etc.
    - Respect for woman's autonomy, dignity, feelings, and choices
    - 100% Maternal Death Reporting and Reviews (MDRs)
    - Grievance redressal mechanism
    - Client feedback mechanism
    - Awards to SUMAN champions
    - Community level maternal death reporting
    - Community engagement and mega Information-Education-Communication (IEC)/Behavior-Change-Communication (BCC)
    - Intersectoral convergence

OSCE 5. Sushila is an ASHA worker. She has brought a laboring woman, Mahua and her husband Ashok from a nearby village to a community health centre in Jharkhand for delivery.
1. Are Sushila and Mahua eligible for a cash incentive? If yes, how much?
2. If Mahua belonged to Kerala, how much incentive money she would receive under the JSY scheme?

Ans.

1. Mahua belongs to rural area in a low performance state (Jharkhand). Hence, Sushila and Mahua are eligible for cash incentives of ₹ 600 and ₹ 1400, respectively.[2]
2. Kerala is a high performing state. Hence a woman delivering in a rural area of Kerala will receive ₹ 700 and the ASHA will receive ₹ 600.

Chapter 23: Maternal and Neonatal Health Programs | **323**

OSCE 6. Mahua has come to the CHC at 6 weeks of childbirth. She has two children now and is confused if she should use an IUCD or go for tubal ligation.
1. Mahua wants to know how much incentive she will get for IUCD insertion and tubectomy. What will you tell her?
2. Within how much period, compensation to client should be applied under the Family Planning Indemnity Scheme?

Ans.
1. Mahua will receive a cash incentive of ₹ 2,000 for interval ligation. She will receive ₹ 300 for postabortal IUCD insertion.[2]
2. All claims of death/complications/failure should be filed by the beneficiary with the District Indemnity Sub-Committee (DISC) within 90 days of occurrence.

OSCE 7.
1. Aim of Mission Parivar Vikas?
2. What was the total fertility rate above which this scheme was applicable?
3. What is *Extended Mission Parivar Vikas*?
4. Name Promotional Schemes under Mission Parivar Vikas.
5. The Government of India recently added a contraceptive to the basket of contraception in March 2023. Name the method.

Ans.
1. *Mission Parivar Vikas* was rolled out in 2016 as a stratified approach to increase access to contraceptives and family planning services.
2. Total fertility rate of 3 or more.
3. It was latter extended to six North Eastern states (Arunanchal Pradesh, Manipur, Mizoram, Nagaland, Tripura, Meghalaya) in 2021 as *Extended Mission Parivar Vikas*.[2]
4. Promotional Schemes under Mission Parivaar Vikas:
    (1) *Nayi pahel kits for Newly Weds:* These family planning kits are distributed to newly wed couples by the ASHAs at a price not exceeding Rs 250/kit.
    (2) *Saas Bahu Sammelan:* The ASHAs are responsible for mobilizing mothers-in-law and daughters-in-law for the Saas Bahu Sammelan.
    (3) *Saarthi: Awareness on Wheels*—A bus/van is operationalized to sensitize and disseminate family planning messages in hard-to-reach areas fortnightly in the months of April, July, November, and January from 11th to 25th of the designated months. The vehicle is equipped with IEC materials, family planning commodities and interactive communication devices.
    (4) *Local radio spots* with messages from local actors
5. The Government of India has recently added the single rod subdermal implant, Implanon NXT to the basket of contraception in March 2023.

OSCE 8. The hon'ble Prime Minister highlighted the aims and purpose of introduction of a Single Window System for reducing maternal and neonatal deaths in India through public private partnership in the July 31st, 2016, episode's Mann Ki Baat.
1. The Prime Minister was referring to which national programme?
2. Write the three salient features of this programme?
3. What do you understand from Mother and Child Protection Cards and Safe Motherhood booklets?

Ans.

1. The Prime Minister in this talk highlighted the aims and objectives of the *Pradhan Mantri Sushrakshit Matritivya Abhiyaan (PMSMA)* in this episode of Mann Ki Baat.[2]
2. *Key features of PMSMA:*
   (1) Antenatal checkup services by an Obs/gyne Specialist/Radiologist/Physicians.
   (2) Voluntary engagement of private practitioners for antenatal care.
   (3) A minimum package of antenatal care (investigations/medicines) should be provided to the pregnant woman on the 9th day of every month at designated government health facilities (PHCs or CHCs, district hospitals, urban healthcare centers) in both rural and urban areas. This will be in addition to the routine outreach at these health facilities.
   (4) A minimum package of investigation that includes a second trimester ultrasound and medicines (iron and calcium supplements) would be provided to all women in the PMSMA clinics.
   (5) Special efforts are made to reach out to all pregnant women not registered for ANC and to those already registered but not availed ANC services, in addition to high-risk cases.
   (6) Provision of Mother and Child Protection Cards (MCP) and Safe Motherhood booklets.
   (7) *IPledgeFor9* awards for individuals and teams for voluntary contributions to the PMSMA programme.
3. Each pregnant woman under the PMSMA programme will be given a MCP card and Safe Motherhood booklet for documentation of ANC services provide to them. Each MCP card will have a sticker at each visit indicating high risk (red sticker) or no risk (green sticker).

OSCE 9. Meenakshi has delivered her second child at a very busy Government hospital of Delhi. Her past childbirth experience at the same hospital was not very satisfactory and she was very apprehensive this time during her admission to the hospital. However, to her surprise, it was a lot better. The doctor had allowed her a companion, the nurses as well as the doctors were very polite and the labor room was very clean, well maintained and allowed much privacy.
1. The following changes are secondary to the implementation of which government programme?
2. What are the three key objectives of this programme?
3. Quality standards of the programme implementation are monitored by which body?

Chapter 23: Maternal and Neonatal Health Programs

Ans.

1. The changes could be due to the implementation of the *LaQshya initiative* or the *Labor Room Quality Improvement Initiative*.
2. The key objective of the programme is to ensure quality of care during intrapartum and immediate postpartum period, stabilization of complications arising during this time, ensuring timely referrals, and enabling an effective two-way follow-up system. It also envisages to enhance the satisfaction of beneficiaries visiting health facilities and provide respectful maternity care (RMC) to all pregnant women attending public healthcare systems.[2]
3. The quality improvement in labor rooms and operation theaters under the LaQshya initiative are monitored by the *National Quality Assurance Standards (NQAS)*. This think tank was established by the Ministry of Health and Family Welfare for quality checks at primary and secondary public healthcare facilities. NQAS recommends internal assessments, state assessments (at least once a year) and national assessments (when the facility scores 70% or more in State assessments).

OSCE 10. Nitya, who is a primigravida at 6 weeks of gestation was infected with HIV I during her childhood. She is an antiretroviral therapy naïve and visits a PHC for antenatal care.
1. Which antiretroviral therapy (ART) will you prescribe?
2. Which phase of National AIDS Control Programme (NACP) is operational as of now?
3. What is 95-95-95 target for Elimination of Mother to Child Transmission (EMTCT) of HIV infection?
4. What are the four prongs of National PPTCT programme?

Ans.

1. Nitya should be started on TLD regimen (Tenofovir (TDF) 300 mg+ Lamivudine (3TC) 300 mg + Dolutegravir (DTG) 50 mg) once a day irrespective of her CD4+ status and the stage of HIV infection.[4]
2. As of now the fourth phase of National AIDS Control Programme is operational.
3. The government of India has set a target of 95-95-95 for EMTCT to be maintained for at least 2 years. This means that more than 95% of all estimated pregnant women are registered for antenatal care and receive at least one antenatal check-up; more than 95% of all estimated pregnant women are tested for HIV; and more than 95% of all HIV positive pregnant women are on ART.[4]
4. The four prongs of the National PPTCT programme are:
    i. Primary prevention of HIV, especially among women of childbearing age
    ii. Prevention of unintended pregnancies among women living with HIV/AIDS
    iii. Prevention of HIV transmission from pregnant women infected with HIV to their children
    iv. Provide care, support and treatment to women living with HIV AIDS and to their children and families[4]

OSCE 11. Mira is a 10-year-old girl and a ninth grader who goes to a government school. She has come to visit her doctor because she is feeling weak. On examination, she was found anemic. Mira discloses that she was given some pills at school that she was not consuming.
1. What could be the pills?
2. What is 6 × 6 × 6 strategy in the Anemia Mukt Bharat? Name only
3. Who all are included in first 6

Ans.
1. Mira is supposed to receive iron and folic acid (IFA) tablets at her school. She is also supposed to take deworming tablets twice in a year along with fortified mid-day meals.[5]
2. The 6 × 6 × 6 strategy in the Anemia Mukt Bharat programme stands for 6 beneficiaries, 6 interventions and 6 institutional mechanisms.
3. 6 beneficiaries include:

> **Beneficiaries**
> - Children between 6 and 59 months of age
> - Adolescents boys (school-going) and girls between 15 and 19 years of age
> - Women of reproductive age
> - Pregnant women
> - Lactating women

OSCE 12.
1. What does NDD programme?
2. What is the objective of the programme?

Ans.
1. NDD programme is National Deworming Day (NDD) programme.
2. According to the programme, bi-annual mass deworming of women and children is done on 10th February and 10th August each year.[6]

OSCE 13.
1. Name two topics for intensified year-round behavioral change communication campaign under Anemia Mukt Bharat programme to help prevent infant anemia.

Ans.
1. a. Delayed cord clamping by at least 3 minutes or until the pulsations in the cord cease in all healthcare facilities.
   b. Initiation of breastfeeding within 1 hour of birth
   c. Following appropriate Infant and Young Child Feeding Practices (IYCF)[6]

OSCE 14. Anemia Mukt Bharat Scheme is also known as Intensified-National Iron Plus Initiative.
1. What are the prophylactic dosages of Iron and Folic acid (IFA) supplementation under the Anemia Mukt Bharat scheme for nonpregnant women?

2. What are the therapeutic dosages of IFA supplementation in adolescent girls under the scheme?

Ans.

1. *Prophylactic dose of IFA:*

	Elemental iron	Folic acid	Dose
Women of reproductive age 20–48 years (nonpregnant, nonlactating); Adolescents 10–19 years	60 mg/tablet	500 µg/tablet	Prophylactic dose: One tablet in a *week* throughout the year

2. *Therapeutic dose of IFA:*

Beneficiaries	Dose	Frequency	Duration	When to refer to FRU/DH
Adolescent girls: Mild and moderate anemia (Hb 8–11.4 g/dL)	120 mg elemental iron and 1000 µg folic acid (i.e., 2 tablets at a time)	Daily	3 months	• No improvement in Hb after 3-month of treatment. • All cases of severe anemia (Hb <8g/dL)

OSCE 15. Anemia Mukt Bharat also covers the control and prevention of non-nutritional anemia in women and children.

1. What are the causes of non-nutritional anemia as highlighted in the I-NIPI?

Ans.

1. The causes of non-nutritional anemia in women and children are malaria, hemoglobinopathies, fluorosis, deficiencies of zinc, copper, vitamin B_{12} and vitamin A.[6] An excess of fluoride in water and food can damage the gastric mucosa and cause malabsorption of iron and other vitamins and minerals leading to anemia.

OSCE 16. The Government of India launched the MAA programme in 2016 to promote breastfeeding.
1. What does MAA stand for?
2. What are the 4 Bs of the scheme?

Ans.

1. The Mother's Absolute Affection (MAA) programme was launched in 2016. It is an intensified programme designed to bring undiluted attention to breastfeeding. The goal of the programme is to 'revitalize efforts towards promotion, protection and support of breastfeeding practices through health systems to achieve higher breastfeeding rates.'[7]
2. The 4 Bs or four components of MAA scheme are:
   B1: Awareness generation
   B2: Community level interventions (capacity building of community healthcare workers (ANM's/ASHAs/AWWs), community health dialogues by ASHAs through the mother' meeting, lactation support and interpersonal communication by skilled ANMs.

B3: Health facility strengthening.
B4: Monitoring

OSCE 17. Institutional mechanisms form one of the 6 × 6 × 6 strategy under the Anemia Mukt Bharat Programme. One of the institutional mechanisms is NCEAR-A.
1. What does NCEAR-A stand for?
2. Where is it located and what is its purpose?

Ans.

1. NCEAR-A stands for National Centre of Excellence and Advanced Research on Anemia Control.[8]
2. It is located at the Centre of Community Medicine at the All India Institute of Medical Sciences, New Delhi, India. It was established with the aim of providing technical support to the Ministry of Health and Family Welfare, Government of India for *'Incorporating Scientific, Policy and Community Perspective in Policy and Programmatic Decisions for the Control of Anemia'*.

OSCE 18.
1. What is POSHAN Abhiyaan? When is the POSHAN MAAH celebrated and what is its slogan?

Ans.

1. POSHAN stands for PM Over-reaching Scheme to Holistic Nourishment. It is a flagship programme to improve nutritional status and outcomes in women and children. It is overseen by the Ministry of Women and Child Development.[9]
   POSHAN MAAH is celebrated every year from 1st to 30th September. The Motto is: *'Suposhit Bharat, Sakshar Bharat, Sakshat Bharat'*.

OSCE 19. India is the most populous country in the world with a population of 1.432 billion. This is despite the implementation of national population policies from time to time.
1. What are the objectives of National Population Policy 2000?

Ans.

1. The medium-term objective of National Population Policy was to reduce the TFR to replacement levels (2.1 per children per woman) by 2010. The long-term objective of the policy is *'to achieve a stable population growth by 2045, at a level consistent with the requirements of sustainable economic growth, social development, and environmental protection'*.[10]

OSCE 20. The Jansankhaya SthirthaKosh (JSK) was a registered society of MoHFW. Before 2003, it was known as the National Population Stabilization Fund.
1. What schemes were implemented by the JSK?
2. Who headed the JSK?

Ans.

1. The JSK implemented three schemes:
   (1) *Prerna Scheme:* For delaying marriage, childbirth and promoting spacing
   (2) *Santushti scheme:* Public private partnership for sterilization services
   (3) National helpline for information on family planning services
   The JSK was discontinued in 2019.[11]
2. JSK was headed by Union Health Minister.

REFERENCES

1. Ministry of Health and Family Welfare. National Health Mission. [Internet]. New Delhi. [Cited 2023 October 30]. Available from: https://nhm.gov.in/.
2. Ministry of Health and Family Welfare. National Health Mission-RMNCH+A [Internet]. New Delhi. [Cited 2023 October 30]. Available from: https://nhm.gov.in/index1.php?lang=1&level=1&sublinkid=794&lid=168.
3. Ministry of Health and Family Welfare. National Health Mission: RMNCH+A: Maternal Health: Dakshta implementation package [Internet]. New Delhi. [Cited 2023 October 30]. Available from: https://nhm.gov.in/index1.php?lang=1&level=3&sublinkid=838&lid=449.
4. National AIDS Control Organization (NACO). National Guidelines for HIV Care and Treatment 2021. [Internet]. New Delhi: Ministry of Health and Family Welfare, Government of India; 2021. [Cited 2023 October 30]. Available from: https://www.aidsdatahub.org/resource/national-guidelines-hiv-care-and-treatment-2021.
5. Ministry of Health and Family Welfare. Anaemia Mukt Bharat. [Internet]. New Delhi: PIB; Feb 2022; [Cited 2023 October 30]. Available from: https://pib.gov.in/PressReleasePage.aspx?PRID=1795421.
6. Kapil U, Kapil R, Gupta A. National Iron Plus Initiative: Current status and future strategy. Indian J Med Res. 2019;150(3):239-47. doi: 10.4103/ijmr.IJMR_1782_18. PMID: 31719294; PMCID: PMC6886130.
7. Ministry of Health and Family Welfare. National Health Mission. MAA (Mothers' Absolute Affection) Programme Promotion of Breastfeeding and IYCF [Internet]. New Delhi. [Cited 2023 October 30]. Available from: https://nhm.gov.in/index1.php?lang=1&level=4&sublinkid=1413&lid=330.
8. Ministry of Health and Family Welfare. Initiatives to tackle anemia in women and children [Internet]. New Delhi: PIB; Mar 2023; [Cited 2023 October 30]. Available from: https://pib.gov.in/PressReleaseIframePage.aspx?PRID=1910377.
9. Ministry of Women and Child Development. Poshan Abhiyaan-Jan Andolan [Internet]. New Delhi. [Cited 2023 October 30]. Available from: https://poshanabhiyaan.gov.in/.
10. Department of Health and Family Welfare. Ministry of Health and Family Welfare. Government of India. National Population Policy 2000. [Internet]. New Delhi: 2002. [cited 2023 October 30]. Available from: https://main.mohfw.gov.in/sites/default/files/26953755641410949469%20%281%29.pdf.
11. Department of Health and Family Welfare. Ministry of Health and Family Welfare. Government of India. Population stabilisation. Annual report 2017–2018 [Internet]. New Delhi. [cited 2023 October 30]. Available from: https://main.mohfw.gov.in/sites/default/files/08Chapter.pdf.

CHAPTER 24

Abortion

Shobha N Gudi

OSCE 1. A 21-year-old, primigravida at 2 and 1/2 months of amenorrhea, presents to the casualty with complaints of severe pain abdomen, fever, and foul smelling vaginal discharge since 2 days. She gives history of passage of a fleshy mass 10 days back and persistent bleeding p/v since then.
1. What is the diagnosis?
2. What is the definition?
3. Enumerate two common pathogens responsible for this condition.
4. What are the antimicrobials used to treat this condition?
5. Enumerate two complications.

Ans.
1. Septic abortion
2. Abortion which is spontaneous or induced when complicated by infection of uterus (endometritis, endomyometritis) and product of conception is called septic abortion.
3. Most of the bacteria causing septic abortion are part of normal vaginal flora—group A beta-hemolytic *Streptococcus*, *E. coli*, *Chlamydia trachomatis*, *Neisseria gonorrhoeae*, *Clostridium*.
4. Clindamycin + Gentamycin + Ampicillin or Metronidazole + Ampicillin + Gentamycin.
5. Parametritis, peritonitis, septicemia, toxic shock syndrome.

OSCE 2. A 25-year-old primigravida at 9 weeks of gestation has come with history of bleeding per vaginum for one day, not associated with pain abdomen. Her USG picture is shown below.

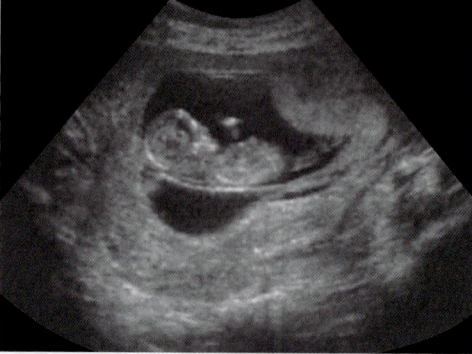

1. What is the diagnosis?
2. What are the clinical findings expected on examination?
3. If her pregnancy continues, what are the complications that are more common in such a condition?

Ans.

1. Threatened abortion
2. Clinical findings:
   - Uterine size corresponds to period of amenorrhea
   - Per speculum—os closed, no products of conception felt
   - Bleeding usually small in quantity
   - Not associated with cramping, colicky pain in abdomen
3. a. Preterm labor
   b. Placental abruption
   c. Fetal growth restriction
   d. Low-lying placenta

OSCE 3. A 22-year-old primigravida at 3 months of amenorrhea with Rh negative status, comes to the casualty with spotting per vaginum since 2 days.
1. What is the risk of alloimmunization in first trimester?
2. Enumerate two indications for anti-D prophylaxis in the case of bleeding in early pregnancy.
3. What is the dose of anti-D depending on gestational age?

Ans.

1. <10% (before 28 weeks)
2. a. Ectopic pregnancy
   b. All abortions >12 weeks of gestation
   c. After surgical evacuation
   d. Molar evacuation
3. *Anti-D dose:*
   - <12 weeks of gestation—50 microgram
   - ≥12 weeks of gestation—100 microgram

OSCE 4. A 20-year-old unmarried girl was referred from PHC with 5 days of high grade fever and chills. She had received 2 days of oral antibiotics initially and was sent home. Her Hb at that time was 10 g/dL and TLC was 10,000/uL.

Her fever worsened at home and she developed progressive vomiting, diarrhea, and abdominal pain. She was then admitted at the PHC, where she was given IV fluids and empirical IV antibiotics for typhoid. USG was not performed as it was not available.

There were no signs of improvement, and she was referred to a higher center after 3 days of inpatient care.

***On examination*:** She looks extremely pale.
- PR 110/min
  RR 28/min
  BP 80/50 mm Hg
- **Abdominal is distended with guarding, tenderness and rigidity.**
- *Local examination:* Foul smelling vaginal discharge.

1. What is your likely diagnosis?
2. How would you manage this patient?
3. What is the microbiology of the given scenario?
4. What are the clinical grades?
5. Enumerate two early complications.
6. What are the antibiotic regimens in use?

Ans.

1. Septic abortion
2. Take complete history of the patient including menstrual history and period of amenorrhea. Do a urine pregnancy test and an ultrasound pelvis.
3. Septic abortion is usually a mixed infection from:
   - Gram-negative bacilli— *E. coli, Klebsiella, Pseudomonas*
   - Gram-positive— *Staphylococcus and Streptococcus*
   - Anerobes— *Clostridium, Bacteroides*
4. a. *Grade-I:* The infection is restricted to the uterus.
   b. *Grade-II:* The infection has spread beyond the uterus to pelvic organs like the parametrium, tubes, and ovaries.
   c. *Grade-III:* The infection has spread beyond pelvis into general peritoneum.
5. a. Perforation of uterus and injury to the adjacent structures like intestines.
   b. Generalized peritonitis
   c. Endotoxic shock
   d. Adult respiratory distress syndrome
   e. Disseminated intravascular coagulation
   f. Acute renal failure.
   g. Maternal mortality
6. *Regimen A:*
   - Injection aqueous Penicillin 5 million units IV 6 hourly after sensitivity test or injection Ampicillin 500 mg to 1 g IV 6 hourly
   - Injection Gentamicin 60–80 mg IV 8 hourly after ruling out renal failure
   - Injection Metronidazole 500 mg IV 8 hourly

   Regimen B:
   - Injection Ciprofloxacin 500 mg IV 12 hourly
   - Injection Metronidazole 500 mg IV 8 hourly

   Regimen C (for severe infection)
   - Injection Cefotaxime 1 g IV 12 hourly or Injection Ceftriaxone 1 g IV 12 hourly

OSCE 5. A young married lady came with 3 months of amenorrhea and complaints of bleeding per vaginum since 1 day along with passage of a fleshy mass and severe abdominal pain. She gives history of taking drugs to induce abortion. On ultrasound, an irregular, tubular distorted sac is seen in the lower uterine segment with no fetal pole.
1. What is your likely diagnosis?
2. Which surgical procedure is done?
3. What is the management postsurgical procedure and advice on discharge?

Ans.
1. Incomplete abortion
2. Suction and evacuation or manual vacuum aspiration (MVA).
3. a. Antibiotics, anti-inflammatory agent/pain killer, and hematinics are prescribed.
   b. Anti-D prophylaxis is given in Rh negative patients
   c. She may be prescribed oral contraceptive pills/contraceptive advice given
   d. She should report in case of bleeding, fever, or pain in the lower abdomen. Otherwise, she should be followed-up after 6 weeks.

OSCE 6.

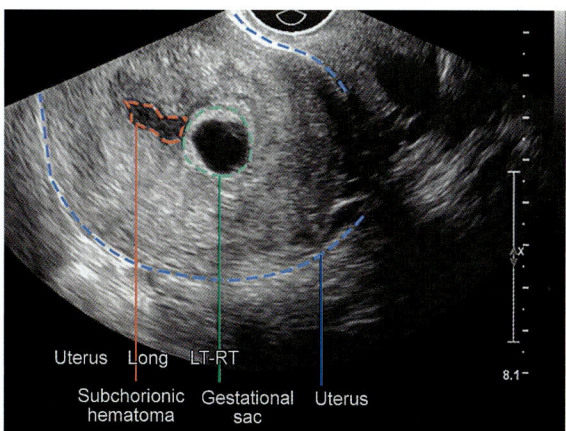

1. With reference to the above USG picture, what is your likely diagnosis?
2. How do you confirm it?
3. Enumerate two findings that suggest a poor outcome on ultrasound.
4. What is the management?

Ans.
1. Threatened miscarriage
2. Ultrasound pelvis (Transvaginal sonography)
3. a. FHS <90 bpm
   b. Small MSD (Mean sac diameter) for gestational age
   c. Irregular gestational sac
   d. Absent or poor decidual reaction
   e. Small SCH (subchorionic hemorrhage)

4. a. Reassurance
   b. Avoidance of strenuous activity
   c. There is no definitive role of medical management

OSCE 7. A 25-year-old pregnant woman with 1.5 months of amenorrhea walks into the OPD with complaints of mild bleeding PV for 2 hours and cramping lower abdominal pain. Her vitals are stable.
1. What is your likely diagnosis?
2. How do you define it?
3. What are the expected pelvic examination findings?

Ans.

1. Inevitable abortion
2. Abortion that has progressed to the extent that expulsion of the products of conception is inevitable with no chance of continuation of pregnancy.
3. a. Per speculum examination—os open, clots and POC (products of conception) may be seen protruding through os with bleeding.
   b. Per vaginum examination—internal and external os open, through which POC may be felt. Size of uterus may be smaller than the period of gestation.

OSCE 8.

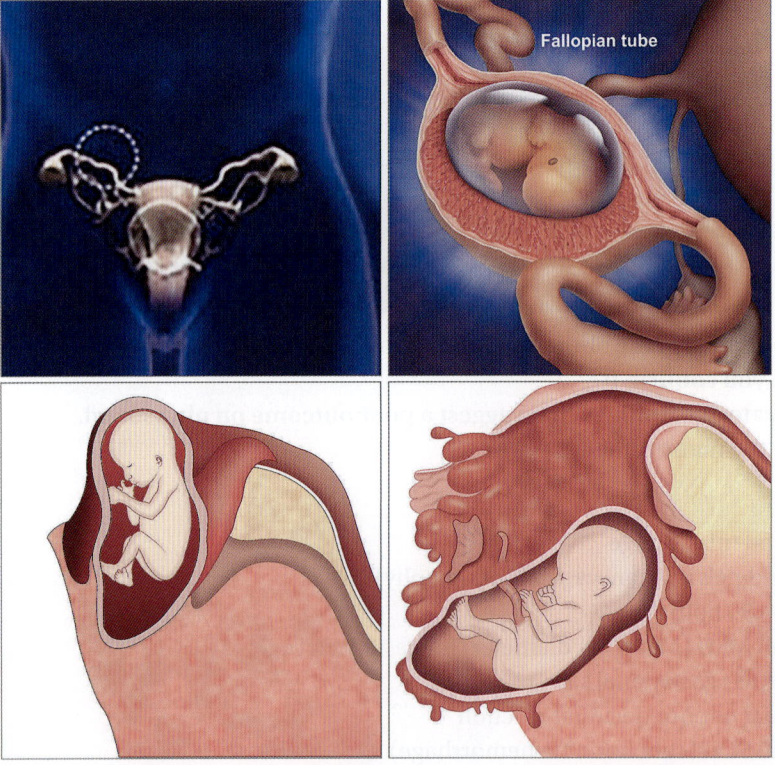

1. Identify the picture.
2. What is the commonest site of ectopic pregnancy in the fallopian tube?
3. Write the incidence of ectopic pregnancy in various parts of the fallopian tube.
4. Enumerate two complications.
5. What is the drug used in medical management of ectopic?
6. Name the various surgical procedures for management of ectopic?

Ans.

1. Ruptured tubal ectopic
2. Ampulla (55%)
3. Ampulla (55%), Isthmus (25%), Infundibulum (18%), Interstitial (2%)
4. a. Tubal rupture causing intraperitoneal hemorrhage and shock
   b. Chronic ectopic pregnancy
5. Injection Methotrexate
6. Laparoscopy/Laparotomy:
   - Salpingostomy
   - Salpingotomy
   - Salpingectomy

OSCE 9.

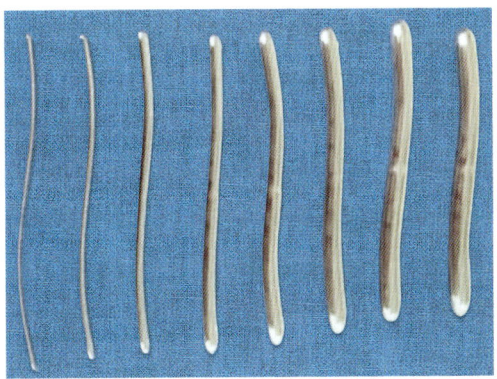

1. Identify the instrument.
2. Enumerate two indications for its use.
3. Enumerate two complications associated while using it.
4. What is the method of its use?

Ans.

1. Hegar dilator
2. a. Used in dilatation and evacuation
   b. To diagnose cervical incompetence in interpregnancy interval
3. a. Vasovagal shock if forcefully used without anesthesia
   b. Uterine perforation
   c. Cervical injury
4. Start with lowest number first and proceed serially till one size smaller than the period of gestation.

OSCE 10.

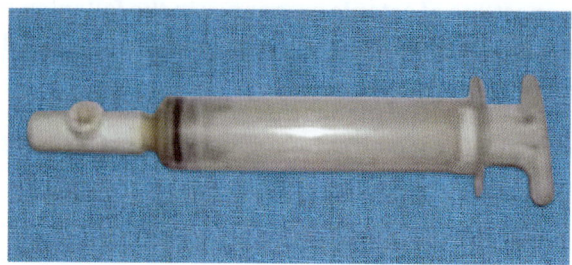

1. Identify this instrument.
2. Name the parts of this instrument.
3. Enumerate the indications for its use.
4. What is the method of sterilization of this instrument?
5. What is the advantage of this instrument over mechanical curette?

Ans.

1. Manual vacuum aspiration syringe
2. Parts—valve button, hinged valve with valve liner, collar stop, cylinder, plunger, plunger handle
3. a. Incomplete abortion/missed abortion (up to 12 weeks)
   b. Molar pregnancy
4. Autoclaving
5. Simple, safe, less traumatic. Can be done in local anesthesia in outpatient basis.

OSCE 11.

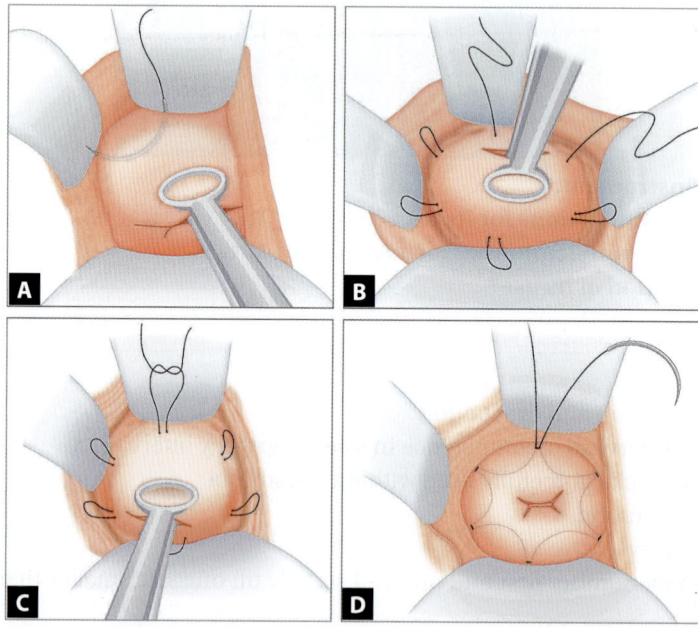

1. What is the name of the procedure shown?
2. Enumerate two indications for the procedure.
3. Define recurrent pregnancy loss.
4. Enumerate two endocrine causes for RPL.

Ans.

1. Shirodkar's cervical cerclage
2. a. *USG indicated cerclage*: Cervical length ≤2.5 cm and history of 1 second trimester abortion.
   b. *History indicated cerclage:* History of two previous second trimester abortions.
3. a. Three or more consecutive pregnancy losses at <20 weeks' gestation or with a fetal weight <500 g (Williams).
   b. Two or more losses of clinical pregnancy, USG or HPE confirmed (ASRM American Society for Reproductive Medicine).
   c. Two pregnancy losses (ESHRE, European Society of Human Reproduction and Embryology).
4. a. Overt hypothyroidism
   b. Uncontrolled diabetes mellitus
   c. Hyperprolactinemia

OSCE 12.

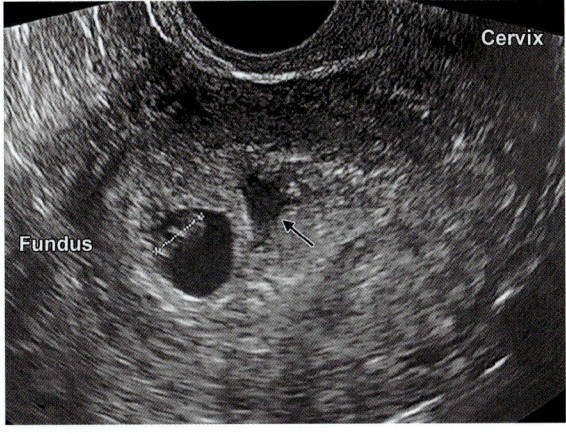

1. What does the black arrow show?
2. What is the clinical diagnosis?
3. Enumerate three USG criteria to define miscarriage.
4. Enumerate two methods to manage missed abortion.

Ans.

1. Retroplacental hemorrhage
2. Threatened miscarriage
3. USG criteria to define miscarriage are:

a. CRL (crown-rump length) ≥7 mm and no cardiac activity
b. MSD (mean sac diameter) ≥25 mm and no embryo
c. Gestational sac + yolk sac present but ≥11 days, no embryo and no cardiac activity

4. a. Medical management with prostaglandin E1 (Misoprostol)
   b. Surgical management—suction and evacuation

OSCE 13.

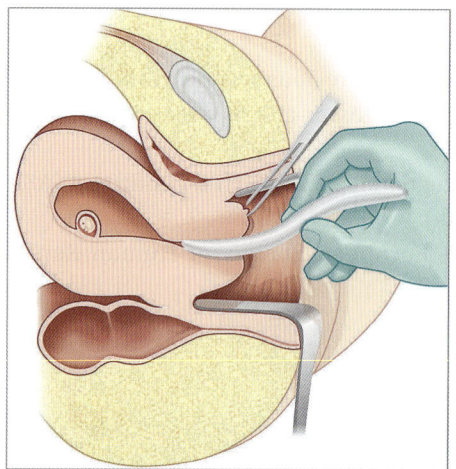
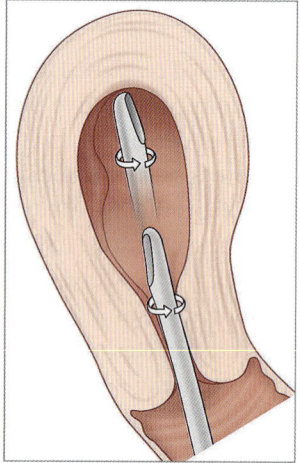

1. What is the procedure shown in the first picture?
2. Enumerate four indications for the procedure.
3. Name the instrument in the second picture.
4. How is appropriate size of this instrument chosen?
5. Enumerate two complications if the size is not accurate.

Ans.

1. Suction curettage
2. a. Missed abortion
   b. Incomplete abortion
   c. Molar pregnancy
   d. Retained placenta after vaginal delivery
3. Karman's cannula
4. Size of Karman's cannula is usually the gestational age-1
5. a. Small cannulas carry the risks of a longer surgery and of missed intrauterine tissue.
   b. Large cannulas risk cervical injury and more discomfort.

OSCE 14.
A 28-year-old, G3P1L1A1 with A-negative blood group presents with complaints of spotting PV at 11 weeks of gestation.

1. Define inevitable abortion.
2. Enumerate two causes of bleeding P/V in early pregnancy.
3. What is the recommended role of anti-D in this case?

Ans.

1. Abortion that has reached a stage of irreversibility
2. a. Miscarriage
   b. Ectopic pregnancy
   c. Molar pregnancy
   d. Implantation bleeding
   e. *Cervical or vaginal pathology:* Erosions, polyp, cancer or trauma
3. *Anti-D to be given:*
   - For threatened abortion and complete abortion if >12 weeks.
   - For inevitable/missed/incomplete abortion, even if <12 weeks.

OSCE 15. A 32-year-old, G4A2D1, known case of hypothyroidism on treatment presents at 7 weeks of gestation to OPD with home UPT positive.

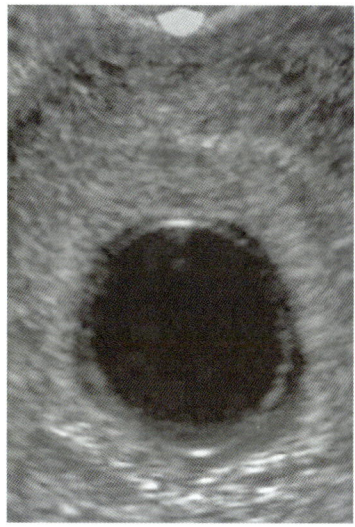

1. Define missed abortion.
2. What is your plan of care?
3. What is the most common metabolic cause of RPL.
4. Mention the Sydney criteria for diagnosing APLA.

Ans.

1. A nonviable pregnancy which has been retained in the uterus with MSD ≥25 mm with no fetal pole/cardiac activity OR if CRL ≥7 mm with no cardiac activity.
2. a. Repeat scan after 2 weeks.
   b. Repeat scan is recommended 2 weeks from visible gestation sac/11–12 days from visible yolk sac without embryo. In this case, the scan doesn't show a yolk sac, only gestational sac is visible. Hence scan should be repeated after 2 weeks.
3. Hypothyroidism.

4.

Clinical criteria	Laboratory criteria
1. *Vascular thrombosis* – Venous, arterial or microvascular – Confirmed by objective validated criteria – No evidence of inflammation in vessel wall	1. *Lupus anticoagulant* present in plasma on ≥2 occasions, at least 12 weeks apart
and/or	and /or

2. *Pregnancy morbidity*
– ≥1 unexplained fetal death ≥10th week of gestation or
– ≥1 premature birth <34th week of gestation because of:
  - Eclampsia or severe pre-eclampsia
  - Features of placental insufficiency
  - ≥3 unexplained consecutive abortions <10th week of gestation
	2. *Anticardiolipin antibody IgG and/or IgM* in serum or plasma, present in medium or high titer (>40 GPL or MPL, or >99th percentile), measured by a standardized ELISA on ≥2 occasions, at least 12 weeks apart

	and/or
	3. *Anti-β2-glycoprotein I antibody IgG and/or IgM* in serum or plasma, present in titer >99th percentile, measured by a standardized ELISA on ≥2 occasions, at least 12 weeks apart

(ELISA: enzyme-linked immunosorbent assay; GPL: IgG phospholipid units; MPL: IgM phospholipid units)

OSCE 16.

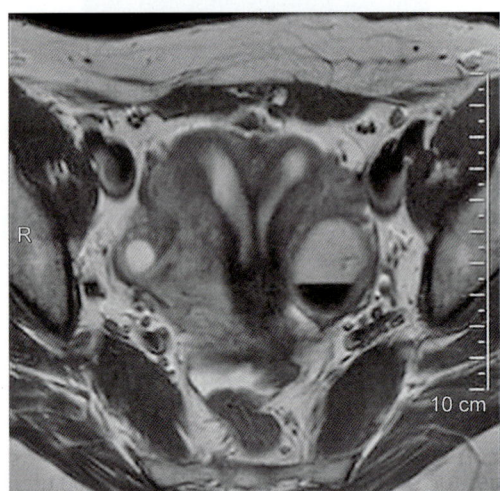

1. **Identify the above MRI image.**
2. **Classify uterine anomalies.**
3. **Which anomaly is associated with pregnancy loss?**
4. **What is the management of septate uterus?**

Ans.

1. MRI is showing septate uterus
2.

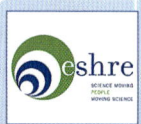 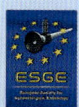

ESHRE/ESGE classification
Female genital tract anomalies

Name: .... **Birth Date:** ....
Diagnostic Method:

	Uterine anomaly			Cervical/Vaginal anomaly	
	Main class	**Sub-class**		**Co-existent class**	
U0	Normal uterus		C0	Normal cervix	
U1	Dysmorphic uterus	a. T-shaped b. Infantilis c. Others	C1	Septate cervix	
			C2	Double "normal" cervix	
			C3	Unilateral cervical aplasia	
U2	Septate uterus	a. Partial b. Complete	C4	Cervical aplasia	
U3	Bicorporeal uterus	a. Partial b. Complete c. Bicorporeal septate	V0	Normal vagina	
U4	Hemi-uterus	a. With rudimentary cavity (communicating or not horn) b. Without rudimentary cavity (horn without cavity/no horn)	V1	Longitudinal non-obstructing vaginal septum	
			V2	Longitudinal obstructing vaginal septum	
			V3	Transverse vaginal septum and/or imperforate hymen	
U5	Aplastic	a. With rudimentary cavity (bi- or unilateral horn) b. Without rudimentary cavity (bi- or unilateral uterine remnants/aplasia)	V4	Vaginal aplasia	
U6	Unclassified malformations				
U			C	V	

3. Septate uterus is associated with RPL, followed by bicornuate uterus
4. Septal resection is beneficial in RPL.

Associated anomalies of non-Müllerian origin:

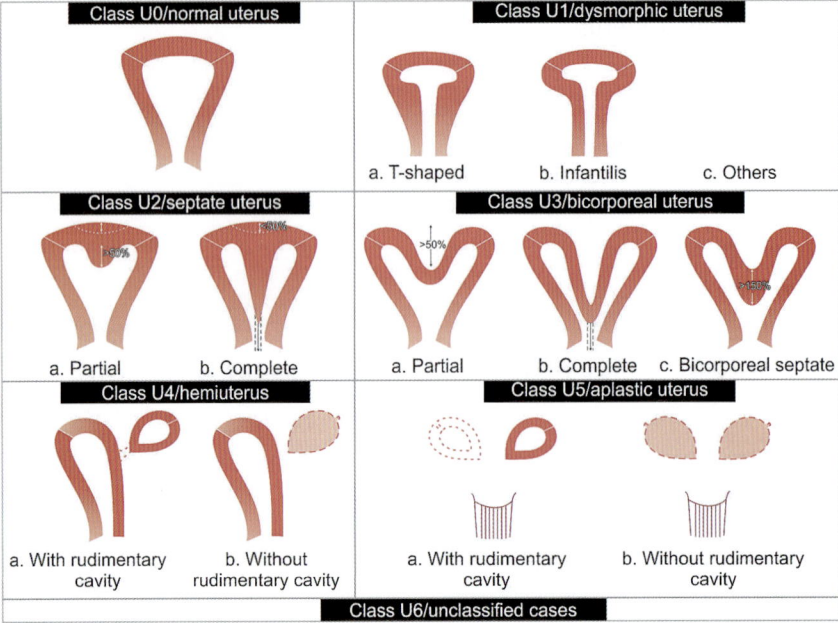

OSCE 17.

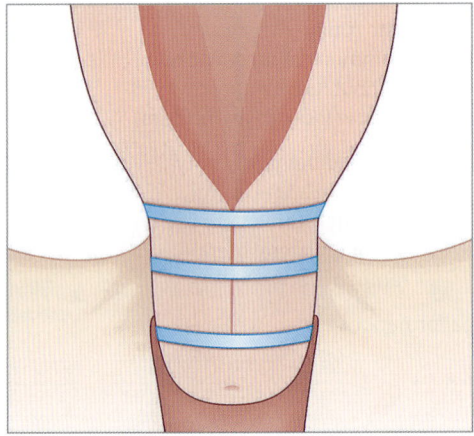

1. Enumerate different types of cerclage.
2. What is Wurm stitch?
3. Enumerate two contraindications of cervical cerclage.
4. What is the name of transabdominal cerclage method?

Ans.
1. a. Abdominal method—Benson and Durfee laparoscopic cerclage
   b. Transvaginal method—Shirodkar and McDonald cerclage

2. *Wurm stitch*: Two mattress sutures with no. 1 proline or silk—horizontal and vertical through substance of cervix with entry points 1 cm apart. It is used as a rescue cerclage when cervix is >3 cm dilated and >80% effacement.
3. Cervical dilatation >4 cm, uterine bleeding, chorioamnionitis, fetal death, congenital anomaly of the fetus, current pelvic infection and placenta previa.
4. Benson and Durfee's abdominal method.

OSCE 18.

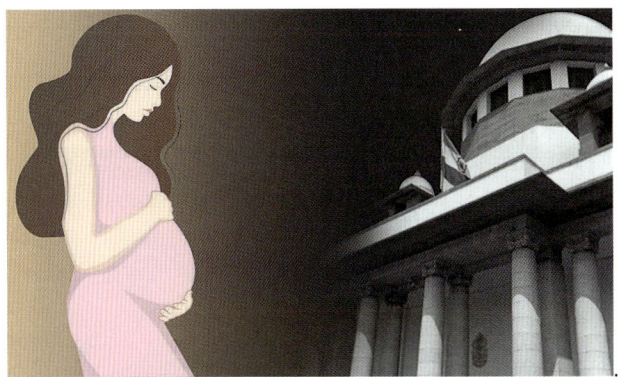

1. When was the MTP Act amended?
2. Mention the only criteria for MTP for which there is no gestational age limitations.
3. A medical board for MTP comprises of?
4. Mention the key amendments made.

Ans.

1. 2021
2. Substantial fetal anomalies
3. Medical board for MTP comprises of :
   - One gynecologist
   - One pediatrician
   - One radiologist
   - Other number of members as notified by Gazette according to the case.
4. Safe abortion services available for unmarried women.

Gestational limits	MTP Act 1971	MTP amendment Act 2021
Till 12 weeks	Advice of 1 doctor	Advice of 1 doctor
12 to 20 weeks	Advice of 2 doctors	Advice of 1 doctor
20 to 24 weeks	Only to save life of the pregnant woman	Advice of 2 doctors only if pregnant woman comes under described categories
After 24 weeks	Only to save life of the pregnant woman	Approval of Medical Board and only if there is substantial Fetal anomalies

CHAPTER 25

Recurrent Pregnancy Loss (I)

K Aparna Sharma, Richa Vatsa

OSCE 1. A 28-year-old lady presented with a history of four 1st trimester abortions. This is the 3D picture of the USG pelvis of the patient.

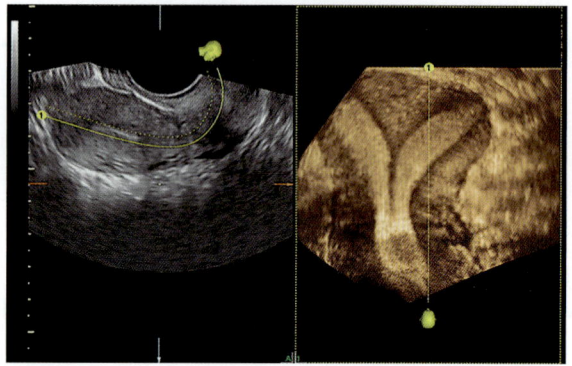

1. What is the diagnosis?
2. What will be the treatment for her recurrent pregnancy loss?

Ans.

1. Septate uterus
2. Hysteroscopic septal resection

OSCE 2. A 28-year-old lady presented with a history of four 2nd trimester abortions. You ordered hysterosalpingography for her and below is her HSG image.

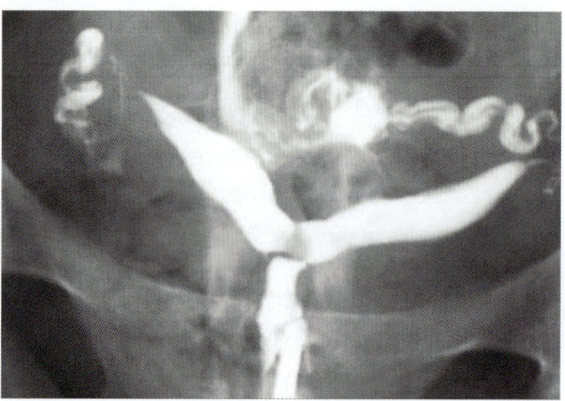

1. What are the differential diagnoses?
2. What will be the noninvasive methods to confirm the diagnosis?

Ans.

1. a. Bicornuate uterus
   b. Septate uterus
2. 3D-USG, MRI

OSCE 3. A 34-year-old, P3L0 presented to you in OPD with complaints of recurrent preterm deliveries at 5 months, 5.5 months, and 6 months. During her evaluation you performed a 3D-USG and following is the USG picture.

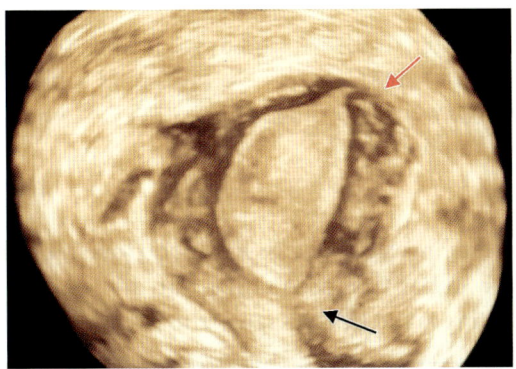

1. What is the diagnosis?
2. What is the available treatment option to manage her RPL?

Ans.

1. Unicornuate uterus
2. Lateral metroplasty

OSCE 4. A 33-year-old, P6L0 lady presented to you with RPL. She had three mid-trimester losses at 3.5 months, 4 months, and 4.5 months; and three preterm vaginal deliveries at 5 months, 5.5 months, and 6 months.

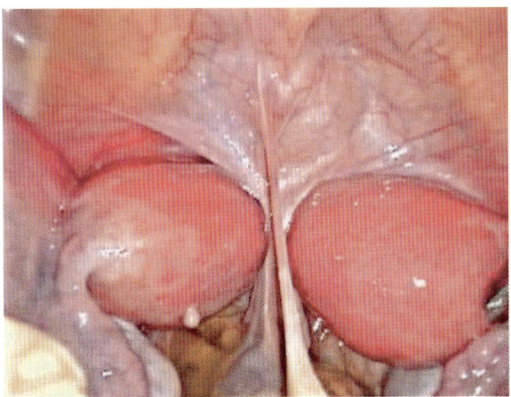

1. What is the diagnosis?
2. What is the treatment option to manage her RPL?

Ans.

1. Bicornuate uterus
2. Strassman metroplasty

OSCE 5. European Society of Human Reproduction and Embryology gave guidelines for Recurrent Pregnancy Loss in 2017. According to that:
1. What is the definition of RPL?
2. Which lifestyle interventions can improve outcomes in cases of unexplained RPL?

Ans.

1. Loss of two or more pregnancies.
2. a. Maintaining optimum weight
   b. Limit alcohol consumption
   c. Limit smoking

OSCE 6. A 29-year-old lady presented with four 1st trimester miscarriages. She underwent surgical evacuation in her first pregnancy. You advised her HSG for evaluation of her uterine cavity. Following is the HSG image of the lady.

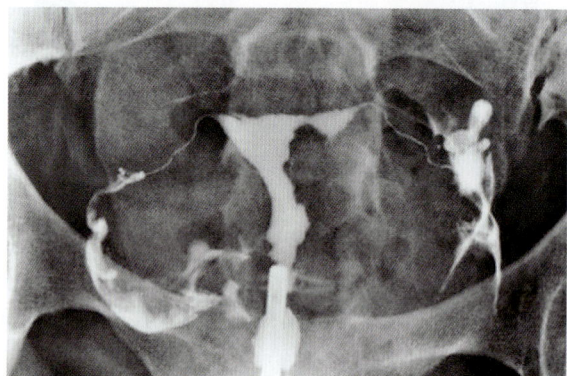

1. What is the diagnosis?
2. What is the treatment option for her?

Ans.

1. Asherman syndrome
2. Hysteroscopic adhesiolysis

OSCE 7. A 35-year-old P1L0A3 presented to you for preconceptional counseling. She had a history of severe fetal growth restriction followed by an intrauterine fetal death (IUFD) in first pregnancy. Following that she had three 1st trimester missed miscarriages. You ordered a few blood investigations. Her anti-β2 glycoprotein is 60 U/mL.

1. What is the reason for her RPL?
2. What is the treatment option to improve her RPL and when to start that?

Ans.

1. APLA syndrome
2. a. *Ecosprin:* Preconceptional
   b. *Prophylactic dose heparin:* At the date of positive urine pregnancy test

Reference

1. Recurrent Pregnancy Loss, Guideline of European Society of Human Reproduction and Embryology Update 2022.

OSCE 8. A 38-year-old lady presented to you with a history of recurrent miscarriages. Other than blood investigations, the USG pelvis was done. Following is the picture of USG.
1. What is the most probable cause of her RPL?

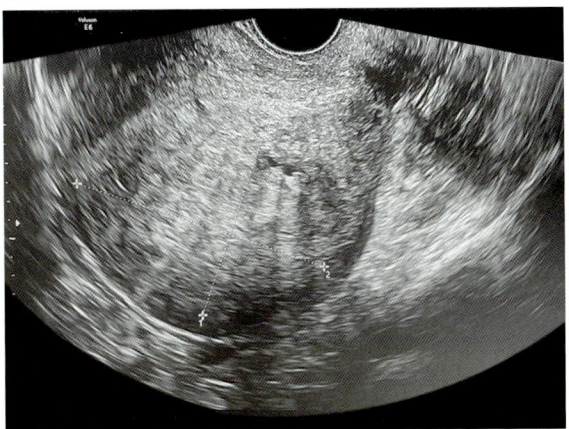

2. What is the treatment option to improve her RPL?

Ans.

1. Adenomyoma
2. Adenomyomectomy

Reference

1. Recurrent Pregnancy Loss, Guideline of European Society of Human Reproduction and Embryology Update 2022.

OSCE 9. A 38-year-old, $G_4P_0L_0A_3$ lady presented to you with bleeding per vaginum. Following are her investigations:
- **Ultrasound:** Single live intrauterine fetus of 8 weeks POG, closed internal OS
- **LAC:** 35 seconds
- **Anticardiolipin antibody IgG:** 2.2 U/mL
- **Anticardiolipin antibody IgM:** 2.6 U/mL
- **3D USG:** Normal cavity

1. What is the treatment option for her?
2. What will the dose of the drug?

Ans.

1. Vaginal progesterone
2. 400 mg two times a day

Reference

1. Recurrent Pregnancy Loss, Guideline of European Society of Human Reproduction and Embryology Update 2022.

OSCE 10. A 38-year-old, $G_4P_0L_0A_5$ lady presented to you at 5 weeks POG. Following are her investigations:
- *Ultrasound:* Single intrauterine fetus of 5 weeks POG
- *LAC:* 35 seconds
- *Anticardiolipin antibody IgG:* 2.2 U/mL
- *Anticardiolipin antibody IgM:* 2.6 U/mL
- *3D USG:* Normal cavity

1. What is the treatment option for her?
2. When should you start the treatment?

Ans.

1. IVIg
2. In early pregnancy

Reference

1. Recurrent Pregnancy Loss, Guideline of European Society of Human Reproduction and Embryology Update 2022.

OSCE 11. A 34-year-old $P_0L_0A_4$ lady presented to you with a history of recurrent midtrimester abortion at around 3–4 months POG. In her last pregnancy, she had cervical cerclage at 13 weeks POG, but she aborted again at 19 weeks POG. She came to you for preconception counseling. You examined her and on per speculum examination, her cervix was deficient at 9 O'clock position.

1. What will be the treatment option for her now?
2. What will the time of this intervention be?

Ans.

1. Interval abdominal cervical cerclage
2. Preferably before planning next pregnancy

OSCE 12. A couple came to you with eight miscarriages. A karyotype was advised for both partners. The karyotype of the male partner showed unbalanced translocation.

1. What are the chances of having a healthy baby for the couple?
2. What will be the treatment option available to the couple for RPL?

Ans.
1. Negligible chance of a live born child
2. PGT, adoption, gamete donation

Reference
1. Recurrent Pregnancy Loss, Guideline of European Society of Human Reproduction and Embryology Update 2022.

OSCE 13. See the image given below.

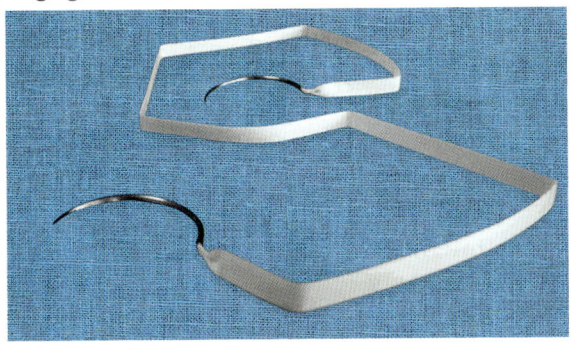

1. Identify the image.
2. Name a condition where it can be used in cases of recurrent pregnancy loss.

Ans.
1. Mersilene tape
2. Abdominal cerclage in cases of failed vaginal cerclage

OSCE 14. A 33-year-old, $P_1L_0A_3$ lady presents for preconceptional counseling. She had preterm cesarean section for breech presentation in labor. Followed by that she has three first-trimester miscarriages.

Following are her investigation results:
- *LAC: 35 seconds*
- *Anticardiolipin antibody IgG: 2.2 U/mL*
- *Anticardiolipin antibody IgM: 2.6 U/mL*

1. What is the most likely diagnosis?
2. Which investigation will you do to confirm the diagnosis?

Ans.
1. Müllerian uterine malformation (septate/bicornuate uterus)
2. 3D-USG

OSCE 15. A 33-year-old, P6L0 lady presented to you with RPL. She had three mid-trimester losses at 3.5 months, 4 months, and 4.5 months; and three preterm vaginal deliveries at 5 months, 5.5 months, and 6 months.

Her 3D-USG: Uterus showing two cavities. The fundal depression was >50% of wall thickness below the interostial line.

1. What further abnormality needs to be ruled out in this case?
2. What will be the treatment for her?

Ans.

1. USG for renal abnormalities
2. Strassman metroplasty

OSCE 16. A 27-year-old lady presents to you with infertility of 5 years. She has irregular cycles occurring on only progesterone withdrawal. Her hormone profile is normal.

Following is the report of her 3D-USG:
- *Right ovary:* 15 antral follicles of 2–7 mm size
- *Left ovary:* 10 antral follicles of 2–7 mm size
- *Uterus:* Septate

1. What is the cause of her infertility?
2. What treatment will you offer her?

Ans.

1. Anovulation due to polycystic ovary syndrome
2. Ovulation induction

OSCE. 17. See the surgical image given below.

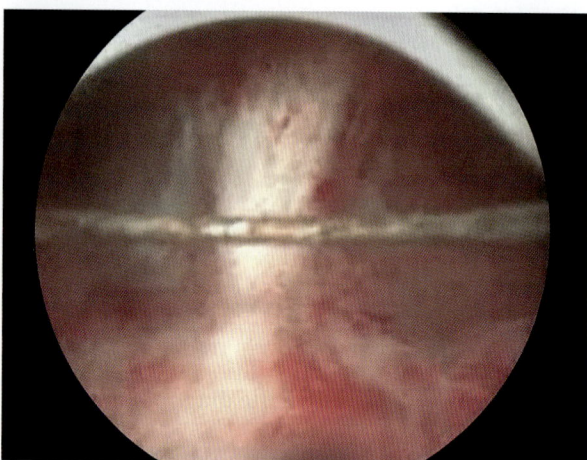

1. Identify the surgical procedure being done.
2. What is the indication of the procedure?

Ans.

1. Hysteroscopic septal resection
2. Recurrent pregnancy loss in a patient with uterine septum

OSCE 18. See the surgical image given below.

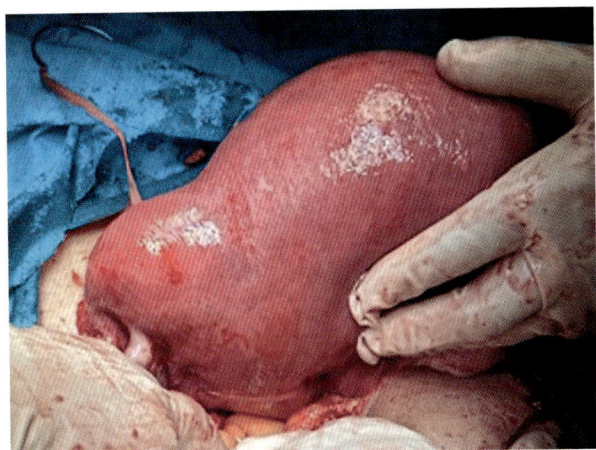

1. Identify the surgical procedure.
2. Write the indication of the procedure.

Ans.

1. Abdominal cervical cerclage
2. Pervious failed vaginal cerclage

OSCE 19. A 41-year-old, $P_0L_0A_3$ presents to you for secondary infertility of 4 years. Her workup for recurrent pregnancy loss (RPL) is normal. She had an anti-Müllerian hormone level of 0.6 ng/dL. You counsel her for in vitro fertilization.
1. What choice can you give her for her RPL?
2. What is the major limitation of this procedure in Indian setting?

Ans.

1. Preimplantation genetic testing for aneuploidy (PGT-A)
2. Cost

OSCE 20. A 33-year-old, $G_5P_0L_0A_4$ lady presents to you at 8 weeks POG with an ultrasound report showing a single intrauterine gestational sac of size 30 mm without any fetal pole. She already had her workup for recurrent pregnancy loss which has ruled out antiphospholipid antibody syndrome and Müllerian uterine malformations. She is very anxious and distressed and wants to know about the cause of her RPL.
1. What investigation can you offer her?
2. What will be the use of this investigation?

Ans.

1. Genetic analysis of pregnancy tissue
2. It could be performed for explanatory purposes.

CHAPTER 26

Recurrent Pregnancy Loss (II)

Sneha Bhuyar

OSCE 1. A young couple comes with history of spontaneous abortion immediately after 2 months of marriage. Six months later, she had another episode of spontaneous abortion of 2 months POG. She again aborted next year, at a POG of 6 weeks.
1. What is your diagnosis?
2. How do you define it?
3. How will you evaluate it?

Ans.

1. Primary RPL
2. According to the European Society for Human Reproduction and Embryology and the Royal College of Obstetricians and Gynecologists, RPL refers to three consecutive pregnancy losses, including nonvisualized ones. However, according to the American Society for Reproductive Medicine it is defined as two or more clinical pregnancy losses (documented by ultrasonography or histopathologic examination).
3. Evaluate first whether it's aneuploid or euploid. If aneuploid, parental karyotype and genetic counseling should be done. If euploid, then further RPL work-up is advised.

OSCE 2. A 32-year-old, G4P1L1A2, with one live child of 7 years, followed by two spontaneous abortions, has come to you for preconception counseling.
1. What is your diagnosis?
2. Enumerate two tests which should be advised.
3. Can male factor be one of the causes here?
4. Can she have a normal viable pregnancy again?

Ans.

1. Secondary RPL
2. Sperm DNA fragmentation, screen for infections, serum progesterone level, qualitative semen analysis
3. Yes
4. Yes

OSCE 3. A patient of RPL has come in the OPD.
1. What specific clinical examination should be done?

2. Enumerate the blood tests which are recommended.
3. Enumerate the imaging investigation which should be advised.

Ans.
1. A complete physical examination, especially to detect any features suggestive of chromosomal aberrations, infections, galactorrhea, etc. should be done.
2. Blood tests to detect problems with the immune system and hormonal assay should be done. Test to detect genetic causes of repeated miscarriages is parental karyotype.
3. Ultrasound pelvis to detect any uterine pathology.

OSCE 4. A couple with previous three spontaneous abortions has come for pre-conceptional counseling. All the investigations advised were normal. The couple has the following queries:
1. Whether they can take a chance to conceive?
2. Whether the pregnancy will continue?
3. What additional investigations can be done?

Ans.
1. Yes
2. If all anatomical, endocrinological, infective, and genetic aspects [Robertsonian translocation—parental karyotype, product of conception (POC) karyotype for aneuploidy] investigated are normal, couple has a chance to have a normal pregnancy with proper supplementation, precautions, and tender loving care.
3. NIPT (Noninvasive prenatal testing), cell-free fetal DNA (cffDNA) test

OSCE 5. A couple with previous two spontaneous abortions has come for preconception counseling. Wife is 35-year-old and husband is 42-year-old.
1. How do you explain the risk with regards to their age now?
2. Do you label mother as elderly?
3. Does paternal age also affect pregnancy outcome?
4. Enumerate two abnormalities associated with paternal aging.
5. How should we counsel such a couple?

Ans.
1. Basically, a couple who has already had two spontaneous abortions is at a very high risk of subsequent abortions. Maternal age above 35 predisposes to chromosomal aberrations and advanced paternal age has definite adverse effect on the pregnancy.
2. Yes
3. Yes
4. Increased risk of miscarriages, congenital malformations like congenital heart disease (CHD), cleft lip/cleft palate, autism, schizophrenia, etc.
5. They can be counseled for IVF with donor gametes.

Section 1: Obstetrics

OSCE 6. A couple with two consecutive abortions has come to you for preconception evaluation and insists for parental karyotype, as suggested by someone else.
1. What investigations should the couple undergo primarily for RPL?
2. If POC karyotype suggests euploidy then what is advised further?
3. What do you look for as causes of RPL in parental karyotype?

Ans.

1. Endocrinological, APLA, and POC karyotype.
2. All other tests should be offered
3. Balanced translocation, inversions, and Robertsonian translocations.

OSCE 7. A hypothyroid lady comes to you with previous three spontaneous abortions. POC karyotype was not done. She also has hyperprolactinemia.
1. Should you re-evaluate her thyroid status and prolactin levels?
2. Would you do parental karyotype?

Ans.

1. Yes—Hypothyroidism and hyperprolactinemia can be the reason for RPL per say but when we are going for preconception evaluation, it's always better to go for all the necessary investigations including karyotype of parents as multiple factors can be present simultaneously.
2. Yes

OSCE 8.
1. Enumerate four endocrinological causes causing RPL.
2. How does prolactin lead to RPL?
3. In PCOS women, what is the contributing factor for RPL?

Ans.

1. Endocrinological causes are implicated for approximately 17–20% of RPL. These include luteal phase insufficiency, androgen disorder, thyroid disorders, and increased serum levels of prolactin. Also, metabolic diseases such as polycystic ovarian syndrome (PCOS) and diabetes mellitus.
2. Hyperprolactinemia causes thin endometrium and luteal phase inadequacy
3. Hyperandrogenism

OSCE 9. We have a patient of RPL with POC karyotype report showing aneuploidy and now she wants to get evaluated for RPL?
1. What is the most important investigation that should be done?

Ans.

1. *Parental karyotyping:* RCOG recommends that karyotype testing of the abortus should be the first cost-effective step in the evaluation of RPL. If the products are euploid other

tests should be offered. If aneuploidy is detected, evaluation of such a loss should be followed by parental karyotyping to detect balanced reciprocal, Robertsonian translocations or mosaicism in parents.

OSCE 10. Answer the following questions regarding a patient of RPL with diagnosed uterine septum.
1. Does every uterine septum lead to RPL?
2. Can it solely lead to RPL?
3. What is the role of uterine anatomy for RPL?

Ans.
1. No
2. Yes—Implantation on the septum or lesion, reduction in capacity to hold and incompetence of os can lead to RPL in case of a uterine septum.
3. Anatomical abnormalities in uterus may be congenital like bicornuate and septate uterus along with acquired causes like intrauterine adhesions and polyp which can cause repeated first as well as second trimester abortions.

OSCE 11.
1. Enumerate two investigations for the diagnosis of uterine pathologies.
2. How do you decide which investigation will be best for which lesion?

Ans.
1. The modalities include hysterosalpingography or sonohysterography, hysteroscopy, and laparoscopy
    Direct visualization which is both diagnostic and therapeutic is by hysterolaparoscopy.
    MRI is a useful noninvasive investigation.
    Ultrasound helps in the diagnosis of uterine myomas, septate uterus, and renal abnormalities.
    Sonohysterography (SIS) delineates the internal contours of the uterine cavity and provides concomitant sonographic visualization of the outer surface and wall of the uterus, the tubal patency and can distinguish between septate and bicornuate uterus that are responsible for second trimester losses.
2. *Intracavitary lesions:* Saline infusion sonography (SIS) is recommended. However, for diagnostic as well as therapeutic purpose, hysterolaparoscopy is advised.

OSCE 12. A woman comes to you with RPL. Her first abortion was after a fall at 16 weeks, second was unexplained loss at 18 weeks and now she is 16 weeks pregnant. She has no congenital uterine malformations; no space-occupying lesions and endocrine profile was normal. Quadruple marker was normal. Cervix is 2.5 cm. How should she be managed?
1. What is the diagnosis?
2. What is the accepted cut-off for labeling short cervix?
3. What are the treatment options?

Ans.
1. Short cervix
2. 2.5 cm
3. *Cervical cerclage and vaginal micronized progesterone:* This is genuinely short cervix as accepted by FOGSI, FIGO, and all the international organizations but the treatment modalities may differ. For a singleton midtrimester pregnancy with short cervix, vaginal micronized progesterone works equally effectively as compared to cervical cerclage, as endorsed by FOGSI.

OSCE 13. A couple comes to you in early pregnancy. She had history of RPL. First pregnancy was 11 weeks missed abortion, second loss was at 5 months, morphologically normal fetus, severe Doppler changes and IUFD. What investigation do you want to do for this patient?
1. What is the diagnosis of this patient?
2. What are the criteria for diagnosis?
3. Should we start low molecular weight heparin (LMWH) alone or in combination with low dose Aspirin?

Ans.
1. APLA syndrome
2. *Revised SAPPORO criteria:* According to this criteria—one clinical and one laboratory criteria is needed for diagnosis of APLA—even one fetal loss of >10 weeks, morphologically fetus, we should subject the patient for lupus anticoagulant (LA), anticardiolipin antibodies and beta-2-glycoprotein.
3. In combination

OSCE 14.
1. In a patient of RPL with all investigations normal including APLA and parental karyotype, is screening for hereditary thrombophilia recommended.
2. Is it recommended routinely in all cases of RPL in general?
3. Does ESHRE recommend thromboprophylaxis in all patients of hereditary thrombophilia?

Ans.
1. Yes
2. No—Screening for hereditary thrombophilia is not recommended routinely in all cases of RPL. However, when APLA and all other tests are negative, then it has to be done for further evaluation.
3. No—Only in view of deep vein thrombosis (DVT)/venous thromboembolism (VTE)

OSCE 15. A 30-year-old with previous two abortions and last product of conception (POC) suggestive of aneuploidy has come for counseling.
1. How to proceed?
2. Suppose one of the parents has significant karyotype abnormality what should we suggest?

3. **Suppose the parents are not willing for donor gamete, do we have some tests to confirm?**

Ans.

1. Karyotype of parents
2. Donor gamete after genetic counseling
3. Preimplantation genetic diagnosis (PGD)—single cell, multiple trophectoderm or blastocyst biopsy.

OSCE 16.
1. **A 28-year-old lady with six spontaneous abortions has come for counseling. Her endocrinological, anatomical, and genetic factors are normal. Some immunological problem is being suspected. What is the role of immunoglobulins?**

Ans.

1. IVIG are being used but evidence does not support its efficacy.

OSCE 17.
1. **What are intralipids?**

Ans.

1. Intralipids are fat emulsions known to have immunomodulatory property and act by inhibiting uterine NK cell activity. This is useful for both recurrent miscarriage and recurrent implantation failure in artificial reproductive treatment (ART). It is given as soon as the urine pregnancy test is positive and continued up to the end of first trimester once in a month.

OSCE 18.
1. **G-CSF is quite promising, how does it act?**

Ans.

1. Granulocyte colony-stimulating factor (G-CSF) is a cytokine which is produced by decidual cells and it is found to have a positive impact on trophoblast and has anti-abortive action. Recent studies indicate possible effects of TNF-α blocker and G-CSF in improving the live birth rate in recurrent miscarriage.

OSCE 19.
1. **You have a patient of RPL, evaluated thoroughly and still no cause could be found. How would you manage her?**

Ans.

1. Lifestyle modification by improvements in diet, exercise, abstinence from drugs, and stress reduction improve pregnancy outcomes. The strategy of emotional support and reassurance works well in unexplained cases as even no treatment shows a good prognosis in 60–80% cases in addition to the supportive medication.

CHAPTER 27

Bad Obstetric History

Juhi Bharti, Supriya Kumari, Akanksha Gupta

OSCE 1. A patient G3P1L0A1 at 32 weeks period of gestation presented with complaint of itching all over body since last 5 days. On evaluation her liver function tests were found to be deranged. She gives a history of similar experience in her last pregnancy following which she had sudden intrauterine death at 36 weeks.
1. What could be the diagnosis?
2. What could be the cause of sudden IUFD?
3. Which drug is used to control this condition?

Ans.
1. Intrahepatic cholestasis of pregnancy
2. SA node inhibition by bile salts
3. Ursodeoxycholic acid

Reference
1. Cunningham F, Leveno KJ, Dashe JS, Hoffman BL, Spong CY, Casey BM. Williams Obstetrics, 26th edition.

OSCE 2. A patient G3P2L0A0 presented to the OPD for preconception counseling. She gives history of intrauterine fetal demise in both her previous pregnancies.
1. Which of these can probably not be a cause of her bad obstetric history?
   - Rh isoimmunization
   - Toxoplasmosis
   - Gestational hypertension
   - Intrahepatic cholestasis of pregnancy

Ans.
1. Toxoplasmosis

Reference
1. Cunningham F, Leveno KJ, Dashe JS, Hoffman BL, Spong CY, Casey BM. Williams Obstetrics, 26th edition.

OSCE 3. USG findings of a patient G2P1L0 are suggestive of absent end-diastolic flow at 30 weeks period of gestation. She is a known hypertensive, on antihypertensive medications and had a similar history in previous pregnancy.

1. How frequently should the Doppler be followed?
2. At what period of gestation should she be terminated?
3. What should be the route of delivery?

Ans.

1. Twice weekly
2. 32–34 weeks or SOS
3. LSCS

Reference

1. Cunningham F, Leveno KJ, Dashe JS, Hoffman BL, Spong CY, Casey BM. Williams Obstetrics, 26th edition.

OSCE 4. A woman G2P1L0 presented to emergency with seizures during pregnancy. On stabilization and evaluation, her BP was found to be 190/120 mm Hg. On detailed evaluation, the husband gives history of similar episode in past pregnancy which had resulted in intrauterine fetal death.
1. What could be the diagnosis of present condition?
2. What percent of women with chronic hypertension land up in eclampsia?
3. What should be administered in raised BP along with antihypertensives to prevent this condition?

Ans.

1. Eclampsia
2. 15%
3. Magnesium sulfate

Reference

1. Cunningham F, Leveno KJ, Dashe JS, Hoffman BL, Spong CY, Casey BM. Williams Obstetrics, 26th edition.

OSCE 5. A patient G2P1L0 was referred from a periphery hospital in view of the present ultrasonography findings and bad obstetric history. Her blood group is A negative, Hb 12.1 g/dL, liver function tests are normal. The ultrasonography reveals collection of fluid around the lungs, and peritoneal cavity in the fetus. On asking, she gives history of previous fetal death and the fetus on delivery looked pale, white and edematous.
1. What could be the diagnosis?
2. What is the treatment for the fetus?

Ans.

1. Rh isoimmunization
2. Intrauterine transfusion

Reference

1. Cunningham F, Leveno KJ, Dashe JS, Hoffman BL, Spong CY, Casey BM. Williams Obstetrics, 26th edition.

Section 1: Obstetrics

OSCE 6. A 30-year-old, G6P4L1A1 female with Rh negative pregnancy with history of fetal hydrops in previous two pregnancies presented to you in 1st trimester.
1. Identify cause of BOH for this patient.
2. Enlist the plan of management for the patient.

Ans.

1. Rh isoimmunized pregnancy
2. Planning for MCA PSV-based fetal monitoring from 16 weeks onwards

OSCE 7. A 24-year-old P2L1A1 female with previous 1 baby with thalassemia major presented to you for preconceptional counseling.
1. Enlist the tests to be done for the couple.
2. What are the chances of fetal affection in subsequent pregnancy if both have thalassemia trait?
3. What is the type of inheritance of Beta thalassemia?

Ans.

1. HPLC for couple
2. 25% if both parents are heterozygous
3. Autosomal recessive pattern

OSCE 8.
1. Identify the fetal anomaly presented in the Figure below.
2. What is the risk of recurrence of the anomaly in subsequent pregnancy?
3. What is the drug of choice and recommended dose for prevention of this condition in fetus?

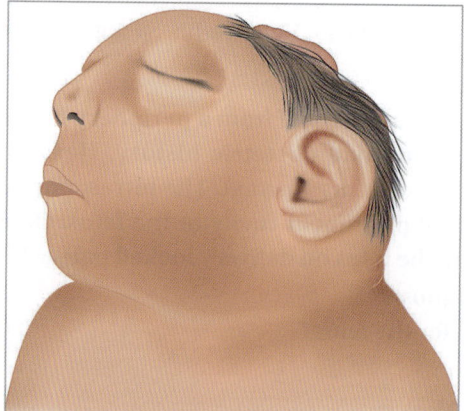

Ans.

1. Anencephaly
2. 2–5%
3. Folic acid 400 mcg OD

Reference

1. Mai CT, Isenburg JL, Canfield MA, Meyer RE, Correa A, Alverson CJ, Lupo PJ, Riehle-Colarusso T, Cho SJ, Aggarwal D, Kirby RS. National population-based estimates for major birth defects, 2010–2014. Birth Defects Research. 2019; 111(18): 1420-35.

OSCE 9. A 36-year-old, G8P5L1A1 female giving history of painless, spontaneous preterm labor in five pregnancies presented to you at 14 weeks POG.
1. Identify the cause of BOH.
2. Discuss the management of this patient.

Ans.
1. Cervical incompetence
2. Elective McDonald's vaginal cerclage

OSCE 10. A 36-year-old, G4P2L1A1 female has the following obstetrics history:
- G1—Spontaneous conception, preterm labor (PTL) at 20 weeks gestation resulting in abortion
- G2—PPROM at 24 weeks POG resulting in expulsion
- G3—PTL at 28 weeks POG resulting in preterm delivery
- G4—Present pregnancy

1. Identify the cause of BOH.
2. Discuss the management of this patient.

Ans.
1. Maternal syphilis infection
2. Injection penicillin 1.2 mIU IM one dose

OSCE 11. A woman presented to you at 29 weeks POG with sudden IUFD.
1. Name the protocol used in medicine for breaking bad news.
2. Elaborate the components of the protocol.

Ans.
1. SPIKES protocol
2. S—Setting, P—Perception, I—Invitation, K—Knowledge, E—Emotions, S—Strategy and summary

OSCE 12. Identify the procedure in Figure.

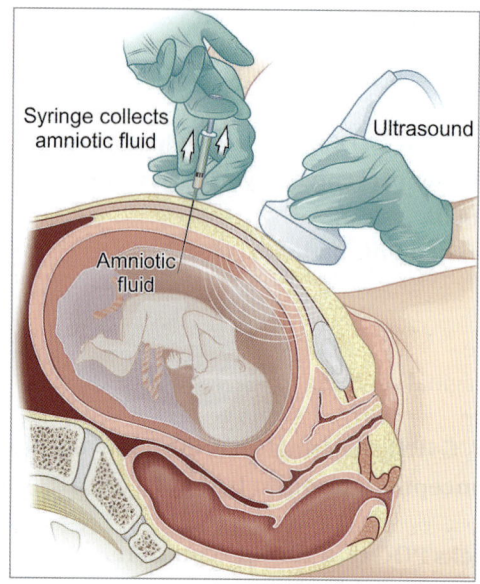

1. Identify the procedure.
2. Name two complications associated with the procedure.

Ans.

1. Amniocentesis
2. Abortion, limb defects

OSCE 13. A P1L0 woman with history of one unexplained full-term IUFD came to you for preconceptional counseling.
1. Enumerate the investigations you would like to order for her.

Ans.

1. GTT, TORCH, VDRL, thyroid, APLA profile, karyotyping, fetal autopsy

OSCE 14. A woman with family history of hemophilia presented to you with BOH.

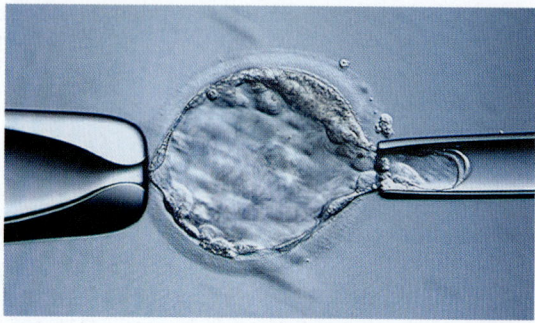

1. Identify the procedure that can be offered to the above woman.

Ans.

1. Preimplantation—genetic diagnosis—monogenic gene defect (PGT-M)

OSCE 15.
1. What is the definition of bad obstetric history?
2. Enumerate five causes of BOH.

Ans.

1. Any untoward past pregnancy outcomes that have an adverse pregnancy implication on the subsequent pregnancies of a woman.
2. Pre-eclampsia, APLA, diabetes, thyroid disorders, genetic diseases, chromosomal translocations.

OSCE 16.
A woman G2P1L0 came to the labor room with pain abdomen and leaking per vaginum. On history taking, she said that her previous vaginal delivery was difficult, the doctor had told her that the head had delivered but there was a delay in the delivery of the shoulder. The fetus weighed 4.5 kg and had expired on day 2 in NICU.
1. What is this condition called as?
2. What is the sign called when the head is delivered but the shoulder is still stuck inside?
3. What medical disorder the woman would be having in this case?

Ans.

1. Shoulder dystocia
2. Turtle sign
3. Diabetes mellitus

Reference

1. Cunningham F, Leveno KJ, Dashe JS, Hoffman BL, Spong CY, Casey BM. Williams Obstetrics, 26th edition.

OSCE 17.
A woman G2P1L0 with pre-eclampsia had an episode of convulsion during this pregnancy. On evaluation, she gives history of raised blood pressure in her previous pregnancy also.
1. What is this condition called as?
2. Which neurotransmitter plays a major role in eclampsia?
3. What percent of women develop blindness following eclamptic convulsion?

Ans.

1. Eclampsia
2. Glutamate
3. 10–15%

Reference

1. Cunningham F, Leveno KJ, Dashe JS, Hoffman BL, Spong CY, Casey BM. Williams Obstetrics, 26th edition.

Section 1: Obstetrics

OSCE 18. A patient G2P1L0 gives history of pain abdomen and bleeding per vagina during her last pregnancy. On examination, the abdomen was woody hard, tense and tender. She was diagnosed to be having intrauterine fetal death and then she delivered vaginally.
1. What do you think she might be having?
2. Which layer of decidua does the bleeding starts in?

Ans.
1. Abruptio placentae
2. Decidua basalis

Reference
1. Cunningham F, Leveno KJ, Dashe JS, Hoffman BL, Spong CY, Casey BM. Williams Obstetrics, 26th edition.

OSCE 19. A woman G2P1L0 presents to your OPD for preconceptional counseling. She gives history of diagnosis of type 1 diabetes.
1. What is the incidence of major malformation in woman with type 1 diabetes?
2. Which is the most common anomaly in fetus of woman with type 1 diabetes?
3. Which is the anomaly most specific to this condition in mothers?

Ans.
1. 11%
2. Cardiovascular anomaly
3. Caudal regression sequence

Reference
1. Cunningham F, Leveno KJ, Dashe JS, Hoffman BL, Spong CY, Casey BM. Williams Obstetrics, 26th edition.

OSCE 20. A woman G2P1L0 came at 42 weeks period of gestation and delivered vaginally. The baby had wrinkled, patchy skin with peeling, the infant was open eyed and appeared old and worried.
1. What is the diagnosis in this case?
2. What is the most common cause of postmaturity?

Ans.
1. Postmaturity syndrome
2. Oligohydramnios

Reference
1. Cunningham F, Leveno KJ, Dashe JS, Hoffman BL, Spong CY, Casey BM. Williams Obstetrics, 26th edition.

CHAPTER 28

Contraception

Pikee Saxena, Shweta Prasad

OSCE 1.

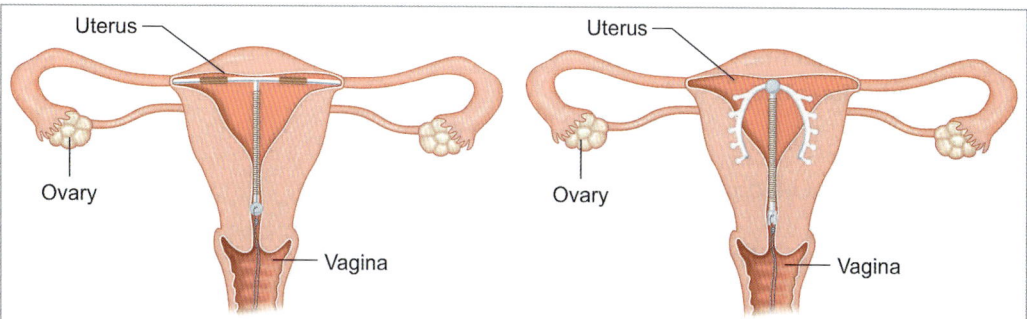

1. Identify the types of contraceptive devices.
2. What is the duration of action of each one?
3. What is its mechanism of action?
4. What are the different time interval when this device can be inserted?

Ans.

1. CuT 380A and CuT 375
2. 10 years, 5 years
3. *Mechanism of action:* Copper ions enhance the inflammatory response and reach concentrations in the luminal fluids of the genital tract that are toxic for spermatozoa.
4. An informed consent needs to be taken for IUCD insertion by a trained healthcare worker.
   - *Interval IUCD:* During menstrual cycle after pregnancy is ruled out/after 6 weeks of delivery/immediately after menstruation
   - *Postpartum IUCD (PPIUCD):* Immediately after delivery of placenta in cesarean section/within 48 hours after vaginal delivery/concurrent with cesarean section
   - *Postabortion IUCD:* Immediately postsurgical abortion. If medical abortion is done, abortion is said to be completed after day 12 of second pill or day 15 of first pill.

OSCE 2.

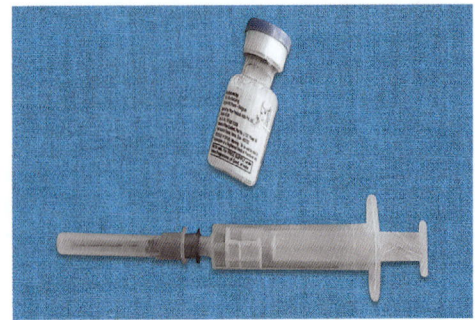

1. Antara Programme is for which contraceptive device?
2. What is its dose and site for injection?
3. What are its benefits?
4. How to give its subsequent doses?

Ans.

1. Injectable Depot Medroxyprogesterone acetate 150 mg
2. a. *Dose:* 150 mg
   b. *Site:* Intramuscular in the upper arm, buttocks or thigh, according to the patient preference
3. Benefits of injection DMPA:
   - No hindrance with sexual intercourse
   - Confidential and private
   - Can be adopted as postpartum (breastfeeding—after 6 weeks of delivery and non-breastfeeding—after 4 weeks after delivery) or postabortal contraception (within 7 days after completion of abortion)
   - Lactation is not affected
   - Decreases dysmenorrhea and menorrhagia
   - Improves anemia
   - Protects against endometrial and ovarian cancer
   - Prevents ectopic pregnancy
4. Woman must follow-up on the scheduled date for subsequent doses, i.e., 3 months after the previous dose. She can come 2 weeks before or 4 weeks after the scheduled date.

OSCE 3.

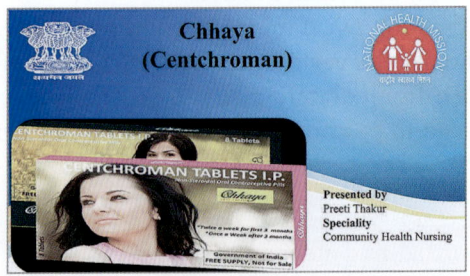

Chapter 28: Contraception

1. What is Chhaya?
2. What is its dosage schedule?
3. What are the benefits of Chhaya?
4. What are the conditions where Chhaya should not be prescribed?

Ans.

1. *Centchroman pills:* It is a nonhormonal and nonsteroidal pill suitable for nearly all women of reproductive age group.
2. It contains 8 tablets per strip. For initiation, the first pill is to be taken on the first day of period and the next pill 3 days later for the first 3 months; starting from fourth month, the pill is to be taken weekly.
3. Benefits of Chhaya are:
   - No hormonal side effects
   - No effect on sexual intercourse
   - Can be used as postpartum (earlier than 4 weeks of delivery) or postabortion contraception (within 7 days after the completion of abortion)
   - No effect on lactation
   - Fertility returns immediately on discontinuation
   - Prevents or improves anemia.
4. Chhaya should be avoided in the following:
   Polycystic ovarian disease, recent history of jaundice, liver impairment, kidney impairment, abnormal growth of cervix, pregnancy, lactation and hypersensitivity.

OSCE 4.

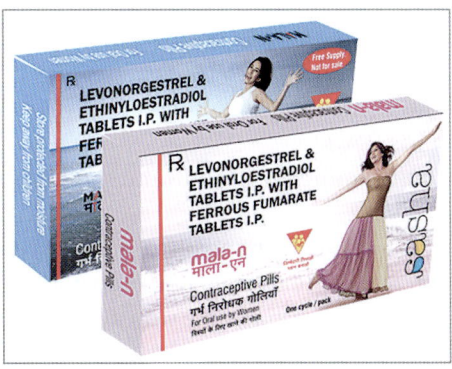

1. What is the composition of MALA-N?
2. What are its noncontraceptive benefits?
3. How to manage when ≥3 pills missed in 1/2nd week?
4. Who is not eligible to use COCs?

Ans.

1. Levonorgestrel (0.15 mg) + Ethinyl estradiol (30 micrograms)
2. Noncontraceptive benefits:
   - Improves dysmenorrhea and menorrhagia

- Regularization of menstrual cycle
- Decreases formation of ovarian cysts
- Reduces benign breast lumps
- Protects against both ovarian and endometrial cancer
- Protects against ectopic pregnancy
- Fertility returns immediately after its discontinuation
- Management of PCOS as it decreases insulin resistance
- Treatment of acne.

3.

How to manage missed pills.	
Missed 1 or 2 pills	Take one hormonal pill as soon as possible/two pills at scheduled time
Missed 3 or more pills in 1st/2nd week	• Take one hormonal pill as soon as possible and continue scheduled pill • Use back up method (condom) for next 7 days
Missed 3 or more pills in 3rd week	• Take one hormonal pill as soon as possible and finish all hormonal pills as scheduled • Start new pack next day • Use back up method (condom) for next 7 days
Missed any nonhormonal pills (Iron pills)	• Discard the missed nonhormonal pill(s) • Continue taking COCs. Start new pack as usual

4. Contraindications of COC:
   - Lactating women who are <6 months postpartum
   - Nonlactating women who are <3 weeks postpartum
   - Women with age ≥35 years who smoke >15 cigarettes/day.
   - Women with the following medical conditions:
     - Deep vein thrombosis (DVT)
     - Heart diseases like Eisenmenger syndrome, pulmonary arterial hypertension, aortic dissection
     - Bleeding disorders like von Willebrand disease, sickle cell disease
     - Liver diseases like active fulminant hepatitis, hepatocellular carcinoma
     - Recurrent migraine headaches, migraine with aura
     - Unexplained abnormal vaginal bleeding
     - Breast cancer
     - On anticonvulsant pharmacotherapy for epilepsy
     - Women with hypertension (BP 140/90)
     - Diabetes, (advanced or long standing) associated with vascular problems, or central nervous system, kidney, or visual disease

OSCE 5.
1. What is the full form of FP-LMIS?
2. Enumerate four salient features of FP-LMIS.

Chapter 28: Contraception

Ans.

1.

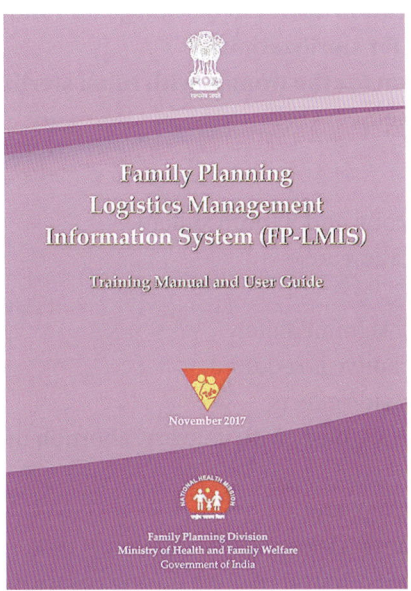

Family Planning Logistics Management Information System: It is a user-friendly web-based, mobile app-based, and SMS-based application for maintaining and strengthening the supply chain of FP commodities. It monitors and manages the family planning commodities at all levels. The application calculates annual demand, enables online indenting, distribution and stock management and provides critical information on stock outs, over stock, expired and damage stock in the form of reports and graphs to decision makers to assist in monitoring of the family planning commodities supply chain system.

2. Salient features of FP-LMIS:
   - Web-based, mobile app-based, and SMS-based application
   - Instant access to stock information from national level to ASHA level
   - Autoforecasting of contraceptives
   - SMS alerts for key indicators
   - Autogenerated reports for program review

OSCE 6.

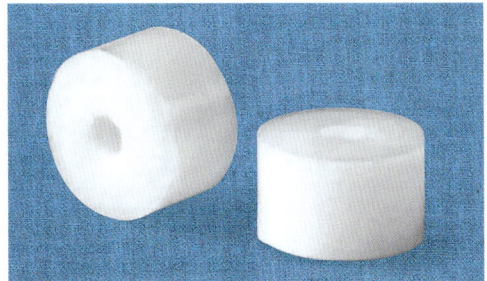

1. Identify the device and what is its chemical composition?
2. What are the benefits of female sterilization?
3. What are the poststerilization advice at discharge for follow-up?
4. What are the incentives for sterilization?
5. What is the compensation for the woman with tubal sterilization failure under Family Planning Indemnity Scheme?

Ans.

1. Falope ring, contains Silicone and Barium sulfate
2. Benefits of female sterilization are:
   - Highly effective
   - Permanent and effective immediately
   - No additional contraceptive is required
   - No long-term harmful side effects
   - Can be adopted simultaneously with delivery/abortion or within 7 days
   - No effect on lactation
3. Follow-up advice at discharge are:
   - After 48 hours (first contact is established)
   - On the 7th day for stitch removal (if done during cesarean section)
   - After 1 month or first menstrual period, whichever is earlier
   - Any time after missing periods or irregular periods
4. After 1 month of the procedure, the sterilization certificate can be collected from the health facility.

	Public health facility	Acceptor	ASHA/Health worker	Others	Total
High focus states (OD, UK, HR, GJ)	• Male sterilization	2,000	300	400	2,700
	• Female sterilization	1,400	200	400	2,000
	• Postpartum sterilization	2,200	300	500	3,000
Mission Parivar Vikas	• Male sterilization	3,000	400	600	4,000
	• Female sterilization	2,000	300	500	2,800
	• Postpartum sterilization	3,000	400	600	4,000
Other high focus (SK, Ladakh, J&K, HP)	Male sterilization	1,100	200	200	1,500
	Female sterilization	600	150	250	1,000
Nonhigh focus states	• Male sterilization (All)	1,100	200	200	1,500
	• Female sterilization (BPL/SC/ST)	600	150	250	1,000
	• Female sterilization (APL)	250	150	250	650

Private accredited health facility		Acceptor	ASHA/Health worker	Others	Total
High focus states (OD, UK, HR, GJ)	• Male sterilization • Female sterilization	1,000 1,000		2,000 2,000	3,000 3,000
Mission parivar vikas	• Male sterilization • Female sterilization • Postpartum sterilization	1,000 1,000 1,000		2,500 2,500 3,000	3,500 3,500 4,000
Other high focus (SK, Ladakh J&K, HP)	• Male sterilization • Female sterilization		200 150	1,300 1,350	1,500 1,500
Nonhigh focus states	• Male sterilization (All) • Female sterilization (BPL/SC/ST)		200 150	1,300 1,350	1,500 1,500

5. ₹ 30,000

The available benefits under the Family Planning Indemnity Scheme are as under.		
Section	Coverage	Limits
SECTION I (A-D): For Beneficiaries		
I A	Death following sterilization (inclusive of death during process of sterilization operation) in hospital or within 7 days from the date of discharge from the hospital	Rs. 2 lakh
I B	Death following sterilization within 8–30 days from the date of discharge from the hospital	Rs. 50,000/-
I C	Failure of sterilization	Rs 30,000/-
I D	Cost of treatment in *hospital and up to 60 days* arising out of complication following sterilization operation (inclusive of complication during process of sterilization operation) from the date of discharge	Actual not exceeding Rs. 25,000/-
SECTION II: Empanelled Doctors under Public and Accredited Private/NGO Sector and Health Facilities under Public and Accredited Private/NGO Sector		
II*	Indemnity coverage up to 4 cases of litigations per doctor and per health facility in a year	Upto Rs. 2 Lakh per case of litigation

OSCE 7.

1. **What is dual method of contraception?**

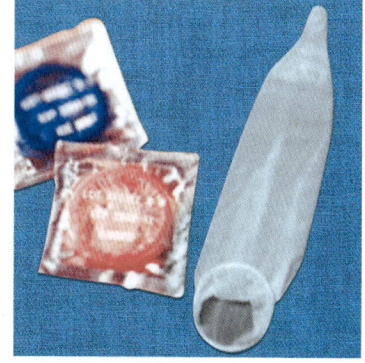

2. What are the benefits of condom?
3. What are the failure rate after perfect and typical use?

Ans.

1. Usage of two contraceptive methods at the same time is known as dual method of contraception. For example, condom can be used with any other method for prevention of STIs and HIV.
2. Benefits of condom:
   - Nonhormonal
   - Only contraceptive that provides dual protection (from unwanted pregnancy and STI/HIV infection)
   - No interaction with any drug
   - No effect on lactation
   - Can be used immediately after delivery or abortion
   - No effect on fertility
   - No need of follow up
3. Failure rate for perfect use (i.e., a condom used correctly at every act of intercourse is approximately 3%, and for typical use (condoms not used for every act of intercourse) the failure rate is 12%.

OSCE 8.

1. What are different methods of emergency contraception?
2. Within how much duration LNG-EC and Cu-IUD is effective as EC?
3. A woman of BMI 30 Kg/m² came after 24 hours of UPSI (unprotected sexual intercourse) and wants contraception. What is the most effective emergency contraceptive for her? What is the effect of weight or BMI on different emergency contraceptives?

Ans.

1.

Method	Class	Recommended dose/use	Indications
Copper intrauterine device (Cu-IUD)	Intrauterine contraceptive method	IUD retained until pregnancy excluded (e.g. onset of next menstrual period) or can be kept for ongoing contraception	Within 5 days (120 hours) after the first UPSI in a cycle or within 5 days after the earliest estimated date of ovulation
Levonorgestrel EC (LNG-EC)	Progestogen	1.5 mg single oral dose*	Licensed for use within 72 hours after UPSI or contraceptive failure
Ulipristal acetate EC (UPA-EC)	Progesterone receptor modulator	30 mg single oral dose	Licensed for use within 5 days (120 hours) after UPSI or contraceptive failure

*A double dose (3 mg) of LNG-EC is recommended if a woman is taking an enzyme-inducing drug. A double dose (3 mg) of LNG-EC should be considered if a woman has a body mass index >26 kg/m² or weight >70 kg

2. a. Cu-IUD is the most effective method of emergency contraception whose effectiveness lies for up to 120 hours after unprotected sexual intercourse (UPSI)

b. UPA-EC is also effective for up to 120 hours after UPSI
c. Effectivity of LNG-EC is up to 72 hours after UPSI. According to evidences, LNG-EC is ineffective if taken after 96 hours of UPSI.
3. a. Effectiveness of the Cu-IUD is not affected by weight or BMI.
b. Women with higher weight or BMI reduces the effectivity of oral EC, particularly LNG-EC. LNG-EC is found to be less effective in women weighing >70 kg or with a BMI >26 kg/m^2.
c. UPA-EC should not be prescribed in women with BMI >30 kg/m^2.

OSCE 9.
1. Name different progestins used in POPs.
2. How effective are POPs?
3. How are they taken in case pills are missed?

Ans.

1. Different progestins used in POPs are:
   - Desogestrel (DSG) 75 µg
   - Drospirenone (DRSP) 4 mg
   - *Traditional POPs:* Levonorgestrel (LNG) 30 µg and norethisterone (NET) 350 µg.
2. After 1 year of typical POP use, the risk of pregnancy is about 9%. If used perfectly, POPs are 99% effective.
3.

Recommendations following incorrect progestogen-only pill use.			
	Traditional POP	**DSG POP**	**DRSP POP**
When is a pill missed?	A pill is missed if taken >3 hours late (>27 hours after last pill taken)	A pill is missed if taken >12 hours late (>36 hours after last pill taken)	A pill is missed if taken >24 hours late (>48 hours after last pill was taken or >24 hours after a new packet should have been started after an HFI)
Action if pill(s) missed	• Take the most recent missed pill as soon as possible • Take the next pill at the usual time (this may mean taking two pills in 1 day) • Use additional contraceptive precautions (eg, condoms) for 48 hours after correct pill-taking has restarted • Consider EC		• Take the most recent missed pill as soon as possible • Take the next pill at the usual time (this may mean taking two pills in 1 day) • Use additional contraceptive precautions (eg, condoms) for 7 days after correct pill-taking has restarted • Consider EC • OMIT THE HFI (PLACEBO PILLS) IF ANY OF THE LAST 7 ACTIVE PILLS ARE MISSED
Is EC required?	EC should be considered if there was UPSI from the time that the first pill was missed until correct pill-taking had resumed for 48 hours		EC should be considered if: • Any active pill(s) were missed and there was UPSI from the time that the first pill was missed until correct pill-taking had resumed for 7 days • Pill(s) were missed on days 1–7 of the packet and there was UPSI during the HFI or week 1
Follow-up	Consider pregnancy test 21 days after last UPSI		

DRSP: drospirenone; DSG: desogestrel; EC: emergency contraception; HFI: hormone-free interval; POP: progestogen-only pill; UPSI: unprotected sexual intercourse)

OSCE 10.

1. **When should contraception after childbirth be discussed/provided?**
2. **What is the ideal interpregnancy interval between two childbirths?**

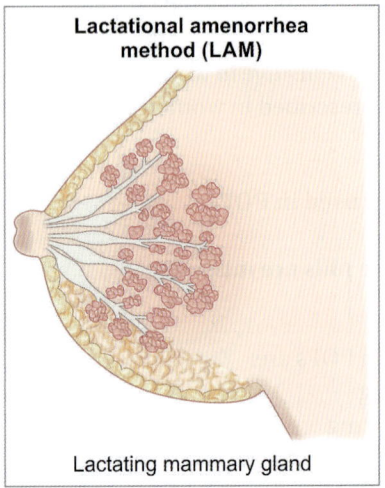

Lactational amenorrhea method (LAM)

Lactating mammary gland

3. **What are the criteria for LAM?**
4. **What is GATHER approach in contraceptive counseling?**

Ans.

1. a. Discuss women fertility intentions, contraception and preconception planning.
   b. During contraceptive counseling, women should not feel any pressure to choose a particular method of contraception.
   c. Since, sexual activity and ovulation may resume very soon afterwards, optimum contraception after childbirth should be initiated by both breastfeeding and nonbreastfeeding women as soon as possible.
   d. It should be ensured that all women after delivery have access to the full range of contraceptives, including the most effective LARC methods, to start immediately after childbirth.
   e. Information regarding the effectiveness of the different contraceptive methods should be provided to all women when they are choosing an appropriate method to use after childbirth.
   f. A person-centered approach should be adopted during the contraceptive counseling.
   g. Information provided by the clinicians regarding contraception should be timely, up-to-date and accurate. This information should be made available in different languages and in audio-visual formats too.
   h. Women should be given contraceptive counseling in the antenatal period itself so that they can choose the method they wish to use after childbirth.
2. An interpregnancy interval (IPI) of less than 12 months between childbirth and conceiving again is associated with an increased risk of preterm birth, low birthweight and small for gestational age (SGA) babies. So, women should be informed regarding the risks associated with short interpregnancy interval.

3. Criteria of LAM:
   - Baby is under 6 months
   - Mother is still amenorrheic
   - Mother practices exclusive or quasi-exclusive breastfeeding on demand, day and night.
4. GATHER approach:
   - *G*reet the client respectfully.
   - *A*sk them about their family planning needs.
   - *T*ell them about different contraceptive options and methods.
   - *H*elp them to make decisions about choices of methods.
   - *E*xplain and demonstrate about choices of methods.
   - *R*eturn for follow-up.

OSCE 11.

1. What is the initial line of management in women with problematic bleeding on hormonal contraceptives?
2. What are the treatment options for problematic bleeding in women on hormonal contraceptives?

Ans.

1. Following history should be taken in women using hormonal contraception with problematic bleeding:
   - Take a clinical history
   - Sexually transmitted infections (STIs)
   - Cervical screening history
   - Pregnancy test
   - Exclude underlying pathology.

> **Points to cover in the clinical history from a woman using hormonal contraception who presents with problematic bleeding.**
>
> *Clinical history taking should include an assessment of a woman's:*
> - Own concerns
> - Current method of contraception and duration of use[a]
> - Compliance with the current contraceptive method[b]
> - Use of any medications (including over-the-counter preparations) which may interact with the contraceptive method
> - Illness/condition that may affect absorption of orally administered hormones
> - Cervical screening history[c]
> - Risk of sexually transmitted infections (i.e. those aged <25 years, or at any age with a new partner, or more than one partner in the last year)
> - Bleeding pattern before starting hormonal contraception, since starting and currently
> - Other symptoms suggestive of an underlying cause (e.g. abdominal or pelvic pain, postcoital bleeding, dyspareunia, heavy menstrual bleeding)
> - Possibility of pregnancy

[a]Progestogen-only methods are more likely to result in problematic bleeding than combined hormonal methods.
[b]For example, missed pills.
[c]A woman presenting with abnormal bleeding who is participating in a National Cervical Screening Programme does not require a cervical screen unless one is due.

2. Medical pharmacotherapy options for women using hormonal contraceptives with problematic bleeding are:
   - Continue with the same COC for at least 3 months as bleeding may settle in this time.
   - Use a COC with increased dose of EE (up to a maximum of 35 microgram)
   - Supplementation with tranexamic acid may also help in reducing bleeding.
   - If women are using injectable DMPA or MIRENA, a first line COC (30–35 micrograms EE) can be considered up to 3 months continuously or in the usual cyclical regimen.

OSCE 12.
1. What contraceptive would you like to offer in a woman with heart disease?
2. What are the risks during IUCD insertion in a woman with heart disease?
3. For how much time pregnancy should be avoided after solid organ transplantation?

Ans.
1.

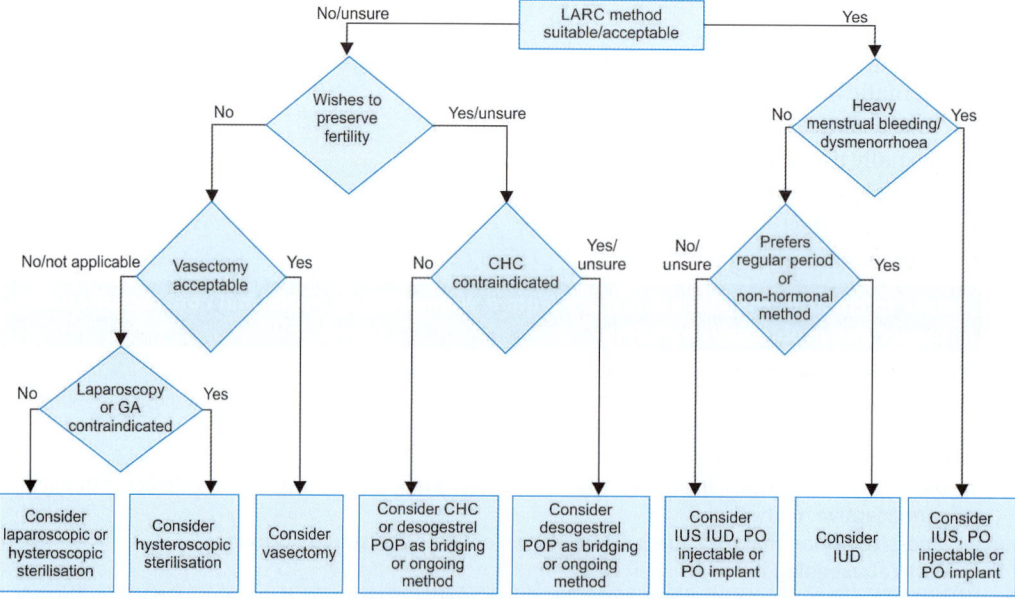

2. Risks during IUCD insertion in heart disease patient:
   - Infection
   - *Vasovagal reaction:* It should be inserted under supervision with aseptic precautions
3. Pregnancy should be avoided for at least 12 months after solid organ transplantation.

OSCE 13.

1. What are the UKMEC category of different contraceptives in a woman with BMI ≥30?
2. When should OCPs be stopped before a major surgery?
3. What are the risks in women with obesity for CHCs?
4. What is the effect of weight/BMI on effectiveness of POPs?

Ans.

1.

Method	BMI (kg/m^2)	UKMEC category* (BMI alone)	UKMEC category if obesity is one of multiple risk factors for cardiovascular disease	History of bariatric surgery
Combined hormonal contraception (COC, vaginal ring, patch)	≥30–34	2	3	2
	≥35	3		3
Progestogen-only pill	≥30–34	1	2	1*
	≥35			
Progestogen-only implant	≥30–34	1	2	1
	≥35			
Progestogen-only injectable (DMPA or NET-EN)	≥30–34	1	3	1
	≥35			
Copper intrauterine device	≥30–34	1	1	1
	≥35			
Levonorgestrel-releasing intrauterine system	≥30–34	1	2	1
	≥35			

(BMI: body mass index; COC: combined oral contraceptive; DMPA: depot medroxyprogesterone acetate; NET-EN: norethisterone enanthate)
*it is important to note that UKMEC categories for contraceptive use after bariatric surgery relate to safety of use rather than effectiveness. Safety considerations after bariatric surgery relate to ongoing high BMI.

2. OCPs should be stopped 4 weeks before a major surgery, lower limb surgery or surgery involving prolonged immobilization in postoperative period. It should be restarted after total mobilization or at least 2 weeks after surgery.
3. Women with obesity should be informed regarding:
   - Risk of thrombosis
   - Risk of dyslipidemia
   - Small increased risk of MI and ischemic stroke.
4. Effectivity of POP is not affected by body weight or BMI.

OSCE 14.

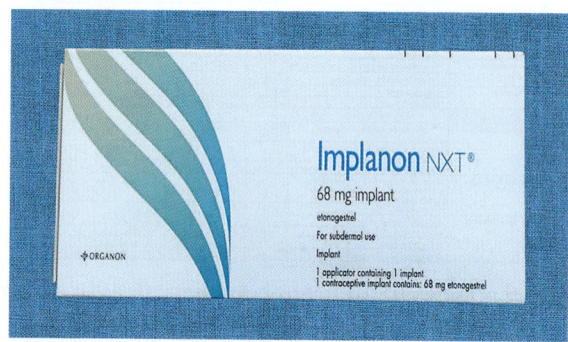

1. Identify the contraceptive device and what are its benefits?
2. When can these implants be inserted?
3. What are the complications of implants insertion?
4. When should an implant be removed?

Ans.

1. Etonogestrel Implant (ENG- IMP). Its benefits are:
   - Effective for 3 years and is not user-dependent.
   - Decreases endometriosis-associated symptoms.
   - No increased risk of venous (VTE) or arterial thromboembolism (ATE).
2. a. Days 1–5 of a natural menstrual cycle
   b. Day 5 after abortion
   c. Day 21 after childbirth without requirement for additional contraceptive precautions.
   d. Nexplanon is inserted subdermally in the inner upper arm, avoiding the sulcus between biceps and triceps muscle. The point of insertion is 8–10 cm proximally from the medial epicondyle along the sulcal line and then 3–5 cm posteriorly (over triceps), perpendicular to the sulcal line.
3. Complications of implant insertion are:
   - Implant migration
   - Intravascular insertion of implants
   - If users cannot feel their implant at any time, its presence should be confirmed by a healthcare professional.
   - Impalpable and deeply sited etonogestrel implants
   - Attempt should not be made to remove an impalpable ENG-IMP which is not localized.

- If an implant is impalpable, additional contraceptive precautions should be advised.
- Removal of a deeply sited implant should only be done by a specialist trained in complex implant removal techniques.

4. Removal of implants can be done any time within 3 years of its insertion without any additional contraception or abstinence prior to its removal.

OSCE 15.

1. **Enumerate the methods of contraception which come under LARC.**

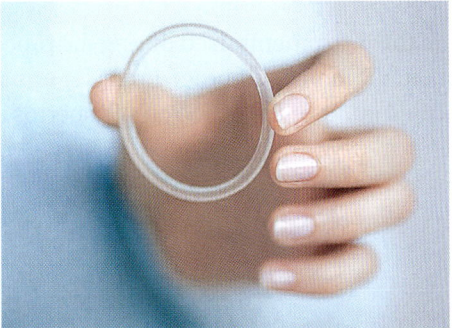

2. **Identify the contraceptive method.**
3. **What is its constituents and how is it used?**

Ans.

1. Intrauterine device, LNG-IUS, vaginal ring, injectable contraceptives—Inj. DMPA and Inj. NET EN, implants.
2. Combine hormonal vaginal ring
3. It contains Ethinylestradiol 15 microbe and Etonogestrel 120 micrograms. Used for 3 weeks and then removed for 7 days. Hormone released is ENG 120 µg/day and EE 15 µg/day over 21 days of use.

OSCE 16.

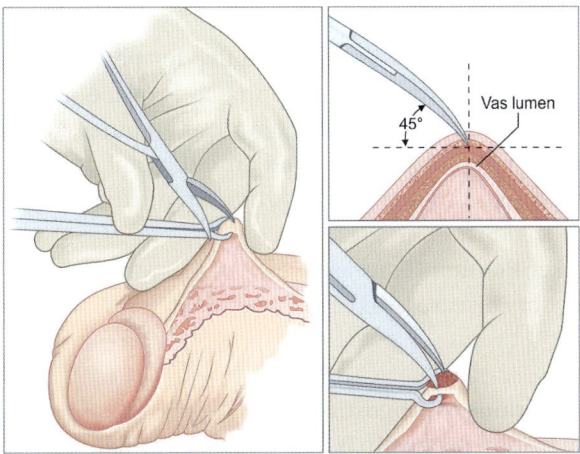

1. What is NSV?
2. When was the procedure incorporated in the National Family Welfare Programme?
3. What are the instruments used during the procedure?
4. After how much time semen analysis is performed and how to diagnose NSV failure?
5. What is its failure rate?

Ans.

1. Nonscalpel vasectomy
2. Incorporated in 1992
3. Vas hook and scissors are the instruments used during the procedure.
4. Semen analysis is done after 3 months of procedure. If sperms are still seen, then repeat semen analysis is performed at 7 months of NSV; if still sperms are present, it is called NSV failure.
5. Failure rate of vasectomy is 1/2000 procedures.

OSCE 17.

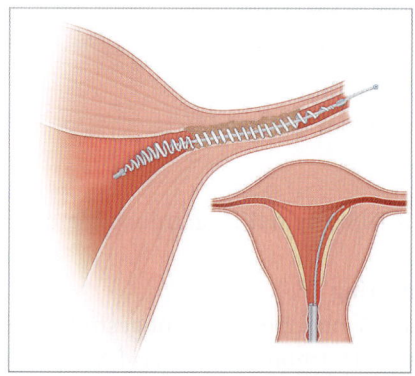

1. Name the device shown in the picture.
2. What are its absolute contraindications?

Ans.

1. Essure system is a minimally invasive alternative for permanent female sterilization. It utilizes a transcervical hysteria optic approach to place a permanent micro insert into the fallopian tube ostia bilaterally. It comprises an inner coil composed of stainless steel/polyethylene terephthalate fibers and an outer coil of nitinol, a nickel titanium alloy. The nitinol coil deploys and expands to anchor into the proximal fallopian tube.
2. Absolute contraindications:
   - Allergies to nickel, titanium, contrast dye
   - Pelvic inflammatory disease (PID)

OSCE 18.

1. Name all four generations of progestins.
2. Which fourth-generation progestin is also known as Millennium molecule?

Ans.

1. a. *First-generation:*
      - Estranes derived from testosterone —norethindrone, norethynodrel, norethindrone acetate, ethynodiol diacetate
      - Pregnanes derived from 17-OH progesterone—medroxyprogesterone acetate, chlormadinone acetate
   b. *Second-generation:* Gonanes derived from testosterone—levonorgestrel, norgestrel
   c. *Third-generation:* Gonane (Levonorgestrel) derivatives—desogestrel, gestodene, norgestimate/norelgestromine, etonorgestrel
   d. *Fourth-generation:*
      - *Nonethylated estranes*: Dienogest, drospirenone
      - Pregnanes (19-norprogesterones), nestorone, nomegestrol acetate, trimegestone
2. Dienogest (17α-cyanomethyl-17β-hydroxy-estra-4,9-dien-3-one) is a fourth-generation progestin with potent oral progestational activity without any systemic androgenic activity.

OSCE 19.

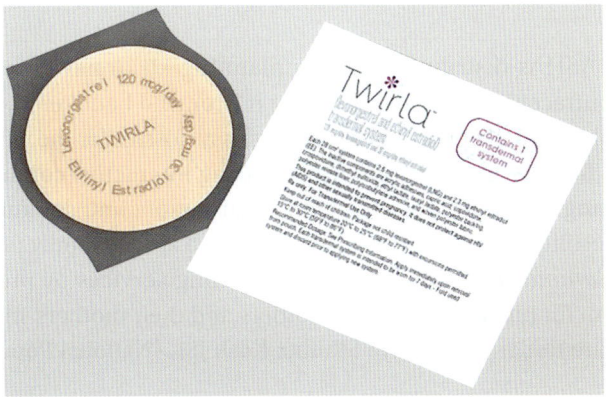

1. **Identify the contraceptive device.**
2. **Which layer contains active ingredients?**
3. **If it is detached for 48 hours, then how to follow such patients?**

Ans.

1. Contraceptive patch
2. It has total 5 layers and inner, out two layers contains active ingredients.
3.
   - If detached ≤48 hours-apply new patch asap keep same patch change day
   - If detached >48 hours-apply new patch asap keep same patch change day
     Additional protection for 7 days
   - If in 1st week of patch use + unprotected sex in last 5 days-consider EC
   - If in 3rd week of patch use-omit patch free week by finishing 3rd week use and starting new patch immediately

OSCE 20.

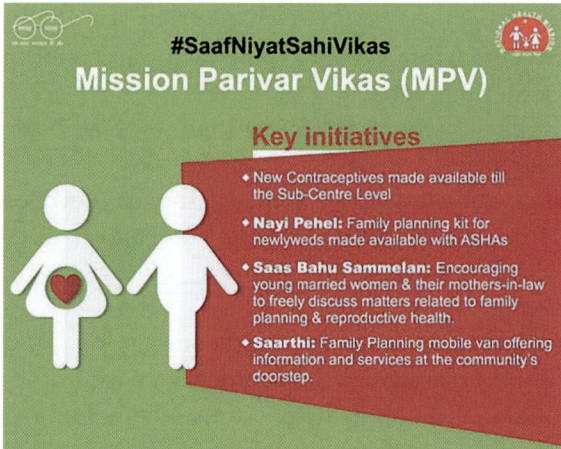

1. What are the initiative under Mission Parivar Vikas?
2. What are the components of Prerna strategy under JSK programme?

Ans.

1. a. *Nayi Pehal:* ASHAs distribute a family planning kit to newlyweds which includes condoms, contraceptive pills, two towels, a mirror, and handkerchiefs for the husband. It includes a bindi, nail cutter, comb, and a glossy dossier for the wife.
   b. *SAARTHI:* A fully customized van or bus having interactive communication devices, family planning commodities, education, information, and communication materials in the high-fertility districts to raise awareness and spread family planning messages
   c. *Saas Bahu Sammelan:* Promotes family planning services by providing an engagement platform for pregnant and new mothers and their mothers-in-law.
2. These schemes are under Jansankhya Sthirata Kosh JSK (National Population Stabilization Fund):
   - PRERNA strategy is for BPL families
   - Meant for helping to push up the age of marriage of girls and delay in first child and spacing in second child birth in the interest of health of young mothers and infants.

   PRERNA strategy recognizes and awards couples who have broken the stereotype of early marriage, early childbirth and repeated child birth and have helped change the mindsets of the community.
   - In order to become eligible for award, the girl should have been married after 19 years of age and given birth to the first child after at least 2 years of marriage.
   - The couple will get an award of ₹ 10,000/- if it is a boy child or ₹ 12,000/- if it is a girl child.
   - If birth of the second child takes place after at least 3 years of the birth of first child and either parent voluntarily accept permanent method of family planning within 1 year of the birth of the second child, the couple will get an additional award of ₹ 5,000/- (boy child)/ ₹ 7,000/- (girl child).

REFERENCES

1. The male latex condom. 10 condom programming fact sheets. Available from: http://whqlibdoc.who.int/hq/1998/WHO_RHT_FPP_98.15_factsheets.pdf [cited in 2009].
2. Faculty of Sexual & Reproductive Healthcare (FSRH). Contraception after prgnancy. England: Faculty of Sexual & Reproductive Healthcare (FSRH); 2023.
3. Faculty of Sexual & Reproductive Healthcare (FSRH). Problematic Bleeding with Hormonal Contraception. England: Faculty of Sexual & Reproductive Healthcare (FSRH); 2015.
4. Faculty of Sexual & Reproductive Healthcare (FSRH). Combined hormonal contraception. England: Faculty of Sexual & Reproductive Healthcare (FSRH); 2023.
5. Faculty of Sexual & Reproductive Healthcare (FSRH). Progestogen only Implant. England: Faculty of Sexual & Reproductive Healthcare (FSRH); 2023.
6. Faculty of Sexual & Reproductive Healthcare (FSRH). Progestogen only Injectable. England: Faculty of Sexual & Reproductive Healthcare (FSRH); 2014.
7. Faculty of Sexual & Reproductive Healthcare (FSRH). Progestogen only Pills. England: Faculty of Sexual & Reproductive Healthcare (FSRH); 2022.
8. Faculty of Sexual & Reproductive Healthcare (FSRH). Emergency Contraception. England: Faculty of Sexual & Reproductive Healthcare (FSRH); 2017.
9. Faculty of Sexual & Reproductive Healthcare (FSRH). Overweight, Obesity and contraception. England: Faculty of Sexual & Reproductive Healthcare (FSRH); 2019.
10. Faculty of Sexual & Reproductive Healthcare (FSRH). Intrauterine contraception. England: Faculty of Sexual & Reproductive Healthcare (FSRH); 2019.
11. Family Planning Guidance booklet for community health officers. National health mission. Ministry of Health and Family Welfare, 2023.

SECTION 2

Gynecology

29. **Pediatric and Adolescent Gynecology**
    Mukta Agarwal
30. **Abnormal Uterine Bleeding**
    Sharda Patra
31. **Endometriosis (I)**
    Ashis Kumar Mukhopadhyay
32. **Endometriosis (II)**
    Juhi Bharti, Vandana Agarwal
33. **Ectopic Pregnancy**
    Sandhya Jain, Pooja Sharma
34. **Uterine Fibroid**
    Jai Bhagwan Sharma, Richa Vatsa
35. **Genitourinary Infections and STDs**
    Niharika Dhiman, Shreshtha Gupta
36. **Pelvic Inflammatory Disease**
    Leena Wadhwa, Sneh Yadav, Deval Rishi Pandit
37. **Polycystic Ovarian Syndrome**
    Seema Grover
38. **Pelvic Organ Prolapse (I)**
    Panchanan Das
39. **Pelvic Organ Prolapse (II)**
    Reena Wani, Krutika Ramdin
40. **Reproductive Medicine and Surgery**
    Fessy Louis T
41. **Amenorrhea**
    Vidya A Thobbi
42. **Endometrial Carcinoma**
    Seema Singhal, Saroj Rajan
43. **Cervical Carcinoma**
    Kasturi V Donimath
44. **Gestational Trophoblastic Neoplasia**
    Neha Mishra
45. **Hysterectomy**
    Nilanchali Singh, Nisha, Deepika Kashyap
46. **Menopause**
    Madhavi M Gupta, Ankita Chonla
47. **Urinary Incontinence and Vesicovaginal Fistula**
    Ajit Kumar Nayak
48. **Gynecological Endoscopy**
    Aswath Kumar
49. **Infertility**
    Shikha Seth, Shristi Jaiswal

CHAPTER 29

Pediatric and Adolescent Gynecology

Mukta Agarwal

OSCE 1. A mother brought a 10-day-old neonate to the hospital showing concerns that her baby is having milky discharge from the breast and blood-stained vaginal discharge.
1. How will you treat this?
2. What is the pathophysiology behind this condition?
3. How long does it take for this to subside on its own?

Ans.

1. Reassurance to the mother
2. Circulating maternal estrogen crosses the placenta and acts on the internal and external genital organs and breast tissue of the neonate.
3. 2 weeks

OSCE 2.

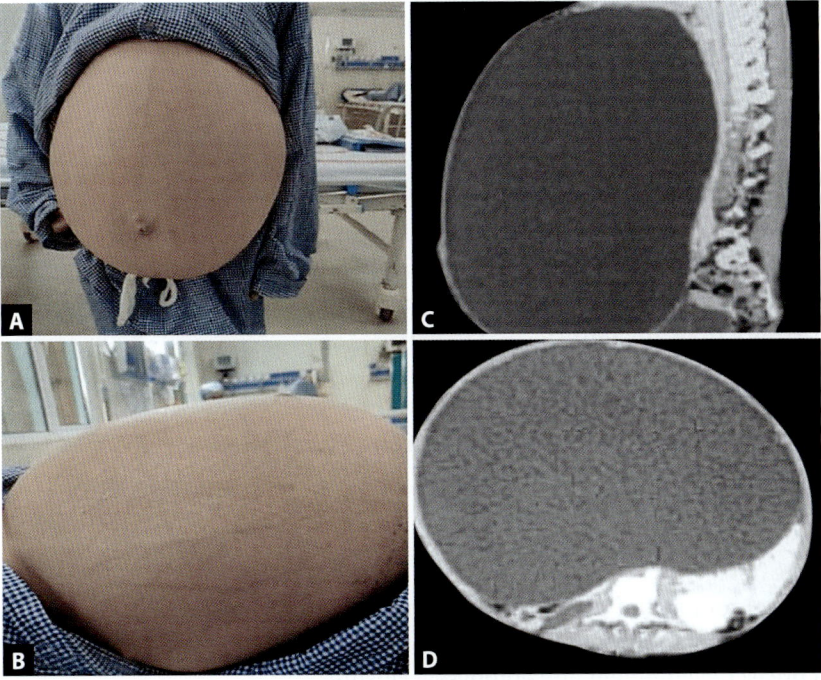

A 17-year-old, girl presented with increasingly gross distension of abdomen for one year associated with vague abdominal pain and respiratory discomfort. All tumor markers were negative. CT scan showed a large, well-defined, uniloculated, homogeneously cystic lesion 37 cm × 31 cm × 22 cm arising from left ovary with no features of malignancy as shown in the above image.
1. What is the most likely diagnosis?
2. Enumerate four radiological features of benign adnexal mass.
3. How will you treat this patient?

Ans.

1. Benign ovarian epithelial tumor—most likely serous cystadenoma.
2. Size <7 cm, anechoic cystic lesions, no solid areas, no papillary excrescences, thin walled, uniloculated, if multiloculated—thin septae, unilateral, no ascites/retroperitoneal nodes, no metastases.
3. Ovarian cystectomy—laparoscopic/open.

OSCE 3.

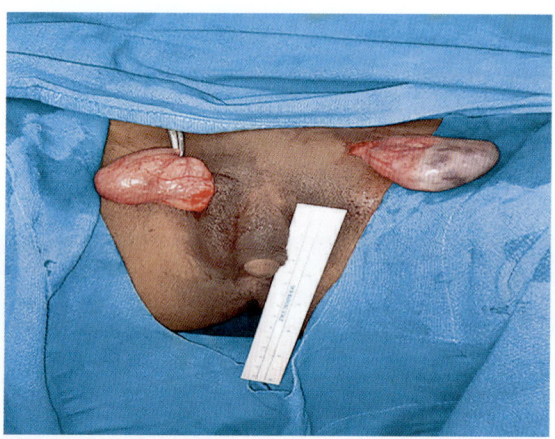

An 18-year-old girl presented with primary amenorrhea and normal breast development. On USG, uterus was absent. Gonads were visualized in labia majora with clitoromegaly and a short and blind vagina. Pubic and axillary hair were scanty and serum testosterone levels were more than 200 ng/mL.
1. What is the most likely diagnosis?
2. What is the karyotype in such cases?
3. Should the gonads be removed? If yes, why and when should it be done?

Ans.

1. Androgen insensitivity syndrome
2. Karyotype is XY
3. Yes, surgical removal of gonads is mandatory as chances of malignancy developing in gonad with Y chromosome are 2–5%; but gonadectomy can be delayed till 18 years to permit breast development and epiphyseal closure.

OSCE 4.

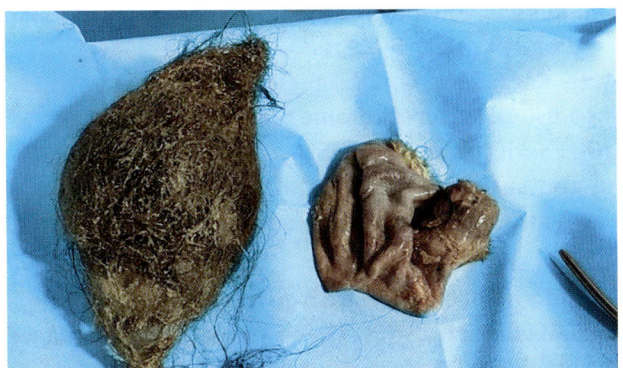

A teenage girl underwent laparoscopic cystectomy for benign ovarian tumor. Cyst wall and its contents are shown in the image above.
1. What is the diagnosis?
2. What are its components?
3. Enumerate four complications.

Ans.

1. Benign (mature) cystic teratoma—dermoid cyst—germ cell tumor of ovary.
2. Ectoderm (skin, hair, teeth, sebaceous material), endoderm (thyroid, bronchus) or mesoderm (bone, smooth muscle).
3. Torsion (10%), rupture, infection, granulomatous if ruptures, rarely malignant transformation.

OSCE 5.
A 5-year-old girl is brought by her mother with complains of development of breasts, pubic, and axillary hair.
1. What is precocious puberty?
2. How will you differentiate between central and peripheral precocious puberty?
3. How will you manage central precocious puberty?

Ans.

1. When onset of puberty is 2 SD earlier than mean age of puberty (8 years)—it is called precocious puberty.
2. Central—LH, FSH elevated, and LH rises on GnRH stimulation. Peripheral—FSH, LH levels low; no LH rise on GnRH stimulation.
3. GnRH agonist 3 weekly to suppress GnRH production till normal age of puberty and surgery for intracranial tumors if required.

OSCE 6.
An 18-year-old girl presented with primary amenorrhea, normal height, and secondary sexual characteristics. External genitalia was normal with vaginal dimple of around 1.5 cm. USG showed normal ovaries with rudimentary uterus.
1. What is the diagnosis?

2. What will be the karyotype and FSH levels in this case?
3. What other anomalies will you look for in this patient and why?

Ans.

1. Mayer-Rokitansky-Küster-Hauser syndrome
2. Karyotype—46, XX. FSH levels are normal
3. Associated renal and skeletal anomalies should be looked for as MRCS association (Müllerian aplasia, renal anomalies, cervical somite anomalies) is common.

OSCE 7. A 15-year-old girl presented with primary amenorrhea, short stature, and absent secondary sexual characteristics. The examination revealed webbed neck, widely spaced nipples, and shield chest. External genitalia is normal.
1. What is the diagnosis?
2. What will be the karyotype and FSH levels in this case?
3. What are the other risks associated with this syndrome?

Ans.

1. Turner syndrome
2. Karyotype—45,X and FSH levels elevated in menopausal range
3. Women with Turner syndrome are at high risk of developing diabetes, hypertension, aortic enlargement, autoimmune thyroiditis, sensorineural hearing loss.

OSCE 8. A 17-year-old girl presented with secondary amenorrhea for 3 months while she was preparing for her higher secondary board examinations. Her UPT is negative and USG is normal. TSH and prolactin levels are normal.
1. What do you think is the diagnosis?
2. What is the mechanism behind secondary amenorrhea in such cases?
3. What will be the values of FSH and LH?

Ans.

1. Functional hypothalamic amenorrhea due to stress of examinations.
2. Stress activates the hypothalamic-pituitary-adrenal axis leading to release of CRH, ACTH, and cortisol. Cortisol suppresses GnRH secretion, leading to decreased pulsatile secretion of LH, absence of mid-cycle surge and anovulation leading to secondary amenorrhea.
3. LH and FSH values will be low.

OSCE 9. An adolescent girl presented with secondary amenorrhea, galactorrhea, and visual problems. Her TSH is normal, and prolactin is 600 ng/mL.
1. What is the most likely diagnosis?
2. What are the other causes of hyperprolactinemia?
3. What further investigations will you advise in this patient?

Ans.
1. Pituitary adenoma leading to hyperprolactinemia.
2. Physiological (stress, pregnancy, lactation, chest wall irritation), drug induced, hypothyroidism, chronic renal failure, hypothalamic or pituitary tumors.
3. MRI to rule out pituitary adenoma and visual field evaluation.

OSCE 10. A 17-year-old girl, presented with oligomenorrhea for 3 years, acne, and hirsutism. USG shows PCOM.
1. Why cannot the PCOS diagnostic criteria for adults be applied to adolescents?
2. Enumerate four long-term consequences of PCOS?

Ans.
1. Irregular and anovulatory cycles are normal in adolescents, acne and mild hirsutism are physiological, polycystic ovaries are common and considered normal, testosterone levels interpretation poses problems.
2. Metabolic syndrome (T2DM, dyslipidemia), infertility, coronary heart disease, endometrial and breast CA, NAFLD, obstructive sleep apnea, depression, anxiety, pregnancy complications (GDM, pre-eclampsia, preterm birth).

OSCE 11. An 18-year-old student presented with 2-year history of weight gain, irregular cycles, severe hirsutism, and clitoromegaly.
1. Enumerate two differential diagnoses.
2. What investigations will you like to order to reach a diagnosis?
3. What are the management options?

Ans.
1. PCOS, nonclassic congenital adrenal hyperplasia, androgen secreting adrenal or ovarian tumor.
2. USG to rule out PCOS, testosterone, 17-OH-P, DHEA.
3. Medical management (COC, spironolactone, cyproterone acetate, flutamide, finasteride GnRH agonist, eflornithine cream) or surgical management in cases of clitoromegaly, adrenal or ovarian tumors.

OSCE 12. A 3-year-old was brought by her mother with complaints of vaginal bleeding for 3 months. On examination of the genitalia; polypoid, friable mass of 5 cm × 6 cm was seen arising from the vagina.
1. What is your most likely diagnosis?
2. What other sites can be involved?
3. What are the histological features?

Ans.

1. Sarcoma botryoides
2. It is a subtype of embryonal rhabdomyosarcoma, that can be observed in walls of hollow, mucosa-lined structures such as nasopharynx, common bile duct, urinary bladder or vagina.
3. Spindle-shaped tumor cells that are desmin positive (rhabdomyoblasts) are crowded in a distinct layer beneath the vaginal epithelium (cambium layer).

OSCE 13. A teenage girl presented with painful labial swelling. On vulval examination, tense, tender, fluctuant swelling of around 5 cm diameter was palpated along left inferior labia minora.
1. What is your diagnosis?
2. What are its causes?
3. How will you manage this case?

Ans.

1. Bartholin gland abscess
2. Obstruction of gland's duct, infection, trauma, mucus changes or congenitally narrowed ducts
3. Incision and drainage or marsupialization

OSCE 14. A teenage girl presented to the emergency with 6 weeks amenorrhea, intermittent worsening pain in left iliac fossa, vaginal spotting and history of one fainting episode. She gives history of self-intake of MTP kit after her overdue of menses 2 weeks back. On examination, she is pale, pulse is 120 bpm, BP is 86/54 mm Hg. Per vaginal examination revealed left adnexal palpable mass with cervical motion tenderness.
1. What is your diagnosis?
2. How will you confirm your diagnosis?
3. How will you manage this patient?

Ans.

1. Ruptured ectopic pregnancy.
2. Ultrasonography to confirm adnexal mass with gestational sac and hemoperitoneum.
3. Resuscitation (IV access, blood transfusion) and taken up for salpingectomy.

OSCE 15. A 15-year-old student presented with heavy menstrual bleeding for 2 weeks following a period of 3 months amenorrhea. She attained menarche at 13 years of age and previous cycles were prolonged in duration and infrequent. Clinically she is pale:
1. What is the diagnosis?
2. How will you evaluate this patient?
3. How will you manage this patient?

Ans.
1. AUB in adolescent— puberty menorrhagia.
2. Detailed family history of bleeding disorders, CBC, coagulation profile, TSH, USG pelvis.
3. Treatment of anemia by blood transfusion or iron therapy, tranexamic acid, hormonal therapy—COC or progesterone alone, hematologist consultation if coagulopathy.

OSCE 16. A 14-year-old presented with recurrent, crampy lower abdominal pain during menses.
1. What points will you ask in history of this patient?
2. What investigations will you do?
3. What are the management options in this patient?

Ans.
1. Age at menarche, age of onset of pain, type of pain, timing, duration, severity, other associated symptoms, impact on day-to-day activity, medications.
2. Ultrasonography to rule out any pelvic pathology.
3. Medical management with NSAIDS, COCs, progestins.

OSCE 17. A 16-year-old girl presents with amenorrhea for 8 months, low-grade fever, weight loss, and weakness. She gives history of contact with pulmonary TB patient (father). On examination, her BMI is 17. Ultrasound of pelvis revealed a tubo-ovarian mass of 5 cm × 6 cm.
1. What is your provisional diagnosis?
2. What investigations will you order?
3. How will you manage this patient?

Ans.
1. Genital tuberculosis leading to tubo-ovarian abscess.
2. CBC, ESR, CXR, Menstrual blood for TB-PCR/CBNAAT
3. Antitubercular drugs for 6–9 months

OSCE 18. A 19-year-old girl has come to you for contraceptive advise.
1. Which contraceptive would you suggest to her and why?
2. If COCs is advised, what will she do in case she misses a single pill?
3. When does fertility return after stopping OCPs?

Ans.
1. OCPs would be ideal for her as it is reversible form of contraception.
2. Single pill missed—forgotten pill to be taken when noticed, next pill taken when due.
3. In majority of women, menses and fertility return to normal within 90 days.

OSCE 19.

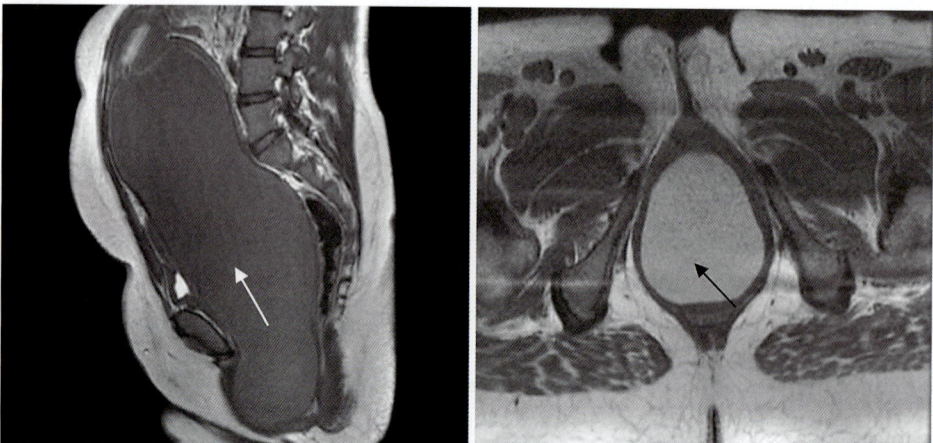

A 16-year-old girl presented with primary amenorrhea and cyclical abdominal pain for two years. Her height is normal and secondary sexual characteristics are well developed. On vaginal examination, bluish bulging membrane was seen at the introitus. MRI showed normal uterus, ovaries and massive hematocolpos as shown in the above image.
1. What is the diagnosis?
2. What are the possible complications?
3. How will you treat this?

Ans.

1. Cryptomenorrhea due to imperforate hymen leading to hematocolpos.
2. Urinary retention, hydroureteronephrosis, bilateral ovarian endometriosis.
3. Hymenotomy—cruciate shaped incision on hymeneal membrane and drainage of hematocolpos.

OSCE 20.
A 6-year-old girl was brought by her mother with complaints of dribbling of urine and burning micturition for 2 months. On examination, labia majora was normal, whereas labia minora were fused with distinct line of demarcation between them and a ventral pinhole meatus between the labia.
1. In what different positions can you examine the external genitalia of this pediatric patient?
2. What is the diagnosis?
3. How will you treat this?

Ans.

1. Frog-leg or knee-chest position or sitting in parent's lap with the child's legs straddling the parent's thighs.
2. Labial adhesion or agglutination.
3. Local estrogen cream therapy followed by separation of adhesion. If adhesion persists, introitoplasty under general anesthesia.

CHAPTER 30

Abnormal Uterine Bleeding

Sharda Patra

OSCE 1.

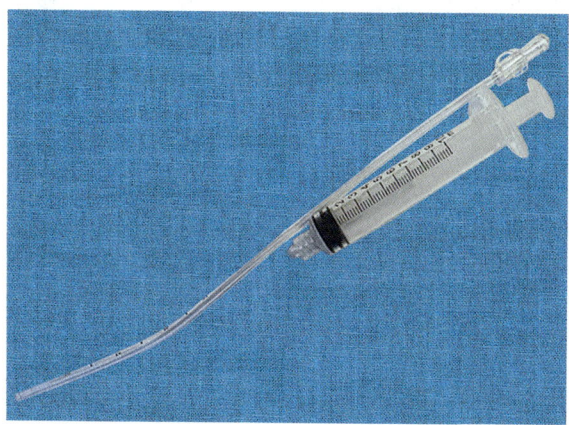

1. Identify the instrument and what is the name of the procedure where it is used?
2. Enumerate two indications for performing the procedure.
3. State two absolute contraindications of endometrial biopsy.
4. Mention two abnormal findings of endometrial biopsy in AUB.
5. What is the right time to perform this procedure?

Ans.

1. Endometrial biopsy cannula for endometrial sampling
2. a. Abnormal uterine bleeding
   b. Evaluation for endometrial neoplasia or precancerous hyperplasia
3. a. Pregnancy
   b. Acute PID
4. a. Endometrial hyperplasia
   b. Endometrial carcinoma
5. Premenstrually

OSCE 2.

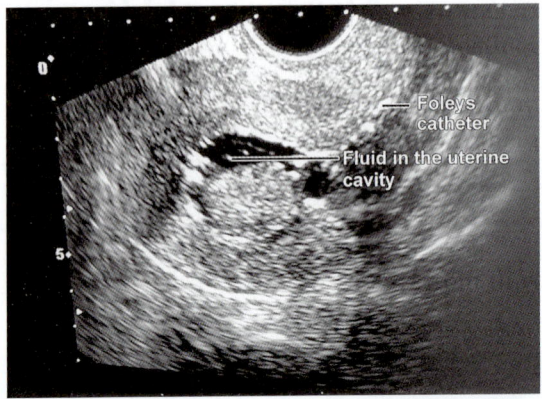

1. What does the USG film depict?
2. What is the abnormality shown?
3. Match the following:

Procedure	Media
a. Hysterosalpingogram	(A) Glycine
b. Saline infusion sono-salpingography	(B) Methylene Blue
c. Chromopertubation	(C) Iodinated contrast
d. Hysteroscopic septal resection	(D) Saline

Ans.

1. Saline infusion sono-salpingography
2. Endometrial polyp
3. a. (C), b. (D), c. (B), d. (A)

OSCE 3.
A 45-year, P2L2 had undergone abdominal hysterectomy. The picture shows the gross anatomy of the specimen.

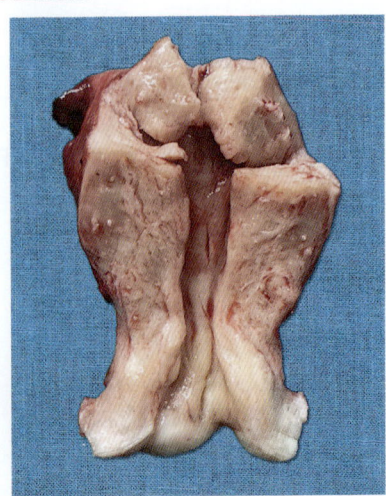

1. Identify the condition.
2. Enumerate two clinical presentations.
3. Enumerate three sonographic findings.
4. What is the possible complication which can occur if it is not treated?

Ans.

1. Adenomyosis
2. Heavy menstrual bleeding and severe dysmenorrhea
3. a. Myometrial cysts
   b. Subendometrial lines and buds
   c. Enlarged globular/asymmetrical enlargement of uterus
4. Anemia

OSCE 4.

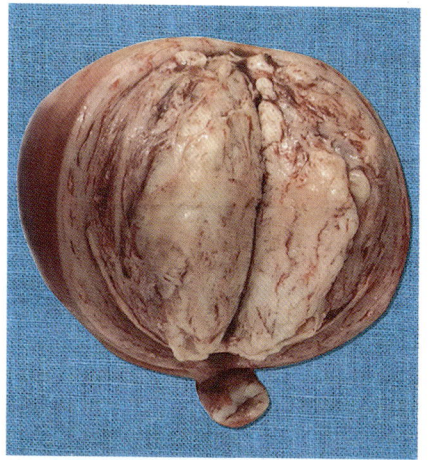

1. Identify the condition as depicted in the specimen picture.
2. What could be the most probable clinical profile of the patient?
3. Enumerate three possible complications during the surgical procedure.
4. What is the incidence of malignant transformation of the uterine fibroid?
5. What is the best modality for imaging preoperatively?

Ans.

1. Uterine fibroid
2. Age between 45–50 years, family complete, presented with heavy menstrual bleeding and mass per abdomen.
3. Bleeding, injury to bladder or bowel injury to ureter
4. 0.1%
5. MRI

OSCE 5.

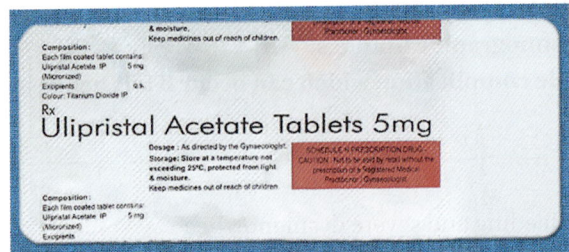

1. Mention two conditions where this drug is indicated?
2. What is its mechanism of action in uterine fibroid?
3. Mention two absolute contraindications.
4. What is the maximum duration for which it can be used?

Ans.

1. a. Medical management of uterine fibroid
   b. Emergency contraception
2. Selective progesterone receptor modulator. It prevents tumor proliferation, induces cell apoptosis and death, hence eventually reducing the size of the fibroid and bleeding.
3. Severe liver disease, severe asthma on steroids
4. 3 months

OSCE 6.

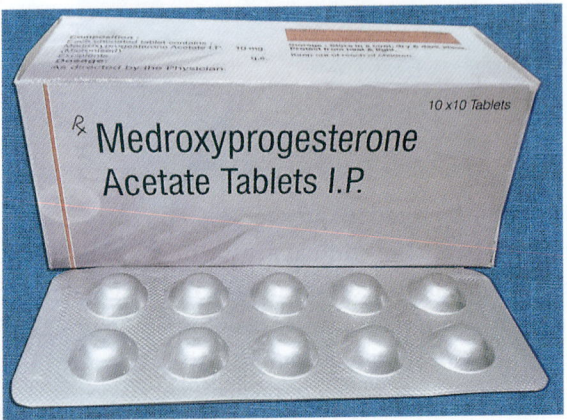

1. Enumerate three clinical uses.
2. Mention one contraindication of the drug.
3. What is its injectable form used for?
4. What is the dose in women with endometrial intraepithelial neoplasia?

Ans.

1. Anovulatory bleeding in AUB, women with amenorrhea for withdrawal bleeding, atypical endometrial hyperplasia

2. Women with history of venous thromboembolism
3. Injection Depo Medroxyprogesterone acetate is used as a contraceptive.
4. 600 mg in divided doses.

OSCE 7.

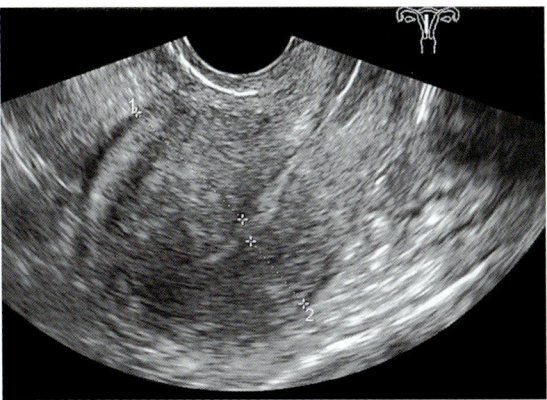

1. Identify the USG picture.
2. Mention two conditions mimicking adenomyosis.
3. Enumerate two medical lines of treatment.
4. Mention one associated condition.

Ans.

1. Diffuse adenomyosis
2. Uterine fibroid and anovulatory bleeding with myohyperplasia
3. Combined oral contraceptives, LNG-IUD (Levonorgestrel intrauterine device)
4. Pelvic endometriosis

OSCE 8.

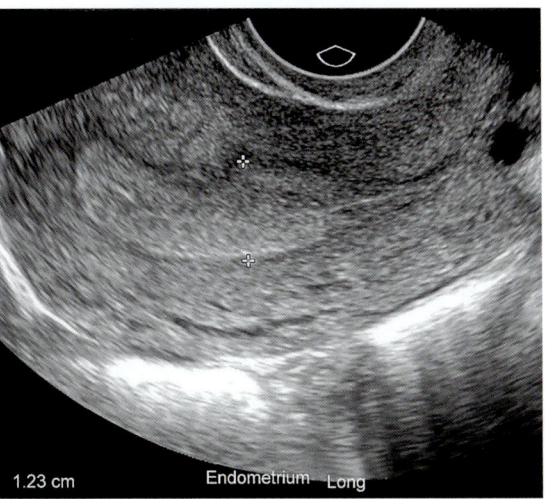

A 48-year-old, P3L3 with heavy menstrual bleeding, comes with the above shown ultrasound report.
1. What is the abnormality shown in the picture?
2. What is the normal endometrial thickness in the premenstrual phase?
3. Mention two risk factors associated with this condition.
4. With this finding what is the next step to confirm the abnormality?
5. Mention two options of medical management.

Ans.
1. Thickened endometrium
2. 10–12 mm
3. Obesity, diabetes mellitus
4. Endometrial biopsy
5. LNG-IUD, oral medroxyprogesterone

OSCE 9.

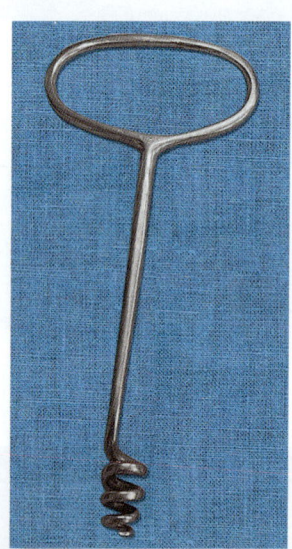

1. Identify the instrument and name the surgery where it is used.
2. State two complications of myomectomy.
3. Enumerate two methods of reducing bleeding during myomectomy.
4. Enumerate two postoperative complications of myomectomy.

Ans.
1. Myoma screw for myomectomy
2. Hemorrhage and infection
3. Injection Vasopressin, Injection Tranexamic acid, tourniquet, use of cautery at the myoma bed
4. Bleeding at the myoma bed, Infection

OSCE 10.

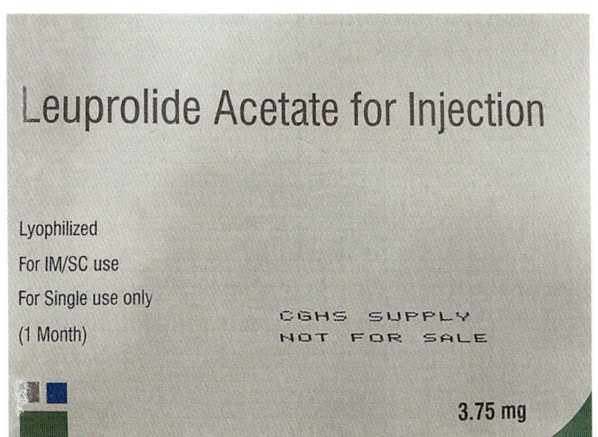

1. Mention the constituent of this drug and its mechanism of action.
2. State its use in abnormal uterine bleeding.
3. Mention two contraindications of this drug.
4. Mentions two adverse effects of the drug.

Ans.

1. Leuprolide acetate is a GnRH analog. It acts on the GnRH receptors, inhibiting the release of FSH and LH.
2. For shrinkage of fibroid size, decreasing bleeding and correction of anemia preoperatively.
3. Pregnancy and breastfeeding
4. Hot flashes, migraine, and weight gain

OSCE 11.

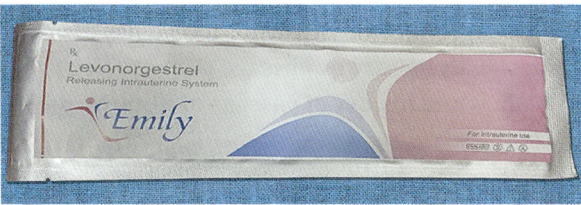

1. Mention two noncontraceptive uses of the above.
2. Enumerate two contraindications.
3. What is the preferred timing of its insertion?
4. Mention two important postinsertion counseling points.

Ans.

1. Endometrial hyperplasia, endometrial intraepithelial neoplasia
2. Undiagnosed genital tract bleeding, distorted uterine cavity (multiple fibroids)
3. Within 4–5 days of menstruation
4. Breakthrough bleeding for 3–4 months, amenorrhea may occur.

OSCE 12.

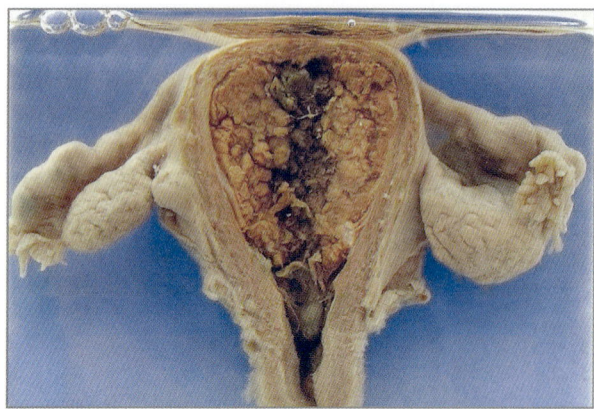

1. Identify the structures and the uterine abnormality.
2. What would have been the most probable clinical profile of this patient?
3. What is the definitive approach to diagnose this condition?
4. What is the definite treatment of endometrial cancer?

Ans.

1. Uterus with bilateral adnexa and cervix, endometrial cancer
2. Postmenopausal women with bleeding
3. Transvaginal ultrasound and endometrial biopsy
4. Surgical staging—hysterectomy with bilateral salpingo-ophorectomy with retroperitoneal lymph-node dissection

OSCE 13. A 43-year, P3L3 presents in G-OPD with complaints of menorrhagia with severe dysmenorrhea, dyspareunia, and increased frequency of urine for 2 years. It occurs for 10–12 days in 28 days, with history of passage of clots. Her previous cycle lasted for 3–4 days occurring in 28 days and history of passage of clots. No personal or family history of cancer.

O/E: Patient is conscious, oriented, and obese. Pallor was present, pulse rate 92/min, BP 130/80 mm Hg, no lymphadenopathy, P/S (per speculum): Cervix, vagina healthy, P/V (per vaginal examination): Uterus 16 weeks, mid position, symmetrically enlarged, firm, nontender with restricted mobility. Bilateral fornices were clear.

1. Mention two differential diagnoses.
2. What are the two most differentiating points between adenomyosis and uterine fibroid?
3. What is the choice of imaging modality?
4. Mention two nonsurgical management of this condition.
5. What are the surgical management options?

Ans.

1. Adenomyosis and uterine fibroid
2. Menorrhagia with severe dysmenorrhea and symmetrical enlargement of uterus is seen in adenomyosis.
3. Transabdominal and transvaginal ultrasound
4. OCPs and LNG-IUD
5. Abdominal hysterectomy and bilateral salpingectomy

OSCE 14. A 35-year, P1L1, presented to GOPD with complaints of menorrhagia of eight months duration. On per abdominal examination, uterus was enlarged to 20 weeks size, firm in consistency, irregularly enlarged, nontender, mobility present from side to side, lower limit of mass could not be reached, P/S: Cervix and vagina healthy, P/V: Cervix firm and regular, pointing downwards, uterus corresponding to 20 weeks, irregularly enlarged, firm, mobility present from side to side, nontender, cervical movements transmitted to mass. Bilateral fornices were free and nontender.
1. What is the probable diagnosis?
2. Name the imaging modality to know the exact site of fibroid.
3. Considering her parity which surgery is advised?
4. Mention two degenerative pathologies associated with this condition.

Ans.

1. Fibroid uterus
2. MRI
3. Myomectomy
4. Hyaline and cystic degeneration

OSCE 15. A 36-year, P2L2 presents to GOPD with complaint of irregular cycles since last 6 months occurring at an interval of 45–60 days lasting for 10–12 days associated with passage of clots. Her previous cycles were normal. She has gained 7 kg weight in the last 6 months. Her examination findings are normal.
1. What is the relevant history to be elicited in the present case?
2. What is the probable diagnosis as per PALMCOEIN?
3. Enumerate four causes of ovulatory dysfunction.
4. Mention the specific hormonal investigations which should be done for the diagnosis.
5. What is the management of AUB due to PCOS?

Ans.

1. History of contraception, IUCD insertion, family history of diabetes mellitus
2. Ovulatory dysfunction
3. PCOD, hypo/hyperthyroidism, diabetes mellitus, obesity, hyper prolactinemia
4. Serum FSH, LH, Prolactin, TSH, T3, T4
5. Oral cyclical combined hormonal pills

Section 2: Gynecology

OSCE 16. A 58-year, postmenopausal woman presents with postmenopausal bleeding since four months. Irregular episodes of bleeding last for 3 to 4 days. She attained menopause 8 years ago. On examination, general examination was normal. P/S: Cervix flushed with vagina, healthy with atrophic changes. P/V: Uterus retroverted, bulky in sizes, bilateral fornices-free, nontender. Per rectal examination was normal.
1. What is the probable diagnosis?
2. Enumerate two risk factors associated with this condition.
3. Mention the condition mimicking endometrial cancer.
4. Mention one diagnostic modality for the confirmation of diagnosis.
5. Mention the imaging modality to know the extent of disease.

Ans.
1. Endometrial carcinoma
2. Obesity, diabetes mellitus, hypertension
3. Endometrial hyperplasia, endometrial fibroid polyp
4. Diagnostic hysteroscopy and biopsy
5. MRI abdomen and pelvis

OSCE 17. A 40-year, P2L2 presents to GOPD with complaint of heavy menstrual bleeding since 8–9 months. Her cycles occur at an interval of 28–30 days, lasting for 10–12 days. Her previous cycles were regular. On examination, pallor was present, general physical examination was normal. P/S: Cervix and vagina healthy. P/V: Uterus was 12 weeks in size, regularly enlarged, bilateral fornices free and nontender.
1. Mention two medical history which should be elicited.
2. Which investigation should be ordered for anemia?
3. Enumerate two differential diagnoses.
4. What is the drug of choice for the medical management of this case.
5. What would be the indication for hysterectomy?

Ans.
1. Hypothyroidism, diabetes mellitus
2. CBC with peripheral blood smear
3. AUB-O, adenomyosis
4. Medroxy progesterone from day 15-day 25, LNG-IUD
5. If she is refractory to medical management.

OSCE 18. A 45-year, multiparous lady presents with complaints of irregular bleeding for the past 4 months. She also complaints of vaginal discharge and intermenstrual bleeding for almost the same duration. O/E: General condition was normal, vitals stable and pallor was present. Systemic examination was normal. P/S: 6 × 6 cm mass seen at the cervical os. Vagina was healthy. P/V: Uterus multiparous, mobile, 6 × 6 cm mass felt coming from cervical os, bled on touch.

Chapter 30: Abnormal Uterine Bleeding

1. What additional points should be elicited in history?
2. What is the differential diagnosis?
3. Match the following:
    a. Cervical cancer   (A) Smooth mass, regular surface, entire cervical lip felt
    b. Fibroid polyp   (B) Soft mass, bleeds on touch, cervical lips felt, absent uterine fundus in P/V examination
    c. Uterine inversion   (C) Hard-indurated ulcerated mass, bleeds on touch, cervical lip involved
4. What is the management of this case?

Ans.

1. History of postcoital bleeding, past menstrual cycles, History of any hormone intake (OCPs)
2. Cervical cancer, fibroid polyp, uterine inversion
3. a. (C), b. (A), c. (B)
4. Vaginal myomectomy

OSCE 19. A 13-year-old girl who attained menarche 9 months back, presents with chief complaints of heavy bleeding (10–12 days) during her menstrual cycles for past 6 months. There is no history of TB. No history of easy bruisability.

O/E: Vitals normal, average built, moderate pallor present, systemic examination was normal. P/A: Soft, nontender. Secondary sexual characters were normal. Per rectal examination was normal.

1. Identify the condition.
2. What are the two most common causes of this condition?
3. Enumerate two blood investigations which should be done.
4. How should anemia be investigated further?
5. How to manage puberty menorrhagia in this case?

Ans.

1. Puberty menorrhagia
2. Anovulatory bleeding, coagulation disorder
3. CBC with peripheral smear, BT, CT, PT, INR, and thyroid function test
4. Iron studies, HPLC
5. Cyclical medroxyprogesterone from Day 15–25.

OSCE 20. A 47-year, P3L3 undergoes hysteroscopy for evaluation of menorrhagia. The histology of endometrial biopsy shows endometrial atypical hyperplasia.
1. What is the probability of concurrent endometrial cancer in such a scenario?
2. What treatment option should be offered to the woman?
3. What is the risk of endometrial cancer in atypical endometrial hyperplasia?
4. Name two conditions which predispose endometrial hyperplasia.
5. What is the indication of hysterectomy in a woman on progesterone therapy?

Ans.
1. 30%
2. Continuous high-dose progesterone, cyclical progesterone, Inj MPA, LNG-IUD, hysterectomy
3. 29%
4. PCOD, diabetes mellitus
5. Persistent endometrial hyperplasia and endometrial intraepithelial neoplasia on follow-up endometrial biopsy

REFERENCES
1. Berek JS. Benign diseases of the female reproductive tract. Berek and Novak's Gynecology, 16th edition. Philadelphia: Lippincott Williams & Wilkins; 2019.
2. Abnormal uterine bleeding. In: Hoffman BL, Schorge JO, Bradshaw KD, Halvorson LM, Schaffer JI, Corton MM (Eds). *Williams Gynecology, 3rd edition*. McGraw Hill; 2016.

CHAPTER 31

Endometriosis (I)

Ashis Kumar Mukhopadhyay

OSCE 1. An 18-year-old unmarried girl with regular cycles, progressive dysmenorrhea, taking analgesics off and on:
1. What is the first line of management?
2. What is the indication of COC pills in this case?
3. What is the role of laparoscopy in this patient?
4. What is the role of postoperative hormone therapy?

Ans.
1. First line of management in this case is analgesics and antispasmodics.
2. If it fails, COC pills (LDP, low dose pills) are recommended.
3. Laparoscopy is no longer recommended for diagnosis, but for treatment in obstinate cases which are not responding and when pain is not relieved with medical treatment.
4. Since fertility is not the issue in this particular patient. Postoperative hormone therapy for a short period in the form of GnRH is recommended—this will delay the appearance or recurrence of pain.

OSCE 2.
1. Write in brief the staging scores of endometriosis. What are the organs used for staging?

Ans.
1. Organs used are peritoneum, ovary, fallopian tube, posterior Cul-de sac obliteration and adhesions.
   Stage I (Minimal): 1–5
   Stage II (Mild): 6–15
   Stage III (Moderate): 16–40
   Stage IV (Severe): >40

OSCE 3.
1. Mention the management plan in order of progress in a case of pelvic endometriosis with subfertility of 5 years duration.

Ans.
1. a. Thorough history, general physical examination, and a detailed pelvic examination to diagnose uterine size, mobility, and retroversion of the uterus.

b. Husband's semen analysis as per WHO 2010 parameters
   c. Pelvic ultrasound to define the adnexa, ovarian endometrioma, and tubal assessment by SIS.
   d. If the endometrioma is/are >5 cm, laparoscopic cyst excision/aspiration. If cysts are <5 cm, then COH followed by IUI if tubes are freely patent. Else, ovum pick-up, cryopreservation followed by IVF and ET.

OSCE 4.

Label the structures (1–6) identifiable in the picture below:

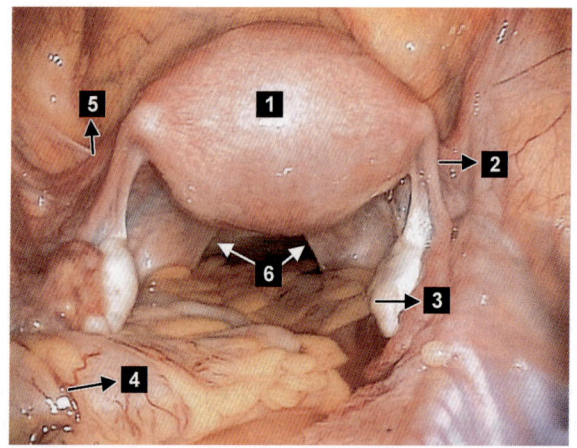

Courtesy: Atlas of Endometriosis, Caroline Overton & Colin Davis.

Ans.

1. Uterus
2. Fallopian tubes
3. Both ovaries
4. Intestine covered with omentum
5. Round ligaments
6. Uterosacral ligaments

OSCE 5.

Enumerate top five conditions associated with chronic pelvic pain in females.

Ans.

a. Endometriosis
b. Leiomyoma
c. Adenomyosis
d. Pelvic inflammatory disease
e. Ovarian remnant syndrome

Level A evidence of a causal relationship to CPP.

OSCE 6.

Match the left side with the right side:

Left side	Right side
Cyclical pain with menses	Endometriosis, adenomyosis
Acyclical pain with no relation with menstrual cycle	Malignancy
Burning pain	IBS, interstitial cystitis
Cramp-like pain	UTI, nerve entrapment pain
Pain onset after menopause	Spasmodic dysmenorrhea, IBD, ureteric stone

Ans.

Left side	Right side
Cyclical pain with menses	Endometriosis, adenomyosis
Acyclical pain with no relation with menstrual cycle	Spasmodic dysmenorrhea, IBD, ureteric stone
Burning pain	UTI, nerve entrapment pain
Cramp-like pain	IBS, interstitial cystitis
Pain onset after menopause	Malignancy

OSCE 7.

Match the following:

Blue domed cyst	Endometriosis of ovary
Powder burn or black lesion	Endometriosis of uterosacral ligament
Chocolate cyst	Endometriosis of post-fornix
Sampson's theory	Lymphatic or vascular spread of endometriotic tissues
Halban's theory	Retrograde menstruation

Ans.

Blue domed cyst	Endometriosis of post-fornix
Powder burn or black lesion	Endometriosis of uterosacral ligament
Chocolate cyst	Endometriosis of ovary
Sampson's theory	Retrograde menstruation
Halban's theory	Lymphatic or vascular spread of Endometriotic tissues

OSCE 8.

1. A 35-year-old, multiparous lady complains of extremely painful menses with heaviness in the lower abdomen. Examination reveals bulky tender uterus with restricted mobility. Write the differential diagnosis.

Ans.

1. a. Adenomyosis
   b. Leiomyoma
   c. Pelvic endometriosis
   d. Endometrial CA
   e. PID

OSCE 9.
1. Write the difference between ovarian remnant syndrome and residual ovary syndrome.
2. What is standard management?

Ans.

1. a. Ovarian remnant syndrome is the part of the apparently healthy ovary retained after an ovarian cystectomy by laparoscopy or laparotomy.
   b. Residual ovary syndrome (also known as ovarian retention syndrome) is the symptom complex arising out of an ovary intentionally left behind during previous gynecological surgery.
2. a. In both cases, standard evaluation is by thorough history taking, detailed operative notes of previous surgery, careful pelvic examination followed by imaging studies by USG and/or CT/MRI.
   b. Surgical excision is often needed.

OSCE 10. An educated 32-year-old refused to take 6 months of GnRH treatment after surgery for severe endometriosis, saying she had read that it can cause weakness of bones.
1. Is it true?
2. How much is the bone loss?
3. What advice can be given to prevent bone loss?
4. Which additional drugs are needed?

Ans.

1. Yes, it is true.
2. Six months of GnRH will cause, 8.2% decline in density of lumbar spine.
3. We can prevent this by Add-back therapy: E plus P (estrogen + progesterone) and shorter duration of treatment with GnRH.
4. Bisphosphonates and calcium

OSCE 11. A 30-year-old, Para 1 with secondary infertility of 5 years along with severe dysmenorrhea and sonographic evidence of a right endometriotic cyst of 10 cm.
1. What are the treatment options?

Ans.

1. *Surgery:*
   - Laparotomy or Laparoscopy (preferred)
   - Salpingo-ovariolysis, cystectomy, fulguration

- Unilateral salphingo-oophrectomy
- Drainage of cyst followed by GnRH analog

OSCE 12.

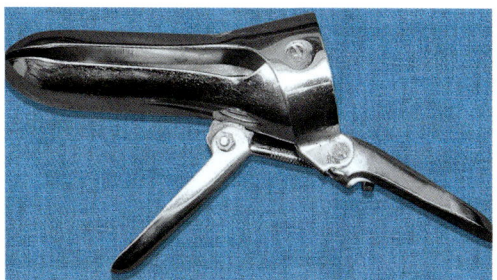

1. Identify the instrument.
2. Write about two advantages and two disadvantages of this instrument.
3. Name two procedures that can be done with this instrument.

Ans.

1. Cusco's bivalve self-retaining vaginal speculum
2. *Advantages:*
   - Self-retaining does not need assistance.
   - Visualizes two walls of the vagina simultaneously together.

   Disadvantages:
   - Skewed view
   - Lack of liberal access for operative procedures
3. *Two procedures:*
   a. LNG-IUS insertion in OPD
   b. Taking vaginal cytology

OSCE 13.

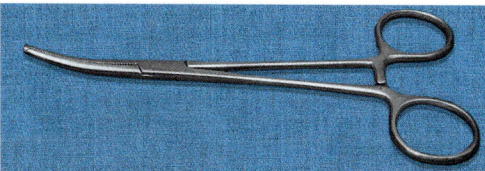

1. Identify and describe the instrument.
2. Enumerate two uses of the instrument in gynecology.

Ans.

1. Kocher's hemostatic clamp. Business end has transverse serrations on it with rat teeth at its tip.
2. *Uses:*
   - To clamp pedicle during hysterectomy (abdominal/vaginal)
   - To clamp pedicle of pedunculated fibroid in myomectomy

- To clamp pedicle of ovarian tumor/cyst
- To steady the uterus and giving traction during abdominal hysterectomy

OSCE 14.

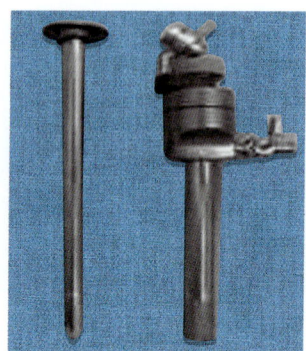

1. Identify the instrument.
2. Where is the primary trocar placed?
3. Where and how are the secondary trocars placed?
4. Enumerate the structures pierced by the trocar starting from skin inwards.
5. Enumerate two dangers of using this instrument.

Ans.

1. 11-mm primary trocar and canula (metallic). Used for 10 mm scopes.
2. Primary trocar is usually placed umbilical or just infraumbilical and it holds the telescope.
3. Secondary ports are placed at both sides of the camera port at suitable places under vision of the camera for insertion of hand instruments.
4. Skin, subcutaneous tissue, rectus sheath, fascia transversalis, and parietal peritoneum
5. *Dangers:*
   a. Injury of the transverse colon and small gut
   b. Vascular injury like abdominal aorta
   c. Other visceral injuries.

OSCE 15.

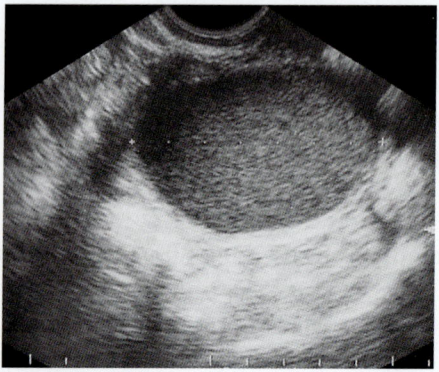

Courtesy: Atlas of Endometriosis, Caroline Overton & Colin Davis.

1. What is the imaging diagnosis?
2. What are the additional investigations to be done?
3. What is the management plan in an unmarried girl with severe dysmenorrhea and this USG finding?

Ans.

1. Transvaginal ultrasound scan showing the typical ground-glass appearance of an endometrioma.
2. Serum CA125, CBC
3. Analgesic and antispasmodic followed by laparoscopic conservative surgery.

OSCE 16.

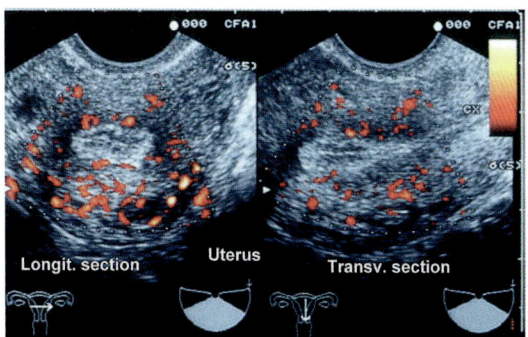

Courtesy: Atlas of Endometriosis, Caroline Overton & Colin Davis.

1. What is the color Doppler picture diagnosis?

Ans.

1. Increased myometrial vascularity is clearly demonstrated in the color Doppler examination. This feature is often associated with pelvic endometriosis and remains very suggestive of adenomyosis.

OSCE 17.

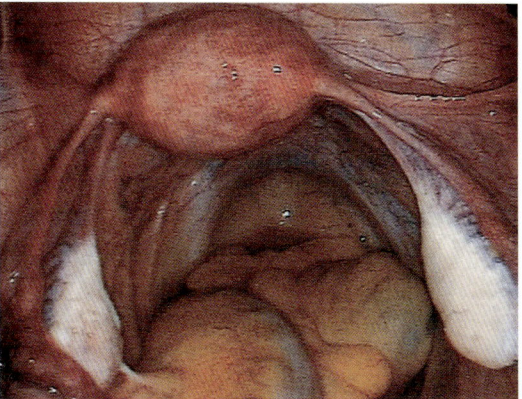

Courtesy: Atlas of Endometriosis, Caroline Overton & Colin Davis.

1. **Identify the pathology.**
2. **Grade the endometriosis.**
3. **Enumerate the principles of management in a 33-year-old, parous woman with this lesion presenting with acute stabbing, cyclical, lower abdominal pain.**

Ans.

1. Laparoscopic view of endometriosis of pelvis
2. Grade I
3. Trial of medical management followed by laparoscopic adhesiolysis, and presacral neurectomy or laparoscopic uterosacral nerve ablation (LUNA).

OSCE 18.

1. Enumerate five differences between spasmodic and congestive dysmenorrhea.

Ans.

Features	Spasmodic or primary	Congestive or secondary
Type of pain	Spasmodic	Colicky discomfort
Age of onset	Adolescents and young adults	Older reproductive years
Relationship with menses	Starts acutely just before menses and stays 1–2 days of menses	Starts with menses; discomfort stays throughout the cycle
Physical examination	Almost normal	Organic pelvic pathology like adnexal mass, enlarged uterus with restricted mobility, tenderness
Investigations	Normal	Ultrasound and laparoscopy detects pathology

OSCE 19.

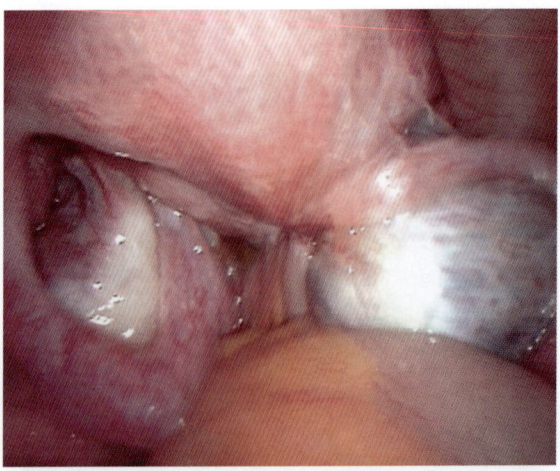

Courtesy: Atlas of Endometriosis, Caroline Overton & Colin Davis.

1. Describe the pathology.
2. Which surgery is recommended?
3. Which energy source is preferred?

Ans.

1. Bilateral ovarian endometrioma with gross pelvic adhesions and obliteration of POD.
2. Adhesiolysis and bilateral ovarian cystectomy
3. Harmonic scalpel and bipolar energy sources

OSCE 20.

1. **IVF and ET (embryo transfer) are recommended treatments for which cases of endometriosis with infertility?**

Ans.

1. IVF and ET is recommended in the following cases of endometriosis with infertility:
   - Women with substantially damaged or blocked tubes
   - Women with moderate or severe endometriosis
   - Women with minimal or mild endometriosis but with a partner who has oligoasthenozoospermia.
   - Women who have failed to conceive by IUI.

CHAPTER 32

Endometriosis (II)

Juhi Bharti, Vandana Agarwal

OSCE 1. A 30-year-old, nulliparous lady presents you with infertility. You advised her ultrasound which suggests left ovarian cyst.

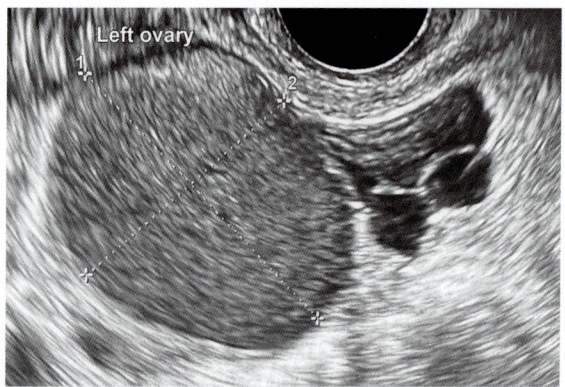

1. Identify the nature of cyst.
2. Enumerate three typical clinical features at presentation.

Ans.

1. Endometrioma
2. Dysmenorrhea, deep dyspareunia, dysuria, dyschezia and/or infertility

Reference

1. Becker CM, Bokor A, Heikinheimo O, et al. ESHRE guideline: endometriosis. Hum Reprod Open. 2022;2022(2):hoac009. Published 2022 Feb 26. doi:10.1093/hropen/hoac009.

OSCE 2.

1. Enumerate two theories about the etiology of endometriosis.
2. What is the most common site of endometriosis?
3. Enumerate two other sites of endometriosis.

Ans.

1. a. Sampson's retrograde implantation theory
   b. Coelomic metaplasia theory
   c. Metastatic theory—vascular and lymphatic metastases

d. Hormonal influence—mainly estrogen
e. Immunological factors—impaired T-cell and NK (natural killer) cells
2. Ovary
3. a. Cul de sac
   b. Uterosacral ligaments
   c. Broad ligament
   d. Fallopian tube
   e. Bowel
   f. Urinary bladder, etc.

OSCE 3.
1. What are the typical findings which can be seen during the clinical examination of a patient with endometriosis?
2. What is the first imaging tool of choice for diagnosis of endometriosis?

Ans.

1. Tenderness on vaginal examination, palpable nodules in the posterior fornix, adnexal mass, restricted mobility of the uterus are suggestive of endometriosis.
2. Pelvic ultrasound

OSCE 4.
1. What is the classic ultrasound finding of an endometriotic cyst?
2. Enumerate four differential diagnoses in a patient with chronic pelvic pain.

Ans.

1. Endometriomas appear as homogeneous formations with a classic ground-glass appearance and low-level internal echoes.
2. a. Endometriosis
   b. Pelvic inflammatory disease
   c. Adenomyosis
   d. Leiomyoma
   e. Irritable bowel syndrome

OSCE 5.
1. Name three standard classification systems of endometriosis.
2. Which classification predicts pregnancy outcome?

Ans.

1. Revised ASRM (rASRM), ENZIAN Classification, Endometriosis Fertility Index (EFI)
2. Endometriosis fertility index (EFI)

Reference
1. Johnson NP, Hummelshoj L, Adamson GD, et al. World Endometriosis Society consensus on the classification of endometriosis. Hum Reprod. 2017;32(2):315-24. doi:10.1093/humrep/dew293.

OSCE 6.
1. Is there any specific tumor marker for the diagnosis of endometriosis?
2. Enumerate two benign conditions where CA125 may be raised.
3. Enumerate two malignant conditions where CA125 may be raised.

Ans.
1. No
2. Endometriosis, acute peritonitis, acute PID
3. Epithelial ovarian carcinoma, endometrial carcinoma, breast cancer

OSCE 7.
A 33-year-old, nulliparous lady presented to you with heavy menstrual bleeding, severe dysmenorrhea, and severe dyspareunia. Following is her intraoperative picture.

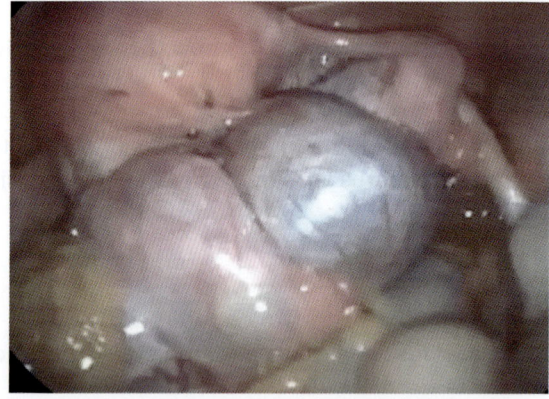

1. What is the grade of endometriosis as per revised ASRM classification?
2. What will be the best surgical treatment option for her pain?

Ans.
1. Grade IV
2. Endometriotic cystectomy

OSCE 8.
A 35-year-old lady presented with severe, noncyclical dysmenorrhea and dyspareunia. She was diagnosed of deep infiltrating endometriosis and is not desirous of future fertility. Her pain did not respond to NSAIDs, and she does not want to take oral medications further for pain.
1. What are the first line options of nonoral medical management?

Ans.
1. Levonorgestrel-releasing intrauterine system (LNG-IUS) or etonorgestrel-releasing subdermal implant.

Reference
1. Becker CM, Bokor A, Heikinheimo O, et al. ESHRE guideline: endometriosis. Hum Reprod Open. 2022;2022(2):hoac009. Published 2022 Feb 26. doi:10.1093/hropen/hoac009.

Chapter 32: Endometriosis (II)

OSCE 9. An adolescent girl of age 17 years presented with history of severe cyclical dysmenorrhea with dyschezia leading to impaired quality of life. Her pain is not responding to NSAIDs. MRI suggests 3 cm endometrioma with deep infiltrating endometriosis.
1. What are the options of medical management?
2. What will be the next step if medical management fails?

Ans.

1. *Hormonal treatment:* Combined hormonal contraceptives/Progestogens (Dienogest/LNG IUS)
2. Laparoscopy and excision of endometriotic lesions

Reference
1. Becker CM, Bokor A, Heikinheimo O, et al. ESHRE guideline: endometriosis. Hum Reprod Open. 2022;2022(2):hoac009. Published 2022 Feb 26. doi:10.1093/hropen/hoac009.

OSCE 10. A 36-year-old lady was prescribed GnRH agonist injections while awaiting surgery for endometrioma. She could not come for surgery due to personal reasons and decided to continue monthly injections for 6 months on her own.
1. What is the side effect profile after long-term use?
2. What can be given in order to avoid side effects?
3. Name one oral GnRH antagonist.

Ans.

1. Bone loss and hypoestrogenic symptoms (Hot flashes/vaginal dryness)
2. *Add back therapy:* Progestin monotherapy/Combined hormonal contraceptives/Selective Estrogen Receptor Modulators (SERMs)/ Bisphosphonates/Tibolone
3. Oral Elagolix.

Reference
1. Sauerbrun-Cutler MT, Alvero R. Short- and long-term impact of gonadotropin-releasing hormone analogue treatment on bone loss and fracture. Fertil Steril 2019;112:799-803.

OSCE 11.
1. What is the gold standard in the diagnosis of endometriosis?
2. What is the role of laparoscopy in endometriosis?

Ans.

1. Laparoscopy
2. a. To detect and diagnosis pelvic endometriosis
   b. Locate the site of endometriosis and staging
   c. To take biopsy
   d. To surgically treat endometriosis by ablation, excision.

OSCE 12.
1. What does DIE stand for?
2. Name the sites of DIE.

Ans.
1. DIE = Deep infiltrating endometriosis
2. *Anterior compartment:* Vesicovaginal septum, bladder
   Posterior compartment: Rectovaginal septum, bowel

OSCE 13.
A 32-year, P2L2 was planned for laparoscopy for endometriosis associated pain.
1. Which is the ideal method of dealing with endometriotic lesions with least recurrence?
2. What should be prescribed in postoperative period for secondary prevention of recurrence of pain? Mention the drug and duration.

Ans.
1. Laparoscopic excision of endometriosis.
2. LNG-IUS or combined hormonal contraceptives for minimum 18–24 months.

OSCE 14.
1. What does LUNA stand for?
2. Name two conditions where it may be performed?

Ans.
1. Laparoscopic uterosacral nerve ablation
2. Unexplained chronic pelvic pain, endometriosis

OSCE 15.
A 40-year-old lady with endometriosis has failed to respond to conservative medical methods and is not desirous of future fertility.
1. What will be the next line of management?

Ans.
1. Hysterectomy and removal of endometriotic lesions with or without ovariotomy.

Reference
1. Becker CM, Bokor A, Heikinheimo O, et al. ESHRE guideline: endometriosis. Hum Reprod Open. 2022;2022(2):hoac009. Published 2022 Feb 26. doi:10.1093/hropen/hoac009.

OSCE 16.
A 25-year-old, nulliparous woman underwent endometriotic cystectomy for severe pain, she is trying to conceive for past 4 years. She has been advised for ART for pregnancy.
1. What is the role of postsurgical hormone treatment for ovarian suppression before ART?
2. What are the indications for surgery for endometrioma prior to ART?

Ans.

1. Should not be provided to improve pregnancy rates.
2. To improve pain or accessibility of follicles

OSCE 17. A 26-year-old lady with 5 cm endometrioma conceived after ART. She was presented at 16 weeks with acute pelvic pain.
1. What could be the possible causes related to endometrioma?
2. What is SHiP?
3. What is the usual clinical presentation of SHiP?

Ans.

1. Infected, enlarged, or ruptured endometrioma
2. Spontaneous hemoperitoneum in pregnancy
3. Acute abdominal pain, hypovolemic shock, signs of fetal distress

References

1. Maggiore ULR, Ferrero S, Mangili G, Bergamini A, Inversetti A, Giorgione V, Vigano P, Candiani M. A systematic review on endometriosis during pregnancy: diagnosis, misdiagnosis, complications, and outcomes. Hum Reprod Update. 2016;22:70-103.
2. Becker CM, Bokor A, Heikinheimo O, et al. ESHRE guideline: endometriosis. Hum Reprod Open. 2022;2022(2):hoac009. Published 2022 Feb 26. doi:10.1093/hropen/hoac009.

OSCE 18. A 49-year-old, postmenopausal lady comes to you with chronic pelvic pain and ultrasound suggestive of endometrioma.
1. What will be the first line management for her?
2. Which is the preferred drug therapy in postmenopausal women, if indicated?

Ans.

1. Surgery is the first-line management in postmenopausal women for endometriosis.
2. Aromatase inhibitor, if surgery is not feasible.

OSCE 19.
1. To which group of drugs does Dienogest belong to?
2. Name two aromatase inhibitors used in endometriosis.

Ans.

1. Dienogest is a SPRM (selective progesterone receptor modulator)
2. Letrozole, Anastrozole

OSCE 20. A 35-year-old lady underwent hysterectomy and ovariotomy for severe endometriosis. She has developed hot flashes in the postoperative period.
1. What is the preferred regimen of menopausal hormone therapy (MHT)?

Ans.

1. Continuous estrogen-progestogen

CHAPTER 33

Ectopic Pregnancy

Sandhya Jain, Pooja Sharma

OSCE 1. A 25-year-old lady presents to the emergency department with complaints of vague pain in the right iliac fossa and vaginal bleeding. She has a history of 6 weeks of amenorrhea. Her urine pregnancy test was positive.
1. What are your differential diagnoses?
2. How will you confirm your diagnosis?
3. Which points in examination suggest a diagnosis of ectopic pregnancy?

Ans.
1. a. Ectopic pregnancy
   b. Missed abortion
   c. Incomplete/threatened abortion
2. Transvaginal ultrasonography
3. a. Hemodynamically unstable
   b. Pelvic/adnexal tenderness
   c. Cervical motion tenderness
   d. Abdominal distension

OSCE 2. A transvaginal USG was performed for the above-mentioned patient to confirm the diagnosis.
1. What is the sensitivity and specificity of USG to diagnose an ectopic pregnancy?
2. Which signs in USG indicate towards an ectopic pregnancy?
3. What is the condition called if a gestational sac is found both in the uterus and fallopian tube on ultrasound?

Ans.
1. *Sensitivity:* 81%, *specificity:* 79.5%
2. a. An adnexal mass moving separate to the ovary comprising a gestational sac containing yolk sac or fetal pole.
   b. An empty uterus
   c. Free fluid in peritoneal cavity
3. Heterotopic pregnancy

OSCE 3.

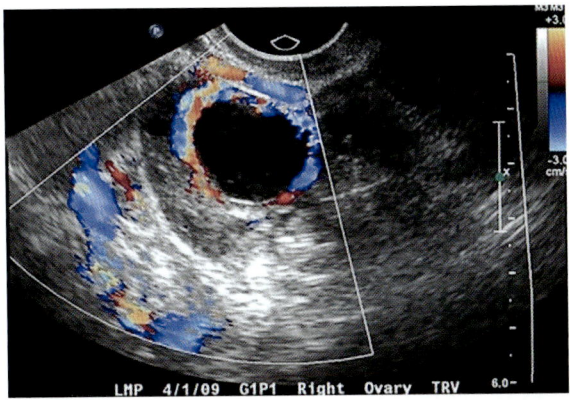

1. Identify the radiological sign depicted above.
2. What are your differential diagnoses based on the above image?
3. What are the risk factors of ectopic pregnancy?

Ans.

1. Ring of fire sign seen on color Doppler because of hypervascular lesion.
2. *Differential diagnosis:*
   - Ectopic pregnancy
   - Corpus luteal cyst
3. Risk factors of ectopic pregnancy are:
   - Previous ectopic pregnancy
   - Prior fallopian tube surgery
   - Pelvic inflammatory disease (PID)
   - Endometriosis

OSCE 4.
A 29-year-old lady presents with a 1-week history of left lower abdominal pain and vaginal spotting. She is sexually active, and her last menstrual period was 7 weeks ago. The patient's vital signs are normal. On physical examination, she appears uncomfortable and there is left adnexal tenderness, closed cervix, and scant blood in the vaginal vault. The patient had a positive urine pregnancy test and a serum β-hCG resulted at 1472 mIU/mL (negative is <5 mIU/mL). The patient's transvaginal ultrasound (TVUS) is shown here:

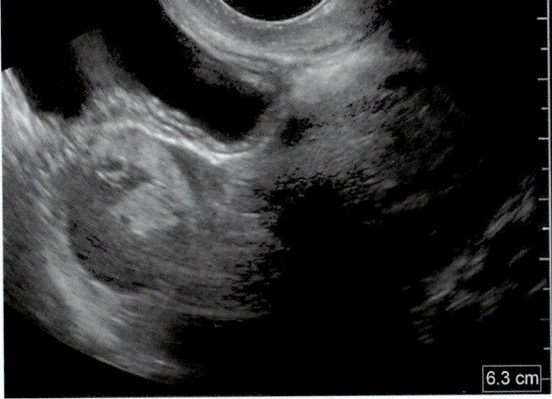

1. How will you describe the USG findings?

2. What is the discriminatory level of β-hCG to diagnose an intrauterine pregnancy?
3. How will you follow-up this case with β-hCG levels?

Ans.
1. Transvaginal ultrasound of the uterus demonstrates an extrauterine gestational sac and yolk sac with a fetal pole in the left fallopian tube. No fetal cardiac activity noted.
2. 1,500 mIU/mL.
3. β-hCG levels are obtained 2 days after initial evaluation. In a normal pregnancy, β-hCG is expected to at least double in 2 days. In an early abortion, β-hCG decreases during repeat testing, while in an ectopic pregnancy, β-hCG does not rise appropriately.

OSCE 5. For the above-mentioned case:
1. How will you manage the patient?
2. How will you decide the mode of management for a patient with ectopic pregnancy?
3. What are the criteria for medical management of ectopic pregnancy?

Ans.
1. Since the patient in the above-mentioned case is hemodynamically stable with β-hCG levels below 1500 mIU/mL, medical management with Inj. Methotrexate 50 mg/m² body surface area should be offered.
2. Management of an ectopic pregnancy is based on patient stability, characteristics of the ectopic mass, desire for future fertility, and understanding of risks and benefits of each therapeutic option. Possibilities include expectant management, medical management, and surgical management, with either a salpingectomy or salpingostomy.
3. Medical management should be offered to patients who:
   - Have no significant pain.
   - Have an unruptured tubal ectopic pregnancy with an adnexal mass smaller than 35 mm with no visible heartbeat.
   - Have a serum hCG level less than 1500 IU/liter.
   - Do not have an intrauterine pregnancy (as confirmed on an ultrasound scan)
   - Are able to return for follow-up. (NICE 2022)

OSCE 6. A patient with an unruptured ectopic pregnancy with stable vitals was administered Inj. Methotrexate as medical management. Next day, she developed a rash on her arms and neck as shown here:
1. What could be the possible cause?
2. What are the side effects of methotrexate?
3. What are the contraindications of methotrexate?

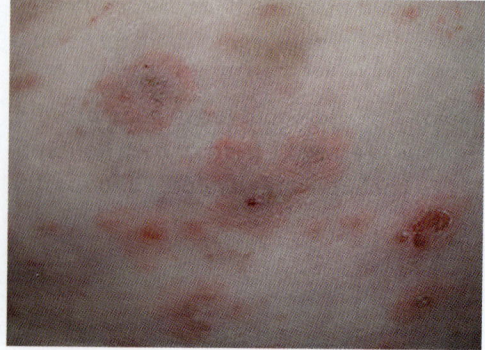

Ans.
1. Methotrexate-induced photosensitivity skin rash
2. Side effects of methotrexate are:
   - Nausea and vomiting
   - Diarrhea, and abdominal discomfort
   - Photosensitivity skin reaction
   - Impaired liver function test
   - Neutropenia
3. Contraindications of methotrexate are:
   - Hemodynamically unstable patient
   - Ruptured ectopic.
   - Immunodeficiency
   - Chronic liver disease
   - Breastfeeding women

OSCE 7. A patient with unruptured ectopic pregnancy was managed medically with systemic methotrexate.
1. How will you follow-up this patient?
2. What are the different dosage protocols of methotrexate?
3. What is surgically administered medical management (SAM)?

Ans.
1. Repeat serum β-hCG levels are done on day 4 and 7. Typically, the levels rise up to day 4, and then start to fall. By day 7, β-hCG level should be at least 15% lower than pretreatment levels. Weekly β-hCG levels are done till it reaches <25 IU/L.
2. a. *Single-dose protocol:* Calculated as 50 mg/m² body surface area, given IM
   b. *Multi-dose protocol:* IM methotrexate in a dose of 1 mg/kg on day 1, 3, 5, 7 along with 0.1 mg/kg folinic acid on day 2, 4, 6, 8.
3. Under USG guidance, direct injection of a drug is given into the ectopic. Methotrexate, KCl (potassium chloride), hyperosmolar glucose can be used.

OSCE 8.

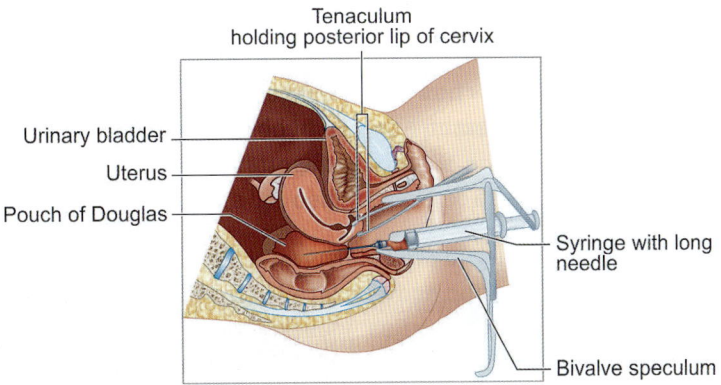

1. Name the procedure depicted in the above image.
2. How do you perform the above procedure?
3. What is the sensitivity and specificity of the above procedure in diagnosing ruptured ectopic pregnancy?

Ans.

1. Culdocentesis, done to identify hemoperitoneum.
2. Posterior lip of the cervix is pulled towards the symphysis with a tenaculum or vulsellum and along needle (16–18 gauge) is inserted through the posterior fornix into the cul-de-sac. The presence of blood indicates hemoperitoneum.
3. *Sensitivity:* 66%
   Specificity: 80%

OSCE 9. A 30-year, G3P2L2 presented to the emergency department complaining of acute onset of lower abdominal pain and vaginal bleeding associated with a history of amenorrhea for three months. Upon clinical examination, the patient looked pale and distressed. Her blood pressure was 90/42 mm Hg, with a pulse rate of 110 beats per minute. Her abdomen was generally distended and tender on both superficial and deep palpation. The digital vaginal examination was positive for cervical motion tenderness. TVS-USG was performed and a diagnosis of left tubal ruptured ectopic pregnancy was made.
1. How will you manage the above patient?
2. What surgical procedure will be performed for the patient?
3. What are the definite indications for laparotomy?

Ans.

1. As the patient is hemodynamically unstable, emergency laparotomy after taking informed, written consent, and arranging adequate blood products should be done.
2. Emergency laparotomy with left salpingectomy
3. Definite indications for laparotomy are:
   - Hemodynamically unstable patient
   - Cornual ectopic
   - Dense abdominal and pelvic adhesions making laparoscopy difficult

OSCE 10.

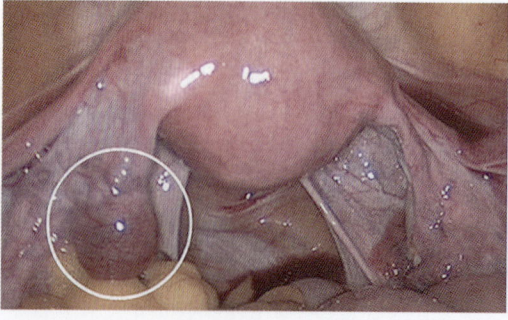
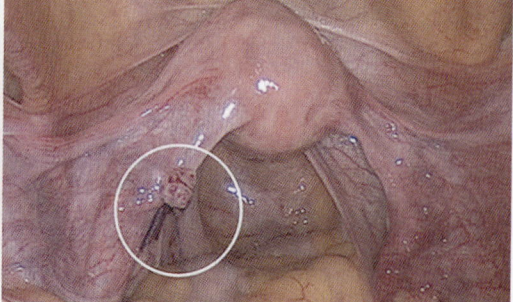

1. Identify the above images.
2. What are the criteria to offer surgical treatment for ectopic pregnancy?
3. Name the conservative surgeries for ectopic pregnancy.

Ans.

1. a. left unruptured tubal ectopic pregnancy
   b. Tubal ectopic pregnancy removed laparoscopically by salpingectomy
2. Criteria for offering surgery as a first-line treatment are:
   - An ectopic pregnancy and significant pain
   - An ectopic pregnancy with an adnexal mass of 35 mm or larger
   - An ectopic pregnancy with a fetal heartbeat visible on an ultrasound scan
   - An ectopic pregnancy and a serum hCG level of 5,000 IU/liter or more. (NICE 2022)
3. Conservative surgeries are:
   - Salpingotomy
   - Salpingostomy

OSCE 11.

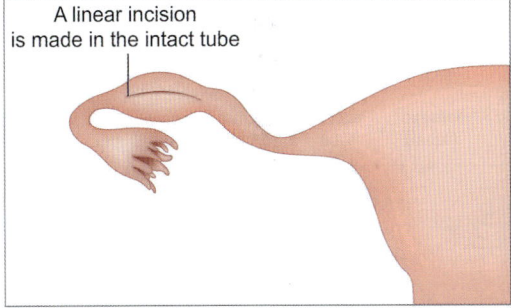

A linear incision is made in the intact tube

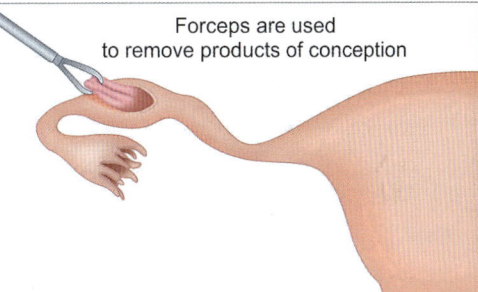

Forceps are used to remove products of conception

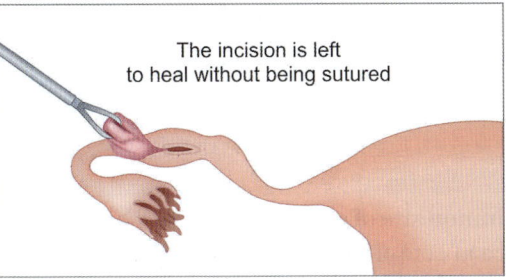

The incision is left to heal without being sutured

1. Identify the above procedure.
2. What is the difference between salpingotomy and salpingostomy?
3. When do you consider conservative surgeries in a case of ectopic pregnancy?

Ans.

1. Salpingostomy
2. In salpingotomy, the incision on the fallopian tube is closed with a fine suture whereas in salpingostomy, it is left unstitched.

3. Conservative surgeries are considered for women with risk factors for infertility such as contralateral tube damage.

OSCE 12. A patient who underwent salpingostomy comes to OPD after two weeks with a β-hCG report of 5430 IU/L. Her pretreatment β-hCG level was 3500 IU/L.
1. What is your probable diagnosis?
2. What factors could be associated with the above condition?
3. How will you manage the patient?

Ans.
1. Probable diagnosis is persistent ectopic pregnancy (PEP). It occurs due to incomplete removal of trophoblasts during salpingostomy.
2. Factors increasing the risk of PEP are:
   - Small pregnancies (<2 cm)
   - Early therapy (before 6 weeks gestation)
   - Implantation medial to the salpingostomy site
3. Additional surgical (salpingectomy) or medical therapy (single-dose methotrexate) is offered to the patients with PEP.

OSCE 13.

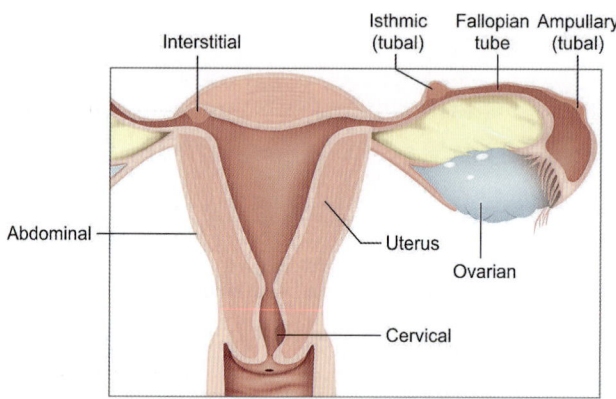

1. What is the most common site of ectopic pregnancy out of the above?
2. What is the incidence of ectopic pregnancy in India?
3. What are the reasons behind increasing rates of ectopic pregnancy?

Ans.
1. Ampulla (80%)
2. 1 in 150 normal pregnancies
3. a. Increase in prevalence of sexually transmitted diseases
   b. Assisted reproductive techniques
   c. Tubal surgeries include salpingostomy for tubal pregnancy and tuboplasty for infertility.

Chapter 33: Ectopic Pregnancy

OSCE 14. A 30-year, G3P0L0A2, a known case of chronic liver disease is diagnosed with left unruptured ectopic pregnancy as per USG report. Her β-hCG report is 1486 IU/L. She is not eligible for medical management and refuses to undergo surgery for the same.
1. How will you manage the patient?
2. What are the criteria for expectant management of ectopic pregnancy?
3. How will you follow this patient?

Ans.
1. Expectant management
2. Expectant management should be offered to the patients who:
    - Are clinically stable and pain free
    - Have a tubal ectopic pregnancy measuring less than 35 mm with no visible heartbeat on transvaginal ultrasound scan
    - Have serum hCG levels below 1,500 IU/L
    - Are able to return for follow-up. (NICE 2022)
3. Repeat hCG levels are done on days 2, 4 and 7 after the original test and:
    - If hCG levels drop by 15% or more from the previous value on days 2, 4 and 7, then repeat weekly until a negative result (less than 20 IU/L) is obtained, or
    - If hCG levels do not fall by 15%, stay the same or rise from the previous value, review the woman's clinical condition to help decide further management. (NICE 2022)

OSCE 15. A 26-year-old lady presents to the emergency department with painless vaginal bleeding. Her last menstrual period was 6 weeks ago. Her vitals are stable. On vaginal examination, the external os is partially open, cervix is soft and enlarged equal to the size of the fundus. β-hCG report is 1678 IU/L. Her transvaginal USG is as depicted here:

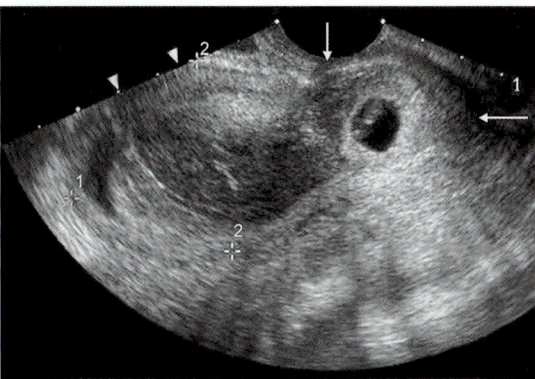

1. What is your diagnosis?
2. What are the USG criteria to diagnose the above condition?
3. What are the management options for the patient?

Ans.
1. Cervical ectopic pregnancy

2. USG criteria to diagnose cervical pregnancy are:
   - Empty uterus
   - Hour-glass shape of the uterus
   - Ballooned out cervical canal
   - Gestational sac and placental tissue in the cervical canal
3. Management options are:
   - Medical treatment with methotrexate
   - Cervical cerclage
   - Curettage and tamponade
   - Uterine artery embolization
   - Hysterectomy in case of profuse bleeding

OSCE 16. A 25-year-old lady presented to the Emergency Department of Gynecology with chief complaints of two-month amenorrhea with bleeding per vaginum on and off for 10–12 days. She was G3P2L2 with previous two cesarean deliveries. The general physical examination was normal. On per speculum, cervix was normal, no discharge or bleeding per vaginum was seen. On bimanual examination, cervix pointed upward, uterus was bulky, retroverted and bilateral fornices were free with no tenderness. Her β-hCG level was 7118 IU/L. Transvaginal ultrasound is as shown here:

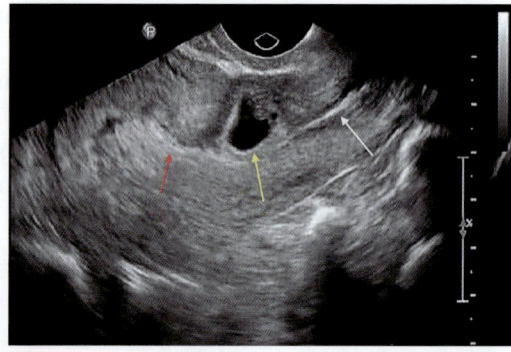

1. What is your diagnosis?
2. Identify the red, yellow, and white arrows.
3. What are the diagnostic criteria on USG for the above condition?

Ans.

1. Cesarean scar ectopic pregnancy
2. *Red arrow:* Uterine cavity
   Yellow arrow: Gestational sac
   White arrow: Cervical canal
3. Diagnostic criteria of cesarean scar pregnancy on USG:
   - Empty uterine and endocervical canal
   - Placenta, gestational sac or both embedded in the hysterotomy scar
   - A thin (<5 mm) or absent myometrial layer between gestational sac and bladder
   - Increased vascularity in the area of cesarean scar

OSCE 17.

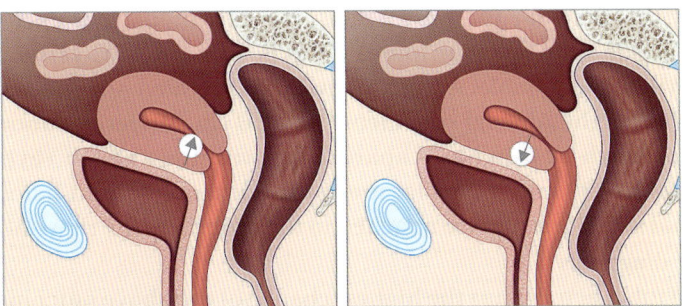

1. Based on the above images, what is the current classification of cesarean scar pregnancy?
2. What are the management options for a patient with cesarean scar pregnancy?
3. How will you follow-up the patient?

Ans.

1. Classification of cesarean scar pregnancy:

On the scar	In the niche
• >2 mm myometrial thickness between placenta or gestational sac and bladder • Progresses towards uterine cavity	• <2 mm myometrial thickness between placenta or gestational sac and bladder • Progresses towards bladder

2. Management options:
   - *Medical:* 25–50 mg Methotrexate (systemic or intragestational)
   - *Surgical:*
     - *Laparotomy:* In patients who are hemodynamically unstable.
     - *Hysteroscopic resection:* Recommended approach for "on the scar" cesarean scar pregnancy that are readily accessible via uterine cavity.
     - *Laparoscopic* excision of cesarean scar pregnancy
     - *Transvaginal* excision of cesarean scar pregnancy
3. *Follow-up:* Weekly β-hCG levels for 3 weeks followed by biweekly till levels <5 IU/L.

OSCE 18.
A 25-year, nulliparous lady was treated with systemic methotrexate for left tubal ectopic pregnancy. She wants to conceive again.
1. What advice will you give her?
2. Which method of contraception would you advise?
3. What are her risks of having an ectopic pregnancy in future?

Ans.

1. She should avoid conception for at least 3 months because of teratogenic effects of methotrexate on the fetus.
2. Depending on the patient's medical history and preference, she can be prescribed any method of contraception immediately after treatment.
3. After one ectopic pregnancy, there is a 10% risk of having a second ectopic pregnancy.

Section 2: Gynecology

OSCE 19. A 25-year-old lady presented to the emergency department with complaints of lower abdominal pain for the past 2 days. Her last menstrual period was 7 weeks ago. Her urine pregnancy test was found to be positive. β-hCG value was 2500 IU/L. She was hemodynamically stable. A transvaginal USG revealed no intrauterine pregnancy with a thick-walled, right adnexal ring measuring 2.6 cm. Moderate amount of free fluid was seen in the pouch of Douglas. Laparoscopy was done which revealed extensive hemoperitoneum of 800 mL, a normal uterus and intact bilateral fallopian tubes and a 2 cm gestational sac-like structure attached to the fimbria of the right fallopian tube.
1. What is your diagnosis?
2. Which site of tubal ectopic has the highest chance of the above outcome?
3. How will you confirm your diagnosis?

Ans.

1. *Tubal abortion:* A rare case of an ectopic pregnancy characterized by the spontaneous expulsion of the products of conception through the fimbriae into the peritoneal cavity.
2. Ampulla
3. Histopathological confirmation of presence of embryonic tissue in the fluid collected during laparoscopy.

OSCE 20. A 24-year-old para 2+2 presented to the outpatient unit with a 4-day history of severe lower abdominal pain associated with mild bleeding per vaginum. On examination, her vitals were stable. There was localized tenderness in the right iliac fossa, there was no guarding or rebound tenderness. Pelvic examination showed a healthy-looking cervix minimally smeared with altered blood, there was no cervical motion tenderness. Her blood results revealed serum β-hCG of 520 IU/L. Transvaginal pelvic ultrasound showed a heterogeneous mass in the right adnexa measuring 61 × 32 × 29 mm, suggestive of a tubo-ovarian abscess/mass, and moderate amount of free fluid. Other tumor markers were done which were normal.
1. What is your probable diagnosis?
2. How will you confirm your diagnosis?
3. How will you manage the patient?

Ans.

1. Chronic ectopic pregnancy
2. Diagnosis can be confirmed by diagnostic laparoscopy or MRI pelvis.
3. The management of choice is laparoscopic right salpingectomy.

CHAPTER 34

Uterine Fibroid

Jai Bhagwan Sharma, Richa Vatsa

OSCE 1. A 26-year-old nulliparous lady presents to you with heavy menstrual bleeding and dysmenorrhea. Multiple medical management has been tried for her heavy menstrual bleeding, but nothing worked. You advised her USG scan and following is the film for review.

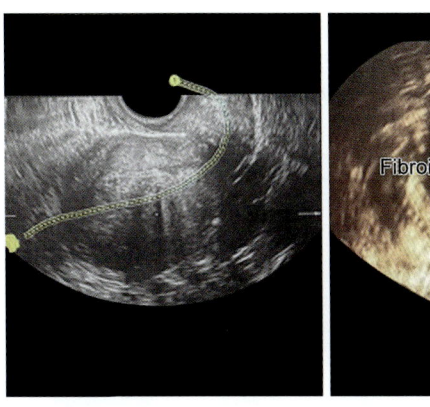
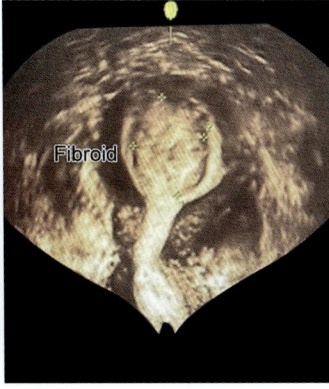

1. What is the type of fibroid?
2. What is the ideal treatment modality for her?
3. What are the problems patients can have due to this condition?

Ans.

1. FIGO grade 0
2. Hysteroscopic myomectomy
3. Infertility, heavy menstrual bleeding, intermenstrual bleeding, recurrent pregnancy loss, infertility.

Reference

1. AAGL Practice Report: Practice Guidelines for the Diagnosis and Management of Submucous Leiomyomas. Journal of Minimally Invasive Gynecology. 2012;19:152-71.

OSCE 2. Hysteroscopic myomectomy has been planned for FIGO grade 0 fibroid of 2 cm size in a 28-year-old healthy nulliparous lady. You planned to use resectoscope with monopolar cutting loop. Answer the following regarding the choice of surgery.

1. What is the distention media of choice?
2. What is the cut off for fluid deficit when the surgery should be stopped?

Ans.

1. Glycine
2. 1,000 mL

Reference

1. Umranikar S, Clark TJ, Saridogan E, et al; British Society for Gynaecological Endoscopy/European Society for Gynaecological Endoscopy Guideline Development Group for Management of Fluid Distension Media in Operative Hysteroscopy. BSGE/ESGE guideline on management of fluid distension media in operative hysteroscopy. Gynecol Surg. 2016;13(4):289-303.

OSCE 3. A 33-year-old, nulliparous lady presented with intermittent sudden onset pain abdomen with spontaneous resolution. She also had episodes of urinary retention, all of which needed catheterization. There were no menstrual complaints. Her USG was done which showed 14 cm solid mass, right ovary was normal and left ovary could not be visualized separately. Her tumor markers were normal. Her laparotomy was planned and following is her intraoperative picture.

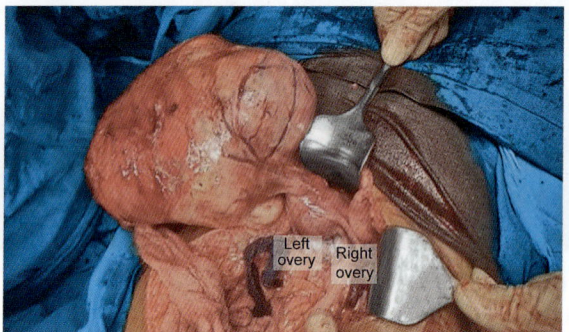

1. What is the diagnosis?
2. What will be the best surgical treatment option for her?

Ans.

1. Pedunculated subserosal fibroid
2. Myomectomy

OSCE 4. European Society of Gynecological Endoscopy has given classification of fibroids. Answer the following question about this classification system.
1. For which type of fibroids this classification system has been given?
2. Grade the fibroids according to this classification system.

Ans.

1. Submucosal fibroids

2. Types:
   - *Type 0:* Entirely within endometrial cavity
   - *Type I:* <50% myometrial invasion
   - *Type II:* >50% myometrial invasion

Reference
1. Wamsteker K, Emanuel MH, de Kruif JH. Transcervical hysteroscopic resection of submucous fibroids for abnormal uterine bleeding: results regarding the degree of intramural extension. Obstet Gynecol. 1993; 82:736-40.

OSCE 5. Lasmar system for presurgical classification of submucous myoma may be useful to consider in planning for hysteroscopic myomectomy. Answer following queries regarding this classification system.
1. Which location of fibroid along uterine wall is most difficult to resect?
2. What extension of myoma base to endometrial surface is most difficult to resect?

Ans.
1. Upper
2. >2/3

Reference
1. Lasmar RB, Barrozo PR, Dias R, Oliveira MA. Submucous myomas: a new presurgical classification to evaluate the viability of hysteroscopic surgical treatment–preliminary report. J Minim Invasive Gynecol. 2005;12:308-11 (II-2).

OSCE 6. A 22-year-old, nulliparous lady presented with heavy menstrual bleeding. Her examination revealed 20-week size, mobile abdominopelvic mass. Following is her magnetic resonance imaging picture.

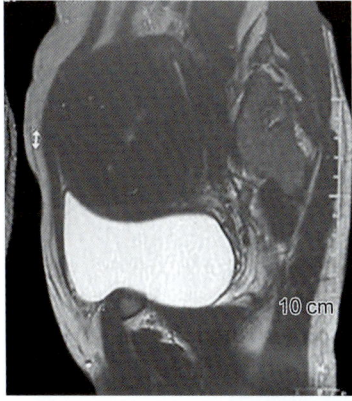
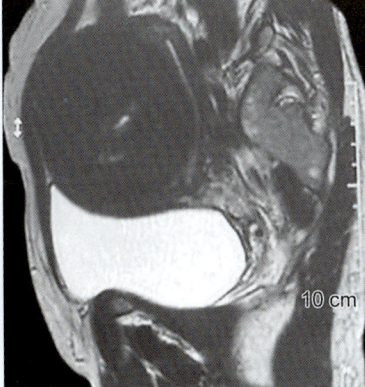
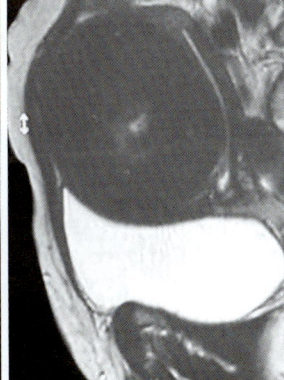

1. What is the most probable diagnosis?
2. What will be treatment for her?

Ans.
1. Fibroid uterus
2. Myomectomy

OSCE 7. A 22-year-old, nulliparous lady presented with heavy menstrual bleeding. Her examination revealed 20-week size, mobile abdominopelvic mass. Her complete blood count showed hemoglobin (Hb) of 6 g/dL. She has been diagnosed with fibroid uterus on imaging. Following is her magnetic resonance imaging picture.

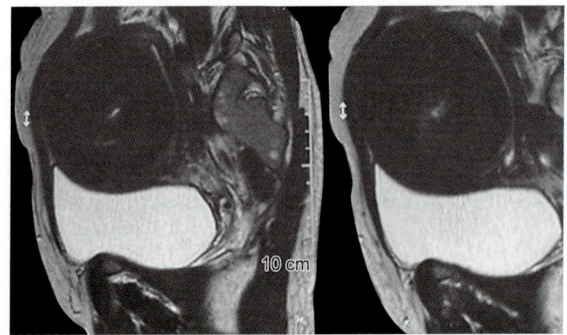

1. What is the location of fibroid?
2. What are the options to increase her Hb before surgery?

Ans.
1. Anterior wall fibroid
2. a. GnRH agonist
   b. Ulipristal acetate
   c. Blood transfusion
   d. Mifepristone

OSCE 8. A 44-year-old, P2L2 was diagnosed with heavy menstrual bleeding. She underwent hysterectomy for the same. This is the specimen sent for histopathology after surgery.

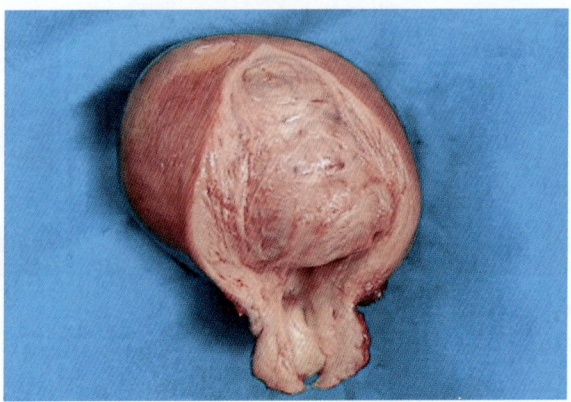

1. What is the most probable diagnosis?
2. What is the FIGO classification of this fibroid?

Ans.

1. Fibroid uterus
2. Hybrid fibroid 2–5

Reference

1. Munro MG, Critchley HO, Broder MS, Fraser IS. The FIGO Classification System ("PALM-COEIN") for causes of abnormal uterine bleeding in non-gravid women in the reproductive years, including guidelines for clinical investigation. Int J Gynaecol Obstet. 2011;113:3-13.

OSCE 9. A 30-year-old, nulliparous lady presented with abnormal uterine bleeding. Her examination revealed 18 week size abdominopelvic mass. Imaging showed 7 cm FIGO grade 2–5 fibroid. She underwent myomectomy. Following is the picture of specimen after surgery.

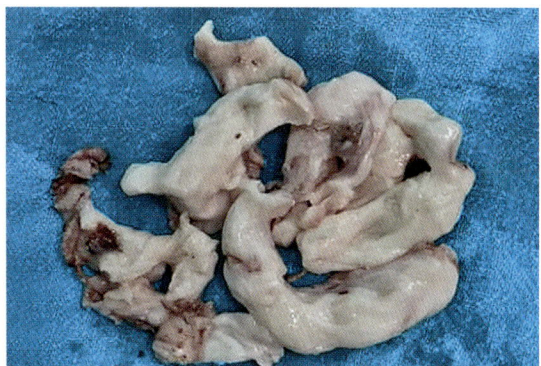

1. What had been the most probable mode of surgery?
2. What is the rare but serious complication of this mode of surgery specific to fibroid?

Ans.

1. Laparoscopic myomectomy with intracorporeal morcellation.
2. Disseminated intraperitoneal leiomyomatosis, dissemination of leiomyosarcoma.

OSCE 10. See the image attached below.

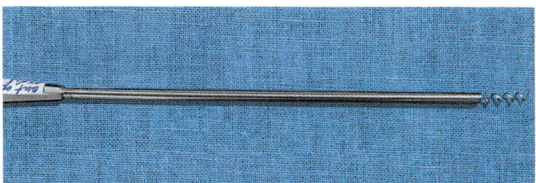

1. Identify the instrument and enumerate its two uses.
2. Enumerate ways to reduce blood loss in myomectomy.
3. Write two complications of myomectomy.

Ans.

1. Myoma screw
   Uses:
   a. Myomectomy
   b. To give traction to uterus in difficult hysterectomy
2. a. Vasopressin injection
   b. Tying torniquet in lower part of uterus during surgery
   c. Preoperative GnRH agonist treatment
   d. Preoperative uterine artery embolization
3. a. Blood loss
   b. Adhesion formation

OSCE 11. A 46-year-old, P3L3 lady presented with heavy menstrual bleeding and dysmenorrhea. She had all her deliveries by LSCS, and during her last child birth she had bladder injury during cesarean. She is a known case of type 2 DM and coronary artery disease. Her BMI was 40 kg/m^2 and examination showed 6-week size uterus. Multiple medical management methods were tried but nothing worked. Following is her USG picture.

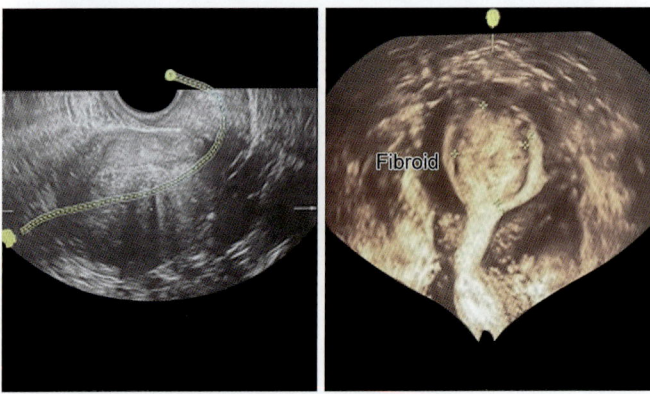

1. What is the next best treatment option for her?
2. What care should be taken during her preferred mode of surgery?
3. What precaution must be taken to prevent the complication?

Ans.

1. Hysteroscopic myomectomy
2. One has to be careful to avoid electrolyte imbalance
3. Stop the procedure when there is fluid deficit of 750 mL for hypotonic solutions and 1500 mL for isotonic solutions.

References

1. Umranikar S, Clark TJ, Saridogan E, et al; British Society for Gynaecological Endoscopy /European Society for Gynaecological Endoscopy Guideline Development Group for Management of Fluid

Distension Media in Operative Hysteroscopy. BSGE/ESGE guideline on management of fluid distension media in operative hysteroscopy. Gynecol Surg. 2016;13(4):289-303. doi: 10.1007/s10397-016-0983-z. Epub 2016 Oct 6. PMID: 28003797; PMCID: PMC5133285.
2. 2013 AAGL Practice Report: practical Guidelines for the Management of hysteroscopic distension media. J Minim Invasive Gynecol. 20:137-48.

OSCE 12. Please answer the questions based on the following drug.

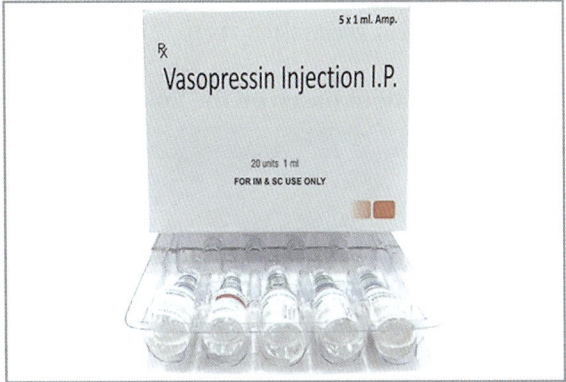

1. Enumerate two uses of this drug in gynecology.
2. What precautions will you take while using this drug?

Ans.

1. a. To decrease blood loss during myomectomy
   b. Vaginal infiltration during vaginal hysterectomy
2. a. Inform anesthetist while giving the injection
   b. Monitor heart rate and blood pressure during injection
   c. Use in dilution (20 IU in 100–400 mL of NS)

OSCE 13. See the tip of instrument given below.

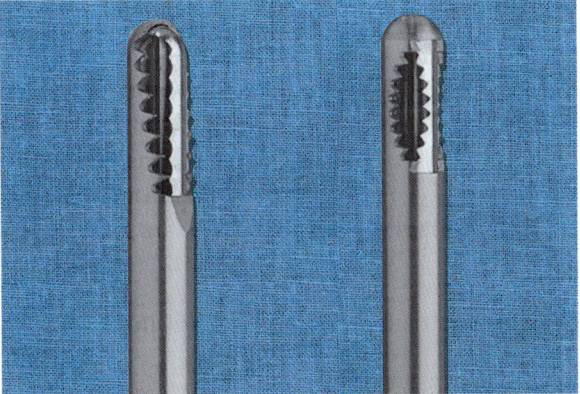

1. Identify the instrument, tip of which is given in the image above.
2. What is the ideal feature of the pathology to be treated by this method?

Ans.

1. Bigatti shaver (Hysteroscopic morcellator device).
2. FIGO 0 and 1 submucosal fibroid of size <2–3 cm.

Reference

1. Van Dongen H, Emanuel MH, Wolterbeek R, Trimbos JB, Jansen FW. Hysteroscopic morcellator for removal of intrauterine polyps and myomas: a randomized controlled pilot study among residents in training. J Minim Invasive Gynecol. 2008;15:466-71 (I).

OSCE 14. Please answer the questions based on the following picture.

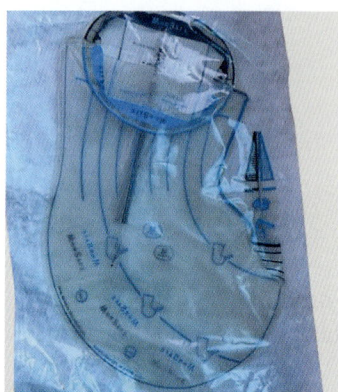

1. Identify the picture.
2. Why is it used and what is it's advantage?

Ans.

1. Bag for in bag morcellation during laparoscopic myomectomy.
2. It is used for in bag morcellation during laparoscopic myomectomy.
   Advantage: It prevents dissemination of fibroid pieces inside abdominal cavity, which can implant and grow later causing peritoneal leiomyomatosis.

OSCE 15. See the instrument given below.

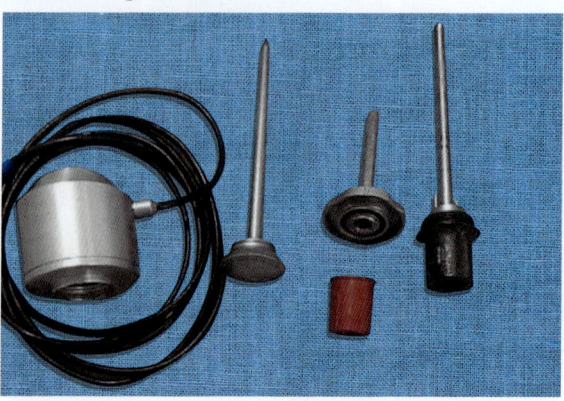

1. Identify the instrument.
2. What complications can happen with the use of this instrument?

Ans.

1. Laparoscopic morcellator
2. a. Dissemination of fibroid pieces inside abdominal cavity, which can implant and grow later causing diffuse peritoneal leiomyomatosis, dissemination of leiomyosarcoma
   b. Bowel injury

OSCE 16. A 49-year-old lady comes with diagnosis of fibroid made during USG done for renal stone workup. She is P3L3, and did not have any gynecological complaint. Her menstrual cycles were regular with average flow. Examination showed a 16-week size abdominopelvic mass. The USG showed 8 cm size subserosal fibroid (FIGO grade 6).
1. What will be the most appropriate management for her?
2. What additional information do you want if you are not planning her for surgery?

Ans.

1. Expectant management, she doesn't need any treatment for her fibroid at present.
2. USG to see for backpressure changes on kidney might be ordered. As ureteric compression can be there causing effect on kidneys. In that case, expectant management might not be appropriate for her.

OSCE 17. Please answer questions based on the following picture showing cut section of a fibroid specimen.

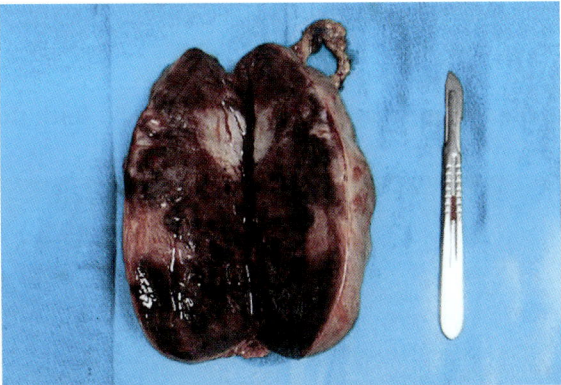

1. Which pathology might have been be there in the fibroid?
2. What is the clinical presentation of this kind of pathology in fibroids and it is common in which condition?

Ans.

1. Red degeneration
2. a. Sudden onset pain abdomen and fever.
   b. Occurs more commonly in pregnancy with fibroid.

OSCE 18. Please answer questions based on the following instrument.

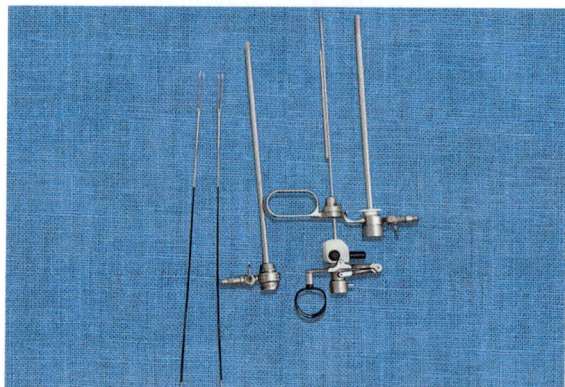

1. What is the instrument in the picture?
2. What are the uses of this instrument?

Ans.

1. Resectoscope with Collin's knife and loop
2. Uses
   a. With loop
      - Hysteroscopic myomectomy
      - Hysteroscopic polypectomy
      - Hysteroscopic isthmocele repair
   b. With Collin's knife
      - Hysteroscopic septal resection
      - Hysteroscopic adhesiolysis

OSCE 19. Below are the intraoperative pictures of a lady. Both the pictures belong to single surgery.

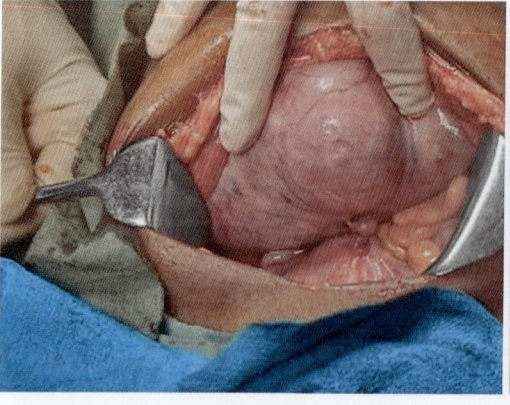 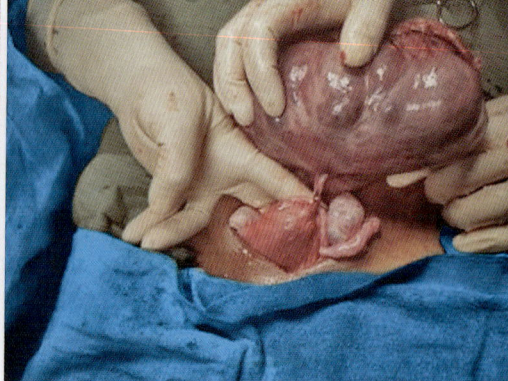

1. What is the intraoperative finding in the pictures?
2. What is the clinical presentation of this condition?

Ans.
1. Torsion of pedunculated subserosal fibroid.
2. Acute onset, severe pain abdomen.

OSCE 20. Please answer questions based on the following image.

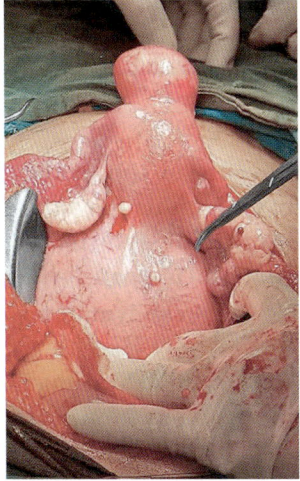

1. What is the most probable diagnosis and the name given to this condition?
2. What the complications of the surgery done for this pathology?

Ans.
1. Cervical fibroid, Lantern on Dome of St. Paul's Cathedral.
2. Bleeding, ureteric injury, bladder injury.

CHAPTER 35

Genitourinary Infections and STDs

Niharika Dhiman, Shreshtha Gupta

OSCE 1. A 28-year-old lady presents to the gynecology OPD with complaints of malodourous vaginal discharge. Often, this becomes more pronounced after sexual intercourse. Additional symptoms include dysuria, dyspareunia, and vaginal pruritus. She has a history of vaginal douching and is also a smoker.
1. Which infection is responsible for these symptoms caused by alteration of normal vaginal flora?
2. Which test is used to identify this infection by using KOH?
3. Name any one pregnancy-related complication caused.
4. Which is the most common aerobic bacteria in normal vaginal flora?
5. Which are the three types of vaginal epithelial cells?
6. What is the normal pH of vagina?

Ans.
1. Bacterial vaginosis
2. Whiff Test
3. Preterm labor, PPROM, Postpartum endometritis
4. *Lactobacillus*
5. a. Superficial cells, the main cell type in women of reproductive age, predominate when estrogen stimulation is present.
   b. Intermediate cells predominate because of stimulation by progesterone.
   c. Parabasal cells predominate in the absence of either hormone, a condition that may be found in postmenopausal women.
6. The pH level of the normal vagina is lower than 4.5, which is maintained by the production of lactic acid.

OSCE 2.

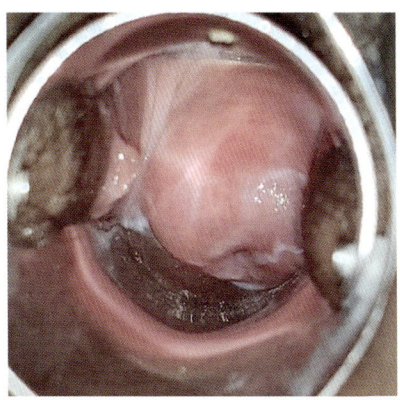

A 23-year-old college student presents to the clinic with a 2-day history of pain on urination, vaginal itching, and thick, white discharge.

She reports she is sexually active with 1 partner and uses latex condoms for birth control.

She recalls having a yeast infection once, a few years ago, which she remembers taking a prescription to treat. This is her per speculum examination.
1. Which is this adherent white discharge?
2. Which is the most common organism responsible for this?
3. Which two conditions lead to higher incidence of this?
4. Which oral drug is given for treatment?

Ans.

1. Candidiasis
2. *Candida albicans*
3. Pregnancy, obesity, diabetes mellitus, immunosuppression (i.e., patients with chemotherapy or antimetabolite medications, HIV infection, or transplant patients), and broad-spectrum antibiotic use are recognized risk factors for acute candidal vulvovaginitis.
4. The oral antifungal agent, fluconazole, used in a single 150-mg dose, is recommended for the treatment of VVC.

OSCE 3.

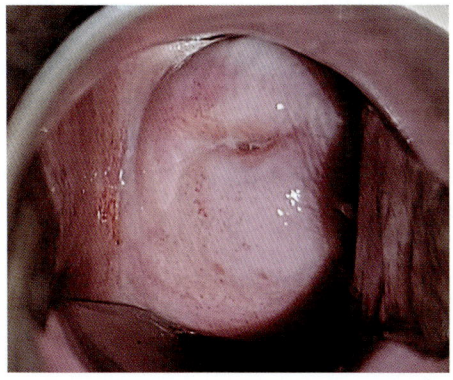

Section 2: Gynecology

1. Which organism is responsible for this patchy vaginal erythema accompanied by vulvar pruritis?
2. What is the drug of choice?
3. Treatment of recurrent infections?

Ans.

1. Trichomonas vaginalis causes strawberry cervix.
2. Metronidazole 200 mg by mouth three times a day for 7 days
3. Recurrent infection is treated with tinidazole 500 mg QID and vaginal pessary 500 mg BD for 14 days.

OSCE 4. A 24-year-old, sex worker presents to the gynecological OPD with mucopurulent discharge and dysuria. Symptoms started after 3 days of unprotected intercourse. On examination of the smear, gram-negative *Diplococcus* was seen.
1. Which organism is responsible for the above complaints?
2. On which media does this organism grow?
3. Which drug is the first line management?
4. Mention any two complications of this infection.
5. Name the syndrome associated with perihepatic inflammation in this infection.

Ans.

1. *Neisseria gonorrhea*
2. Chocolate agar, Thayer–Martin agar
3. A single dose of 500 mg of intramuscular ceftriaxone
4. In women, Gonorrhea can spread to the reproductive organs and cause pelvic inflammatory disease (PID). PID can lead to long-term pelvic pain, ectopic pregnancy, and infertility. During pregnancy, gonorrhea can cause miscarriage, premature labor and birth and neonatal conjunctivitis.
5. Fitz–Hugh–Curtis syndrome is the extra pelvic manifestation of gonorrhea. It represents the spread of *N. gonorrhea* through the peritoneal cavity from fallopian tubes to the Glisson's capsule of the liver.

OSCE 5. STI/RTI syndrome is a combination of symptoms and signs typically associated with sexually transmitted microorganisms, e.g., genital ulcer disease syndrome, which may be due to syphilis, chancroid, herpes simplex, etc. This is important because mixed infections occur frequently in STI/RTI. Syndromic management of STI/RTI can effectively treat cases in settings with limited or no laboratory facilities.
1. Which of the following are known to cause and transmit reproductive tract infections?
    a. Sexual intercourse.
    b. Infected blood.
    c. Overgrowth of normally present organisms in the genital tract.
    d. Breastfeeding.
    e. All the above.

2. **True or False:**
    a. Bacterial infections such as gonorrhea and chlamydia are only a concern for women and do not affect men.
    b. Viral STDs cannot be cured.
    c. Pregnant women with syphilis, HIV and herpes may transmit the infection to their newborns.
    d. The presence of another STD does not increase the risk of HIV transmission.
    e. Consistent and correct use of condoms is the most effective way for sexually active people to prevent the transmission of both bacterial and viral STDs.
3. Public health strategies for reducing the spread of STDs include which of the following?
    a. Promoting consistent and correct condom use.
    b. Targeting core transmitters, such as sex workers, truck drivers and military men.
    c. Using mass media, comic books, posters, and magazines to help change social norms.
    d. Offering STD services through family planning/maternal child health clinics.
    e. All the above
4. Give an example of dual method used to prevent pregnancy and the transmission of STDs?
5. Healthcare providers should emphasize the four Cs of STDs management. What are the four Cs?

Ans.

1. e. All the above.
2. a. Bacterial infections such as gonorrhea and chlamydia are only a concern for women and do not affect men. **False**
    b. Viral STDs cannot be cured. **True**
    c. Pregnant women with syphilis, HIV and herpes may transmit the infection to their newborns. **True**
    d. The presence of another STD does not increase the risk of HIV transmission. **False**
    e. Consistent and correct use of condoms is the most effective way for sexually active people to prevent the transmission of both bacterial and viral STDs. **True**
3. e. All the above
4. Condoms and oral contraceptives. IUD (intrauterine device) and condoms.
5. a. Counseling and education
    b. Condom promotion
    c. Compliance with treatment
    d. Contacting partners for diagnosis

OSCE 6. A 24-year-old lady presents to the office with a 3-month history of tender, itchy "bumps" on her vulva. She had two male sexual partners in the past. On examination, you find multiple papillomatous lesions on her outer labia that are consistent with the appearance of warts.
1. Which is the most common virus causing genital warts?

2. Which are the two common subtypes of this virus?
3. Vertical transmission of this virus causes which disease in newborn?
4. Name any one vaccine used to prevent infection of this virus.
5. Which topical application is used to treat warts?

Ans.

1. Human Papilloma Virus (HPV)
2. HPV 16, 18
3. Laryngeal papillomatosis
4. Cervarix, Gardasil
5. Imiquimod and podophyllotoxin are two new treatments for external genital warts that are less painful and can be applied by patients at home.

OSCE 7.

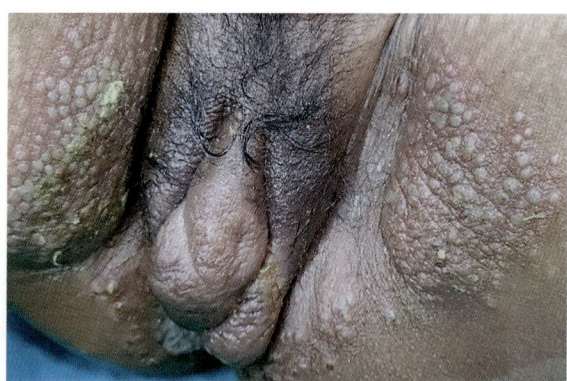

A 24-year-old married lady presented with lesions in the vulval area, preceding which she had malaise, fever and vulval paraesthesia. Within the next 7 days, she noticed coalesced vesicles on the vulva extending up to the medial border of the thigh resulting in painful ulcers.

1. What is your diagnosis?
2. What is the differential diagnosis of painful genital ulcers?
3. How will you manage it?
4. What are the complications?

Ans.

1. Genital Herpes—caused by double-stranded DNA of herpes simplex virus I/II (80% are type-II infections). Incubation period is 3–7 days.
2. Chancroid
3. *Diagnosis:* Diagnosis is mainly clinical, in the presence of active lesions, polymerase chain reaction assay is the preferred test, with sensitivity and specificity of 95%.
   Scenarios to consider herpes simplex virus type—Specific Serologic Testing—History of suggestive symptoms but no lesions are present, or polymerase chain reaction assay results are negative, or when the patient's partner is infected.

Treatment:
  Primary outbreak:
  Oral 200 mg Acyclovir five times daily for 5 days
  Or
  Valacyclovir 500 mg BD or Famciclovir 125–250 mg BD for 7 days.
  Or
  Valaciclovir 250 mg BD for 3–7 days is also effective.

  Severe cases:
  - Acyclovir 5 mg/kg body weight intravenously every 8 hourly for 5 days.
  - Local application of Acyclovir cream on lesions.
  - Counseling of couples for barrier contraception should be done.
4. Encephalitis, urinary tract involvement causing retention of urine, neonatal infection, pelvic inflammatory disease, pneumonitis, hepatitis and disseminated herpes.

OSCE 8. A 32-year-old lady presented with painless papule on both the labia majora with swelling in the inguinal area.

On examination: Bilateral labia majora showed ulcero-granulomatous lesions which were 'beefy-red', nontender and bled on touch. A similar lesion was seen on the anterior lip of cervix between 1 o'clock to 3 o'clock position.
1. What is the provisional diagnosis?
2. What is the differential diagnosis?
3. What is the definitive test for diagnosis?
4. Name the causative organism.
5. What is the cause of inguinal swelling?
6. What is the treatment?

Ans.

1. Granuloma inguinale (Donovanosis).
2. Primary syphilis, secondary syphilis (condylomata lata), lymphogranuloma venereum, cutaneous tuberculosis, neoplasm
3. Demonstration of Donovan bodies which are seen within large, mononuclear cells as gram-negative intracytoplasmic cysts filled with deeply staining bodies. They can have a characteristic "safety pin" appearance on staining with Wright-Giemsa, Warthin-Starry, toluidine blue, or Leishman stain. The stain is prepared by making a smear or by taking a small piece of tissue from the ulcer edge or base.
4. Intracellular gram-negative *Bacterium, Klebsiella granulomatis* formerly known as *Calymmatobacterium granulomatis*.
5. The subcutaneous spread to the inguinal region where it can cause swelling and ulceration and is called pseudobubo, it is not a true adenitis. Inguinal swelling can also occur as extragenital involvement of inguinal lymph nodes seen commonly in patients with HIV infection.
6. *Recommended treatment:*
   - *Azithromycin* 1 g per oral (PO) weekly or 500 mg daily for >3 weeks and until all the lesions have completely healed.

- *Alternate treatment: Doxycycline* 100 mg PO 2 times/day for at least 3 weeks and until all lesions have completely healed
  OR
  Erythromycin base 500 mg orally 4 times/day for >3 weeks and until all lesions have completely healed
  OR
  Trimethoprim-sulfamethoxazole one double-strength (160 mg/800 mg) tablet orally 2 times/day for >3 weeks and until all lesions have completely healed.

OSCE 9. A 25-year-old married lady presented with fever, malaise and myalgia associated with discharge per vaginum and painful swelling in both the groins.

On taking a detailed history, it was found that preceding this swelling, she had noticed a small, painless lesion which had ulcerated. This was also associated with mucopurulent discharge from urethra and vagina. She also had constant pain in the lower abdomen and history was suggestive of tenesmus.

On examination: Multiple small healing ulcer lesions were present on bilateral labia majora, with mucopurulent discharge from the cervix and urethra. Bilateral fluctuant, tender, inguinal lymphadenopathy with overlying skin showing discoloration.

1. What is the clinical diagnosis?
2. Name the causative agent?
3. How is the diagnosis confirmed?
4. What stage of disease does the patient have?
5. What is the reason for lower abdominal pain and tenesmus?
6. What is the recommended treatment for the disease and inguinal swelling?
7. What are the late sequelae?

Ans.

1. Lymphogranuloma Venereum (LGV)
2. *Chlamydia trachomatis* serovars L1, L2, or L3-intracellular gram-negative bacteria.
3. The diagnosis is based on:
   - Clinical suspicion
   - Epidemiologic information
   - Positive *C. trachomatis* NAAT at the symptomatic anatomic site,
   - Exclusion of other etiologies for proctocolitis, inguinal lymphadenopathy, or genital, oral, or rectal ulcers.

   The definitive diagnosis of LGV on any of the following serology tests:
   - Complement fixation (CF)
   - Micro-immunofluorescence
   Or
   Identification of *Chlamydia trachomatis* in genital, rectal, urethral and lymph node specimens (by culture, nucleic acid amplification test or direct immunofluorescence). CF sensitivity is 80% for LGV. A test titer of 1:16 is strongly suggestive of LGV and a titer of >1:64 indicates active LGV.

   On micro-immunofluorescence a titer greater or equal to 1:512 is diagnostic.

4. *The secondary stage or inguinal stage:* The development of unilateral or bilateral, tender inguinal and/or femoral lymphadenopathy also called buboes, which occurs two to six weeks after the primary stage. Anorectal syndrome may also be present which is characterized by proctitis or proctocolitis-like symptoms, dysuria, abdominal pain, or tenesmus. Generalized symptoms such as body aches, headache, and fever can occur during this stage.
5. Proctitis or proctocolitis is the cause of pain.
6. The recommended treatment regimen is doxycycline 100 mg orally twice a day given for 21 days.

    An alternate regimen:
    - Erythromycin 500 mg orally four times a day given for 21 days (preferred during pregnancy)
    - Azithromycin 1 gm orally once weekly for 3 weeks is also an effective alternative regimen.
    - All patients who are suspected to have LGV (either genito-ulcerative disease with lymphadenopathy or proctocolitis) should be empirically treated for LGV before definitive diagnosis is made.

    Fluctuant or pus-filled buboes should be aspirated of the node, incision and drainage of the nodes are not recommended.
7. *Late sequelae:*
    - Necrosis and rupture of the lymph nodes
    - Anogenital fibrosis, and strictures
    - Anal fistulae
    - Elephantiasis of the genital organs.

OSCE 10. A 30-year-old lady presented with a painless lesion.

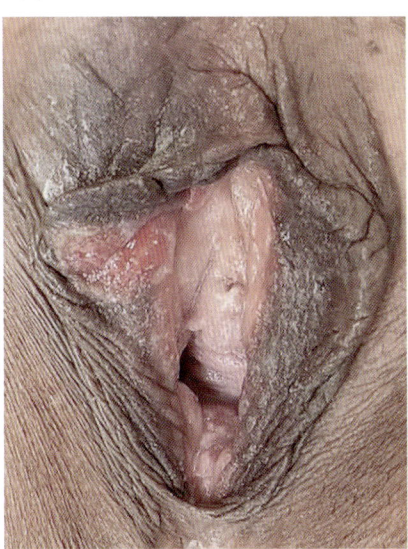

Ulcer: Single, superficial, sharply demarcated, firm, base was red and smooth, non-indurated with serous secretions.

Nontender, firm right inguinal lymphadenopathy was also present.

1. Identify the lesion.
2. What is the diagnosis?
3. Name the causative organism.
4. What is the management?
5. What is the management for the partner?
6. Within 24 hours of initiation of therapy, she develops headache, myalgia, and fever. What is the diagnosis?
7. Match the following:

Disease	Type of ulcer
Granuloma inguinale	The ulcer (also called chancre) is a firm painless ulceration, 5–15 mm and sharply demarcated. Often, a painless inguinal lymphadenopathy
Syphilis	Grouped papules or vesicles on an erythematous base, painful coalesced ulcers
Genital herpes	A genital papule or pustule with tender, fluctuant lymphadenopathy (buboes)
Lymphogranuloma venereum (LGV)	progressive, painless highly vascular genital ulcers without inguinal lymphadenopathy (pseudo-buboes)

Ans.

1. Chancre
2. Primary syphilis
3. Motile spirochete *Treponema pallidum*
4. Management:
   - *Investigations:* Dark field microscopy of chancre scrapings reveals spirochetes. Serological test (VDRL test) at this stage is negative.
   - *Treatment:* Single dose Inj. Benzathine penicillin 2.4 million units intramuscular.
   - Screen both partners for other STDs and HIV
   - Counseling
   - Treating all sexual partners of infected individual
5. Management of sexual partner:
   - Sexual contact with a person with diagnosis of primary, secondary, or early latent syphilis <90 days should be treated presumptively for early syphilis, even if serologic test results are negative.
   - Sexual contact with a person with a diagnosis of primary, secondary, or early latent syphilis >90 days should be treated presumptively for early syphilis if serologic test results are not immediately available. If serologic tests are negative, no treatment is needed. If serologic tests are positive, treatment should be based on clinical and serologic evaluation and syphilis stage.

6. Jarisch-Herxheimer reaction
7.

Disease	Type of ulcer
Syphilis	The ulcer (also called chancre) is a firm painless ulceration, 5–15 mm and sharply demarcated. Often, a painless inguinal lymphadenopathy
Genital herpes	Grouped papules or vesicles on an erythematous base, painful coalesced ulcers
Lymphogranuloma venereum (LGV)	A genital papule or pustule with tender, fluctuant lymphadenopathy (buboes)
Granuloma inguinale	Progressive, painless, highly vascular genital ulcers without inguinal lymphadenopathy (pseudo-buboes)

CHAPTER 36

Pelvic Inflammatory Disease

Leena Wadhwa, Sneh Yadav, Deval Rishi Pandit

OSCE 1.

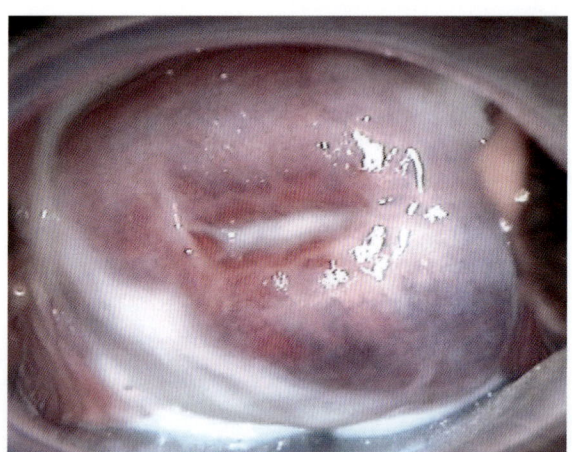

1. A 30-year-old, diabetic woman presents to Gyne OPD with complaints of curdy white vaginal discharge with intense itching. What is the likely causative organism in this condition?
2. How can you confirm the diagnosis?
3. What is the treatment of this condition?

Ans.

1. Candidal infection. Thick white discharge, labial erythema and edema are seen with candidiasis.
2. On KOH preparation, Serpentine pseudohyphae are seen suggestive of *Candida albicans*.
3. *Treatment:* Topical agent clotrimazole 1% vaginal cream once application for 7 days and Tab Fluconazole 150 mg stat.

Reference
1. CDC 2021

OSCE 2.

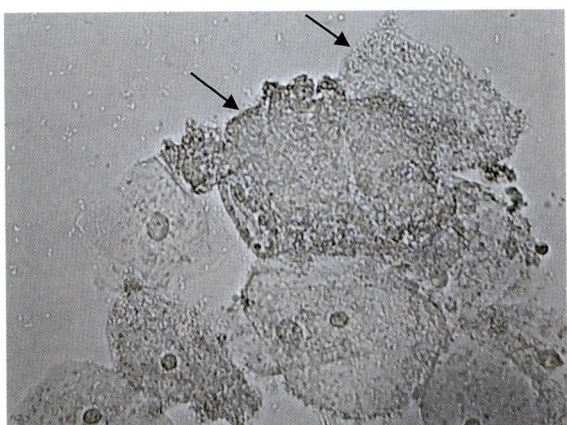

1. What is depicted in this picture?
2. What is Amsel's criteria?
3. What are the organisms responsible for this infection?
4. Describe the treatment of this infection.
5. Which scoring system is used by microbiologist to diagnose this condition?

Ans.

1. Clue cells on saline wet preparation. Several of these squamous cells are heavily studded with bacteria. Clue cells are covered to the extent that cell borders are blurred, and nuclei are not visible.
2. According to Amsel's criteria, if at least three of the following four criteria are fulfilled, it is confirmed to be a case of bacterial vaginosis.
   a. Greyish white, thin, and homogeneous vaginal discharge
   b. Vaginal pH higher than 4.5
   c. Fishy or amine odor after addition of 10% KOH
   d. Presence of clue cells (>20%) on microscopic examination
3. Bacterial vaginosis occurs due to alteration of vaginal flora in which normal flora (Lactobacilli) is replaced by mixed bacterial flora which includes *Gardnerella vaginalis*, *Mobiluncus* species, *Mycoplasma hominis*, *Bacteroides* species, and some other anaerobic bacteria.
4. Tab Metronidazole 500 mg orally 2 times per day for 7 days or metronidazole gel 0.75% one full applicator (5 g) intravaginally, once a day for 5 days or clindamycin cream 2% one full applicator (5 g) intravaginally at bedtime for 7 days.
5. Gram staining is done to determine the Nugent's score by a clinical microbiologist. Nugent's score system was based on the number of different morphotypes of bacteria, viz., Lactobacillus-like (large uniform Gram-positive bacilli), *Gardnerella vaginalis*-like (small pleomorphic Gram–variable bacilli). A Nugent score of 7–10 was interpreted as consistent with BV and a score of 4–6 as intermediate, while a score of 0–3 was interpreted as negative for BV.

Reference
1. CDC 2021

OSCE 3.

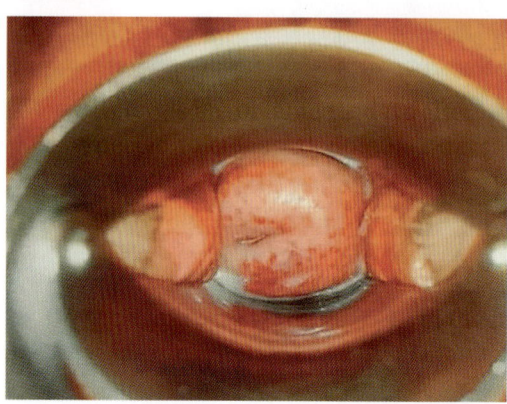
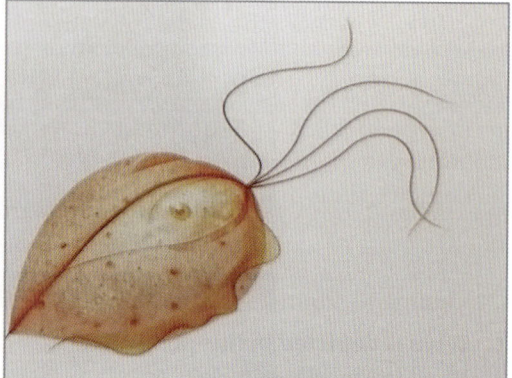

A 36-year-old lady presented to OPD with complaint of discharge per vagina and pain abdomen. On per abdomen examination, abdomen is soft, nontender. On per speculum examination, patient had greenish frothy discharge with punctate hemorrhage on cervix.
1. What is your diagnosis?
2. Name the causative agent.
3. How can you confirm your diagnosis?
4. What treatment will you advise for this patient?

Ans.
1. Strawberry cervix in *Trichomonas vaginalis*
2. *Trichomonas vaginalis*
3. Organism can be detected by *Hanging drop preparation*.
4. Metronidazole 2 g stat or tinidazole 2 g stat or metronidazole 500 mg twice daily for 7 days

Reference
1. CDC 2021

OSCE 4.
A 32-year-old lady presented to OPD with pain in her lower abdomen and purulent white discharge. Her menstrual cycles are regular but associated with increased flow. On per vaginal examination, cervical motion tenderness was present, uterus retroverted, and, bilateral fornices were tender.
1. What is the diagnosis?
2. What are the CDC diagnostic criteria for this condition?
3. What is the best treatment option for her?

Ans.

1. Pelvic inflammatory disease (PID)
2. CDC 2021 criteria for the diagnosis of PID:

   Definitive criteria
   - Laparoscopic evidence of PID
   - Histopathologic evidence of endometritis on biopsy
   - Imaging studies (TVS/MRI) evidence of thickened fluid-filled tubes (tubo-ovarian abscess)

   Minimum criteria
   - Lower abdominal tenderness
   - Adnexal tenderness
   - Cervical motion tenderness

   Additional criteria
   - Oral temperature >38.3°C
   - Raised ESR or CRP
   - Mucopurulent cervical or vaginal discharge and cervical friability
   - Laboratory documentation of positive cervical infection with *Gonorrhea* or *Chlamydia*

3. Treatment of PID: Outpatient treatment of PID (According to CDC 2021 guidelines)
   - A single dose of IM ceftriaxone 250 mg + oral doxycycline 100 mg BD +/– metronidazole 400 mg BD for 14 days
   - A single dose of IM ceftriaxone 250 mg followed by azithromycin 1 g per week for 2 weeks.

OSCE 5. Answer the following:
1. Name two causative organisms of PID.
2. What is the pathogenesis of PID?

Ans.

1. Causes of PID
   - *Neisseria gonorrhoeae* and *Chlamydia trachomatis* are identified as the causative agents of PID.
   - *Gardnerella vaginalis*, anaerobes and other organisms commonly found in the vagina may also be implicated.
   - *Mycoplasma genitalium* has been associated with upper genital tract infections in women and is very likely cause of PID.
   - Insertion of an IUD (intrauterine device) increases the risk and is highest in women with pre-existing *Gonorrhea* or *C. trachomatis*.
   - Genital tuberculosis is one of the causes of PID in India.

Reference
1. CDC 2021

2. *Pathogenesis of PID:*
   - Ascending infection
   - Hematogenous
   - Local spread

   Most cases of PID occur in two stages:

   Stage 1: Acquisition of a vaginal or cervical infection, which is often sexually transmitted and may be asymptomatic.

   Stage 2: Direct ascent of microorganisms from the vagina or cervix to the upper genital tract, with infection and inflammation of these structures causing nonpathogenic organisms to overgrow and ascend.

OSCE 6.

1. **Enumerate four risk factors of PID.**
2. **Enumerate complications of PID.**
3. **Enumerate four differential diagnosis in a young woman with lower abdominal pain.**

Ans.

1. *Risk factors of PID:*
   - Instrumentation of the uterus/interruption of the cervical barrier
   - Termination of pregnancy, insertion of intrauterine device within the past 4 months, hysterosalpingography, in vitro fertilization, intrauterine insemination (IUI), hysteroscopy
   - Young <25 years
   - Menstruating women
   - Multiple sexual partners
   - Recent new partners
   - Past history of sexually transmitted infections (STIs) in the patient or their partner
   - No history of contraception use
   - Living in an area of high prevalence of PID
   - Tampons use (forgotten)
   - Poor menstrual hygiene
   - Bacterial vaginosis
   - However, in Indian scenario the most common causes are abortions, puerperal sepsis, and intrauterine device insertions.
2. *Complications of PID:*
   - *Tubo-ovarian abscess and pelvic peritonitis* is an indication for hospital admission for parenteral antimicrobial therapy with appropriate anaerobic cover.
   - Fitz-Hugh-Curtis syndrome
   - Septicemia
3. *Differential diagnosis of lower abdominal pain in a young woman:*
   - Ectopic pregnancy
   - Acute appendicitis
   - PID

- Complication of an ovarian cyst such as rupture and torsion
- Urinary tract infection
- Endometriosis
- Irritable bowel syndrome
- Functional pain (pain of unknown physical origin)

Reference
1. CDC 2021

OSCE 7. A 26-year-old lady presented with abdominal pain for 10 days and a temperature of 102°F with negative urine pregnancy test. She also had mucopurulent vaginal discharge and cervical motion tenderness.
1. Does she require admission? Enumerate four criteria for hospitalization in PID.
2. What is the treatment of PID in hospitalized patients?
3. Enumerate four criteria for surgery in PID.
4. What are the stages of PID?

Ans.
1. Yes, she requires hospitalization.
   Criteria for hospitalization in PID include:
   - Tubo-ovarian abscess
   - Pregnancy
   - Severe illness, nausea and vomiting, or oral temperature >38.5°C
   - Unable to follow or tolerate an outpatient oral regimen.
   - No clinical response to oral antimicrobial therapy
2. *Treatment of PID in hospitalized patients:*
   - Ceftriaxone 1 g IV every 24 hours plus Doxycycline 100 mg orally or IV every 12 hours plus Metronidazole 500 mg orally or IV every 12 hours
   - Cefotetan 2 g IV 12 hourly + doxycycline 100 mg orally/IV every 12 hourly for 48 hours is given. followed by oral doxycyclin 100 mg +/− metronidazole 400 mg for 14 days.
   - Cefoxitin 2g IV 6 hourly + doxycycline 100 mg IV 12 hourly followed by oral route
3. *Criteria for surgery in PID includes:*
   - Intestinal obstruction
   - Ruptured tubo-ovarian abscess
   - Suspected intestinal injury
   - Drainage of pelvic abscess by colpotomy
   - Dilatation and evacuation of septic products of conception or for hemorrhage in the postabortal period
   - Acute spreading peritonitis resistant to chemotherapy. Presence of pyoperitoneum mandates laparotomy
4. *Stages of PID:*
   - *Stage 1:* Acute salpingitis without peritonitis—no adhesion
   - *Stage 2:* Acute salpingitis with peritonitis—purulent discharge

- *Stage 3:* Acute salpingitis with superimposed tubal occlusion or tubo-ovarian complex
- *Stage 4:* Ruptured tubo-ovarian abscess
- *Stage 5:* Tuberculous salpingitis

Reference

1. CDC 2021

OSCE 8.

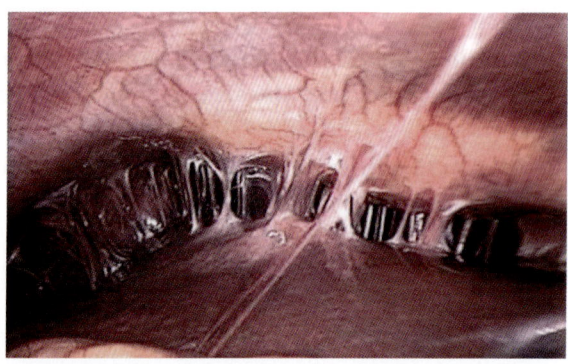

A 32-year-old lady presented to emergency with pain lower abdomen on and off since 6 months with abnormal vaginal discharge. Given picture depicts her diagnostic laparoscopy finding:
1. What is the diagnosis? What does this indicate?
2. Enumerate four pelvic findings of PID in laparoscopy.
3. Enumerate four hysteroscopic findings in chronic endometritis (CE).
4. Write the role of endometrial biopsy in diagnosing chronic endometritis.
5. Enumerate four causative organisms for chronic endometritis.

Ans.

1. *Fitz-Hugh-Curtis syndrome:* Perihepatitis with violine string sign. It is a chronic manifestation of pelvic inflammatory disease (PID). *Neisseria gonorrhoeae* and *Chlamydia trachomatis* are thought to be the primary causative agents of Fitz-Hugh-Curtis syndrome.
2. Laparoscopic findings for diagnosing PID include tubal wall edema, visible hyperemia of tubal surface, adhesions, and presence of exudate on the tubal surfaces and fimbriae. Pelvic masses consistent with miliary tubercles, tubo-ovarian abscess can be directly visualized.
3. Hysteroscopic findings in chronic endometritis includes signs of inflammation as focal or diffuse hyperemia, stromal edema, presence of micropolyps, endometrial polyps, and the typical 'strawberry aspects' on the endometrial surface.
4. Histologically chronic endometritis (CE) is characterized by the presence of ≥1 plasma cell/10 HPF in endometrial stroma with hematoxylin-eosin staining which is the gold standard for the diagnosis. Immunohistochemically staining for CD138 to detect plasma cells is diagnosis of CE.

5. Chronic endometritis (CE) is a persistent inflammation of uterine endometrium. It is caused by a variety of infectious agents including *Gonorrhea, chlamydia, Mycoplasma, Ureaplasma, E. coli, Streptococcus species, Staphylococcus, Enterococcus faecalis*, yeast and tuberculosis.

OSCE 9. Match the following: NACO STI Kits with disease

1.	Kit 1 (Gray)	Genital ulcer disease (Herpetic)
2.	Kit 2 (Green)	Genital ulcer disease (Nonherpetic)
3.	Kit 3 (White)	Genital ulcer disease (Nonherpetic) in patient allergic to penicillin
4.	Kit 4 (Blue)	Lower abdominal pain
5.	Kit 5 (Red)	Inguinal bubo
6.	Kit 6 (Yellow)	Urethral or anorectal or cervical discharge
7.	Kit 7 (Black)	Vaginal discharge (vaginitis)

Ans.

1.	Kit 1 (Gray)	Urethral or anorectal or cervical discharge
2.	Kit 2 (Green)	Vaginal discharge (vaginitis)
3.	Kit 3 (White)	Genital ulcer disease (nonherpetic)
4.	Kit 4 (Blue)	Genital ulcer disease (nonherpetic) in patient allergic to penicillin
5.	Kit 5 (Red)	Genital ulcer disease (herpetic)
6.	Kit 6 (Yellow)	Lower abdominal pain (pelvic inflammatory disease)
7.	Kit 7 (Black)	Inguinal bubo

OSCE 10.

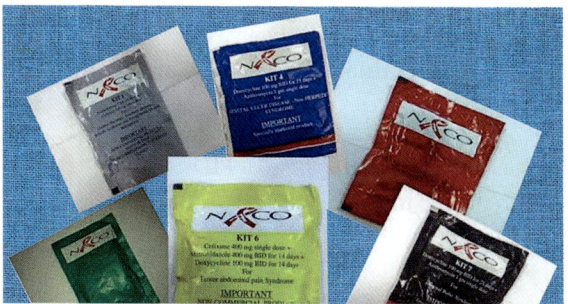

1. What are the drugs included in NACO-STI kits?

Ans.

1. a. *Kit 1:* Tab Azithromycin 1 g (1 tab) and Tab Cefixime 400 mg (1 tab)
   b. *Kit 2:* Tab Secnidazole 2 g (1 tab) and Tab Fluconazole 150 mg (1 tab)
   c. *Kit 3:* Inj Benzathine penicillin 2.4 MU (1 vial) and Tab Azithromycin 1 g (1 tab)
   d. *Kit 4:* Tab Doxycycline 100 mg (1 tab BD for 14 days) tab Azithromycin 1 g (1 tab)

e. *Kit 5:* Tab Acyclovir 400 mg (1 tab) TDS for 7 days
f. *Kit 6:* Tab Cefixime 400 mg (1 tab) + Tab Metronidazole 400 mg BD for 14 days +Tab Doxycycline 100 mg BD for 14 days
g. *Kit 7:* Tab Doxycycline 100 mg BD for 21 days and Tab Azithromycin 1 g (1 tab)

OSCE 11. A 28-year-old lady presented to emergency with complaint of abdominal pain and vaginal discharge and was diagnosed with PID.
1. Should her partner be treated at the same time if he is asymptomatic?
2. What is the management of sex partners of a PID patient?

Ans.

1. Yes, the partner should be treated even if asymptomatic. Sex partner of persons who have PID caused by *C. trachomatis* or *N. gonorrhoeae* are frequently asymptomatic.
2. Persons who have had sexual contact with a partner with PID during the 60 days preceding symptom onset should be evaluated, tested, and presumptively treated for *Chlamydia* and *Gonorrhea*, regardless of PID etiology or pathogens isolated.
    Partner should be instructed to abstain from sexual intercourse until they and their sex partners have been treated (i.e., until therapy is completed, and symptoms have resolved, if originally present).

OSCE 12. Patient with diagnosis of PID. Write True/False:
1. *Neisseria* is the most common cause of PID.
2. Cervicitis is not included in PID.
3. Oral contraceptive pills intake is a risk factor for PID.
4. Fitz-Hugh-Curtis syndrome is a complication of this condition.
5. Bacterial vaginosis is a known etiological factor.
6. Characteristic findings at laparoscopy are diagnostic.
7. Long-term sequelae include preterm delivery.
8. Pelvic abscess results from secondary invasion by anaerobic organisms.

Ans.

1. False. *Chlamydia* is the most common cause of PID.
2. True. Cervicitis is not included in PID.
3. False. OCP is not a risk factor for PID.
4. True
5. False
6. True
7. False
8. True

OSCE 13.

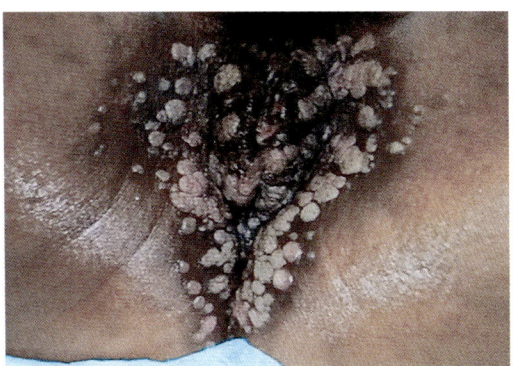

1. What is the name of lesions depicted in this image?
2. Lesions shown in image belongs to which stage of disease?
3. What is the cause of these lesions?
4. Describe the treatment according to stage of disease.
5. Is this disease STD or not?

Ans.

1. Woman with multiple condyloma lata on her labia. Soft, flat, moist, pink-tan papules and nodules on the perineum and perineal area are typical.
2. Secondary syphilis
3. *Treponema pallidum*
4. Treatment (a):
   - Primary, secondary, and early latent syphilis
   - Benzathine penicillin G, 2.4 million units IM single dose

   (b)
   - Late latent, tertiary, and cardiovascular syphilis
   - Benzathine penicillin G, 2.4 million units IM weekly 3 doses
5. Syphilis is a STD.

Reference
1. CDC 2021

OSCE 14.

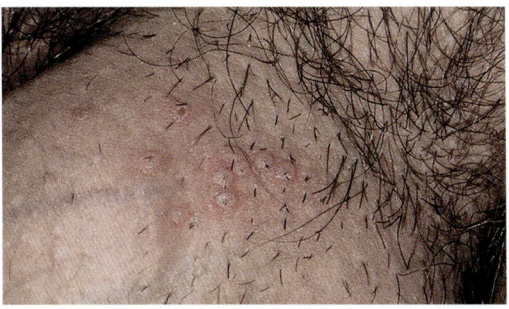

Answer the following as True/False:
1. The lesion shown in image is molluscum contagiosum.
2. The cause of these lesions is pox virus.
3. Doxycycline is used to treat this infection.

Ans.
1. False. Genital herpetic vesicles prior to ulceration.
2. False. Caused by HSV-2 (Herpes simplex virus-2)
3. False. *Treatment:* Tab Acyclovir 400 mg three times daily for 7–10 days.
   or Famcyclovir 250 mg three times daily for 7–10 days
   or Valacyclovir 1 g twice daily for 7–10 days

Reference
1. CDC 2021

OSCE 15.

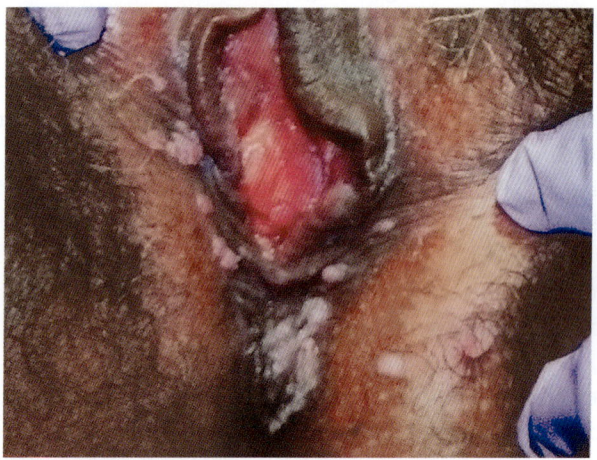

1. Identify the lesions shown in the image.
2. What is the cause of these lesions?
3. What is the mode of spread of these lesions?
4. What is the treatment of these lesions?

Ans.
1. Condyloma acuminata. Multiple exophytic verrucous warts are seen on labia and perineum.
2. Human papilloma virus (HPV). Most common strain of HPV that causes anogenital warts are 6 and 11.
3. Spreads by having unprotected vaginal, anal, or oral sex, skin-to-skin contact (handshakes or hugs)
4. Recommended regimens for anogenital warts (i.e., penis, groin, scrotum, vulva, perineum, external anus, or perianus):

Local application: Imiquimod 3.75% or 5% cream or podofilox 0.5% solution or gel or sinecatechins 15% ointment.

Also: Cryotherapy with liquid nitrogen or cryoprobe or surgical removal by tangential scissor excision, tangential shave excision, curettage, laser, or electrosurgery or trichloroacetic acid or bichloroacetic acid (BCA) 80–90% solution

Reference
1. CDC 2021

OSCE 16.

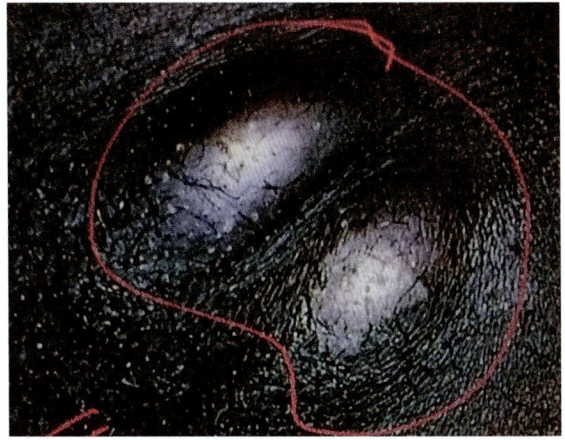

1. Identify the sign shown in the image.
2. Name the causative organism.
3. Name the disease.
4. What is the treatment?

Ans.

1. Groove sign seen with lymphogranuloma venereum. Enlarged lymph nodes matted together on either side of inguinal ligament create this characteristic groove.
2. *Chlamydia trachomatis* serotype L1, L2 and L3
3. Lymphogranuloma venereum
4. Doxycycline 100 mg orally twice daily for 21 days. Alternatively, Erythromycin 500 mg orally four times daily for 21 days

Reference
1. CDC 2021

OSCE 17.

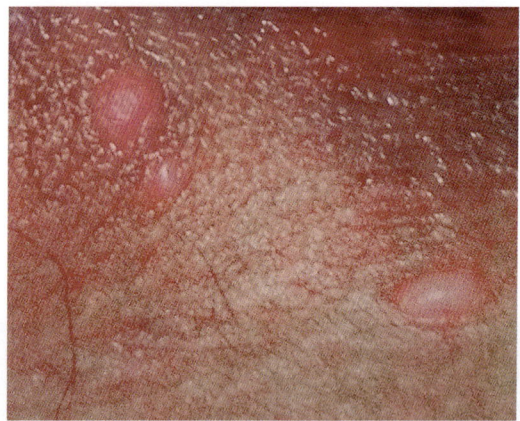

Answer the following as True/false statement:
1. These lesions are caused by sarcoptes scabiei.
2. This is caused by RNA virus.
3. A characteristic appearance of lesion is papules with central umbilication.
4. Lesions contain intranuclear bodies.

Ans.

1. False. Molluscum contagiosum. Labial lesions are flesh colored, dome-shaped papules with central umbilication.
2. False. Molluscum contagiosum is a DNA pox virus.
3. True
4. False. Molluscum bodies are large intracytoplasmic structure.

Reference

1. CDC 2021

OSCE 18. Answer the following:
1. How does genital TB cause infertility?
2. Enumerate four clinical features of female genital TB.

Ans.

1. Causes of infertility in tuberculosis are:
    - Fallopian tubes are involved in almost all cases of female genital TB (FGTB). It is often bilateral causing exosalpingitis and endosalpingitis with tubal blockage.
    - *Uterus:* TB affects endometrial receptivity with damage of endometrium and formation of intrauterine synechiae (Asherman's syndrome). Latent FGTB can cause recurrent implantation failure and recurrent miscarriages due to endometrial hostility through increased TNF-alpha (tumor necrosis factor-alpha) and interleukin 2 (IL-2) levels [17]. It also shifts T-helper cells response from T1 to T2.
    - TB causes oophoritis with poor ovarian reserve and increased need of gonadotropins for ovulation induction. It can also destroy ovaries.

Reference

1. Sharma JB, Sharma E, Sharma S, Dharmendra S. Recent Advances in Diagnosis and Management of Female Genital Tuberculosis. J Obstet Gynaecol India. 2021;71(5):476-87. doi: 10.1007/s13224-021-01523-9. Epub 2021 Aug 28. PMID: 34483510; PMCID: PMC8402974.

2. Female genital TB can have varied presentation as follow:
   - *Menstrual symptoms:* Abnormal uterine bleeding (AUB), oligomenorrhea, dysmenorrhea, amenorrhea
   - Infertility—primary or secondary
   - Lower abdominal pain
   - Pelvic pain
   - Abnormal vaginal discharge

OSCE 19.
1. **Enumerate four differential diagnosis of female genital TB.**
2. **What are the diagnostic modalities of female genital TB?**

Ans.

1. Abdominopelvic TB and FGTB are great mimickers and may be confused with other genital diseases such as ovarian cyst, vulval or vaginal cyst, ectopic pregnancy, endometriosis, genital malignancies, and other intestinal diseases (appendicitis, Crohn's disease), actinomycosis and various miscellaneous conditions (Schistosomiasis, filariasis, silicosis, leprosy, granuloma inguinale).
2. *Diagnostic Modalities for Female Genital Tuberculosis:*
   - Endometrial aspiration for AFB smear and culture, CBNAAT (Cartridge-based nucleic acid amplification test) or Gene Xpert.
   - *Radiological tests:* USG/MRI/CT to rule out tubo-ovarian masses.
   - *Endoscopic modalities:* Laparoscopy and hysteroscopy

OSCE 20.

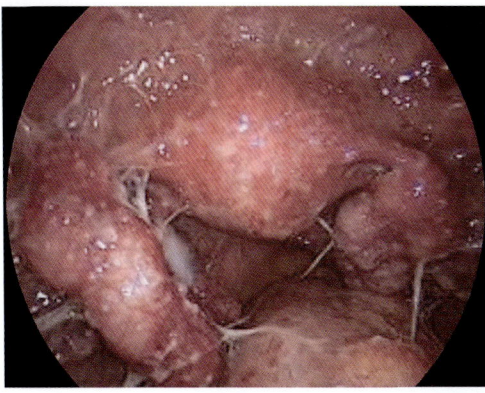 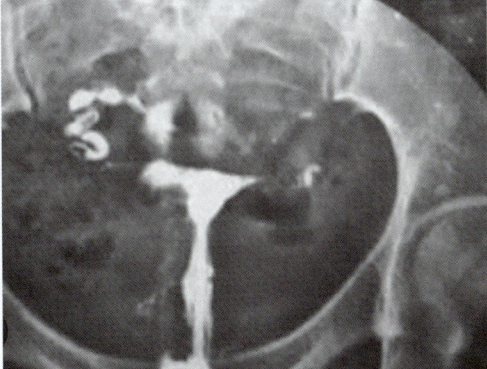

1. **Enumerate four laparoscopic findings of female genital TB.**
2. **Enumerate two hysteroscopic findings of female genital TB.**
3. **Enumerate four hysterosalpingogram findings of female genital TB.**

Ans.

1. Laparoscopic findings suggestive of genital TB may vary from normal appearance to tubercles on the surfaces, fimbrial block, fimbrial phimosis, tubal beading, peritubal adhesions, periovarian adhesion, tubo-ovarian mass, hydrosalpinx, and rigid tubes.
2. Hysteroscopic findings suggestive of genital tuberculosis include tubercles, pale endometrium, and intrauterine adhesions.
3. Hysterosalpingogram is contraindicated in the presence of recent acute pelvic infection. Hysterosalpingographic findings suggestive of female genital TB may be following:
    - Tubal occlusion
    - Tobacco-pouch appearance
    - Leopard skin appearance
    - Rosette appearance
    - Beaded appearance of tube
    - Coiling/calcified shadow
    - Distal tubal obstruction
    - Moth-eaten appearance
    - Bilateral cornual block
    - Irregular, honey-comb appearance of uterine cavity

OSCE 21.

1. What is the treatment of genital TB?
2. What is the treatment of genital TB during pregnancy? Should she be advised MTP?

Ans.

1. *Treatment of genital tuberculosis:*
   Intensive phase: Four drugs (RHZE)—75 mg/150 mg/400 mg/275 mg per FDC Tablet for 2 months and

   Continuation phase: Three drugs (HRE)—75 mg/150 mg/275 mg per FDC Tablet for 4 months
    - Dose depends on weight of the patient.
2. a. Both pulmonary and extrapulmonary TB can occur in pregnancy.
   b. Drug-sensitive TB must be treated with all the four drugs (RHZE) for 2 months and the three drugs (RHE) for 4 months even in first trimester of pregnancy.
   c. Drug-resistant TB patients should not conceive while on reserve drugs.
   d. Medical termination of pregnancy (MTP) is advised for MDR-TB in first trimester as reserve drugs can be teratogenic. If patient refuses MTP, then treatment is modified by excluding injections (kanamycin, amikacin, gentamycin, as they are fetotoxic) avoiding ethionamide till 32 weeks and after counseling the patient. Use of Bedaquiline though safe is still debatable in pregnancy.

CHAPTER 37

Polycystic Ovarian Syndrome

Seema Grover

OSCE 1.

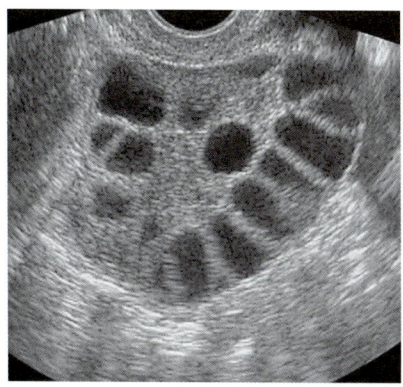

1. Spot the diagnosis.
2. What are the ultrasound criteria for diagnosis?
3. What are the symptoms and clinical signs that you will look for in such a patient?

Ans.

1. Polycystic ovary morphology (PCOM)
2. Ultrasonography indicating the presence of ≥12 follicles with a maximum diameter of 2–9 mm or any ovarian volume >10 mL.
3. Oligomenorrhea/Oligo-anovulation, obesity, hirsutism, acne, acanthosis nigricans.

OSCE 2.

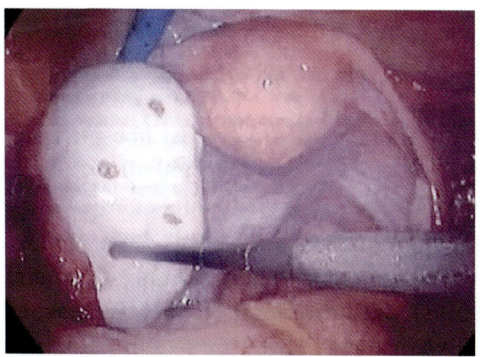

1. What is the surgery being done?
2. What is the instrument used for this procedure and what is rule-of-4?
3. Advantages of this laparoscopic procedure over medical options?

Ans.

1. Laparoscopic ovarian drilling (LOD).
2. LOD needle using monopolar cautery.
   Rule-of-4: Ovarian cortex is punctured at 4 sites, to a depth of 4 mm, for 4 seconds, each at 40 watts.
3. LOD is good for Clomiphene resistant cases. When LOD is compared to gonadotropins. Pregnancy rates are similar but disadvantages like OHSS and multiple pregnancy are minimal. This procedure improves ovarian response to clomiphene citrate in one-third of cases.

OSCE 3.

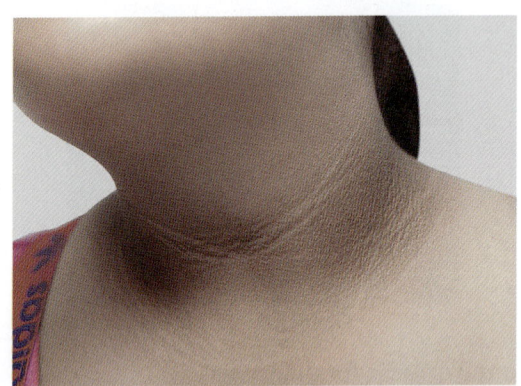

1. Spot the diagnosis.
2. Enumerate four causes for the above condition.
3. What is HAIR-AN syndrome?
4. What are the areas affected by this condition?

Ans.

1. Acanthosis Nigricans (AN)
2. *Causes:* Diabetes mellitus, PCOS, thyroid disorders, adrenal disease, obesity, and stomach cancer.
3. Hyperandrogenism (HA), Insulin resistance (IR) and Acanthosis Nigricans (AN)
4. Areas affected are nape of neck, armpits, groin, elbows, knees, and knuckles.

OSCE 4. A 24-year-old lady, married for 1 year, presented to the OPD with delayed menstrual cycles for last 1 year. She has also gained about 5 kg weight and there is recent hair growth on her chin and chest. She is visibly upset and wants proper evaluation.
1. What are the differential diagnoses in this case?
2. What investigations will you advise for this patient?
3. What are the medical treatment options if the patient fulfills Rotterdam criteria in this case?

Ans.

1. *Differential diagnosis:* Polycystic ovarian syndrome (PCOS), Cushing's syndrome, adult-onset CAH, hypothyroidism, hyperprolactinemia.
2. *Bloods investigations:* Fasting lipid panel, Fasting insulin level, blood sugar level, FSH and LH, testosterone, prolactin, thyroid function tests, DHEAS, dexamethasone suppression test, transabdominal ultrasonography
3. Trial of starting COCP with drospirenone for antiandrogen effects. Can also consider topical eflornithine cream for hirsutism. Addition of metformin if there is evidence of impaired glucose tolerance.

OSCE 5. A 26-year-old, married lady was taking COCP with Drospirenone for PCOS. She returns after one month of treatment, and during this period she had discussed about her PCOS with her local GP, who has told her that this condition can cause serious health issues later in life. She has come to you for expert opinion.
1. What are the pregnancy-related complications that she can develop?
2. Does she have an increased risk of gynecological cancer? Justify your answer.
3. Does she have an increased cardiovascular risk? Justify your answer.

Ans.

1. This patient can have infertility which affects 75% of women with PCOS. Pregnancy-related complications which can occur are spontaneous pregnancy loss, gestational diabetes, and pre-eclampsia.
2. She has an increased risk of endometrial hyperplasia and endometrial cancer because of hyperestrogenism due to oligomenorrhea/amenorrhea.
3. The PCOS patients have a *higher cardiovascular risk profile*, due to metabolic syndrome, insulin resistance, diabetes, hyperlipidemia, NAFLD and hypertension.

OSCE 6. Mrs Sunita, a 32-year-old lady with PCOS, is undergoing treatment for infertility from a specialist and is taking injections as she is planned for IVF in this cycle. One day she presents to her doctor with acute abdominal pain and vomiting. Ultrasound of pelvis was done, and these findings were noted in the ovary.

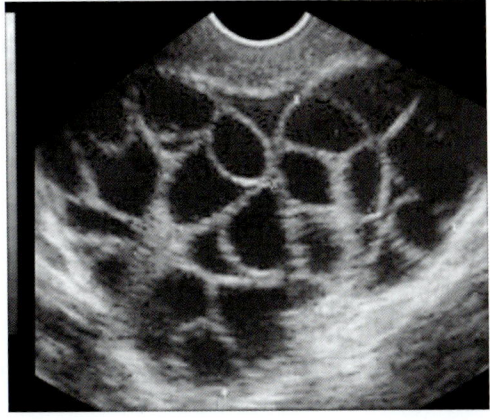

1. What complication has occurred in this case?
2. Enumerate three risk factors for this condition.
3. What are the clinical features if she develops a severe condition?

Ans.

1. Ovarian hyperstimulation syndrome (OHSS)
2. PCOS, high baseline AMH, low BMI, >25 oocytes collected, Elevated serum estradiol concentrations.
3. Clinical ascites, decreased urine output, dyspnea/pleural effusion.

OSCE 7. Mrs Sonia, 28 years, diagnosed with PCOS had been prescribed tablet Metformin by a junior doctor. But Mrs Sonia returns to discuss this treatment issue with the senior doctor since she is not a diabetic, and the chemist told her that Metformin is used to treat diabetes.
1. How will you explain to the patient that this tablet will be helpful for her condition?
2. What is the mechanism of action of Metformin?
3. What are the other insulin sensitizers?

Ans.

1. Tablet Metformin helps in restoring ovulation and helps to reduce weight. It reduces circulating androgen levels, hence for hirsuitism in PCOS patients. It should be used only with clinical evidence of insulin resistance.
2. Metformin reduces hepatic glucose production, stimulates glycolysis in liver, increases peripheral glucose uptake in liver, muscle and adipose tissue and improves insulin sensitivity.
3. Other insulin sensitizers used in PCOS are Pioglitazone, Roziglitazone, D-chiro Inositol and Myoinositol (postreceptor insulin sensitizer)

OSCE 8. An 18-year-old girl got an ultrasound done of whole abdomen, as advised by her doctor for abdominal pain. She is of average build and has regular cycles. Her ultrasound reported polycystic ovaries and subsequently she read about PCOS on the Internet and has become worried. She has come to you for expert opinion.
1. What is the difference between PCO and PCOS?
2. What are the Rotterdam criteria for diagnosis of PCOS?
3. Does PCO alone pose any risk for her future health?

Ans.

1. Around 25% of normal women meet ultrasound criteria of polycystic ovaries. Ovarian changes alone are a sign and not a disease.
2. Rotterdam (2003) Diagnostic criteria for PCOS—two out of three of:
    a. Clinical hyperandrogenism (Ferriman-Gallwey Score >8) or Biochemical Hyperandrogenism (Elevated Total/Free Testosterone) OR

b. Oligomenorrhea (Less than 6–9 menses per year) or oligo-ovulation OR
c. Polycystic ovaries on ultrasound (≥12 antral follicles in one ovary or ovarian volume ≥10 mL^3
3. Even with PCO alone, patients have increased risk of metabolic changes including insulin resistance, and increased risk of OHSS during IVF.

OSCE 9.

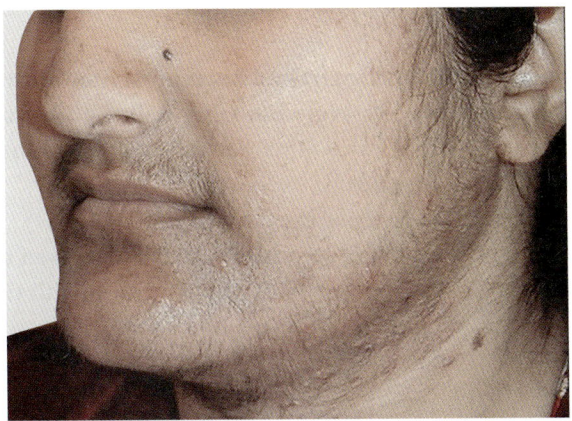

1. Identify and define the above condition.
2. Enumerate the broad causes for this condition.
3. What investigations would you advise in this condition?

Ans.

1. Hirsutism. This is defined as presence of excessive androgen responsive terminal coarse hairs in females and in a male-like distribution.
2. The causes of hirsutism can be ovarian, adrenal, drugs, genetic, or hepatic causes.
3. Investigations advised will be serum testosterone and free testosterone, DHEA levels, 17-OH levels, LH, FSH, LH:FSH ratio, ultrasound abdomen and pelvis.

OSCE 10. A 23-year-old college-going girl, presents with irregular cycles and hair growth on upper lip and chin. She is very concerned about the hair growth on her face and has many queries.

1. What are the various types of hair and how will you describe them?
2. Define hirsutism, virilism and hypertrichosis.
3. What is the association between androgens and hirsutism?

Ans.

1. There are three types of hair namely:
   a. *Lanugo hair:* This is lightly pigmented, covers the fetus and is shed early postpartum.
   b. *Vellus hair:* This is soft, usually nonpigmented and gradually replaces lanugo hair.
   c. *Terminal hair:* Its longer, coarser, darkly pigmented and arises from vellus hair. This is scalp hair, pubic, axillary hair, etc.

2. *Hirsutism* is an increase in transformation of vellus hair to terminal hair.

   Virilism: Extreme hyperandrogenism and apart from hirsutism it includes acne, amenorrhea, alopecia, decreased breast size, hoarseness of voice, increased muscle mass and clitoromegaly.

   Hypertrichosis: A diffuse increase in vellus hair growth which is not androgen dependent.
3. Hirsutism is due to an increase in level of androgen or increase in androgen sensitivity. Androgens convert lanugo hair and vellus hair into terminal hair.

OSCE 11. A 23-year-old college-going girl had been presented with irregular cycles and hair growth on upper lip and chin. On evaluation, her pelvic ultrasound shows polycystic ovarian morphology and LH/FSH ratio is >2. Other investigations are within normal limits. How will you plan her treatment?
1. Which are the drugs available for treatment for hirsutism?
2. What are the combined hormonal preparations that can be used in this case and why?
3. What is the medication available for local application for hirsutism and how does it work?

Ans.
1. a. Hormonal contraceptive
   b. Insulin sensitizers
   c. 5-alpha reductase agonists
   d. Spironolactone
   e. Glucocorticoids
2. Combined oral pills that can be used in this case are those which contain third and fourth generation progestins such as Gestodene, Desogestrel, Norgestimate, and Drospirenone. The advantages of these pills are that they suppress LH, hence reduce androgen production. They also decrease DHEAS from adrenals, and increase SHBG levels, thus they decrease-free testosterone.
3. Eflornithine, it inhibits L-Ornithine decarboxylase, an enzyme of dermal papilla, essential for controlling hair growth and proliferation. Hence, it makes the hair growth slow and much less coarse.

OSCE 12. A 30-year-old lady married for 3 years, is unable to conceive despite taking treatment from her GP. She has irregular and delayed menstrual cycles with scanty, sometimes heavy bleed. She has a family history of diabetes. On examination, she has findings of obesity and hirsutism. Investigations showed her LH/FSH ratio is >2, Serum Prolactin and TSH are within normal, HbA1c is 6.5%. Semen analysis of husband is normal. Her TVS shows multiple hypoechoic follicles in both ovaries. No dominant follicle is seen. She wants treatment for infertility.
1. What other investigations are to be advised?
2. Will you prescribe oral contraceptive pills for this patient? Justify your answer.
3. Which preparations of COC will you prescribe and for how long?

Ans.

1. Lipid profile, AMH, DHEAS, 17OHP, Basal AFC (Antral follicle count)
2. Yes, as Combined Oral Contraceptive (COC) helps to decrease LH surge, improve ovulation, and improve insulin resistance.
3. Preparations containing newer progestogens which are antiandrogenic like Gestodene, Norgestimate, Desogestrel, and Drospirenone are used and can be given for 3–6 months.

OSCE 13. A 30-year-old lady has been evaluated for infertility. She was diagnosed to have PCOS and has been taking combined oral contraceptive pills containing ethinyl estradiol and drospirenone for PCOS, as prescribed, for three months. Her cycles are regular now, and she has lost about 3 kg weight in this period. She wants treatment for conception.
1. What are the drugs you can give to this patient for ovulation induction?
2. Which drug will you prefer and why?
3. Role of laparoscopic ovarian drilling.

Ans.

1. First-line drugs for ovulation induction are clomiphene citrate and letrozole. In clomiphene-resistant cases, low-dose gonadotropins and glucocorticoids are used. Metformin helps as insulin sensitizer.
2. Letrozole is the preferred drug for ovulation induction in PCOS because it is associated with improved ovulation, pregnancy and live-birth rates compared to clomiphene citrate.
3. Laparoscopic ovarian drilling (LOD) is good for clomiphene-resistant cases. When LOD is compared to gonadotropins, pregnancy rates are similar but disadvantages such as OHSS and multiple pregnancy are minimal. This procedure improves ovarian response to CC in one-third of cases.

OSCE 14.

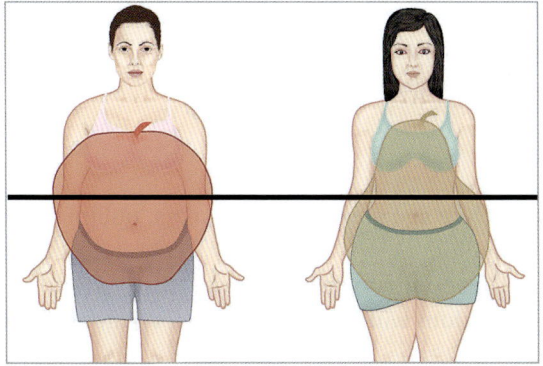

1. Which syndrome is associated with Apple-type obesity?
2. What are the components of this syndrome?
3. What other body measurements/ratio predict greater risk of chronic disease?

Ans.

1. Metabolic syndrome or syndrome X
2. *Metabolic syndrome criteria:* Abdominal obesity, high blood pressure, impaired fasting glucose, high triglyceride levels, and low HDL cholesterol levels. Insulin resistance is thought to be the uniting pathogenic factor.
3. a. *Waist circumference:* A larger waist circumference (>88 cm) in women.
   b. *Waist-to-hip ratio:* A ratio of greater than 0.80 in women.
   c. *Body fat percentage:* This can tell how much fat is stored in the body.

OSCE 15. A 38-year-old lady with a BMI of 33 kg/m² presents with irregular menstrual cycles for last 9 months. Her BP is 144/86 mm Hg, ultrasound shows bilateral bulky ovaries and grade 2 fatty liver.
1. What investigations would you advise in this case?
2. What is the newer medical management of obesity and its dose?
3. What is the cut-off value of BMI for bariatric surgery?

Ans.

1. Investigations required are fasting lipid profile, HbA1c, TFTs, LFTs, S.LH, and S. FSH, free testosterone.
2. New drug approved for obesity includes Orlistat. It promotes weight loss by decreasing fat absorption from the intestine. The dosage is 120 mg twice a day.
3. Cut-off BMI for bariatric surgery is 35 kg/m².

OSCE 16. A 36-year-old nulliparous woman, presented with heavy menstrual bleeding after 2 months of amenorrhea. Her cycles have become irregular for the last year, and she has been evaluated for PCOS and primary infertility. She had an ultrasound done which showed uterus size of 8 × 5 × 4 cm with endometrial thickness of 16 mm and polycystic ovaries.
1. What is your diagnosis?
2. What are the risk factors in this case for this condition?
3. How will you evaluate this patient further?
4. What are the medical management options?

Ans.

1. Endometrial hyperplasia
2. Risk factors in this case are age greater than 35 years, nulliparity, PCOS and unopposed estrogen due to anovulation.
3. Further evaluation will be by endometrial biopsy.
4. Medical management options will be progestogens for 6 months or Mirena IUCD.

OSCE 17.

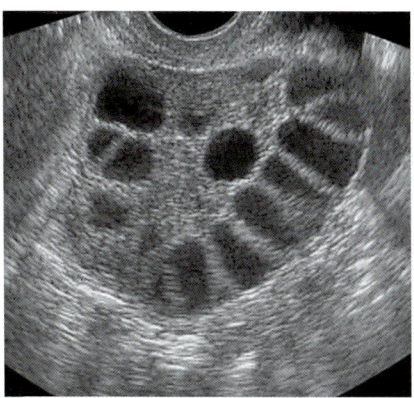

1. Spot the diagnosis.
2. Which sonographic parameter(s) is/are included as specific diagnostic cut-offs?
3. Why should ultrasound not be used for diagnosis of this condition in patients <8 years after menarche?
4. What biochemical markers are tested in this condition?

Ans.

1. PCOM
2. Ultrasound criteria consist of presence of 12 or more follicles within the ovary with a diameter of 2–9 mm and/or ovarian volume 10 cm^3 or greater.
3. Ultrasound should not be used for diagnosis of this disease for patients who present <8 years after menarche (age <20 years) due to the high incidence of multi-follicular ovaries in this stage of life.
4. Biochemical tests done are Serum FSH, LH, Free Testosterone, DHEAS, and AMH levels.

OSCE 18. A 23-year-old unmarried woman works in a computer shop as sales manager. She has been having irregular bleeding since 8 months. Her cycle seems to be always changing, sometimes every 2 weeks, sometimes once in two months. She has some spots on her face due to acne, and coarse hair on upper lip and chest. She has also experienced weight gain and she is upset due to all these symptoms. There is no history of skin changes, weight loss, tiredness, myalgia, constipation. No striae present.

1. What investigations would you advise for this patient?
2. What is the role of lifestyle modifications in an adolescent PCOS patient?
3. What lifestyle changes would you advise?

Ans.

1. *Blood investigations:* Fasting lipid panel, fasting blood glucose, FSH and LH, testosterone, prolactin, TFTs, dexamethasone suppression test—transabdominal USG.
2. *Role of lifestyle modifications:* It reduces insulin resistance, improves menstrual regularity, normalizes hyperandrogenism, improves metabolic rate, reduces incidence of diabetes, and improves pregnancy rate.

3. Lifestyle changes advised would be to eat a balanced diet, low in fat, low in carbohydrate, and high in protein. Emphasis should be on eating at regular intervals in small quantities, increasing fiber intake, increase low glycemic index foods, and decrease refined foods. Exercising 150 minutes per week helps to burn calories and boost metabolism.

OSCE 19. A 30-year-old unmarried lady presented with irregular periods since two years. Her previous menstrual cycles were of variable duration, from one to three months, and she had decreased flow lasting only for two days. There is a history of recent weight gain of about 5 kg. On examination, there was no abnormal finding except for increased BMI of 28 kg/m^2.
1. What is the differential diagnosis in this case?
2. What are other important points to ask in history?
3. What investigations would you advise?
4. How can USG pelvis help in making the diagnosis?

Ans.

1. Hypothyroidism, PCOS, hyperprolactinemia, premature ovarian insufficiency (POI)
2. If there is family history of PCOS, early menopause or autoimmune disorders.
3. CBC, blood sugar, serum TSH, serum prolactin, day 3 serum FSH, serum estradiol, AMH and ultrasound pelvis.
4. If ovarian volume >10 mL and number of antral follicles >12 per ovary: diagnosis in favor of PCOS. If ovarian volume is less than 5 mL and only 1–2 antral follicles per ovary, diagnosis is in favor of POI.

OSCE 20. A young unmarried girl of 16 years presents with history of irregular cycles and heavy menstrual bleeding. On examination, her BMI was 27 kg/sqm, and she had hirsutism on upper lip and chest.
1. What are the causes of puberty menorrhagia?
2. How will you explain the cause of HMB after amenorrheal at this age?
3. How will you investigate this case?
4. How will you manage this case?

Ans.

1. Causes are anovulatory cycles due to immature HPO axis, hypothyroidism, PCOS, von Willebrand's disease.
2. The cause of HMB is anovulation, no progesterone production, excessive proliferation of endometrium, endometrial hyperplasia, and instability. It is associated with stromal breakdown, dilated and unstable venous capillaries and bleeding.
3. Investigations advised are urine pregnancy test, CBC with PBF, ESR, Mantoux and chest X-ray, CT, PTI INR, FSH, LH, TFT, ultrasound pelvis.
4. *Management:* No anemia should be corrected by giving iron tablets. Nonhormonal treatment can be done by giving NSAIDs or tablet tranexamic acid 500 mg thrice a day for 5 days. Hormonal treatment can be by cyclical progesterone 10 mg/day for 21 days or oral contraceptives, continuous or cyclical.

CHAPTER 38

Pelvic Organ Prolapse (I)

Panchanan Das

OSCE 1.

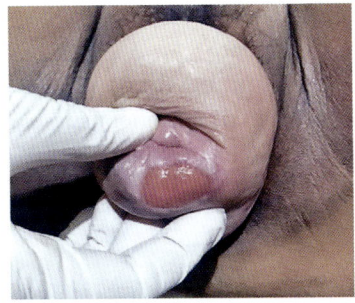

The above picture of POP (pelvic organ prolapse) shows an ulcer over posterior lip of cervix.
1. What is the cause of development of such ulcers?
2. What is the treatment of these ulcers?
3. If the ulcer doesn't heal after conservative treatment, what is the next step?
4. Looking at the margins, can it be a malignant ulcer?

Ans.

1. Due to chronic venous congestion.
2. Reposition of POP with vaginal tampons soaked in antiseptic (acriflavine/povidone-iodine) and hygroscopic solution (glycerine).
3. Biopsy from the ulcer margin
4. No.

OSCE 2.

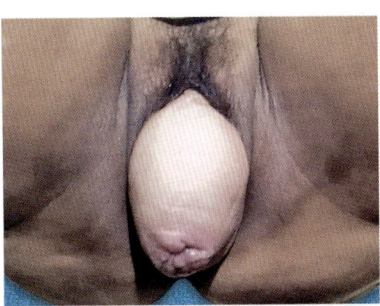

In the above picture of POP:
1. What kind of anterior vaginal wall defect is seen?
2. How do you differentiate between different types of anterior vaginal wall defects in cases of POP?
3. What extra surgical steps need to be done during repair in a case of lateral vaginal wall defect?

Ans.

1. Midline or distension anterior wall defect.
2. a. *Absence of rugosities:* Midline defect
      Presence of rugosities: Lateral defect
   b. On Valsalva after elevating anterior vaginal wall with sponge holder or split speculum:
      - *Midline defect:* Absence of defect
      - *Lateral defect:* Vaginal wall protrudes from both sides.
3. Vaginal wall to be dissected up to arcus tendineous fascia pelvis (ATFP) and paravaginal connective tissue is anchored to it or to obturator internus fascia, if ATFP is not visible.

OSCE 3.

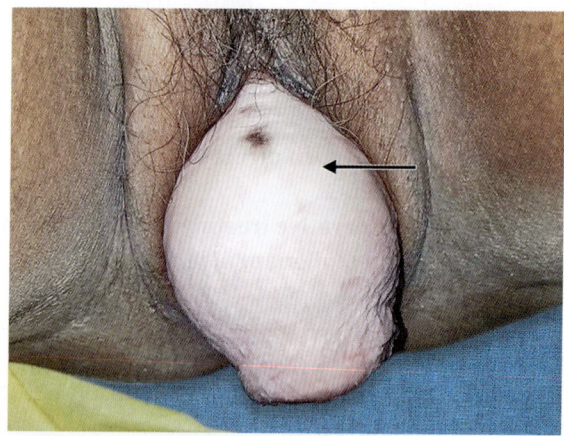

1. How can one say that it is or is not a case of procidentia?
2. Identify the area shown with arrow and the causative pathology behind it.
3. Does this type of area alter the management of POP?

Ans.

1. In procidentia, we can get above the swelling and the entire vagina would be everted.
2. Keratinized area. Its causative pathology is prolonged chronic exposure to atmosphere.
3. No.

OSCE 4. Regarding POP-Q system:
1. Who introduced this system and when?
2. What does point C refer to in pre- and posthysterectomy cases?
3. Point D is omitted in cases of_____.

4. Which point in the POP-Q system can differentiate between uterosacral ligament support failure and cervical elongation?

Ans.
1. International Continence Society in 1996.
2. Prehysterectomy—most distal edge of the cervix and posthysterectomy—leading edge of vaginal cuff.
3. Absence of cervix.
4. Point D.

OSCE 5. The POP-Q findings of a patient is as follows:

Aa	Ba	C
+3	+5	+6
GH	PB	TVL
+5	+2	10
Ap	Bp	D
+3	+5	+4

1. What is the stage of prolapse in this case?
2. All these measurements are done with Valsalva, except.
3. How is genital hiatus measured?
4. How POP-Q is better than other conventional POP classification systems?

Ans.
1. Stage 3
2. TVL
3. Middle of external urethral meatus to midline of posterior hymenal ring.
4. a. High intra- and interexaminer reliability
   b. Measures site-specific components and quantification of different compartments.

OSCE 6. A 65-year-old, obese lady came with complaints of something coming out per vagina since 10 years and involuntary leakage of urine on coughing since two years.
1. What is the type of urinary incontinence and the cause of such incontinence in a case of utero-vaginal prolapse?
2. What is the significance of a positive Bonney's test in a case of SUI?
3. Q-tip testing is done to determine _____.
4. The technique of plicating bladder neck that is traditionally being used for POP with SUI is _____.

Ans.
1. Stress urinary incontinence (SUI). Its cause is anatomical distortion of the angle between the urethra and urinary bladder.
2. Positive Bonney test indicates higher chances of curing SUI following surgical correction.
3. Urethral hypermobility
4. Kelly's plication.

OSCE 7. Answer the following:
1. In absence of POP, the upper vagina lies nearly vertical in standing position—true/false.
2. Name the different components of levator ani muscle.
3. The parietal fascia covering the medial aspects of obturator internus and levator ani muscles is known as _____.
4. The fibromuscular layer of tissues all around the vagina is known as _____.
5. Rectocele occurs due to defect in the De Lancey level _____ support.

Ans.
1. False
2. Pubococcygeus, ischiococcygeus and iliococcygeus
3. Arcus tendineus fascia pelvis
4. Endopelvic fascia
5. Level 2.

OSCE 8.
1. Name two commonly used questionnaires used to assess severity of POP.
2. Which symptom most strongly correlates with POP?
3. Urodynamic testing should be done in all patients of POP with urinary symptoms—true/ false
4. Which type of urinary incontinence is more commonly associated with POP?

Ans.
1. a. Pelvic floor distress inventory (PFDI)
   b. Pelvic floor impact questionnaire (PFIQ)
2. Bulge symptoms
3. False
4. Stress urinary incontinence (SUI)

OSCE 9.
1. Name two surgical procedures that can be done during surgery of POP to prevent vault prolapse.
2. What is the use of Miya hook in prolapse surgery?
3. What is the use of Kelly's plication?
4. What is the complete name of vaginal hysterectomy surgery?

Ans.
1. a. McCall's culdoplasty
   b. Sacrospinous fixation
2. To pass thread in sacrospinous fixation
3. Treatment of SUI
4. Ward-Mayo's vaginal hysterectomy.

OSCE 10.

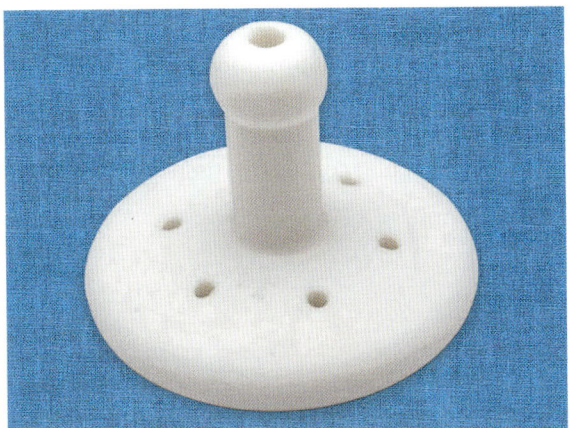

1. Identify the device along with its category.
2. It is used in which stages of prolapse?
3. Mention two complications associated with it.
4. What are the follow-up recommendations?

Ans.
1. Gelhorn pessary, space-filling pessary
2. Stage 3 and 4 prolapse
3. Vaginal discharge, odor, excoriation, irritation, vesicovaginal fistula, small bowel entrapment.
4. After initial fitting, the patient should return after 1–2 weeks and then after 4–6 weeks depending on her independence with pessary and proficiency of use. After this initial follow-up, she should come every 6–12 monthly.

OSCE 11.

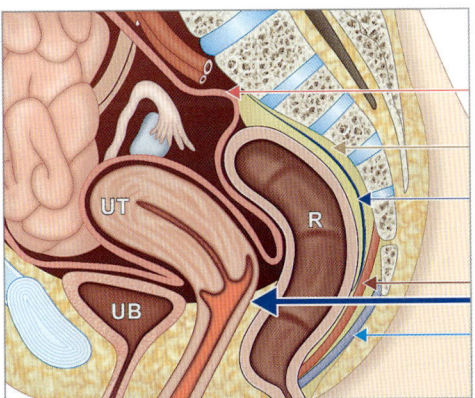

1. Identify the structure marked with dark blue arrow.
2. Mention its composition along with its attachment.
3. What does the apical compartment support include?

Ans.

1. Denonvillier's (pararectal) fascia
2. It is composed of fibromuscular layer of posterior vaginal wall which is laterally attached to the fascia levator ani.
3. a. Cardinal/uteroscaral ligament
   b. Upper paravaginal fibromuscular connective tissue
   c. Paracervical fascia

OSCE 12.

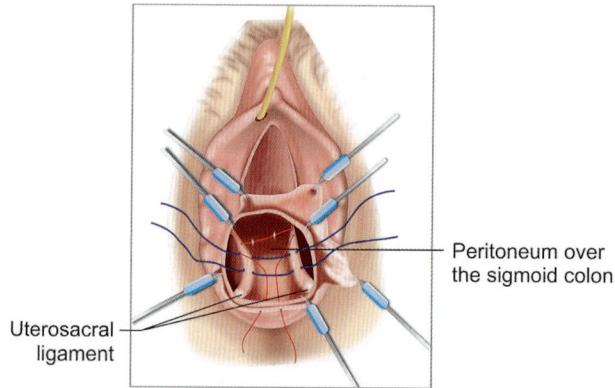

1. Identify the procedure in blue and red stitches.
2. What is the ideal suture material and space between two rows?
3. Mention the advantages of the above procedure.

Ans.

1. a. *Red:* External McCall culdoplasty
   b. *Blue:* Internal McCall culdoplasty
2. 2-0 gauze permanent suture; 0.5–1 cm
3. a. It adds support to posterior vaginal wall prolapse
   b. Prevents enterocele formation

OSCE 13.

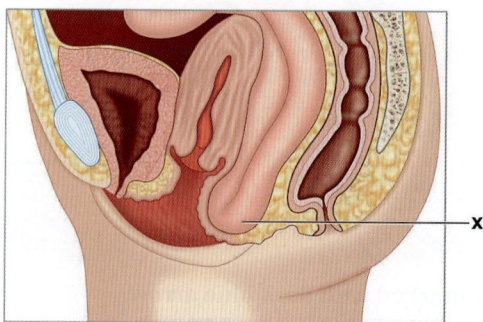

1. What does the area marked (×) in the above picture signify?
2. How do you differentiate it from rectocele?

3. Mention the only true hernia in POP.
4. What are the different reflexes tested in POP examination?

Ans.

1. Enterocele
2. a. *Enterocele:* Apical segment of the posterior vaginal wall bulge is seen and in rectovaginal examination small bowel can be palpated.
   b. *Rectocele:* Bulge in seen in the distal posterior wall and in rectovaginal examination bowel can't be palpated.
3. Enterocele
4. Bulbocavernous reflex and anal wink reflex

OSCE 14. A postmenopausal lady underwent some vaginal operation for POP 10 years ago, now she has come with something coming out per vagina which increases on coughing, standing and decreases on lying down.
1. Enumerate four causes for it.
2. On inspection, how you will differentiate stage three uterovaginal prolapse from vault prolapse?
3. What is the indication of sacrospinous fixation?
4. What is LeForts operation?

Ans.

1. a. Cystocele
   b. Rectocele
   c. Recurrent uterovaginal prolapse
   d. Vault prolapse
2. In UV prolapse, cervical opening is seen, it is absent in vault prolapse.
3. After repair of UV prolapse, if most distal part comes up to the level of hymen.
4. Partial vaginal occlusion.

OSCE 15.

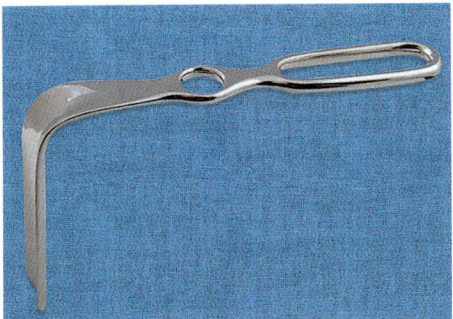

1. Name the instrument.
2. Mention its uses in vaginal hysterectomy.
3. What other instruments can be used in place of it?
4. How is bladder injury detected and repaired during pelvic floor repair surgery?

Ans.
1. Landon vaginal retractor.
2. To retract the urinary bladder.
3. Sim's speculum.
4. Bladder injury is detected by leakage of urine during surgery and is repaired in the same setting. Bladder is repaired in two layers with 2-0 delayed absorbable threads.

OSCE 16.

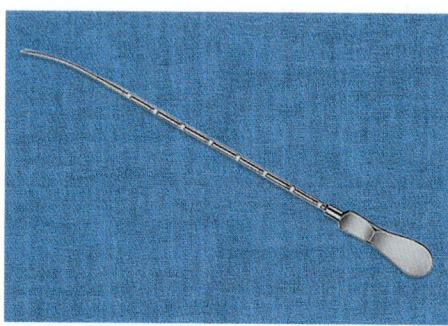

1. Name the instrument.
2. What is its role in prolapse surgery?
3. After operation, if the patient becomes pregnant, what complication she may have in early pregnancy, how is it diagnosed and treated?

Ans.
1. Metallic, graduated, and angulated uterine sound.
2. It will measure the uterocervical canal, length of cervical canal and give measurements as to what cervical length is to be amputated.
3. *Cervical incompetence:* It is diagnosed with ultrasonography if cervical length is <2.5 cm. It is treated with cervical encirclage stitch.

OSCE 17. A 60-year-old, para 4, postmenopausal lady with diabetic nephropathy presents with heaviness in the pelvis. On examination, she is stage 1 POP.
1. What are the nonsurgical treatment options for this patient?
2. Which group of muscle needs training in one of the nonsurgical procedures? How can you evaluate the strength and tone of these muscles?
3. Mention the advantages of the above treatment.

Ans.
1. PFMT (pelvic floor muscle training or Kegel exercise) and pessary
2. *Levator ani:* The strength and tone can be assessed by placing the index finger 2–3 cm inside the hymen at 4 and 8 o'clock. Both resting and contraction tone and strength of levator ani are thus evaluated.
3. a. Prevents further POP
   b. Regular muscle strength training builds permanent muscle volume and structural support.

Chapter 38: Pelvic Organ Prolapse (I)

OSCE 18. A postsacrocolpopexy patient presents to you with complaints of hematuria and occasional vaginal bleeding and pain after 3 months following surgery.
1. What is your provisional diagnosis?
2. What is the role of urologist in this case?
3. What should be the next line of treatment?

Ans.
1. Mesh erosion
2. Cystoscopy to look for bladder erosion and assist in mesh removal.
3. Relaparotomy and removal of the mesh and repair of bladder and pelvic tissue.

OSCE 19.
1. Match the following:

A. 27 years, Para 1, stage 2 POP	i. Ring pessary
B. 87 years, DM, HTN, old MI	ii. Vaginal hysterectomy
C. POP-Q stage 2 with atypical endometrial hyperplasia	iii. Ischial spine
D. Sacrospinous fixation	iv. McCall's culdoplasty
E. Uterosacral ligament stump	v. No.1 prolene suture
	vi. Sling operation

Ans.
1. A (vi), B (i), (C) ii, D (v), (E) iv

OSCE 20. 73-year-old, menopausal lady presents with acute retention of urine, examination reveals procidentia with large cystocele.
1. Mention the immediate measure to relieve her symptoms.
2. If POP is nonreducible, how is it managed?
3. On investigation, her serum creatinine is 3 mg/dL:
   a. Can elevated creatinine be an effect of prolapse?
   b. If yes, where is the pathology?

Ans.
1. Indwelling catheterization to keep the bladder evacuated.
2. To reduce the tissue edema, compress the prolapsed mass with towel soaked in hot water and proper lubrication. Elevated foot end can also help to reduce edema.
3. a. Yes
   b. At the level of uterosacral and cardinal ligament. Elongated uterosacral and cardinal ligament compresses the ureter, causing nephropathy with elevated creatinine level.

Reference
1. William's Gynecology (Indian Edition) Reprint 2020.

CHAPTER 39

Pelvic Organ Prolapse (II)

Reena Wani, Krutika Ramdin

OSCE 1.

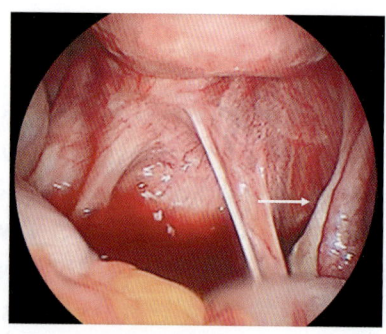

1. Identify the structure.
2. Which level is it of de Lancey levels of support system?
3. List the major supports of the uterus.
4. State the origin and insertion of the structure.

Ans.

1. Uterosacral ligament
2. Level 1
3. Uterosacral ligament, Mackenrodt ligament
4. Origin—posterolateral aspect of cervix at the level of internal os and insertion at anterior aspect of the sacrum.

OSCE 2.

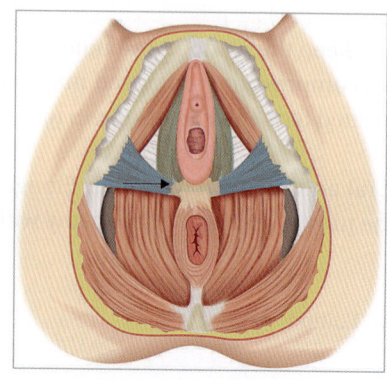

1. Identify the structure.
2. Name the muscles inserting in it.
3. Which defect can be caused if it is damaged?
4. List the options for repair.

Ans.

1. Perineal body
2. Levator ani, bulbospongiosus muscle, superficial and deep transverse perineal muscles, external anal sphincter muscle, external urethral sphincter muscle fiber.
3. Lax perineum, widening of introitus
4. Perineorrhaphy, levator stitch

OSCE 3.

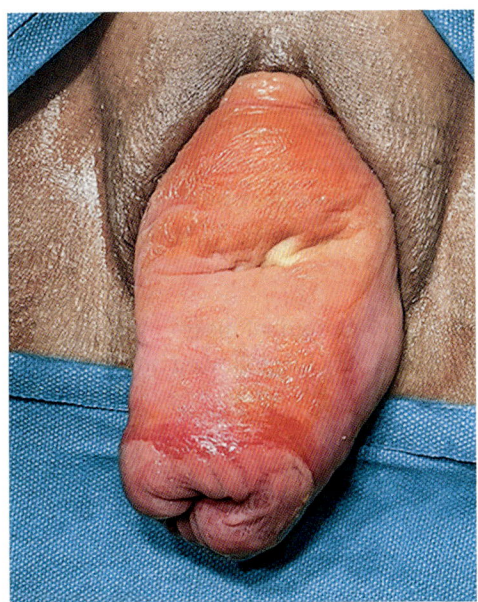

1. State the degree of UV descent.
2. Name one classification system of prolapse.
3. How many grades of cystoceles are listed?
4. What is 4th grade of cystocele?

Ans.

1. Third degree
2. POP Q
3. Four grades
4. Bladder is outside the introitus at rest.

OSCE 4.

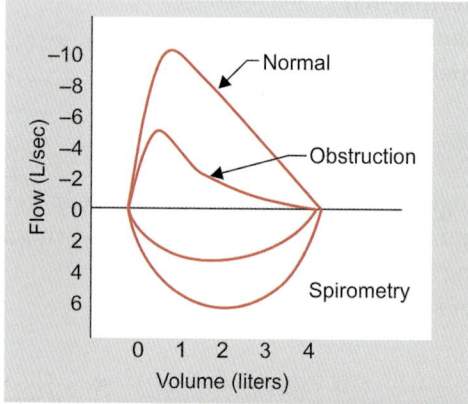

A 67-year-old lady with the above pathological condition came with grade 3 UV descent.
1. Identify the predisposing condition.
2. Enumerate two other predisposing conditions which can cause prolapse.
3. What would be the treatment options?
4. If associated with prolapse would surgery be recommended?

Ans.

1. COPD
2. Previous instrumental delivery, abdominal mass
3. Initial treatment would be cure of COPD followed by repair of prolapse
4. Yes, after cure of COPD

OSCE 5.

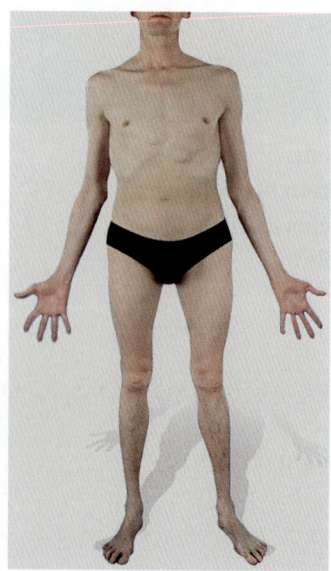

1. Identify the condition.
2. Can the condition lead to prolapse?
3. Enumerate four precipitating factors causing prolapse.
4. What are the other problems associated with this condition?

Ans.

1. Marfans syndrome
2. Yes
3. Postmenopausal atrophy, weight lifting, obesity, COPD, constipation.
4. Mitral valve prolapse, aortic aneurysm.

OSCE 6.

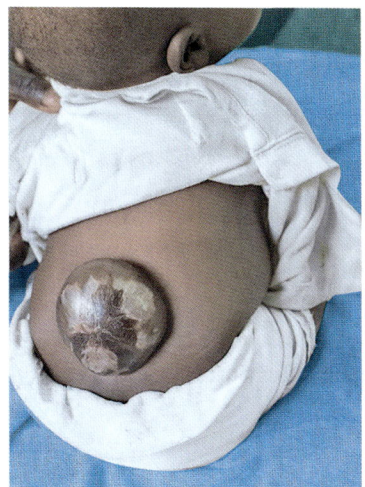

1. Identify the condition.
2. Can it predispose to prolapse?
3. Name two other predisposing factors of prolapse.
4. How can this condition be prevented?

Ans.

1. Spina bifida
2. Yes, in later life
3. Marfans syndrome, abdominal mass
4. Prevention by folic acid consumption

OSCE 7. A multiparous postmenopausal woman has come with a bulge near urinary meatus.

1. Identify the possible condition.
2. Enumerate two differential diagnosis
3. Enumerate two clinical symptoms of the condition.
4. What is the treatment?

Ans.

1. Urethrocele
2. Urethral caruncle, suburethral diverticulum
3. Urinary urgency, nocturnal enuresis
4. Surgical repair

OSCE 8.

Anterior wall Aa	Anterior wall Ba	Cervix or cuff C
Genital hiatus gh	Perineal body pb	Total vaginal length tvl
Posterior wall Ap	Posterior wall Bp	Posterior fornix D

1. What is the name of the classification?
2. What does point Bp signify.
3. State two drawbacks of the classification.
4. What is stage three of this classification?

Ans.

1. POP-Q classification
2. The most distal position of any descending part of the posterior vaginal wall.
3. Reference point is hymen which is not seen in most women with prolapse, staging is complicated.
4. The prolapse extends more than 1 cm beyond the hymenal ring, but there is no complete vaginal eversion.

OSCE 9.

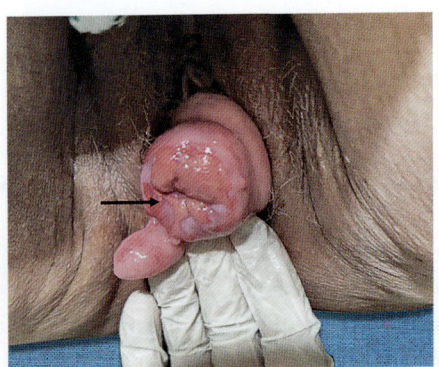

1. State the diagnosis.
2. What is the treatment plan?
3. Enumerate two complications associated with it.
4. What is the definitive management if her family is complete?

Ans.

1. Decubitus ulcer with polyp and 3rd degree UV decent.
2. Biopsy of decubitus ulcer and DnC polypectomy, repair of prolapse.
3. Leukorrhea, irregular bleeding, dyspareunia
4. Vaginal hysterectomy with repair

OSCE 10.

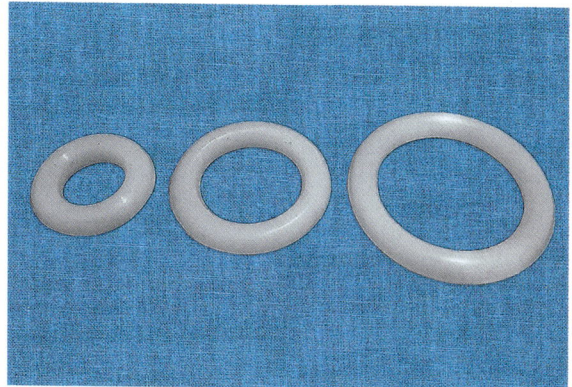

1. Identify the device.
2. Enumerate two indications for its use
3. Enumerate two contraindications of using it.
4. Describe the method of insertion.
5. Enumerate two complications of usage.

Ans.

1. Ring pessary
2. Young women desiring for future pregnancy, patients unfit or unwilling for hysterectomy.
3. Presence of unhealthy cervix, pregnancy, decubitus ulcer
4. Requires initial gynecologist evaluation for size, and then patient can be taught to insert.
5. Erosions, sepsis.

OSCE 11.

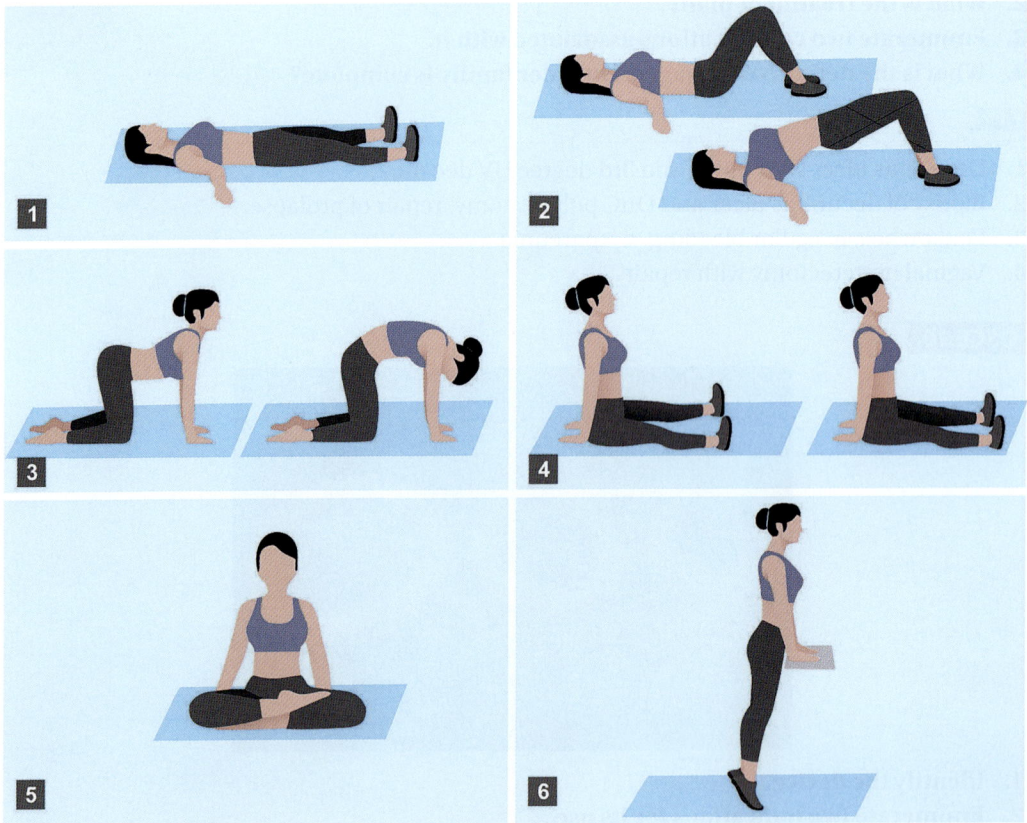

1. Name the exercise.
2. What is the indication for these exercises?
3. What is the benefits of this?
4. What other conservative management is possible?

Ans.

1. Kegels exercise
2. For strengthening the supports of uterus (nonsurgical option)
3. Increasing the strength of supports of uterus thus preventing prolapse
4. Vaginal ring pessary

OSCE 12.

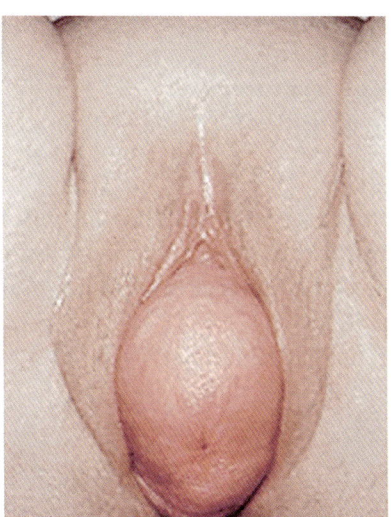

1. Identify the defect.
2. What is the contributary factor for the condition?
3. Name the procedure for correcting it.
4. Enumerate two complications of the procedure.

Ans.

1. Pubocervical fascia defect
2. Presence of uterine descent
3. Anterior colporrhaphy
4. Postoperative bleeding, surgical trauma, urinary urge incontinence.

OSCE 13.

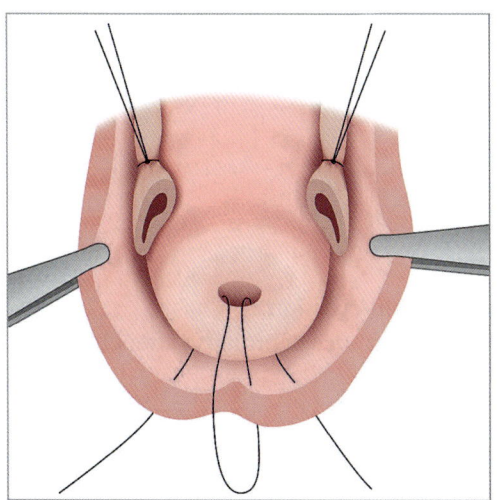 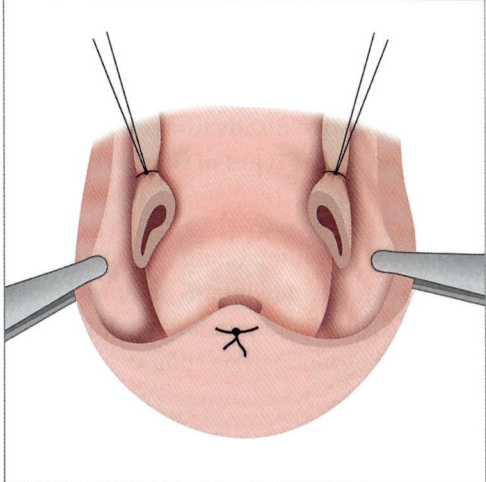

1. What is the indication for the surgery?
2. What are the principles of the surgery?
3. What is the name of the procedure?
4. Enumerate one drawback of the procedure.
5. What is the name of the modification?

Ans.

1. Young patient who wishes to preserve her childbearing function with cervical elongation.
2. Vaginal wall is dissected around the cervix, uterosacral ligament is dissected and brought forward and sutured in front of the cervix after cervical amputation.
3. Fothergill/Manchester operation
4. Cervical amputation thus reducing the fertility
5. Fothergill's modification

OSCE 14.

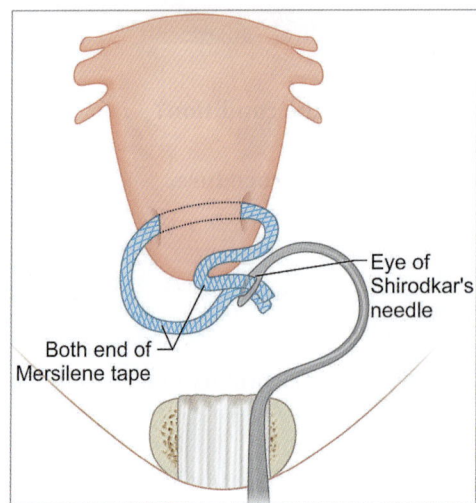

1. What is the name of the procedure?
2. Enumerate two advantages of the procedure.
3. Enumerate two disadvantages of the procedure.
4. Name two other types of sling surgery.

Ans.

1. Shirodkar abdominal sling
2. Fertility sparing, maintains anatomical position and anteversion.
3. Technically difficult, static sling, increased risk of recurrence of prolapse after childbirth.
4. Virkud sling, Soonawala sling

OSCE 15.

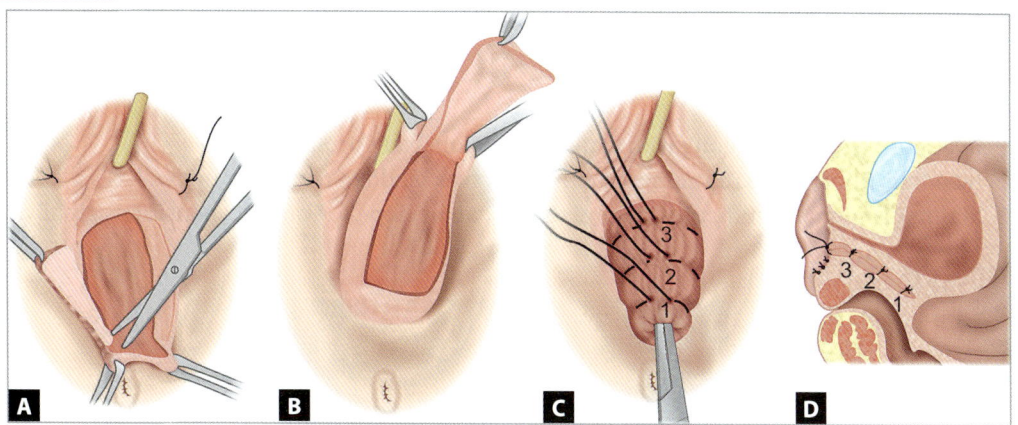

1. What is the name of the procedure?
2. Enumerate two indications for the procedure.
3. Enumerate two advantages of the procedure.
4. Enumerate two disadvantages of the procedure.

Ans.

1. Modified Le Fort's partial procedure.
2. Surgically unfit patients, patient not willing for hysterectomy.
3. Defect of three levels are repaired simultaneously, can be done under short anesthesia/local.
4. Postoperative SUI, sexual dysfunction

OSCE 16.

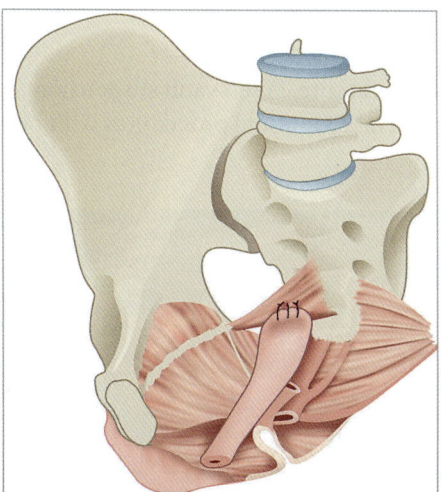

1. Identify the procedure.
2. What is the indication for the procedure?

3. Enumerate two complications of the procedure.
4. Enumerate two advantages of the procedure.

Ans.

1. Sacrospinous fixation
2. In grade 3, UV decent along with vault suspension, vault prolapse.
3. Bleeding, injury to surrounding structures such as bladder, rectum or ureter.
4. Maintains vaginal depth, uses natural tissue, can be done for vault suspension vaginally.

OSCE 17.

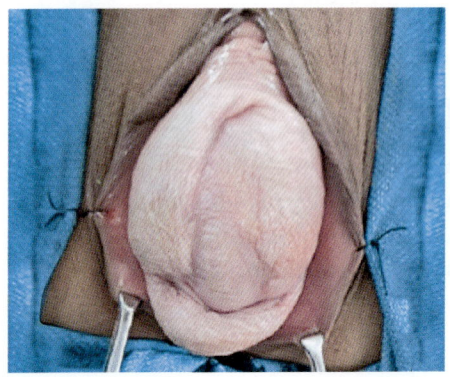

1. Identify the condition.
2. State the previous procedure she underwent.
3. Enumerate two predisposing factors for the condition.
4. What is the management?

Ans.

1. Vault prolapse
2. Hysterectomy
3. Increased intra-abdominal pressure, failed vault suspension.
4. Vault suspension by vaginal or abdominal procedures with perineal repair as needed.

OSCE 18.

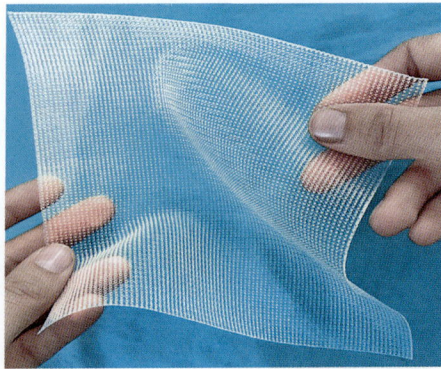

1. Identify the picture.
2. What is the name of the material from which it is made?
3. Enumerate two procedures where it is used.
4. Enumerate two complications.

Ans.

1. Pelvic mesh
2. Polypropylene mesh
3. Hernia repair, pelvic organ prolapse sling surgeries
4. Mesh erosion, infection, sinus formation

OSCE 19. A 60-year-old, P5L4 previous all normally delivered came with complain of something coming out of vagina since 2 years.
1. Enumerate two differential diagnosis.
2. Enumerate two predisposing factors for the condition.
3. How would you manage the case?
4. Do we need any specific local treatment before surgery?

Ans.

1. Polyp, prolapse of uterus, cystocele
2. Previous vaginal deliveries, multiparity
3. Hysterectomy along with colporrhaphy/pelvic floor repair
4. In case of atrophic vaginitis or decubitus ulcer, estrogen cream and packing can be done.

OSCE 20.

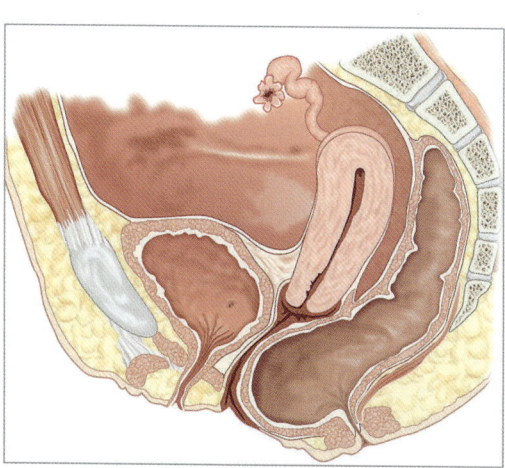
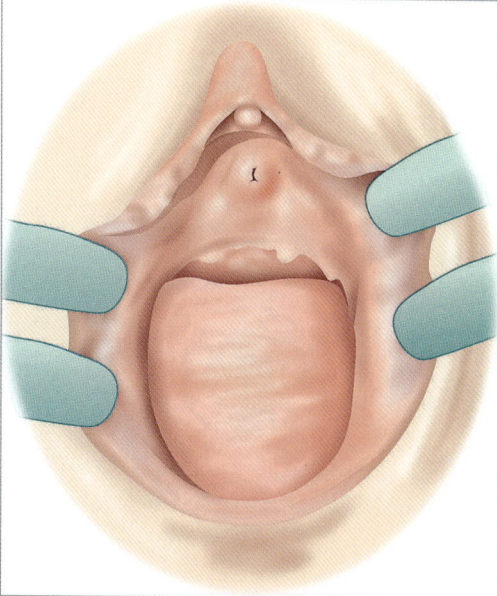

1. What is the defect?
2. Enumerate two clinical symptoms.
3. Name the surgery done for the defect.
4. Enumerate two complications of the procedure.

Ans.

1. Rectocele, defect in middle one-third of posterior vaginal wall
2. Difficulty in passage of stools, local bulge/discomfort, dyspareunia
3. Colpoperineorrhaphy
4. Injury to the rectum, infection

REFERENCES

1. Modern Gynaecology Virkud, 4th edition.
2. 20th edition, Grays anatomy.
3. Te Linde's Operative Gynaecology. Philadelphia, PA: Lippincott Williams & Wilkins, 2003.
4. Berek & Novak's Gynecology. Philadelphia: Wolters Kluwer Health/Lippincott Williams & Wilkins, 2012.

CHAPTER 40

Reproductive Medicine and Surgery

Fessy Louis T

OSCE 1.

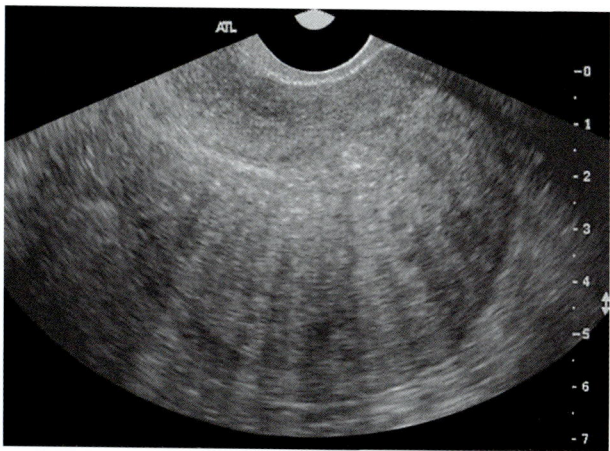

1. Identify the condition.
2. Enumerate ultrasound features of this condition.

Ans.

1. Adenomyosis
2. MUSA (Morphological Uterine Sonographic Assessment) criteria:
   Direct features:
   - Myometrial cysts
   - Hyperechogenic islands
   - Echogenic subendometrial lines and buds

   Indirect features:
   - Fan-shaped shadowing
   - Translesional vascularity
   - Irregular/interrupted junctional zone
   - Asymmetrical myometrial thickening
   - Globular uterus

OSCE 2.

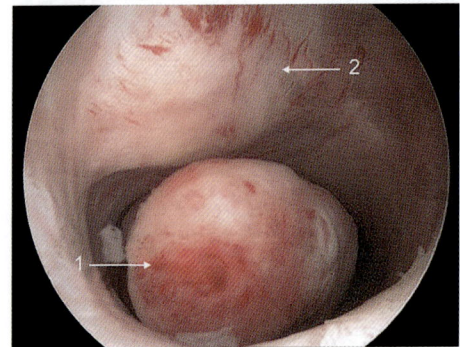

1. Identify the 1 and 2 in the image.
2. Enumerate the different classification systems for this condition.

Ans.

1. a. 1—Type 0—submucous myoma
   b. 2—Type 2—intramural myoma
2. Classification systems for fibroids:
   - FIGO classification
   - LASMAR classification
   - STEP-W classification

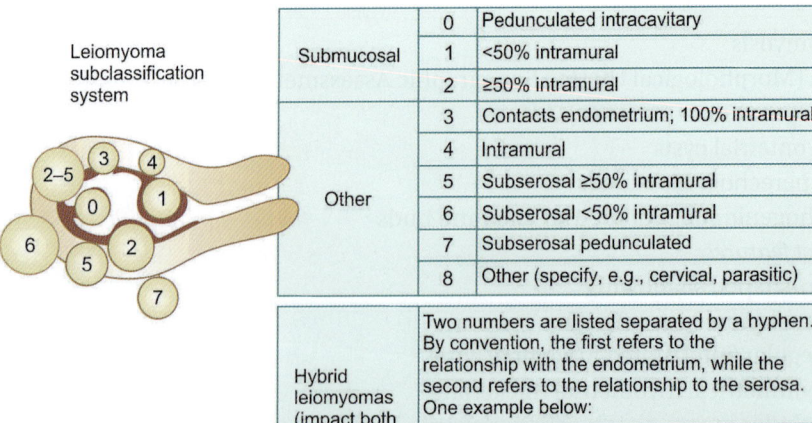

Chapter 40: Reproductive Medicine and Surgery

STEPW submucous fibroid classification.

	Size (cm)	Topography	Extension of the base	Penetration	Lateral wall	Total
0	<2	Low	<1/3	0		
1	>2 and 5	Middle	>1/3–2/3	<50%	+1	
2	>5	Upper	>2/3	>50%		
Score	•	•	•	•	•	

Score	Group	Complexity and therapeutic options
0–4	I	Low complexity hyteroscopic myomectomy
5–6	II	• High complexity hysteroscopic myomectomy, consider GnRH use? • Consider two-step hysteroscopic myomectomy
7–9	III	Consider alternatives to the hysteroscopic technique

Source: Lasmar new classification of submucous myomas. Fetal Steril 2011.

OSCE 3.

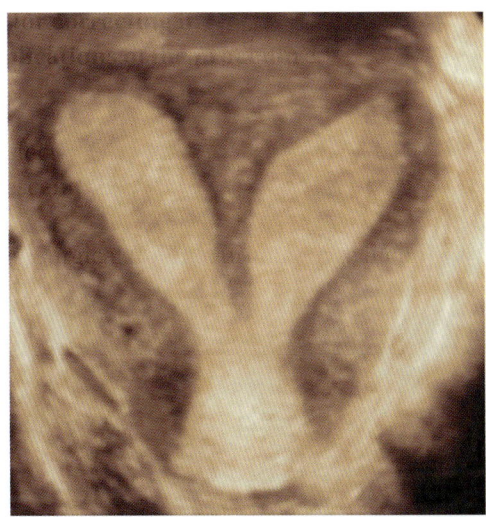

1. A 30-year-old lady presented with history of two, first trimester pregnancy losses. On workup, 3D transvaginal scan showed this picture. Identify the condition.
2. How will you manage this condition?

Ans.
1. Septate uterus
2. Hysteroscopic septal resection

OSCE 4.

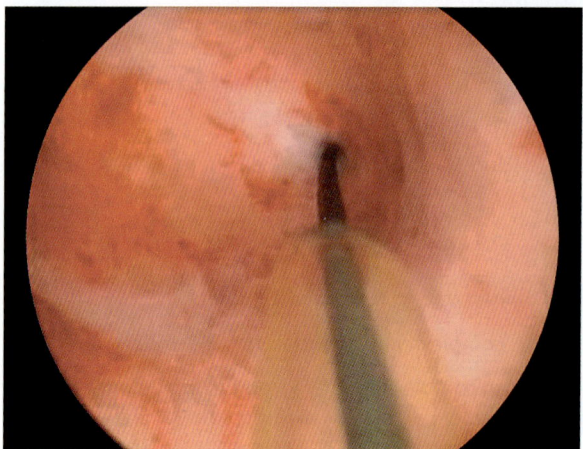

1. Identify the procedure.
2. Indication for this procedure.

Ans.

1. Hysteroscopic tubal cannulation
2. Proximal tubal block

OSCE 5.

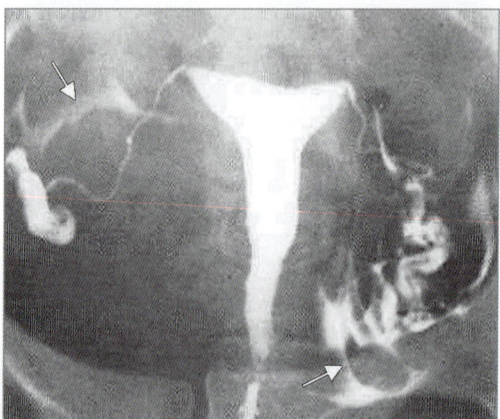

1. Name the investigation shown in the figure and explain the findings.
2. Enumerate one indication of this investigation.

Ans.

1. This is a contrast X-ray hysterosalpingogram showing normal uterine cavity with bilateral peritoneal spill suggestive of patent fallopian tubes.
2. To see the patency of fallopian tubes

OSCE 6.

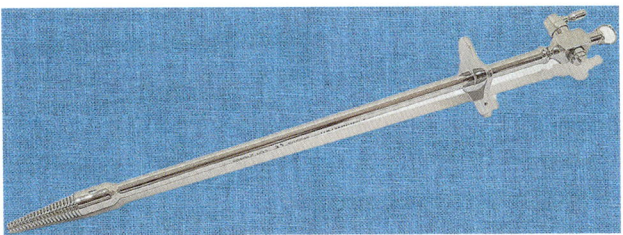

1. What is the name of this instrument?
2. It is used during which investigation?

Ans.

1. Leech Wilkinson cannula
2. Hysterosalpingography/Chromopertubation

OSCE 7. A couple with 32-year-old female and 34-year-old male, married for 3 years, presented with primary infertility. She is having complaints of decreased libido and dryness of vagina. She is having irregular periods for last 2 years (2–3 days/3–4 months). Her last menstrual period was 4 months back. On evaluation, urine pregnancy test is negative. Other reports are as follows:
- S. FSH: 30 mIU/mL
- S. AMH: 0.3 ng/mL

1. What is the diagnosis?
2. What is the treatment option for infertility in this case?

Ans.

1. Premature ovarian insufficiency
2. In vitro fertilization with donor oocyte

OSCE 8. A couple with 26 years female and 28 years male, married for 3 years, presented with primary infertility. She is having regular menstrual cycles (3–4 days/28–30 days). On male examination, bilateral testis normal in volume, epididymis mildly dilated, bilateral vas not palpable, no varicocele, penis and glans normal. Semen analysis showed azoospermia.
1. What is the type of male infertility and the diagnosis in this case?
2. What is the management?

Ans.

1. Obstructive azoospermia, congenital bilateral absence of vas deferens (CBAVD)
2. IVF-ICSI with sperm retrieved by percutaneous epididymal sperm aspiration (PESA) or testicular sperm aspiration (TESA).

Section 2: Gynecology

OSCE 9. A 34-year-old lady was diagnosed with 5 cm size submucous fibroid and admitted for hysteroscopic resection of fibroid. Procedure started with glycine 1.5% at pressure of 80–100 mm Hg. At the end of the procedure, distension media input was 3L and output was 2L.
1. What complication may occur in postoperative period?
2. Enumerate four signs and symptoms of this complication.

Ans.

1. Fluid overload syndrome, hyponatremia
2. *Sign and symptoms:* Headache, nausea, vomiting, blurring of vision, confusion, cardiac arrhythmia, convulsions, coma and death.

OSCE 10. A 32-year-old, recently married lady is diagnosed with breast cancer. The oncologists have planned for chemotherapy and have sent the patient to you for fertility preservation options.
1. What options can be given to her?
2. Postcompletion of chemotherapy, when should she plan pregnancy?

Ans.

1. Options for fertility preservation:
   - Embryo cryopreservation
   - Oocyte cryopreservation
2. One year after completion of therapy

OSCE 11.
1. How many polar bodies are formed in oogenesis cycle?
2. At which stage of oogenesis, first polar body is formed?
3. At which stage of oogenesis, second polar body is formed?

Ans.

1. Two polar bodies
2. At the time of ovulation
3. At the time of fertilization

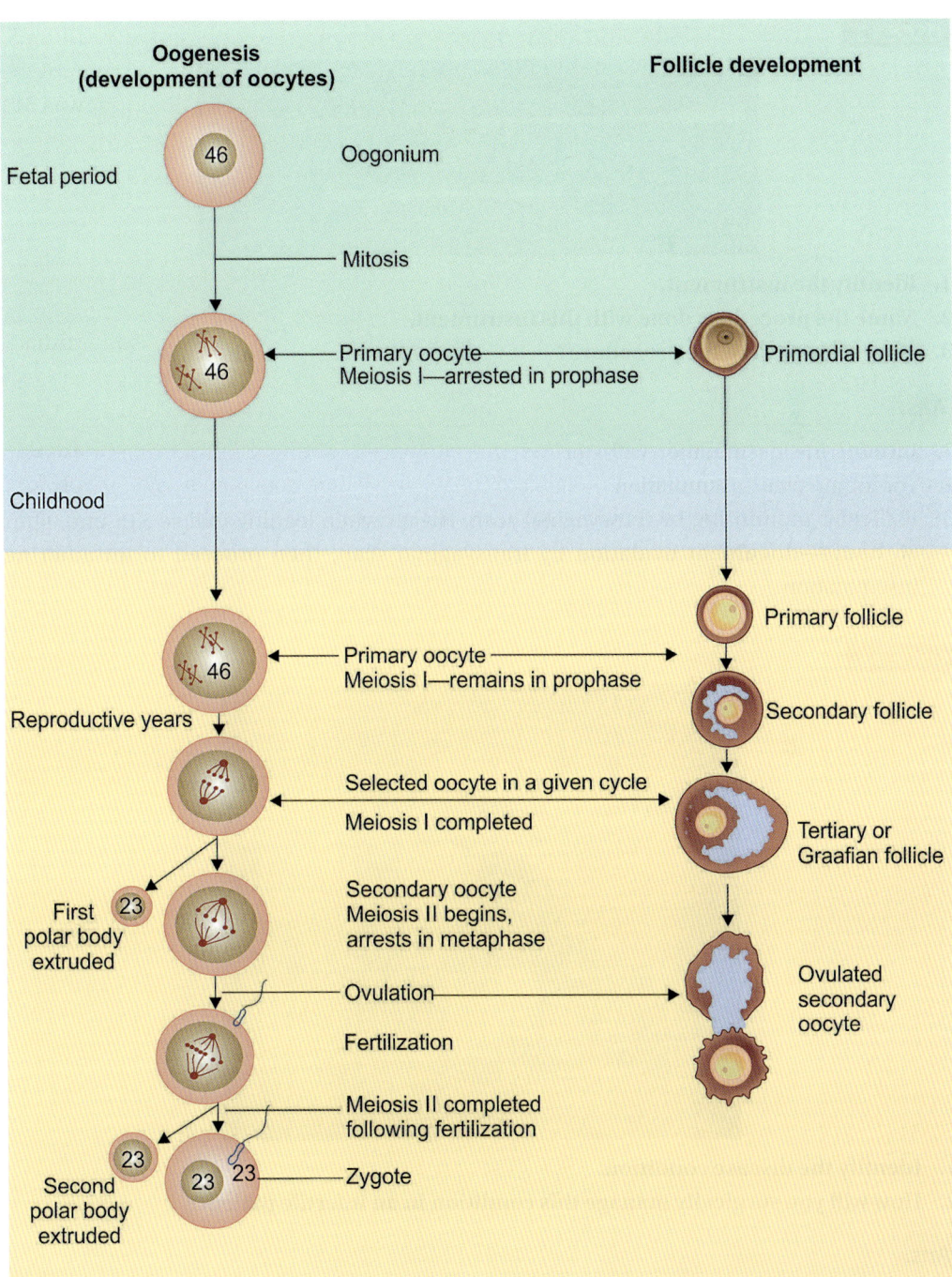

OSCE 12.

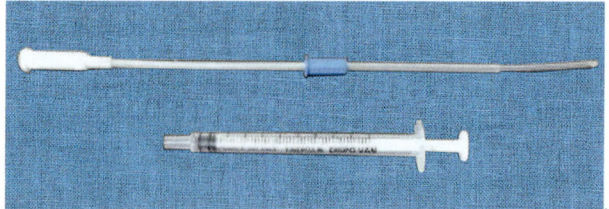

1. Identify the instrument.
2. Name the procedure done with this instrument.
3. How will you time the procedure?

Ans.

1. Intrauterine insemination catheter
2. For intrauterine insemination
3. Follicular monitoring by transvaginal scan, trigger when leading follicle >18 mm, after 36 hours—document ovulation by transvaginal scan, then proceed to intrauterine insemination.

OSCE 13.

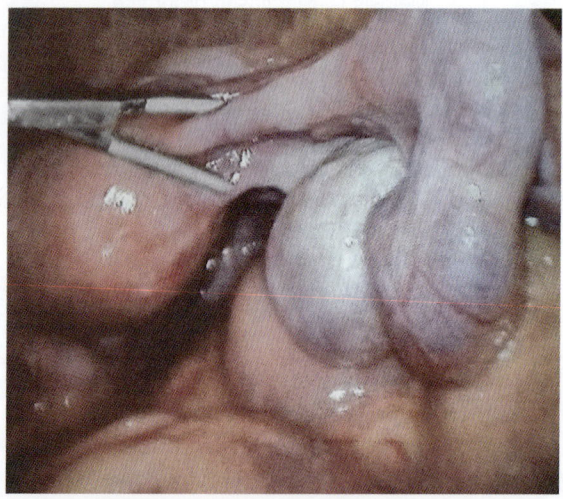

1. Identify the disease condition.
2. How will you surgically manage this condition in an infertile patient?

Ans.

1. Right hydrosalpinx
2. Surgical management options:
   - Salpingectomy
   - Tubal occlusion with electrocautery/clips

OSCE 14.

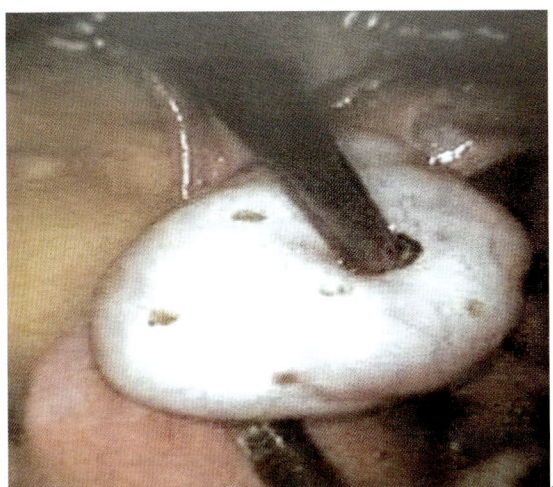

1. Name the procedure.
2. What are the complications of this procedure?
3. What is rule of 4?

Ans.

1. Laparoscopic ovarian drilling
2. Adhesion formation, decreased ovarian function if not following "Rule of 4"
3. *Rule of 4 of ovarian drilling involves*: Four punctures per ovary, each for 4 seconds at 40 Watts

OSCE 15. According to WHO 2021 semen analysis, what are the lower reference limits for the following parameters?
1. Volume
2. Count
3. Progressive motility
4. Morphology

Ans.

1. Volume—1.4 mL
2. Count—16 million/mL
3. Progressive motility—30%
4. Morphology—4%

OSCE 16.

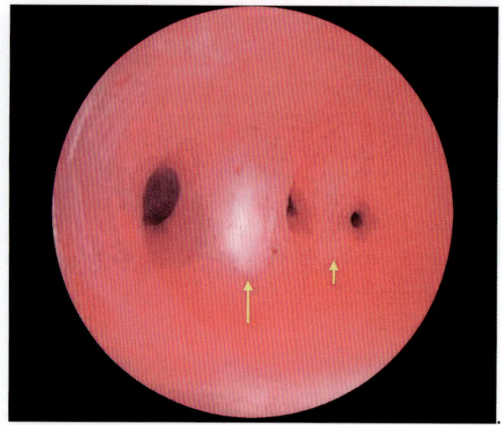

A 28-year-old lady presented with secondary amenorrhea for 4 months. She is P1A1, with history of abortion and D&C 6 months back. Hysteroscopic findings are shown as above.
1. Diagnose the condition
2. What are the management options?

Ans.

1. Asherman's syndrome
2. Hysteroscopic adhesiolysis

Reference

1. Bhandari S, Bhave P, Ganguly I, Baxi A, Agarwal P. Reproductive Outcome of Patients with Asherman's Syndrome: A SAIMS Experience. J Reprod Infertil. 2015 ;16(4):229-35.

OSCE 17.

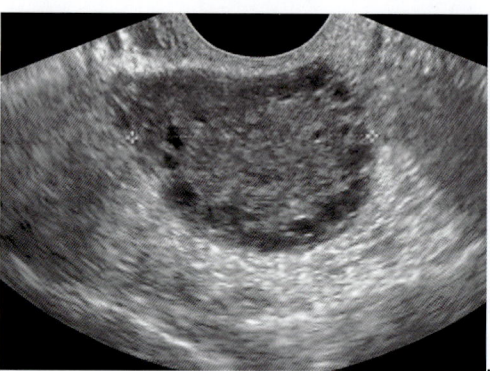

A 34-year-old lady presented with irregular, infrequent cycles. She is married for 7 years. In infertility workup, husband semen analysis was within normal limits. Her transvaginal scan showed this picture. Her fertility specialist advised the couple for IVF treatment.
1. What is the diagnosis?
2. What is the most important complication with this case in IVF cycles?

Ans.
1. Polycystic ovarian syndrome
2. Ovarian hyperstimulation syndrome

OSCE 18.
1. **Match the following:**

Embryonic urogenital structures	Adult homologues in females
a. Genital ridge	1. Uterus, fallopian tubes, upper vagina
b. Urogenital folds	2. Granulosa cells
c. Sex cords	3. Ovary
d. Paramesonephric ducts	4. Labia minora

Ans.
1.

Embryonic urogenital structures	Adult homologues in females
a. Genital ridge	3. Ovary
b. Urogenital folds	4. Labia minora
c. Sex cords	1. Granulosa cells
d. Paramesonephric ducts	2. Uterus, fallopian tubes, upper vagina

Embryonic urogenital structures and their adult homologues.

Indifferent structure	Female	Male
Genital ridge	Ovary	Testis
Primordial germ cells	Ova	Spermatozoa
Sex cords	Granulosa cells	Seminiferous tubules, Sertoli cells
Gubernaculum	Utero-ovarian and round ligaments	Gubernaculum testis
Mesonephric tubules	Epoophoron, paroophoron	Efferent ductules, paradidymis
Mesonephric ducts	Gartner duct	Epididymis, ductus deferens, ejaculatory duct
Paramesonephric ducts	Uterus, fallopian tubes, upper vagina	Prostatic utricle, appendix of testis
Urogenital sinus	• Bladder, urethra • Vagina • Paraurethral glands • Greater (Bartholin) and lesser vestibular glands	• Bladder, urethra • Prostatic utricle • Prostate glands • Bulbourethral glands
Genital tubercle	Clitoris	Glans penis
Urogenital folds	Labia minora	Floor of penile urethra
Labioscrotal swellings	Labia majora	Scrotum

OSCE 19.
A couple presented with infertility for 2 years. Female partner is having regular menstrual cycles. On examination, both partners were normal. On evaluation,

male partner was diagnosed with nonobstructive azoospermia and female partner was normal. Fertility specialist counseled them for IVF treatment.
1. Name the techniques to retrieve sperm in this case.
2. If sperms could not be obtained, what can be the option for infertility treatment?

Ans.

1. Sperm retrieval techniques:
   - Percutaneous Epididymal Sperm Aspiration (PESA)
   - Testicular Sperm Aspiration (TESA)
   - Microsurgical Sperm Aspiration (MESA)
   - Testicular Sperm Extraction (TESE)
   - Microsurgical Testicular Sperm Extraction (Micro-TESE)

Sperm retrieval techniques.

	Advantages	Disadvantages
PESA	• Fast and low cost; no surgery • Minimal morbidity, repeatable	• Few sperm retrieved • Cryopreservation limited • Fibrosis and obstruction at aspiration site • Risk of hematoma spermatocele
MESA	• Large number of sperm retrieved • Sperm cryopreservation • Reduced risk of hematoma	• Increased cost and time-demanding • Microsurgical instruments and expertise • Postoperative discomfort
TESA	• Fast and low cost, no surgery • Repeatable • Minimal/mild postoperative discomfort	• Low success rate/few sperm retrieved in NOA • Cryopreservation limited • Risk of hematoma/esticular atrophy
TESE	• No microsurgical expertise • Fast and repeatable	• Low success rate/few sperm retrieved in NOA • Risk of testicular atrophy (multiple biopsies) • Postoperative discomfort
Micro-TESE	• Higher success rates in NOA • Larger number of sperm retrieved	• Increased cost and time-demanding Microsurgical instruments and expertise • Postoperative discomfort

2. IVF and ICSI with donor semen

OSCE 20.

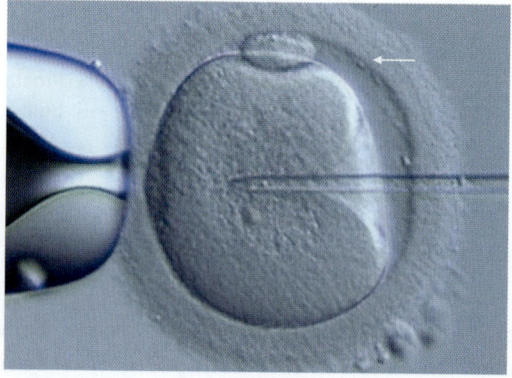

1. Name the procedure.
2. Name the labeled structure.

Ans.

1. Intracytoplasmic sperm insemination
2. First polar body

OSCE 21. A 28-year-old lady presented with pain abdomen, distension of abdomen, vomiting and decreased urine output. She has history of oocyte retrieval 4 days back for IVF, done for polycystic ovarian syndrome with severe male factor.
- *On examination:* Vitals stable, chest—clear, per abdomen—mildly distended.
- *On evaluation:* TLC—14000/mm^3, hematocrit— 42%, LFT—normal, S. creatinine—1.2 mg/dL
- *TVS:* Uterus normal, right ovary—7 cm, left ovary— 6 cm, free fluid in POD and hepatorenal pouch, no fluid in lower pleural region (in sitting position)
1. What is the diagnosis?
2. How to prevent this complication?

Ans.

1. Moderate ovarian hyperstimulation syndrome
2. Preventive measures:
   - Prediction of high risk cases (hyper-responders)
   - GnRH antagonist protocol for COH with GnRH agonist trigger
   - Freeze all—no fresh embryo transfer
   - Avoid hCG for luteal phase support in fresh transfer

Preventive measures for OHSS.		
Preventive measures	**Rationale**	**Level of evidence**
Primary prevention		
Reducing gonadotropin exposure (both dose and duration)	Increased gonadotropins enhance both follicular recruitment and serum estradiol (E2) concentrations with increased risk of OHSS	Grade A
Avoiding adjunct GnRH agonist (GnRHa) utilization	Pituitary downregulation prevents FSH rise in the luteofollicular transition; so no atresia of follicles; hence cohort of follicles recruited for stimulation is more. More gonadotropin requirement, more E2 levels	Grade A
GnRH antagonist protocol	More physiological follicular selection, recruitment of smaller number of follicles, less gonadotropin requirement, less E2 and hence reduced risk of OHSS	Grade A
Avoidance of hCG for luteal phase support	hCG increases the risk for OHSS Progesterone significantly reduces the risk of OHSS without affecting pregnancy rates	Grade B

Contd…

Contd...

Preventive measures	Rationale	Level of evidence
Insulin sensitizing agents (Metformin)	By improving hyperinsulinemia and intraovarian hyperandrogenism, reduces number of nonperiovulatory follicles and hence E2 secretion	Grade A
Secondary prevention		
Alternative agents for triggering ovulation [GnRHa or recombinant LH (rLH)]	GnRHa trigger causes massive luteolysis and thus less E2 levels in luteal phase. Also hCG itself is a risk factor for OHSS	Grade A
Reduced dose of hCG for triggering ovulation	Appears to decrease the risk of severe OHSS	Grade C
Cryopreservation of all embryos	Avoids endogenous hCG rise in fresh transfer cycles which can exacerbate fate onset OHSS	Grade B
Cycle cancellation	Cycle cancellation and withholding hCG is definitive method for preventing OHSS	Grade C
Coasting	Withholding gonadotropins and delaying hCG reduces the risk of OHSS. Also alters the capacity of granulosa cells to produce VEGF	Grade C
Dopamine agonists	Prevents phosphorylation of VEGF receptor-2 and thus reduces the release of vasoactive angiogenic agents	Grade A
Calcium infusion	Inhibition of cAMP dependent renin secretion leading to decreased angiotensin-II production and thus VEGF synthesis	Grade B
Aspirin	Inhibits platelet activation thus inhibiting release of substances that can potentiate OHSS	Grade A
Glucocorticoids	Inhibitory effect on VEGF gene expression	Grade C
Colloid (albumin and hydroxyethyl starch) infusion	Increases plasma oncolic pressure and counteracting the permeability effect of Angiotensin II	Grade C
Aromatase inhibitors	Inhibits aromatase enzyme and prevents excessive synthesis of estrogen	Grade C
Follicular aspiration		Grade C
Experimental		
In vitro maturation	Aspiration of immature oocytes helps in preventing OHSS	
VEGF antagonists	Blocks action of VEGF	
Kisspeptin trigger for oocyte maturation	Stimulates GnRH release and in turn FSH and LH release	
Vasopressin V1a receptor antagonist	Inhibits vasopressin induced VEGF secretion	

OSCE 22. In cases of nonobstructive azoospermia, planned for IVF with surgical sperm retrieval.
1. Which genetic test should be done?
2. Which variant has best chances of obtaining sperms with surgical sperm retrieval?

Ans.

1. Karyotyping, Y-chromosome microdeletion for AZFa/AZF b/AZFc region
2. Best chance of retrieval of sperms with AZFc region Y chromosome microdeletion
   Deletions within the male-specific region of the Y-chromosome, known as Y-chromosome. Microdeletions (YCMs), are present in as many as 5% and 10% of severe oligospermic and azoospermic men, respectively. These microdeletions are distinguished by which segment of the Y chromosome is absent, identified as AZFa (the most proximal segment), AZFb (middle), and AZFc (distal). The reported prevalence of YCMs within the world's populations of infertile men displays vast heterogeneity, ranging from less than 2% to over 24% based on region and ethnicity. AZFc is the most commonly identified YCM, and its phenotypic presentation provides for the highest chance for fertility through artificial reproductive techniques. Conversely, deletions identified in the subregions of AZFa, AZFb, or any combination of regions containing these segments, are associated with low probabilities of achieving pregnancy.

Reference
1. Rabinowitz MJ, Huffman PJ, Haney NM, Kohn TP. Y-Chromosome Microdeletions: A Review of Prevalence, Screening, and Clinical Considerations. Appl Clin Genet. 2021:14:51-9.

OSCE 23. A 28-year-old lady married for 5 years, nulligravida, presented with complains of severe dysmenorrheal and dyspareunia for last 3 years. Her cycles are regular. She is anxious to conceive for which she consulted a gynecologist.
- **O/E:** Per abdomen—Soft. Per vagina— uterus anteverted, firm, normal size, mobility restricted. Right forniceal fullness and tenderness.
- **TVS:** Uterus anteverted, normal in size and echotexture, endometrial thickness 6.3 mm, right ovary with 3.5 X 4 cm cystic mass with ground-glass appearance. Left ovary and adnexa normal. No free fluid in POD.

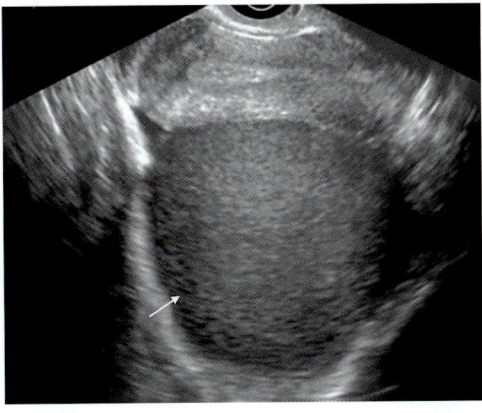

1. What is the diagnosis in this case?
2. Is there any role for medical management in this case?

Ans.

1. Right ovarian endometriotic cyst
2. No role of medical management in endometriosis with infertility per se or either before or after surgery.

OSCE 24.

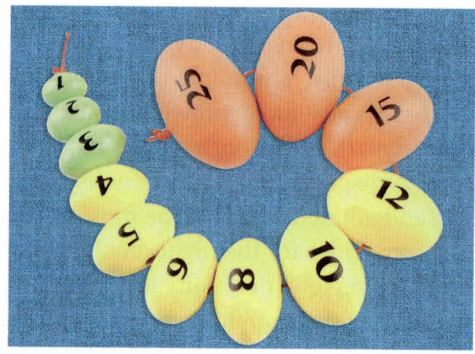

1. What is the name of the instrument?
2. What is the use of this instrument?
3. What is the normal volume of testis?
4. What are the other methods to assess volume of testis?

Ans.

1. Prader orchidometer
2. To assess volume of testis
3. Normal volume of testis: 8–15 mL
4. Other methods to assess volume of testis:
   - Clinical examination
   - Vernier calipers (Length × breadth × width × 0.5)
   - Ultrasound

OSCE 25.

A 28-year-old lady presented with lower abdomen pain. USG scan showed a mixed echogenic cyst in right ovary (as shown in the picture).

1. What is the diagnosis?
2. What is the most common complication?

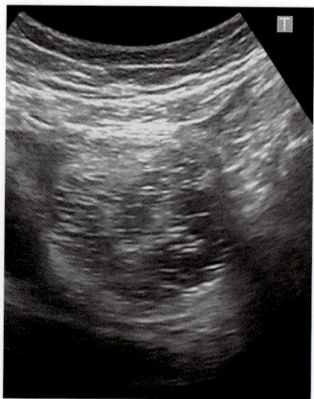

Ans.

1. Mature teratoma or dermoid cyst
2. Torsion of the ovary

CHAPTER 41

Amenorrhea

Vidya A Thobbi

OSCE 1.

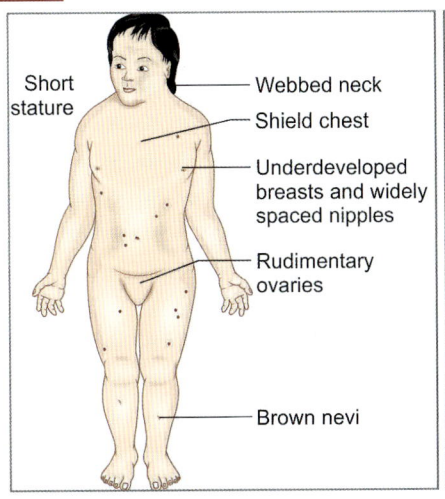
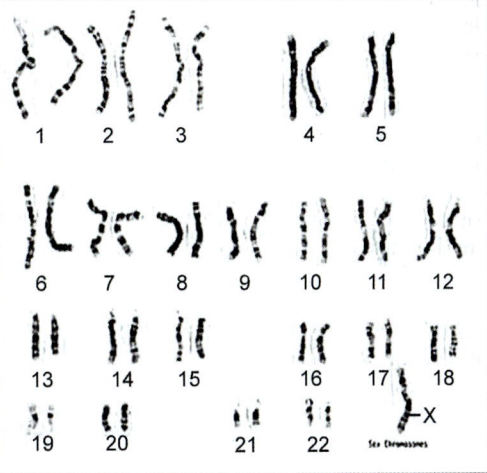

1. Identify the syndrome.
2. Type of amenorrhea seen
3. Karyotype of this syndrome

Ans.

1. Turner syndrome
2. Primary amenorrhea
3. 45XO

OSCE 2.

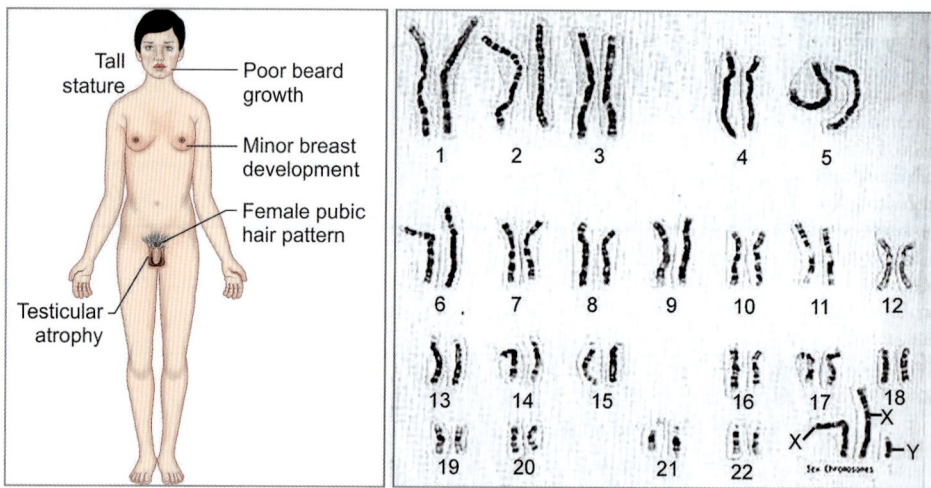

1. Identify the syndrome.
2. Type of amenorrhea seen.
3. Karyotype of the patient.

Ans.

1. Klinefelter's syndrome
2. Primary amenorrhea
3. 47 XXY

OSCE 3. A 20-year-old girl presents with primary amenorrhea with karyotype of 46XY. Her serum FSH and LH are increased but estradiol and progesterone are decreased. Secondary sexual characteristics are absent. Ultrasound shows hypoplastic uterus.
1. What is your diagnosis? Explain your diagnosis.

Ans.

1. Pure gonadal dysgenesis also known as Swyer syndrome. It is a disorder of sexual differentiation. The patients are phenotypically female with a 46XY karyotype and hypoplastic gonads without germ cells. They most often present with primary amenorrhea.

OSCE 4.
1. Match the following:

A	Stage 1	1. Hair is adult pattern
B	Stage 2	2. Hair extend to inner aspect of thigh
C	Stage 3	3. No hair
D	Stage 4	4. Long, coarse, and curly hair seen on labia majora
E	Stage 5	5. Coarse, long, and curly hair on mons pubis

Ans.

1. A (3), B (4), C (5), D (1), E (2)

OSCE 5.
1. Name two syndromes which present as amenorrhea with absence of secondary sexual characters.
2. First line of investigation to be done.
3. Investigation of choice for diagnosis.

Ans.

1. a. Swyers syndrome
   b. Turner's syndrome
2. Measure serum FSH and LH
3. Karyotyping

OSCE 6.

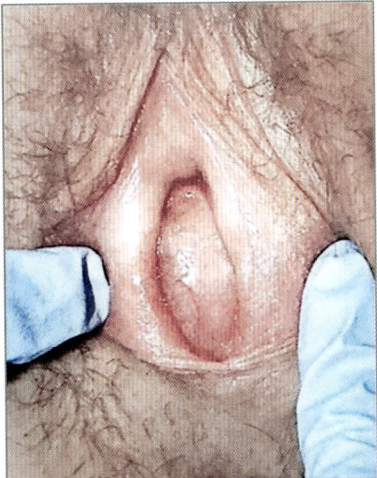 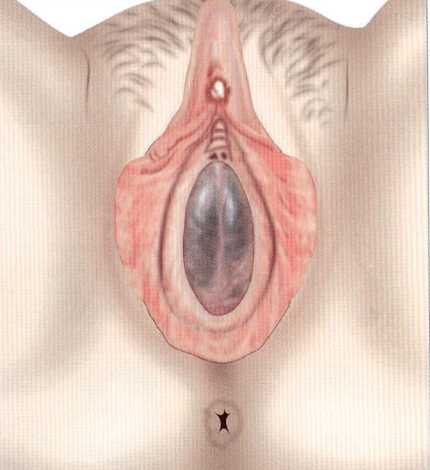

1. Differential diagnosis?
2. Management?

Ans.

1. Transverse vaginal septum and imperforate hymen
2. a. *Transverse vaginal septum:* Excision of septum and drainage of hematocolpos.
   b. *Imperforate hymen:* Hymenotomy (cruciate incision on the hymen).

OSCE 7.

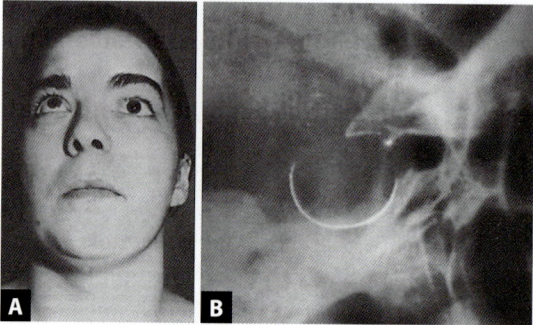

A 24-year-old, primipara presented with 9 months of amenorrhea.

Figure A: Examination revealed fixation of left eye and swelling of lower eyelid.

Figure B: Radiological examination of skull showing grossly enlarged Sella turcica with erosions of bones that outline the fossa.

1. What are the differential diagnoses?
2. Management.

Ans.

1. Pituitary adenoma, craniopharyngioma, and other tumors in and around pituitary gland.
2. Surgical excision of tumor.

OSCE 8.

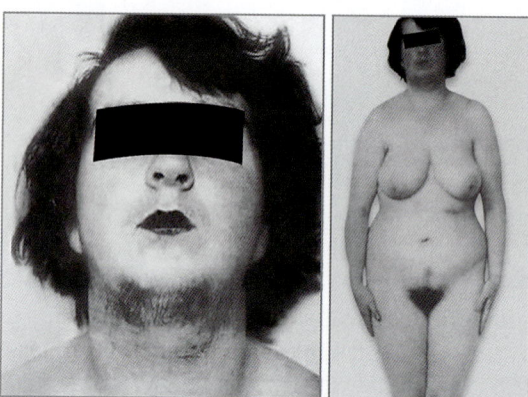

A 21-year-old girl presented with secondary amenorrhea with facial hirsutism.

1. Identify the syndrome.
2. What is the name of the diagnostic criteria and its components?

Ans.

1. PCOS
2. *Rotterdam criteria:* Two of the following three criteria should be fulfilled:
    - Oligo/anovulation

- Hyperandrogenism (clinical hirsutism or less commonly male pattern alopecia) or biochemical (raised FAI or free-testosterone)
- Polycystic ovaries on ultrasound

OSCE 9. A 22-year-old girl complains of secondary amenorrhea and increasing weight, had slight hypertension with striae on hips and flanks. Radiograph shows calcified tumor of the left adrenal displacing the kidney downward.
1. Identify the condition.

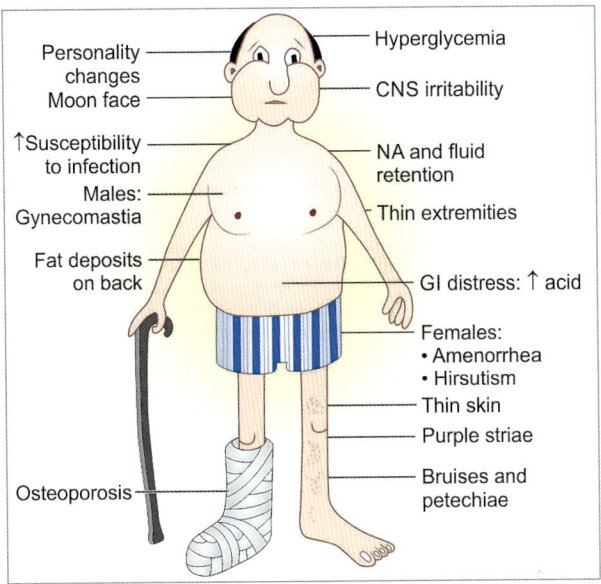

Ans.

1. Cushing syndrome is caused by adrenal cortical tumor.

OSCE 10. Match the following:

1.	Stage 1	A	Adult contour
2.	Stage 2	B	Breast elevation
3.	Stage 3	C	Breast bud
4.	Stage 4	D	Prepubertal
5.	Stage 5	E	Areolar mound

Ans.

1 (D), 2 (C), 3 (B), 4 (A), 5 (E)

OSCE 11. A patient presented with amenorrhea and delayed growth and sexual development with inability to perceive odors along with family history of delayed puberty.
1. Identify the syndrome.

2. **How will you differentiate this from constitutional delay of puberty?**
3. **Cause of anosmia in this syndrome.**

Ans.

1. Kallmann syndrome
2. Presence of pubic hair (adrenarche) is normal in Kallmann syndrome whereas it is delayed in constitutional delay of puberty.
3. Kallmann syndrome is a classical X-linked recessive disorder caused by genetic mutation in kal gene which encodes Ansomin-1, a neural adhesion molecule that promotes migration of GNRH neurons and olfactory neurons from the olfactory placode into hypothalamus during embryonic development.

OSCE 12.
1. **What is the association of BMI (weight) with amenorrhea?**
2. **What is the normal weight to hip ratio?**
3. **What is the critical body fat level for menarche and for regular menstruation?**

Ans.

1. Critical weight hypothesis-onset and regularity of menstrual function require bodyweight to remain above a critical threshold level with corresponding level of body fat.
2. 1.85 or less.
3. *Critical body fat level:* 17% for menarche and 22% for regular menstruation.

OSCE 13.
1. **What is Sheehan syndrome?**
2. **What is clinical presentation?**

Ans.

1. Sheehan syndrome occurs when anterior pituitary gland is damaged due to significant blood loss (PPH).
2. *Clinical presentation:* Failed lactation after delivery followed by amenorrhea.

OSCE 14
1. **An 18-year-old girl came with a history of not having menses ever. On examination, age-appropriate breast and pubic hair development is noted with blind-ending vagina. Urine pregnancy test-negative, hormonal assay was normal. What is the next appropriate investigation?**
2. **Differential diagnosis for blind-ending vagina.**

Ans.

1. Ultrasound pelvis.
2. Imperforate hymen, transverse vaginal septum, Müllerian agenesis, androgen insensitivity syndrome.

Chapter 41: Amenorrhea

OSCE 15.

A 14-year-old girl was presented with severe colicky abdominal pain since 10 days. She had a history of cyclical abdominal pain for 4 months, has not attained menarche but has normal secondary sexual characteristics. On examination, pink membrane seen in vagina not bulging with Valsalva maneuver.
1. What is the diagnosis?

Ans.

1. Transverse Vaginal Septum

OSCE 16. Match the following:

1.	Swyers syndrome	A	Mutation in *Kal1* gene
2.	Kallmann syndrome	B	Mutation in *FMR1* gene
3.	Fragile X syndrome	C	Mutation in *SRY* gene
4.	Turner's syndrome	D	45 XO

Ans.

1 (C), 2 (A), 3 (B), 4 (D)

OSCE 17. Fill in the blanks:

Clinical state	Serum FSH	AMH
Normal adult female	5–20 IU/L (Midcycle)	? (QUESTION 1)
Premature ovarian failure	? (QUESTION 2)	< 0.2 ng/mL

Ans.

1. 2.2 to 4 ng/mL
2. >40 IU/L

OSCE 18. Match the following:

1. 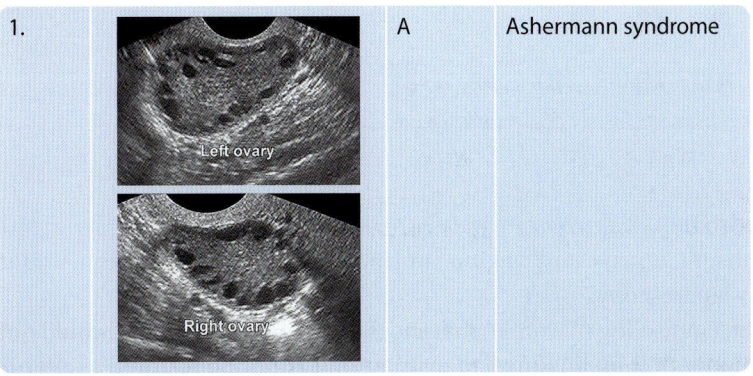 A Ashermann syndrome

Contd…

Contd...

2.	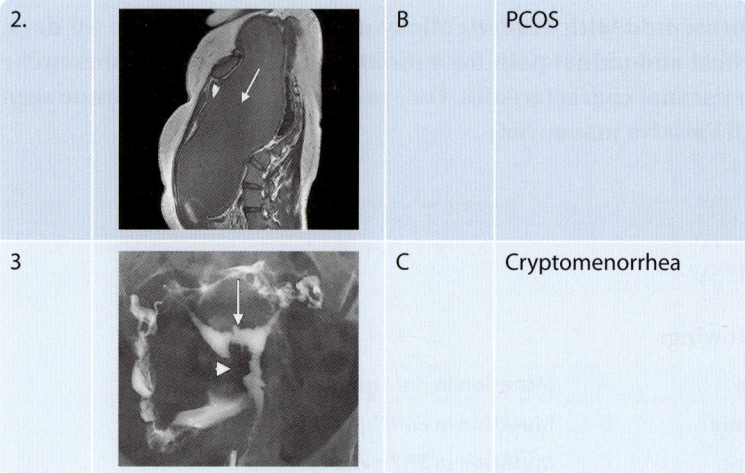	B	PCOS
3		C	Cryptomenorrhea

Ans.

1 (B), 2 (C), 3 (A)

OSCE 19. Karyotype of an 18-year girl who presented with primary amenorrhea is given below. Development of her breast is at Tanner stage 5. She has no other complaints.
1. Diagnosis
2. Test to confirm the diagnosis
3. Treatment options

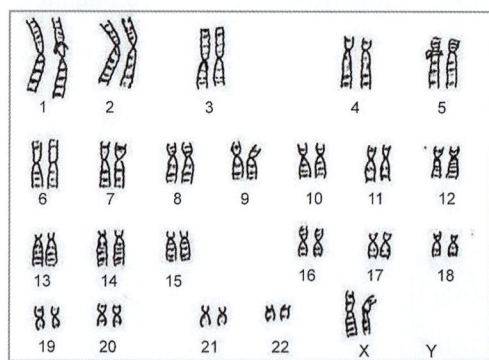

Ans.

1. Mayer-Rokitansky syndrome.
2. Ultrasound pelvis (absent uterus and vagina, normal ovaries), examination under anesthesia followed by laparoscopy.
3. No definitive treatment, counseling of women that she is genetically female and would not have any hormonal changes till menopause, menstruation cannot be restored as uterus is absent.

OSCE 20.

1. A 17-year girl who has not yet started her menstrual periods visits a gynecologist to discuss her concern. During examination, the doctor observes her to have normal external genitalia, but she is unable to locate a cervix or vagina. On further testing, ultrasound shows the following image. What is the differential diagnosis?
2. How can you confirm the diagnosis?

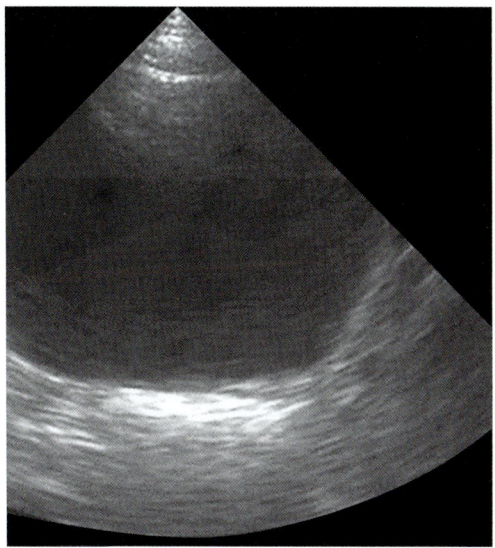

Ans.

1. Androgen insensitivity syndrome and Müllerian agenesis
2. *Karyotyping:* Müllerian agenesis (46XX), androgen insensitivity syndrome (46 XY).

REFERENCES

1. Jeffcoate's Principles of Gynaecology, 8th International Edition.
2. Speroff's Clinical Gynecologic Endocrinology and Infertility, 9th Edition.

CHAPTER 42

Endometrial Carcinoma

Seema Singhal, Saroj Rajan

OSCE 1. A 58-year-old, P3L3 obese, hypertensive woman presented with postmenopausal bleeding for 2 months. On examination cervix, the vagina is healthy. Uterus retroverted normal size, bilateral fornices free and nontender.
1. What is the probability of cancer in woman with postmenopausal bleeding?
2. What is the first ideal investigation?
3. What is the cut-off limit of endometrial thickness on TVS that warrants further evaluation?

Ans.
1. The most common cause of postmenopausal bleeding remains endometrial atrophy (60–80%). Only 10% of cases are due to endometrial cancer.
2. Transvaginal ultrasonography is used to evaluate postmenopausal bleeding initially. A thin endometrial echo (less than or equal to 4 mm) has a greater than 99% negative predictive value for endometrial cancer. Transvaginal ultrasonography is a reasonable alternative to endometrial sampling as the first approach in evaluating a postmenopausal woman with an initial episode of bleeding.
3. The 4 mm endometrial thickness identifies 96% of women with endometrial carcinoma and 92% with benign endometrial pathology.

OSCE 2. Mrs X, a 56-year-old, lean postmenopausal lady with no comorbidities, was advised to undergo USG abdomen and pelvis during the evaluation of gallstones. The USG revealed a normal-sized uterus with an endometrial thickness of 7 mm and normal adnexa.
1. How will you evaluate a woman with incidentally detected thick endometrium without a history of postmenopausal bleeding?
2. What are the causes of recurrent postmenopausal bleeding?
3. How will you investigate a woman with recurrent postmenopausal bleeding?

Ans.
1. An incidentally discovered endometrial measurement ≥4 mm in a postmenopausal patient without bleeding does not necessarily require histological evaluation. However, the approach should be individualized based on the patient's risk factors.
   In a review of 1,750 postmenopausal women without bleeding who were screened with transvaginal USG, an endometrial thickness of ≤6 mm had a negative predictive

value of 99.94% for excluding malignancy. Among 42 women with endometrial thickness ≥6 mm, there was only one case of adenocarcinoma and no hyperplasia (positive predictive value of 2.4%).
2. Women with recurrent PMB have a higher risk of pathology (endometrial polyps, endometrial hyperplasia or cancer) when compared with those with a single episode.
3. Rare cases of endometrial carcinoma (mainly type II) can present with an endometrial thickness of less than 3 mm; hence, persistent or recurrent uterine bleeding should prompt an endometrial aspiration regardless of endometrial thickness.

Reference
1. ACOG Committee Opinion No. 734 Summary: The Role of Transvaginal Ultrasonography in Evaluating the Endometrium of Women with Postmenopausal Bleeding. Obstetrics & Gynecology. 131(5):pp. 945-6, May 2018. DOI: 10.1097/AOG.0000000000002626

OSCE 3.

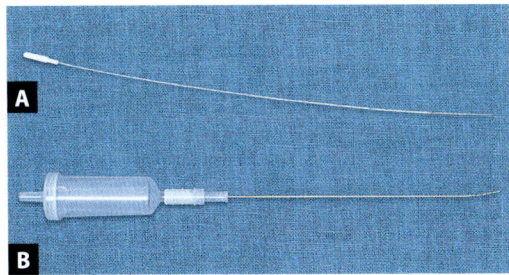

1. Name the devices displayed in the photograph used for endometrial sampling.
2. List three more devices that can be used for endometrial sampling.

Ans.

1. A— Pipelle suction curette. B—Vabra aspirator
2. Tao brush, SAP-1 device, Karman cannula are devices which can be used for endometrial sampling.

OSCE 4.

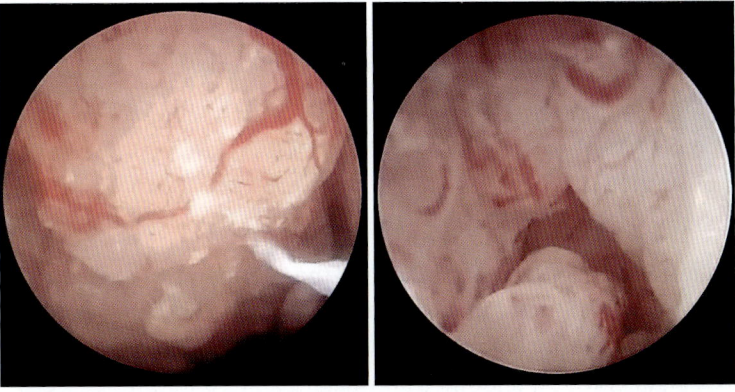

Section 2: Gynecology

1. What are the indications of hysteroscopy in a woman with postmenopausal bleeding?
2. How much intrauterine pressure is preferred while doing hysteroscopy in suspected endometrial carcinoma?
3. What is the impact of hysteroscopy on the course of disease in women with endometrial carcinoma?
4. What are the hysteroscopic features suggestive of hyperplasia or cancer in polyp?

Ans.

1. Hysteroscopy enables direct visualization of the cavity with a sensitivity of 82.6% and specificity of 99.7%.
   Indications:
   - USG suggestive of a focal lesion, e.g., polyp
   - Persistent symptoms of bleeding with inconclusive endometrial aspiration.
2. Intrauterine pressure should be kept below 70 mm Hg as a significantly lower number of endometrial cells were observed in the abdominal cavity below this pressure.
3. No significant impact. Hysteroscopy does not increase the risk of progression of cancer and is not associated with higher rates of positive peritoneal cytology.
4. Polyp size, surface irregularity and vascularity are predictors for harboring malignancy, but hysteroscopic appearance does not provide a safe method of differentiating polyps with hyperplasia and cancer.

Reference
1. Larish A, Kumar A, Weaver A, Mariani A. Impact of hysteroscopy on course of disease in high-risk endometrial carcinoma. Int J Gynecol Cancer. 2020;30(10):1513-9. doi: 10.1136/ijgc-2020-001627

OSCE 5. A 53-year-old, P2L2 lady complained of postmenopausal bleeding for 7 months. On examination, the cervix and vagina were healthy. TVS showed an endometrial thickness of 21 mm. The endometrial biopsy was suggestive of well-differentiated endometrioid adenocarcinoma.

1. Which is the preferred imaging modality for further evaluation?
2. What is the role of tumor markers in the evaluation of suspected carcinoma endometrium?

Ans.

1. Contrast-enhanced MRI is the modality of choice for evaluation.

Parameter	Sensitivity
Myometrial invasion	80–90%
Cervical involvement	56–100%
Lymph node involvement	17–80%

2. There is a limited role of tumor markers in the preoperative evaluation of suspected endometrial cancer. Two tumor markers have been studied in clinical practice:
   - *CA 125:* For extrauterine involvement, type 2 histology, more value in premenopausal women and for follow-up if initially elevated

- *HE4:* Elevated in all the stages but more sensitive in early-stage disease. It is helpful to monitor response to therapy and to detect recurrent disease.

OSCE 6. A 65-year-old, P1L1 lady presented with postmenopausal bleeding for the last 6 months. Her BMI was 32, and she is a known case of hypertension.
- *TVS:* Normal-sized uterus, endometrial thickness of 21 mm, bilateral adnexa normal.
- *Endometrial biopsy:* Endometrioid carcinoma grade 1.
1. Which is the most common histology of endometrial cancer? How is it graded?
2. What is high-risk histology?

Ans.
1. Endometrioid histology is the most common (seen in approximately 80%). It is graded based on the degree of non*squamous* or *nonmorular* solid growth pattern:
    - Grade 1: Less than 5% growth pattern
    - Grade 2: 6–50% solid growth pattern
    - Grade 3: Greater than 50% solid growth pattern.
2. Grades 1 and 2 endometrioid adenocarcinoma are considered low risk histologies. High-grade histologies include grade 3 endometrioid adenocarcinoma, serous adenocarcinomas, clear cell adenocarcinomas, mesonephric-like carcinomas, gastrointestinal-type mucinous endometrial carcinoma, undifferentiated carcinomas, and carcinosarcomas.

OSCE 7.

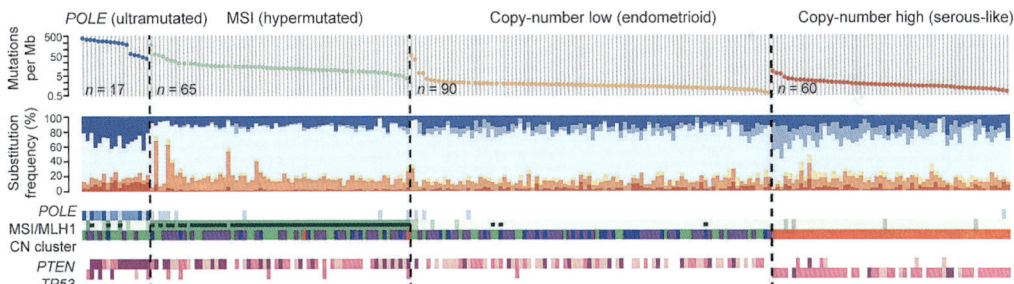

1. What is the molecular classification of endometrial classification?
2. How do molecular subgroups affect prognosis?

Ans.
1. The Cancer Genome Atlas studies have identified four molecular subgroups:
    a. *Group 1 (7%):* Ultramutated group characterized by mutations in the exonuclease domain of the POLE DNA polymerase.
    b. *Group 2 (28%):* Hypermutated group characterized by microsatellite instability and defects in mismatch repair factors.
    c. *Group 3 (39%):* Low copy-number group with microsatellite stability (nonspecific molecular profile)
    d. *Group 4 (26%):* High copy-number group characterized by low mutation rate, chromosomal instability and TP53 mutations.

2. Groups 1 and 2 have a good prognosis, group 3 has an intermediate prognosis, and group 4 has the worst prognosis.

Reference

1. Bhatla N, Aoki D, Sharma DN, Sankaranarayanan R. Cancer of the cervix uteri: 2021 update. International Journal of Gynecology & Obstetrics. 2021;155:28-44.

OSCE 8.

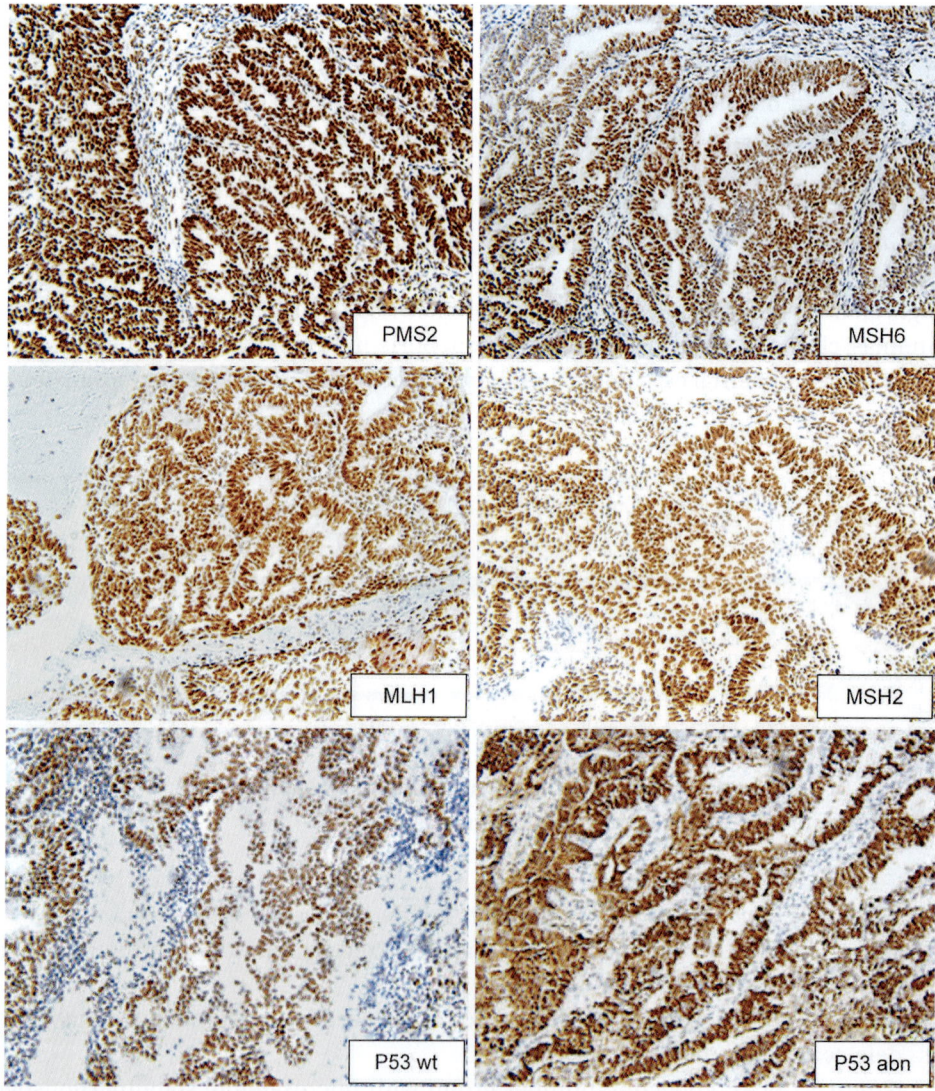

1. What markers applied to the histological specimen are used to determine the molecular subgroup?
2. What are multiple classifiers?

Ans.

1. Three immunohistochemical markers (p53, MSH-6, PMS-2) and somatic mutation analysis of POLE (exons 9, 11, 13, 14) is used to determine molecular subgroup.

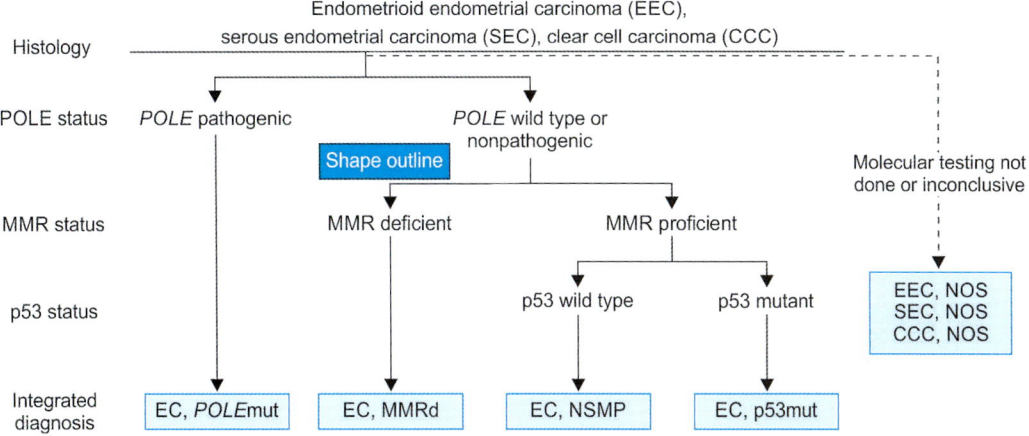

2. Five percent of tumors have more than one molecular feature (e.g., POLEmut and p53abn or MMRd and p53abn) and are called "multiple classifiers."

Reference
1. Vermij L, Smit V, Nout R, Bosse T. Incorporation of molecular characteristics into endometrial cancer management. Histopathology. 2020;76(1):52-63.

OSCE 9.
1. Which patients with endometrial cancer should be suspected of having Lynch syndrome?
2. What additional molecular testing should be formed in the evaluation of Lynch syndrome?
3. How should surveillance be performed for women with Lynch syndrome?

Ans.

1. Lynch syndrome (germline mutation of mismatch repair genes, MLH1, PMS2, MSH2, and MSH6) constitutes 3% of all endometrial carcinomas and 10% of Mismatch repair-deficient (MMRd) endometrial carcinomas. Hence, regardless of patient age, MMR status must be tested in all endometrial carcinoma samples. In addition, Lynch syndrome may be suspected in women with a personal/family history of colorectal, endometrial, gastric, ovarian, pancreas, ureter and renal pelvis, biliary tract, brain (glioblastoma), and small intestinal cancers.
2. MMR deficiency is frequently due to sporadic mutations; hence, when IHC or PCR-based methods detect loss of *MLH1 MMR* gene, MLH1 promoter methylation status analysis is advised (epigenetic modification). In the absence of hypermethylation, a germline mutation should be suspected.

3.

Disorder	Lower age limit (years)	Examination	Interval (years)
Lynch syndrome	20–25 30–35	• Colonoscopy • Gynecological examination, transvaginal ultrasound, aspiration biopsy	1–2 1–2
	30–35 30–35	• Gastroduodenoscopy* Abdominal ultrasound, urinalysis and cytology urine†	1–2 1–2
Familial clustering of colorectal cancer without evidence of MSI‡	45–50 or 5–10 before age at diagnosis of first CRC in family	Colonoscopy	3–5

(CRC: colorectal cancer; MSI: microsatellite instability)
*If gastric cancer runs in the family or in countries with a high incidence of gastric cancer.
†If urinary tract cancer runs in the family.
‡Amsterdam positive families.

OSCE 10. A 65-year-old, P1L1 presented with postmenopausal bleeding for the last 6 months. Her BMI is 32 kg/m², and she is a known case of hypertension.
- *TVS:* Normal-sized uterus, endometrial thickness of 21 mm, normal bilateral adnexa.
- *Endometrial biopsy:* Endometrioid carcinoma grade 1.
- *CEMRI:* Endometrium thickness of 20 mm, no myometrial invasion, pelvic lymph nodes not enlarged, bilateral ovaries normal.

1. What is the subsequent management for this case?
2. What is the preferred route of surgery?
3. Can ovaries be conserved in premenopausal women?
4. When is omentectomy as a part of staging required?

Ans.

1. A staging surgery comprising peritoneal wash cytology, sentinel node biopsy, extra-fascial hysterectomy, and bilateral salpingo-oophorectomy should be performed.
2. The preferred route of surgery is minimally invasive.
3. Ovaries may be preserved in premenopausal women <45 years with low-grade endometrioid endometrial carcinoma with <50% myometrial invasion and no obvious ovarian or other extrauterine disease.
4. Staging infracolic omentectomy should be performed in serous carcinoma, carcinosarcoma, and undifferentiated carcinoma.

Reference

1. Concin N, Matias-Guiu X, Vergote I, Cibula D, Mirza MR, Marnitz S, Ledermann J, Bosse T, Chargari C, Fagotti A, Fotopoulou C. ESGO/ESTRO/ESP guidelines for the management of patients with endometrial carcinoma. International Journal of Gynecologic Cancer. 2021; 31(1).

OSCE 11.

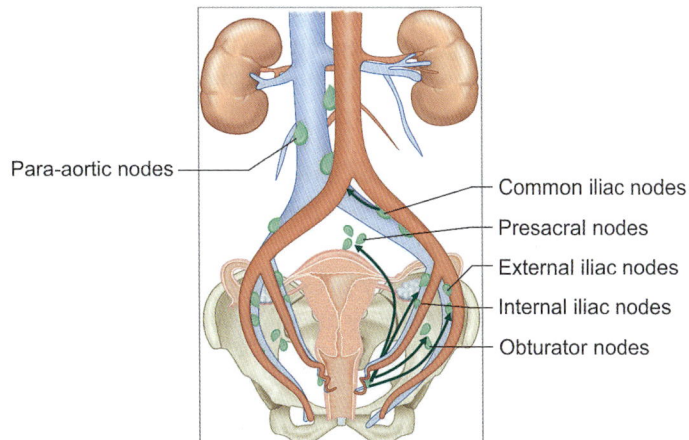

1. How should lymph nodes be assessed in women with endometrial cancer?
2. Which is the most common sentinel node in women with endometrial cancer?
3. Can sentinel node mapping be performed in patients with high-risk histology?

Ans.

1. Sentinel node biopsy is an alternative to systemic lymph node dissection for lymph node staging, associated with lower postoperative morbidity. Prospective studies have confirmed the high sensitivity of sentinel lymph node mapping in patients with early-stage endometrial carcinoma.
2. External iliac and obturator nodes.
3. Sentinel node mapping may be done even in women with high-risk histology.

References

1. Concin N, Matias-Guiu X, Vergote I, Cibula D, Mirza MR, Marnitz S, Ledermann J, Bosse T, Chargari C, Fagotti A, Fotopoulou C. ESGO/ESTRO/ESP guidelines for the management of patients with endometrial carcinoma. International Journal of Gynecologic Cancer. 2021;31(1).
2. Persson J, Salehi S, Bollino M, Lönnerfors C, Falconer H, Geppert B. Pelvic Sentinel lymph node detection in High-Risk Endometrial Cancer (SHREC-trial)—the final step towards a paradigm shift in surgical staging. Eur J Cancer. 2019;116:77-85. doi: 10.1016/j.ejca.2019.04.025.

OSCE 12.

1. According to the revised FIGO 2023 staging of Ca endometrium, how is a woman with carcinoma endometrium with an adnexal mass staged?
2. How is fallopian tubal involvement by tumor staged?

Ans.

1. a. *Stage IA3:* If MI <50%, absence of substantial LVSI, absence of additional metastasis, unilateral ovarian tumor without capsular invasion or rupture.
   b. *Stage IIIA:* Those without these features will be classified as stage IIIA disease.
2. Tumor involvement of the fallopian tube should be staged as IIIA1.

Reference

1. Berek JS, Matias-Guiu X, Creutzberg C, Fotopoulou C, Gaffney D, Kehoe S, Lindemann K, Mutch D, Concin N, Endometrial Cancer Staging Subcommittee, FIGO Women's Cancer Committee, Berek JS. FIGO staging of endometrial cancer: 2023. International Journal of Gynecology & Obstetrics. 2023 Jun 20.

OSCE 13. Mrs X, a 36-year-old nulliparous lady with a BMI of 36 kg/m^2, has presented with heavy menstrual bleeding for the past 6 months. An endometrial biopsy revealed grade 1 endometrioid adenocarcinoma.
1. What is the eligibility criteria for fertility-preserving treatment of endometrial cancer?
2. What medical agents are used for fertility preservation?

Ans.

1. Approximately 5% of endometrial cancers occur in women less than 40 years of age. Women wishing to retain their fertility can undergo fertility-sparing treatments if they have atypical hyperplasia or grade 1 endometrioid carcinoma without myometrial invasion.
2. Medroxyprogesterone acetate (400–600 mg/day), megestrol acetate (160–320 mg/day) or levonorgestrel intrauterine device can be used.

OSCE 14.
1. Which patients with endometrial cancer do not require adjuvant therapy?
2. Can adjuvant treatment be tailored according to the molecular classification of endometrial cancer?

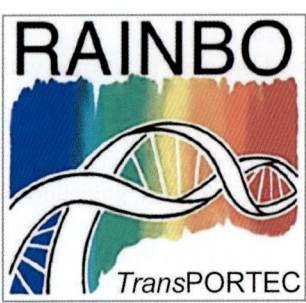

Ans.

1. Women with low-grade (grades 1 or 2) endometrioid adenocarcinoma, with Stage IA disease (<50% myometrial invasion) and no or focal lymphovascular space invasion, are considered low risk and do not require adjuvant therapy.
2. Molecular profiling may enable tailored adjuvant treatment for endometrial cancer. In patients with stage I/II disease with POLE mutation, treatment may be de-escalated as these cases have excellent prognoses. Based on their molecular profiles, the on-going PORTEC-4a study may provide more definitive data on adjuvant treatment options in stage I and II cancers. The RAINBO program of clinical trials has been designed to investigate treatment strategies for each of the four molecular subgroups.

OSCE 15.
There was a 4 cm growth at the uterine fundus, invading 60% of the myometrium. A microscopic examination revealed grade 2 endometrioid adenocarcinoma and extensive lymphovascular invasion. There was no evidence of tumor cells in the sentinel lymph nodes. On immunohistochemistry, expression of all MMR proteins was retained, and p53 expression was wild. There was no POLE mutation.
1. What is the stage?
2. Define the prognostic risk group of the patient.
3. What adjuvant therapy is advisable?

Ans.
1. Stage IIB
2. High-intermediate prognostic risk group
3. External beam radiation therapy is recommended.

Reference
1. Concin N, Matias-Guiu X, Vergote I, Cibula D, Mirza MR, Marnitz S, Ledermann J, Bosse T, Chargari C, Fagotti A, Fotopoulou C. ESGO/ESTRO/ESP guidelines for the management of patients with endometrial carcinoma. International Journal of Gynecologic Cancer. 2021;31(1).

OSCE 16.
1. Name two groups of patients with endometrial cancer most likely to benefit from adjuvant chemotherapy.
2. What agents are used for first-line chemotherapy?

Ans.
1. The most significant overall survival benefit with the addition of adjuvant chemotherapy is seen in stage III carcinomas and serous carcinomas regardless of stage.
2. Carboplatin and paclitaxel

OSCE 17.
1. What is the incidence of recurrence after early stage endometrial cancer?
2. What is the most common site of recurrence?
3. In a radiotherapy-naïve patient, how is recurrence treated?

Ans.
1. 7–15% of early-stage (I/II) patients present with recurrent disease, usually 3 years of primary treatment.
2. Recurrence is confined to the pelvis (local) in 50% of the patients, associated with distant metastases in 25%, and maybe simultaneously local and distant in 25%.
3. Isolated pelvic metastasis in a radiotherapy-naive patient may be treated with radiotherapy. Metastatic disease may be treated with chemotherapy, hormonal therapy or immunotherapy.

Reference

1. Legge F, Restaino S, Leone L, Carone V, Ronsini C, Di Fiore GLM, Pasciuto T, Pelligra S, Ciccarone F, Scambia G, et al. Clinical outcome of recurrent endometrial cancer: Analysis of post-relapse survival by pattern of recurrence and secondary treatment. Int. J. Gynecol. Cancer. 2020;30: 193–200. doi: 10.1136/ijgc-2019-000822

OSCE 18. Mrs Y, 63 years of age, had been diagnosed with stage IIB grade 2 endometrioid adenocarcinoma in 2020 and had undergone surgical staging followed by adjuvant external beam radiotherapy. She has currently presented with enlarged para-aortic lymph nodes and omental and peritoneal deposits.

1. What additional histological markers should be in a case of recurrent endometrial cancer?
2. How do these markers determine the use of therapeutic agents in recurrent disease?

Ans.

1. Histological marker	2. Therapeutic agent
Estrogen and progesterone receptor status	Hormonal therapy: • Pregestational agents (Medroxyprogesterone acetate, Megestrol acetate) • Aromatase inhibitors • Tamoxifen
Mismatch repair deficiency	Immune checkpoint inhibitors
Mismatch repair proficiency	Lenvatinib + Pembrolizumab
HER2 expression in serous cancers	Trastuzumab

CHAPTER 43

Cervical Carcinoma

Kasturi V Donimath

OSCE 1.

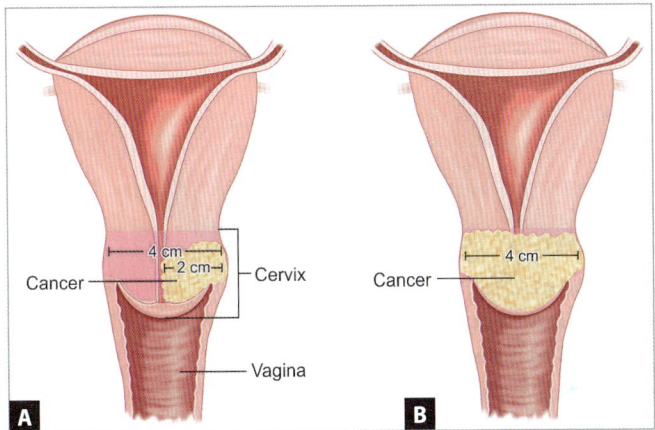

1. What is the stage of carcinoma cervix in the above Figure A and B?
2. In which stage of carcinoma cervix lymph nodes are involved?
3. In which stage of carcinoma cervix parametrium is involved?
4. In which stage of carcinoma cervix distant metastasis is present?

Ans.

1. a. Figure A—1B2
   b. Figure B—1B3
2. Stage 3
3. Stage 2B
4. Stage 4B

OSCE 2.

> **HPV subtypes**
> 6, 11, 16, 18, 31, 33, 35, 39, 42, 43, 44, 45, 51, 52, 56, 58, 59, 68

1. What are the HPV subtypes associated with high risk?
2. What are the HPV subtypes associated with low risk?
3. What is the most common HPV subtype responsible for squamous cell carcinoma cervix?
4. What is the most common HPV subtype responsible for adenocarcinoma of cervix?

Ans.
1. HPV-16, 18, 31, 33, 35, 39, 45, 51
2. HPV-6, 11, 42, 43, 44
3. HPV-16
4. HPV-18

OSCE 3.

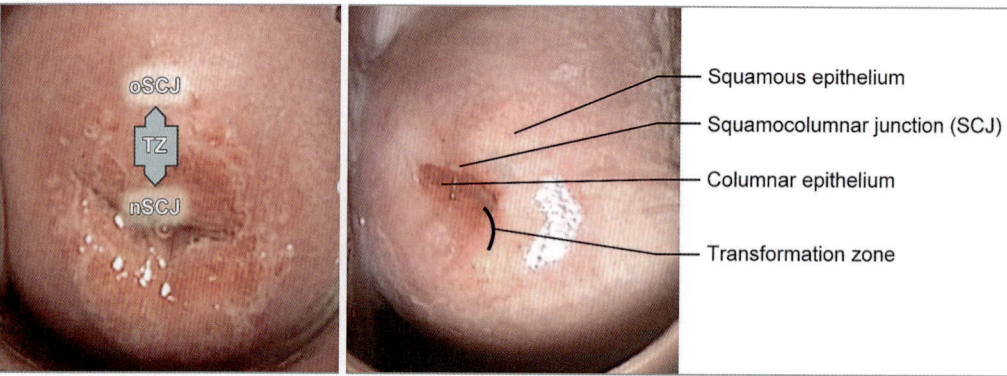

1. What is transformation zone?
2. What is the clinical significance of transformation zone?
3. What is the epithelial histology of ectocervix?
4. What is the epithelial histology of endocervix?

Ans.
1. The place at which columnar epithelium of endocervix changes to squamous epithelium of exocervix.
2. It is the dynamic point where repeated cell division takes place and hence the change in the histology leads to infection with sexually transmitted HPV virus and leads to carcinoma cervix.
3. Single layer of tall columnar epithelium.
4. Stratified nonkeratinized squamous epithelium.

OSCE 4.

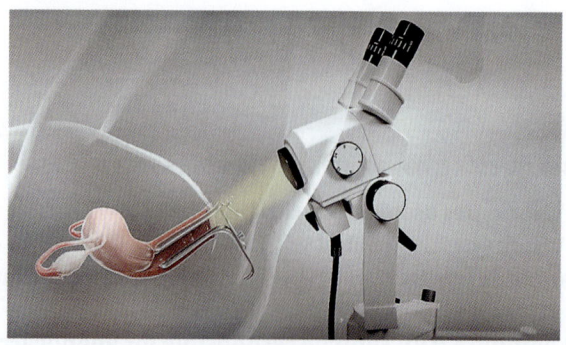

1. Identify the instrument shown.
2. What is the use of the instrument?
3. What are cervical features which indicate neoplasia?
4. What are the disadvantages of the instrument?

Ans.

1. Colposcope
2. Screening for carcinoma cervix and taking colposcopy-guided cervical punch biopsy
3. a. Leukoplakia on cervix
   b. Rough and raised area of cervix
   c. Abnormal vessel pattern like mosaic, reticular, comma-shaped and punctate blood vessels
   d. Acetowhite area on 3% acetic acid application
   e. Unstained area on 5% Lugol's iodine application
4. It cannot be used in low resource setting

OSCE 5.

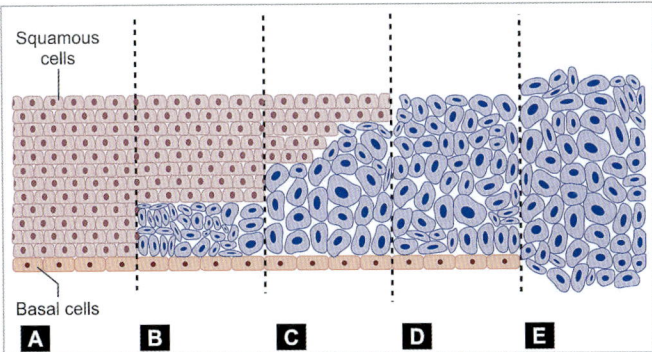

1. Which of the above histopathological areas depicted by alphabets indicates CIN2?
2. Which of the above histopathological area depicted by alphabets indicate LSIL?
3. Which of the above histopathological areas depicted by alphabets indicate HSIL?
4. What is metaplasia?

Ans.

1. C
2. B
3. C and D
4. Physiological, nonpremalignant change in columnar epithelium of endocervix to squamous epithelium exocervix.

OSCE 6.

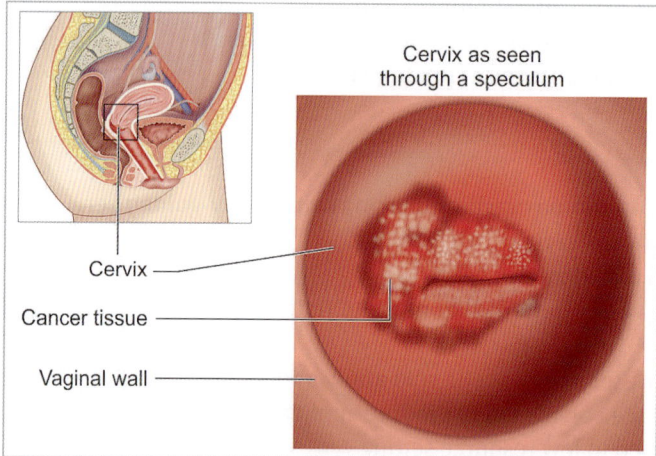

1. Enumerate five risk factors for the disease shown in the above image.
2. Enumerate four specific symptoms of this disease.

Ans.

1. a. Coitus before 18 years of age
   b. Multiple sex partners
   c. Multiparity
   d. Poor personal hygiene
   e. Poor socioeconomic status
2. a. Postmenopausal bleeding
   b. Postcoital bleeding
   c. Foul smelling discharge per vagina
   d. Pelvic pain or low backache

OSCE 7.

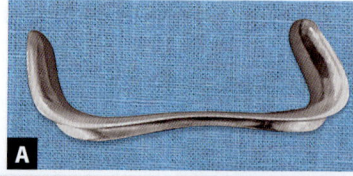

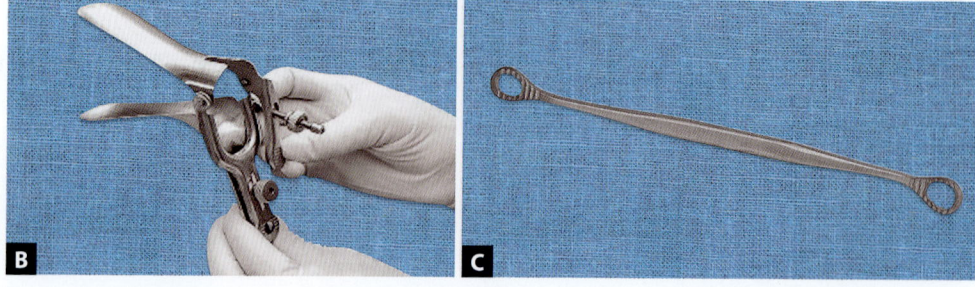

1. Identify the above instruments A, B and C.
2. What are identifying features of these instruments?
3. What is the difference between instruments A and B?

Ans.

1. a. A—Sim's speculum
   b. B—Cusco's speculum
   c. C—Curette
2. a. A—Single blade is used to retract
   b. B—Double bade is used to retract
   c. C—Long slender curved, fenestrated, serrated ends
3.

Sim's speculum	Cusco's speculum
Not self-retaining	Self-retaining
Assistance is needed to retract	No need of assistance

OSCE 8.

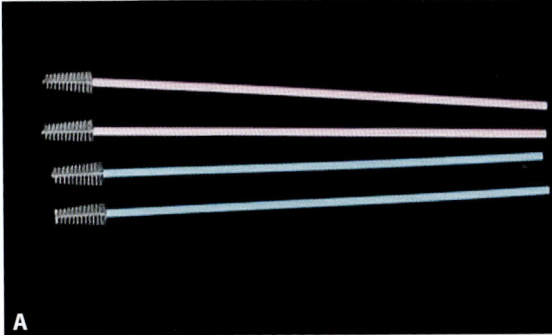

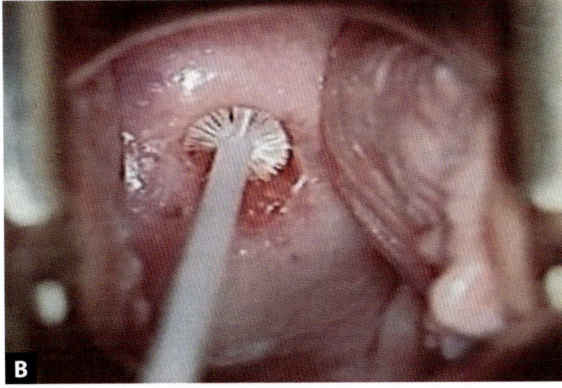

1. Identify the instrument.
2. What is its use?
3. What is the use of the above procedure?
4. What is co-testing?

Ans.
1. Cytobrush
2. To take exfoliated cell sample from cervical canal
3. To screen for carcinoma cervix
4. Co-testing is combination of PAP cytology plus HPV DNA testing.
   - Advantage of this test is that frequency of CA cervix screening can be reduced from 3 to 5 years.
   - It increases the sensitivity and specificity of the screening.

OSCE 9.

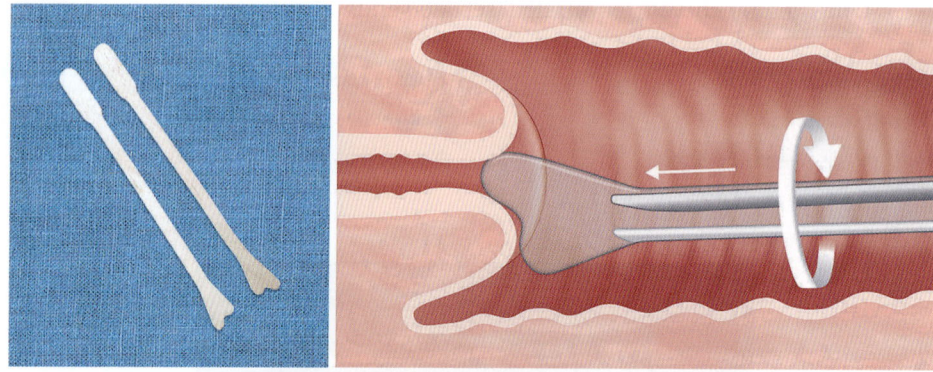

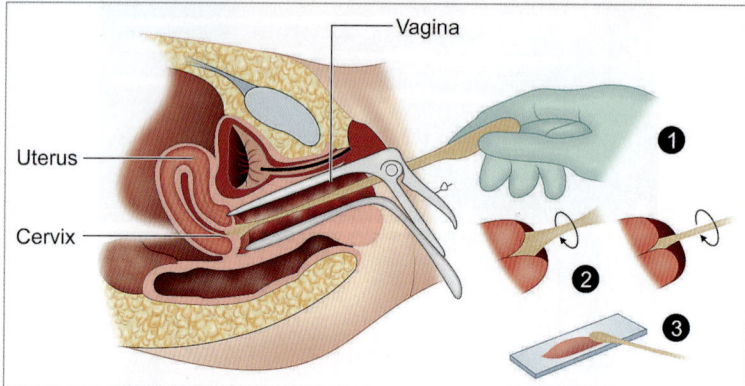

1. Identify the above instrument.
2. What is its use?
3. What is the use of above procedure shown in the image?
4. What is the reagent used to fix the smear?

Ans.
1. Ayres spatula
2. To take the exfoliated cell sample from transformation zone of the cervix
3. a. Screening carcinoma cervix
   b. Infective organisms and inflammatory or atrophic cells can be visualized
4. 95% ethanol

OSCE 10.

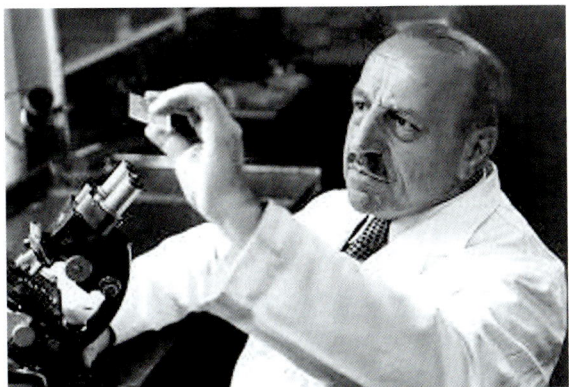

1. Identify the person in the image.
2. What are the guidelines for screening carcinoma cervix?

Ans.

1. Georgios Papanikolaou
2. a. The age to begin Pap smear is 21 years or earlier at the start of sexual activity.
   b. *21–29 years:* Pap smear once in every 3 years.
   c. *30–65 years:* Pap smear once in every 3 years or co-testing once in 5 years.
   d. Screening is stopped at 65 years provided no history of dysplasia, or three negative PAP or two negative co-tests in the row of last 10 years, last one should be done within 5 years.

OSCE 11.

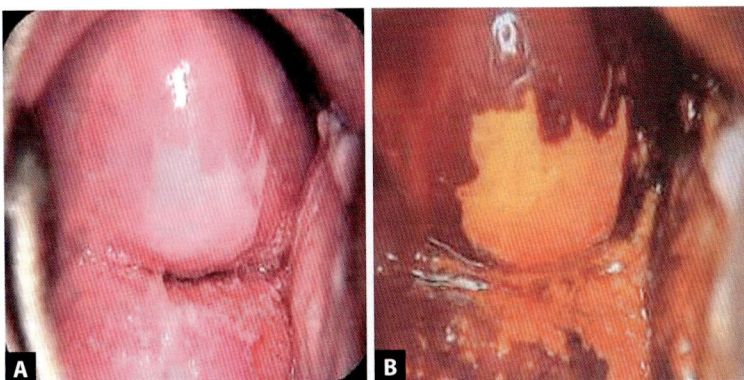

1. What is the method used to identify the abnormal area of transformation zone in A and B?
2. What are the reagents used in above procedure to identify the abnormal area in the transformation zone?
3. What is acetowhite area in the image A?
4. What is the yellow area in the image B indicate?

Ans.
1. A—VIA; B—VILI
2. A—3% acetic acid; B— 5% Lugol's iodine
3. Acetic acid coagulates, the abundant proteins in the large nuclei and cytoplasm, making the proteins opaque and white which are called acetowhite areas.
4. Normal squamous epithelium contains glycogen. It takes up the stain from Lugol's iodine. In case of premalignant cells, lack of glycogen does not take the stain and remains yellow.

OSCE 12.

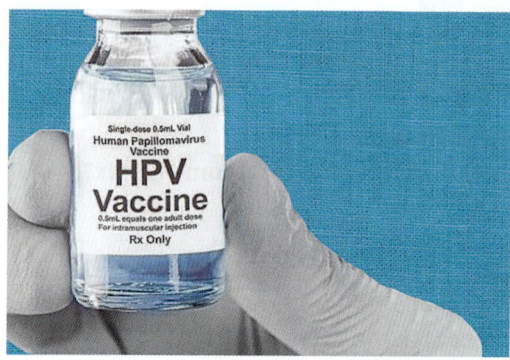

1. Mention the types of vaccines available and the HPV subtypes covered by these vaccines.
2. What are the guidelines for vaccination in prevention of carcinoma cervix?

Ans.
1.

Vaccine	HPV subtype covered
Cervarix bivalent	16, 18
Gardasil quadrivalent	6, 11, 16, 18
Gardasil-9 nonavalent	6, 11, 16, 18, 31, 33, 45, 52, 58

2. a. *Ideal age:* 11–12 years
   b. *Range:* 9–26 years
   c. *In 9–14 years*: Two doses are recommended.
      - The second dose should be given 6–12 months after the first dose (0, 6–12-month schedule).
      - The minimum interval is five months between the first and second dose. If the second dose is administered after a shorter interval, a third dose should be administered a minimum of five months after the first dose and a minimum of 12 weeks after the second dose.
   d. *Above 15 years*: Three doses are recommended.

Reference
1. HPV vaccine schedule and dosing. Centers for Disease Control and Prevention; 2021.

OSCE 13.

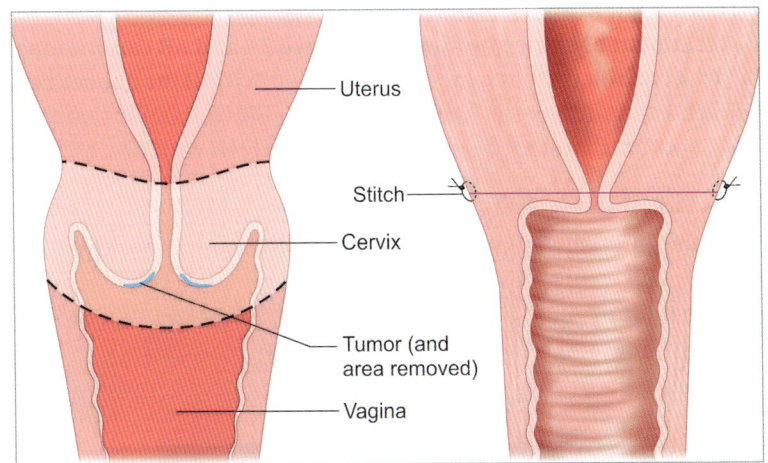

1. What is the procedure depicted in the above image?
2. At what stage and under which circumstances the above procured is done?
3. What is the most common group of lymph nodes involved in carcinoma cervix?
4. What is the 1st lymph node involved in carcinoma cervix?

Ans.

1. Trachelectomy
2. Stage 1A2, 1B1, who desire to uterine preservation and fertility
3. Obturator group
4. Paracervical lymph node

OSCE 14.

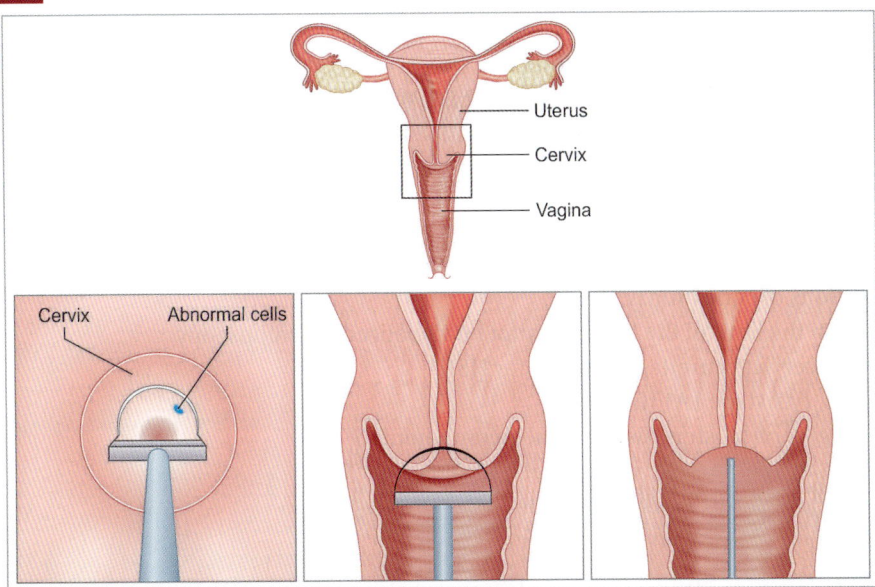

1. What the procedure shown in the above image?
2. What is the indication of above procedure?
3. What is the treatment of choice for the stage above 2A and 3B carcinoma cervix?
4. What is the drug of choice used to increase the sensitivity of the cancer cells of cervix to radiotherapy?

Ans.

1. LLETZ
2. a. CIN-2 in young girls when repeat Pap test plus colposcopy is positive
   b. CIN-3 in any age.
3. Chemoradiation therapy
4. Cisplatin

OSCE 15.

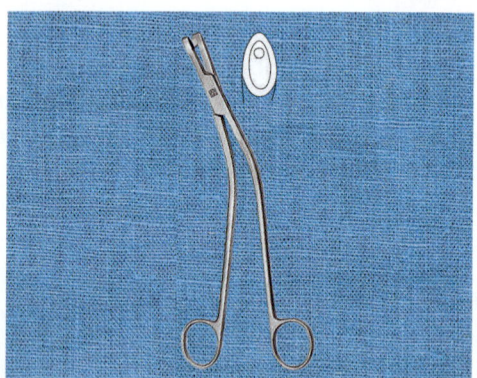

1. Name the instrument.
2. What is the use of this instrument?
3. What is cone biopsy?
4. What is the indication of cone biopsy?
5. Enumerate two complications of cone biopsy.

Ans.

1. Punch biopsy forceps
2. To take biopsy for the diagnosis of carcinoma cervix
3. Removal of a cone of cervix including the exocervix, T-Z zone and part of endocervix.
4. Indications of cone biopsy are:
   - When the limit of the lesion cannot be visualized on colposcopy
   - Endocervical curettage positive for HSIL
   - CA cervix stage 1A1 in young
5. Bleeding, cervical stenosis, cervical incompetence

OSCE 16.

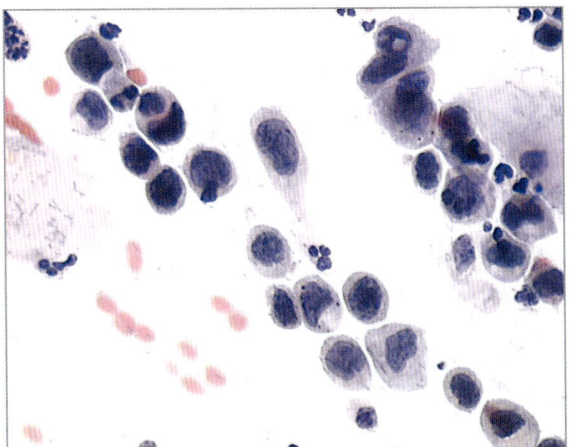

1. What is the class indicated by Bethesda reporting type of classification for above Pap smear image?
2. What is dysplasia and its features?
3. Write the reporting types of Bethesda classification.

Ans.

1. HSIL
2. Pathological premalignant change in the histology. Features—high mitotic activity, large irregular hyperchromatic nuclei, altered N/C (nucleocytoplasmic) ratio, cells vary in size and shape.
3. Normal, ASC-H, ASC-US, LSIL, HSIL.

OSCE 17.

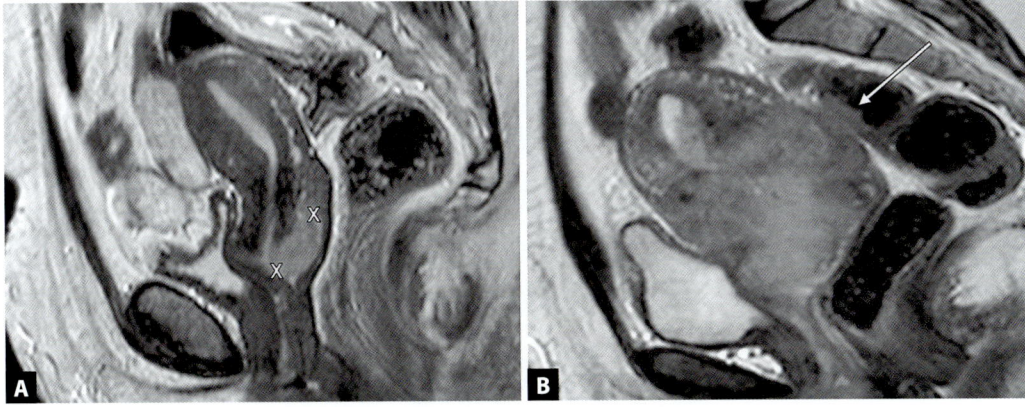

1. What is the imaging modality used in the above pathology?
2. What is the part involved in the malignant pathology in image A?
3. What is the part involving in the malignant pathology of cervix in image B?
4. What is the stage of carcinoma cervix in the image B?

Ans.

1. MRI
2. Posterior cervical lip
3. Anterior rectal wall
4. 4A

OSCE 18.

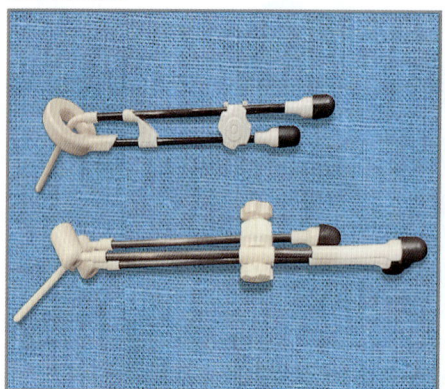
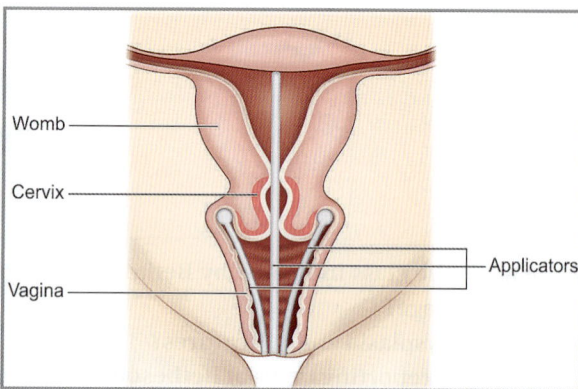

1. **Identify the instruments above.**
2. **What it is used for?**
3. **Enumerate two complications of the above treatment.**

Ans.

1. Brachytherapy uterine applicators
2. A type of radiotherapy used to treat carcinoma cervix
3. Proctitis, radiation cystitis, fistulas, enteritis, femoral head necrosis, rectal strictures.

OSCE 19.

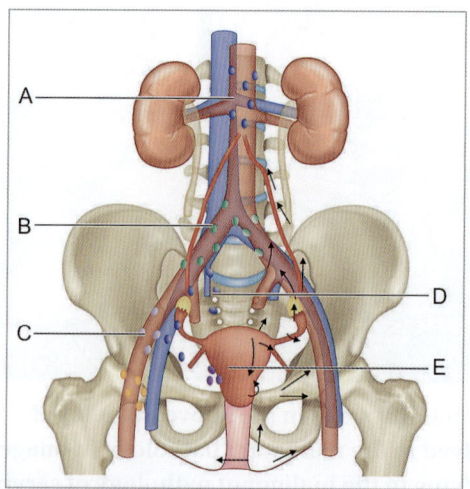

1. **Name the group of lymph nodes from the above picture.**

Ans.

1.
   A—Para-aortic
   B—Common iliac
   C—External iliac
   D—Internal iliac
   E—Obturator

OSCE 20.

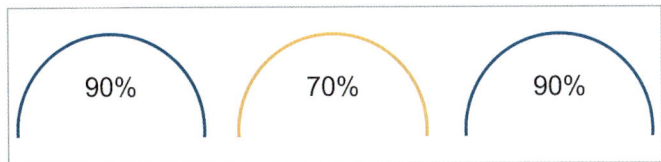

1. What is 90-70-90 strategy?
2. It was initiated by which organization?
3. By when is the target expected to reach?

Ans.

1. Global strategy for elimination of cervical cancer.
   90% screening coverage, 70% HPV vaccination coverage and 90% access to treatment for cervical precancer and cancer including access to palliative care.
2. WHO
3. 2030

CHAPTER 44

Gestational Trophoblastic Neoplasia

Neha Mishra

OSCE 1.

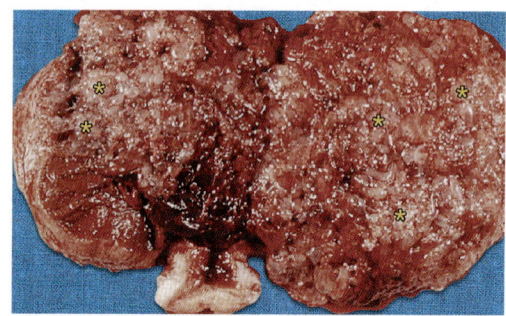

Reprinted with permission from[1] under the terms of the CC BY-NC-ND license.

1. Identify the specimen.
2. Enumerate four risk factors for the above pathology.
3. Compare and contrast between complete and partial mole.
4. Enumerate the oncogenes involved in the development of gestational trophoblastic neoplasia (GTN).

Ans.

1. Complete hydatidiform mole
2. a. Low dietary intake of carotene
   b. Vitamin A deficiency
   c. Higher maternal age >35 years
   d. Previous history of molar pregnancy
3. Compare and contrast complete and partial mole

Features	Complete Mole	Partial Mole
Karyotype	Diploid	Triploid
Gross examination	Diffuse hydropic villi, fetus absent	Patchy hydropic villi, fetus with partial mole exhibits stigmata of triploidy
Trophoblastic hyperplasia	Marked	Mild
Cytologic atypia	Marked	Mild
Progress to GTN	15–20%	0.1–5%

4. Overexpression of Oncogenes like c-myc, m-TOR, MAPK, Mcl-1, and EGFR. Down-regulation of FTL (ferritin light polypeptide) and IGFBP1 (Insulin-like growth factor binding protein 1).

References

1. Lepore A, Conran R. (2021). Educational case: hydatidiform molar pregnancy. academic pathology. 8. 237428952098725. 10.1177/2374289520987256.
2. Berek SJ, Hacker FN. Berek & Hacker's Gynaecologic Oncology, 7th Edition, Wolters Kluwer Health, 2020.

OSCE 2.

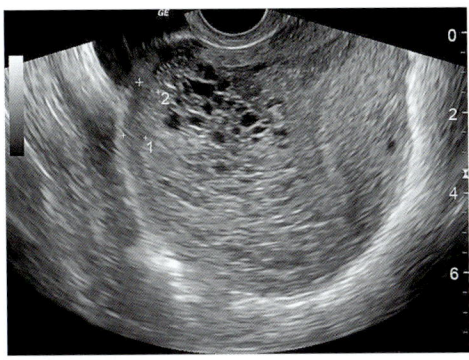

1. **Identify the above USG film?**
2. **Enumerate four radiological features of a complete mole.**
3. **Enumerate four radiological features of partial mole.**

Ans.

1. Ultrasonography appearance—complete mole
2. *USG features:*
    - Complete Mole
    - No fetus
    - Absent amniotic fluid
    - *Central heterogeneous mass with discrete anechoic spaces:* Snowstorm/Swiss Cheese Appearance
    - Ovarian theca lutein cysts
3. *USG features:*
    - Partial mole
    - Fetus identified, often growth restricted, fetal anomalies or demise.
    - Amniotic fluid+, volume reduced.
    - Placenta enlarged, cystic spaces within placenta.
    - Increased transverse diameter of gestational sac.

Reference

1. Berek S Jonathan. Berek & Novak's Gynecology, 16th Edition, Lippincott Williams and Wilkins, 2019.

OSCE 3.

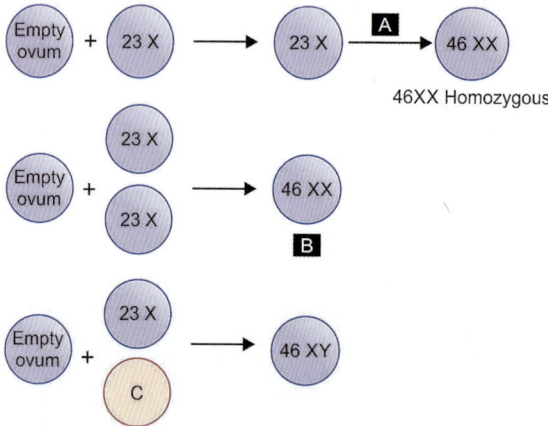

1. Identify A, B and C in above figure.
2. The molar chromosomes are entirely of _____ origin.
3. In molar pregnancy, mitochondrial DNA is of _____ origin.

Ans.

1. A: Endoduplication, B: 46XX Heterozygous, C: 23Y
2. Paternal
3. Maternal

Reference

1. Berek S Jonathan. Berek & Novak's Gynecology, 16th Edition, Lippincott Williams and Wilkins, 2019.

OSCE 4.

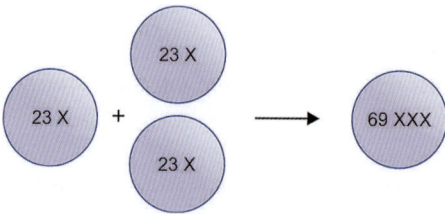

1. Identify above figure.
2. Enumerate two pathological features of partial hydatidiform mole.
3. The karyotype in partial mole is _____.
4. Discuss two stigmata demonstrated by fetus with partial mole.
5. Mutation in _____ gene is responsible for familial recurrent molar pregnancy.

Ans.

1. Formation of partial mole

2. Chorionic villi of varying size with focal hydatidiform swelling, cavitation, and trophoblastic hyperplasia, Marked villous scalloping, Prominent stromal trophoblastic inclusions, Identifiable embryonic or fetal tissues.
3. Triploid (69XXX/69XXY/69XYY)
4. Syndactyly, Fetal Growth Restriction
5. *NLRP7* and *KHD3CL*

References

1. Berek S Jonathan. Berek & Novak's Gynecology, 16th Edition. Lippincot Williams and Wilkins, 2019.
2. Ngan HYS, Seckl MJ, Berkowitz RS, Xiang Y, Golfier F, Sekharan PK, Lurain JR, Massuger L. Diagnosis and management of gestational trophoblastic disease: 2021 update. Int J Gynaecol Obstet. 2021;155(Suppl 1):86-93. doi: 10.1002/ijgo.13877. PMID: 34669197; PMCID: PMC9298230.

OSCE 5.

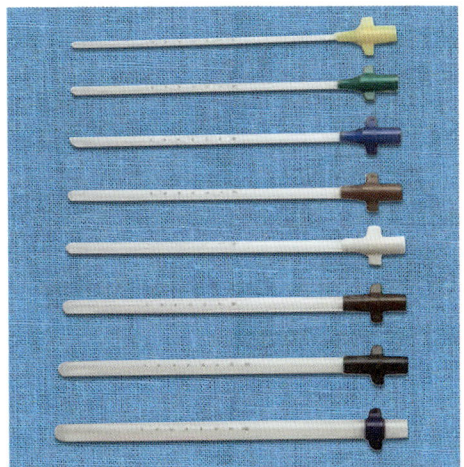

1. Identify the instrument.
2. Which size of the above instrument is used in surgical management of molar pregnancy?
3. Name the procedure used for treatment of molar pregnancy. How is the cervical dilatation done for the above procedure?
4. Should anti-D prophylaxis be given in Rh-negative women after suction and evacuation?
5. What are preferred methods of contraception during the follow-up period?

Ans.

1. Karman's Cannula
2. Karman's Cannula no. 12–14
3. Suction and Evacuation, mechanical dilatation is preferred. Prostaglandins are not used for ripening as it induces uterine contractions increasing risk of trophoblastic embolization to pulmonary vasculature.

4. Yes, as partial molar pregnancy contains fetal tissue and results of histopathology are available later.
5. Hormonal Contraception (Oral Contraceptive pills, Progesterone only pills, and injection Depot Medroxy Progesterone) and Barrier Methods

References

1. Management of Gestational Trophoblastic Disease: Green-top Guideline No. 38 - June 2020. BJOG. 2021 Feb;128(3):e1-e27. doi: 10.1111/1471-0528.16266. Epub 2020 Sep 29. PMID: 32996207.
2. Seckl MJ, Sebire NJ, Fisher RA, et al; ESMO Guidelines Working Group. Gestational trophoblastic disease: ESMO Clinical Practice Guidelines for diagnosis, treatment and follow-up. Ann Oncol. 2013 Oct;24 Suppl 6:vi39-50. doi: 10.1093/annonc/mdt345. Epub 2013 Sep 1. PMID: 23999759.

OSCE 6. A 26-year-old Primigravida was referred to a tertiary center at 18 weeks due to elevated maternal serum alpha-fetoprotein levels (MSAFP, MoM >3.9). Her dates were confirmed. On examination, she was found to be hypertensive and fundal height of 16 weeks with no other remarkable findings. Her β-hCG levels were 345320 mIU/mL. The scan revealed a live 16-week fetus with findings of syndactyly. The placenta was enlarged with focal cystic spaces with bilateral adnexal masses of 6.5 cm × 7 cm each. Amniocentesis was done.

1. What is the most probable diagnosis in the above case?
2. What would be the most probable fetal karyotype in the above case?
3. Enumerate other stigmata seen in affected fetuses.
4. How will you manage the above case?
5. Enumerate four histopathological features of partial mole.

Ans.

1. Partial molar pregnancy
2. Triploidy
3. Fetal growth restriction
4. Medical Termination of Pregnancy followed by follow-up (weekly β-hCG till 3 consecutive normal values followed by 3 monthly for next 6 months)
5. Chorionic villi of varying size with focal hydatidiform swelling, cavitation, and trophoblastic hyperplasia, marked villous scalloping, prominent stromal trophoblastic inclusions, Identifiable embryonic or fetal tissues.

References

1. Ngan HYS, Seckl MJ, Berkowitz RS, Xiang Y, Golfier F, Sekharan PK, Lurain JR, Massuger L. Diagnosis and management of gestational trophoblastic disease: 2021 update. Int J Gynaecol Obstet. 2021;155 (Suppl 1):86-93. doi: 10.1002/ijgo.13877. PMID: 34669197; PMCID: PMC9298230
2. Berek S Jonathan. Berek & Novak's Gynecology, 16th Edition, Lippincot Williams and Wilkins, 2019.

OSCE 7. A patient presents to casualty with complaints of amenorrhea of 4 months and bleeding along with passage of grape-like vesicles per vaginum. Her UPT is positive and serum beta hCG was >10,000 IU/mL.

1. Identify the above condition. Enumerate four common clinical features of the above condition.
2. Which lab investigation is used in diagnosis as well as prognostication of the above disease.
3. What is the prozone phenomenon?
4. Enumerate the imaging modalities used in diagnosis and follow-up of GTN.

Ans.

1. Molar Pregnancy
   Clinical features: Vaginal bleeding (M/C) (46%), Excessive uterine enlargement >POG (28%), Pre-eclampsia (27%), hyperemesis gravidarum (8%), hyperthyroidism (7%), respiratory distress (2%), theca lutein ovarian cysts (50%), anemia (5%)
2. Beta-Human Chorionic Gonadotrophin
3. High analyte concentration saturates the antibody binding sites, preventing formation of Ab-hCG-Ab sandwich leading to hook-like effect.
4. *Imaging in GTN:*
   a. *Pelvic Doppler USG:* Confirm absence of pregnancy, measure uterine size, determine volume and vasculature of tumor.
   b. Chest X-ray—to see metastasis.
   c. *CT chest:* If metastatic lesions >1 cm.
   d. *MRI brain, CT abdomen and pelvis:* If CT chest shows metastatic lesions >1 cm

References

1. Berek S Jonathan. Berek & Novak's Gynecology-16th Edition, Lippincott Williams and Wilkins, 2019.
2. Gestational Trophoblastic Neoplasia, Version 1.2022, NCCN Clinical Practice Guidelines in Oncology.

OSCE 8.

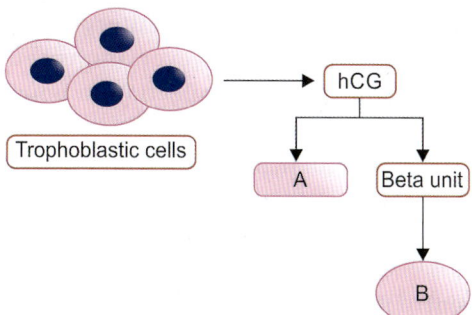

1. Identify A and B in the above figure.
2. Which subunit of hCG is homologous to that of LH, FSH and TSH?
3. Discuss criteria for diagnosis of post molar gestational trophoblastic neoplasia.
4. Which hCG assay should be used for monitoring GTN?

Ans.

1. A—alpha subunit, B—detects pregnancy
2. Alpha subunit
3. Criteria-1 or more of the following:
   - hCG levels plateau (+10%) for 4 consecutive values over 3 weeks
   - hCG levels rise ≥10% for 3 values over 2 weeks.
   - hCG persistence ≥6 months after molar evacuation
   - Histopathologic evidence of choriocarcinoma
   - Presence of metastatic disease
4. Free beta subunit

References

1. Berek SJ, Hacker FN. Berek & Hacker's Gynaecologic Oncology, 7th Edition, Wolters Kluver Health.
2. Seckl MJ, Sebire NJ, Fisher RA, et al; ESMO Guidelines Working Group. Gestational trophoblastic disease: ESMO Clinical Practice Guidelines for diagnosis, treatment, and follow-up. Ann Oncol. 2013;24 (Suppl 6):vi39-50. doi: 10.1093/annonc/mdt345. Epub 2013 Sep 1. PMID: 23999759.
3. Gestational Trophoblastic Neoplasia, Version 1.2022, NCCN Clinical Practice Guidelines in Oncology.

OSCE 9. A 25-year nulliparous lady was referred to a tertiary care hospital, as a case of ruptured ectopic pregnancy. On admission, the patient was conscious but had signs of hypovolemic shock with severe pallor (blood pressure 80/60 mm Hg, pulse rate 140 bpm). Abdominal examination revealed a distended and tense abdomen with lower abdominal tenderness. Vaginal examination showed minimal bleeding, closed external os, and fullness in fornices. Paracentesis showed nonclotting blood. The patient had a history of dilatation and curettage done 2 months back in view of spontaneous abortion and passage of grape like products at 12 weeks gestation in a private hospital. No histopathology had been sent. Patient remained asymptomatic for 1 month and developed bleeding per vaginum, thereafter. She assumed it as menstruation, though pattern of bleeding was different from normal. After 5 days of bleeding, she developed acute pain in abdomen. Ultrasound was done which showed normal size uterus with endometrial thickness of 12 mm. Bilateral ovaries were normal, however, increased vascularity in bilateral adnexa and mild amount of heterogeneous collection in pouch of Douglas was noted. The β-hCG levels came out to be 2,97,198 IU.

1. What percentage of complete molar pregnancy and partial molar pregnancy progresses to GTN?
2. Enumerate the investigations done to diagnose a case of gestational trophoblastic neoplasia.
3. What is the management of the above case?

Ans.

1. *Complete Molar Pregnancy*: 15–20%, partial molar pregnancy—0.5–5%
2. Serial Beta-hCG values, Chest X-ray, abdominal ultrasound and computed tomography (CT), magnetic resonance imaging (MRI) brain, CT Head, CSF hCG level

(metastatic disease or presence of neurologic signs), Stool guaiac tests, selective angiography of abdominal and pelvic organs, if indicated, whole body ^{18}FDG-PET scan to identify occult disease, if indicated, review of all available pathology.
3. *Emergency Exploratory Laparotomy:* To look out for molar tissue invading myometrium and causing uterine rupture. Decision for hysterectomy/preserving the uterus as peroperative findings followed by chemotherapy as this case seems to be of perforating mole.

Reference

1. Ngan HYS, Seckl MJ, Berkowitz RS, Xiang Y, Golfier F, Sekharan PK, Lurain JR, Massuger L. Diagnosis and management of gestational trophoblastic disease: 2021 update. Int J Gynaecol Obstet. 2021;155(Suppl 1):86-93. doi: 10.1002/ijgo.13877. PMID: 34669197; PMCID: PMC9298230.

OSCE 10. A 26-year nulliparous woman presented in casualty with signs and symptoms of hypovolemic shock. She gives history of spontaneous abortion followed by dilatation and evacuation 4 months back. Her UPT was positive. The β-hCG level of the above patient was 3,17,492. On admission, abdomen was distended and tense. On per speculum and per vaginum examination, vagina and cervix were healthy, no bleeding from external os, uterus normal size and fullness of both fornices was noted. She was taken for emergency laparotomy and intraoperative finding are depicted in below image. Bleeding was controlled through hemostatic sutures from bleeding points and uterus was preserved keeping nulliparous state of women in consideration after taking consent.

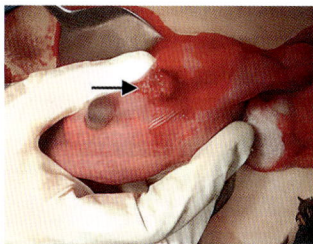 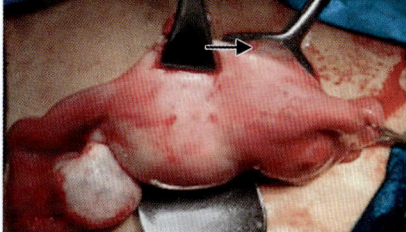 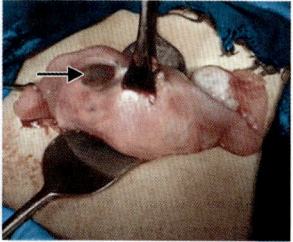

1. What is your provisional diagnosis?
2. Histopathological report of blebs and vesicles came out to be hyperplastic trophoblasts, generalized cystic degeneration of chorionic villi and presence of molar villi within myometrium. Her uterus was conserved. What will be the next line of management?
3. What are histological types of GTN?
4. _____ comprises 80% of all GTN. What is the cure rate of low-risk GTN with chemotherapy?

Ans.

1. The uterus enlarged to 10–12 weeks size with a rent of 2 × 1 cm on fundus with torrential bleeding through it and grape-like vesicles popping from it, most likely perforating mole.
2. After reviewing of all reports and prognostic WHO scoring, multiagent chemotherapy (EMACO) should be started.

3. *Histological types of GTN:*
    - Invasive mole
    - Choriocarcinoma
    - Placental site trophoblastic tumor
    - Epithelioid trophoblastic tumor
    - Atypical placental site nodule
4. Invasive mole, 100%

References
1. Singh N, Singh S, Sharma E, Rajaram S, Mishra N. Perforating Mole in a Nullipara Leading to Massive Hemoperitoneum: Fertility Preservation: a challenge. Ann Clin Case Rep. 2020;5:1806.
2. Berek SJ, Hacker FN. Berek & Hacker's Gynaecologic Oncology, 7th edition, Wolters Kluver Health, 2020.

OSCE 11.

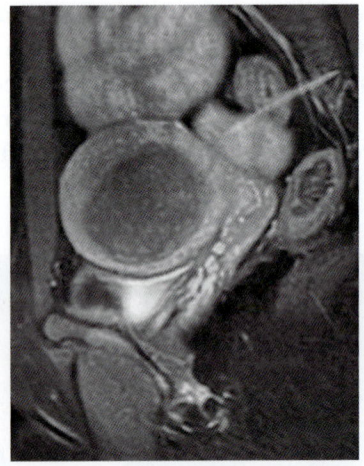

A 25-year-old, P0A4, last pregnancy being molar pregnancy, suction and evacuation was done with histopathological diagnosis of complete hydatidiform mole. During follow-up, she was diagnosed with 5 × 4.4 × 3.7 cm hypo enhancing mass lesion involving more than 50% of myometrium on contrast-enhanced MRI as shown in image above with rising of beta-hCG level.

1. What is the diagnosis?
2. About 50% of GTN occur after _____ pregnancy.
3. Enumerate the sites to which GTN can metastasize? Which is the most common site.
4. What are the most common sites of vaginal metastasis in GTN?
5. Is it recommended to take biopsy of vaginal secondary deposits in a case of GTN? Cite the reasons.

Ans.

1. *GTN:* Invasive mole
2. Molar pregnancy

3. Lungs, vagina, pelvis, brain, liver, bowel, kidney, spleen
4. Fornices or suburethral
5. No, it might bleed profusely

Reference
1. Berek SJ, Hacker FN. Berek & Hacker's Gynaecologic Oncology, 7th Edition. Wolters Kluver Health, 2020.

OSCE 12. A 30-year lady presents to casualty with complaints of excessive vaginal bleeding. She gives a history of dilatation and curettage followed by tubal ligation after spontaneous abortion 4 months ago. Her menstrual cycles were regular last 2 months until this cycle where she is bleeding profusely. Her UPT is positive.
1. What is the most probable diagnosis?
2. Discuss FIGO staging of classification of gestational trophoblastic neoplasia.
3. What are indications of prophylactic chemotherapy in the case of GTN?
4. What factors will you consider choosing chemotherapy in the case of GTN?

Ans.
1. Gestational trophoblastic neoplasia
2. FIGO Stage

   Stage 1: Gestational trophoblastic tumors strictly confined to the uterine corpus.

   Stage 2: Gestational trophoblastic tumors extending to the adnexa or to the vagina, but limited to the genital structures.

   Stage 3: Gestational trophoblastic tumors extending to the lungs, with or without genital tract involvement.

   Stage 4: All other metastatic sites
3. Role of prophylactic chemotherapy is controversial. It might reduce the incidence of post-molar GTN to 3–8%. According to the NCCN Guidelines, it could be considered for high-risk patients such as:
   a. Uterine size > POG
   b. hCG >1,00,000 mIU/mL
   c. Age >40 years
   d. Theca lutein cysts >6 cm
4. We will keep FIGO Staging and GTN-FIGO prognostic scoring in mind along with pre-chemotherapy work-up before starting chemotherapy.

Score	Prognostic Risk	First-line Treatment
FIGO Stages I–III: Score <7	Low-risk GTN	Single-agent chemotherapy
FIGO Stages II–III: Score ≥7 and FIGO Stage IV	High-risk GTN	Combination chemotherapy

Reference
1. Gestational Trophoblastic Neoplasia, Version 1.2022, NCCN Clinical Practice Guidelines in Oncology,

OSCE 13. A 35-year lady with previous full-term normal delivery presents at 12 weeks amenorrhea with excessive vomiting and spotting per vaginum. On examination, her uterus is 16 weeks' size. Pregnancy test is positive. Her β-hCG levels came out to be 14569 mIU/mL. Her ultrasound showed snowstorm appearance and bilateral theca lutein cysts of size 6 cm and 7 cm in right and left ovary respectively.
1. What is spot diagnosis? What is the procedure of choice in the above case?
2. Discuss risk factors for development of GTN.
3. What is the current evidence regarding prophylactic chemotherapy?
4. What is the time required for theca lutein cysts to regress?
5. How will you follow-up above patient?

Ans.

1. Molar pregnancy. Suction and Evacuation
2. Uterus larger than gestation, pre-evacuation hCG >10^5 mIU/mL, Theca lutein cysts >6 cm, Age >40 years
3. It may have a role in women with multiple high-risk factors who are not compliant with hCG surveillance.
4. 2–3 months
5. Follow-up is done with β-hCG. 48 hours after evacuation, weekly thereafter until 3 consecutive normal assays (<5 mIU/mL), and thereafter 3 monthly for 6 months. Contraception is advised till hCG level normalizes and continued for 12 months.

Reference
1. Ngan HYS, Seckl MJ, Berkowitz RS, Xiang Y, Golfier F, Sekharan PK, Lurain JR, Massuger L. Diagnosis and management of gestational trophoblastic disease: 2021 update. Int J Gynaecol Obstet. 2021;155(Suppl 1):86-93. doi: 10.1002/ijgo.13877. PMID: 34669197; PMCID: PMC9298230.

OSCE 14. A 33-year lady underwent suction and evacuation for complete mole 6 months back. She is taking low-dose oral contraceptive pills regularly. On serial follow-up her β-hCG are persisting between levels 50–100 mIU/mL for past 3 months.
1. What do these findings signify?
2. What are the chances of developing active GTN in this case?
3. How can we differentiate between active and quiescent GTN?
4. What are the criteria for development of postmolar GTN?
5. What are the indications of using dactinomycin in a case of low-risk GTN?

Ans.

1. This represents Quiescent Gestational Trophoblastic Disease
2. 10%
3. A variant of β-hCG, hyperglycosated hCG (hCG-H) is produced by invasive trophoblasts and may be used to differentiate between active and quiescent GTN.
4. *FIGO criteria to diagnose GTN:*
   a. When the plateau of hCG lasts for four measurements over a period of 3 weeks or longer; that is, days 1, 7, 14, 21.

b. When there is a rise in hCG for three consecutive weekly measurements over at least a period of 2 weeks or more; days 1, 7, 14.
   c. If there is a histologic diagnosis of choriocarcinoma.
5. Dactinomycin is used as a secondary therapy for patients with methotrexate toxicity or effusions contradicting the use of methotrexate. It is preferred drug is there is hepatic dysfunction. The response of dactinomycin in methotrexate resistant cases is 75%.

References

1. Lakshmi Sesadri, Essentials of Gynecology, 3rd edition, LWW Wolters Kluwer, 2022.
2. Ngan HYS, Seckl MJ, Berkowitz RS, Xiang Y, Golfier F, Sekharan PK, Lurain JR, Massuger L. Diagnosis and management of gestational trophoblastic disease: 2021 update. Int J Gynaecol Obstet. 2021;155 (Suppl 1):86-93. doi: 10.1002/ijgo.13877. PMID: 34669197; PMCID: PMC9298230.

OSCE 15. A 39-year-old lady with three living issues presents to OPD with complaints of irregular vaginal bleeding. She gives history of molar pregnancy 12 months back. She had undergone tubal ligation 6 months back.
1. What are points would you like to elucidate from history and previous records?
2. Her reports after current evaluation are: β-hCG levels are 18932 mIU/mL, uterus size is normal, bilateral theca lutein cysts of 5 cm each, Chest X-ray shows three-coin shaped lesions. What is her Figo staging and risk score?
3. What are the treatment options for the above patient?
4. How will you monitor the above case?
5. Enumerate four investigations which should be done while she is on chemotherapy.

Ans.

1. Presenting symptoms, histopathology report, any requirement of chemotherapy, β-hCG levels during serial follow-up
2. FIGO Stage 3, Risk score 5
3. Since this patient has completed his family, she can be given the option of hysterectomy explaining risks and benefits. If she refuses, primary single agent chemotherapy can also be given.
4. *Monitoring:* Do weekly beta-hCG till 2–3 consecutive hCG values are normal, continue systemic therapy regimen for 2–3 cycles, hCG assay every month for 12 months and contraception for 12 months.
5. Following investigations should be done while patient is on chemotherapy.
   a. Weekly beta-hCG
   b. Weekly CBC with Absolute Neutrophil Count, LFT, KFT
   c. Monthly Chest X-ray (in patient with pulmonary metastases)

References

1. Gestational Trophoblastic Neoplasia, Version 1.2022, NCCN Clinical Practice Guidelines in Oncology.
2. Lakshmi Sesadri, Essentials of Gynecology, 3rd edition, LWW Wolters Kluwer, 2022.

Section 2: Gynecology

OSCE 16. A 36-year-old lady underwent suction and evacuation following diagnosis of complete hydatidiform mole. Her histopathological report states that "Hydropic villi are present. The proliferating cytotrophoblasts and syncytiotrophoblasts invade the myometrium."

1. What is the final diagnosis? What percentage of invasive mole cases demonstrate metastasis?
2. Enumerate four complications that can occur in the above case.
3. What is the most important differentiating feature between invasive mole and choriocarcinoma microscopically?
4. How will you proceed in the above case if FIGO risk scoring is 8?
5. Can patients with GTN get pregnant after treatment and follow-up of GTN?

Ans.

1. Invasive mole, 5%
2. Uterine perforation, intraperitoneal hemorrhage, profuse vaginal bleeding, sepsis
3. Absence of chorionic villi in choriocarcinoma
4. With FIGO scoring 8, this will be a case of high-risk GTN, hence option of multiagent chemotherapy (EMACO/EMAEP) should be given. EMA/CO: Etoposide, Methotrexate, Dactinomycin/Cyclophosphamide, Vincristine (Repeat every 2 weeks until hCG normalizes, then continue for an additional 6–8 weeks).
5. Patients with treated GTN can anticipate normal reproduction in the future.

References

1. Lakshmi Sesadri, Essentials of Gynecology, 3rd edition, LWW Wolters Kluwer, 2022.
2. Berek SJ, Hacker FN. Berek & Hacker's Gynaecologic Oncology, 7th edition, Wolters Kluver Health, 2020.

OSCE 17. A 36-year, P3L3, last full-term normal delivery, 14 months ago presents to casualty with complains of irregular vaginal bleeding since past 3 months, she has cough with occasional hemoptysis, and she had 3 episodes of seizure since past 2 months. Her β-hCG levels came out to be 1,24,356 mIU/mL, her USG followed by contrast-enhanced MRI showed 7 × 8 cm mass lesion involving more than 50% of myometrium. Her chest X-ray showed 4 coin shaped lesions and MRI showed brain secondaries as cluster-enhancing lesions in occipital lobe.

1. What is the most probable diagnosis?
2. What is FIGO stage and FIGO risk score in above case? What is Ultrahigh-risk GTN?
3. How will you manage the above case? What is induction chemotherapy?
4. How will you monitor the above case?

Ans.

1. Choriocarcinoma
2. Stage 4, FIGO risk 14 (>13), Ultrahigh Risk GTN are the ones having FIGO risk score of 13 or higher.

3. Patients with liver, brain, or extensive metastases, to avoid sudden tumor collapse in such patients, use of initial gentle induction chemotherapy rather than full-dose chemotherapy is preferred. For 1–3 courses prior to starting EMA/CO, Induction with Etoposide 100 mg/m^2/day IV and Cisplatin 20 mg/m^2/day IV on Days 1 and 2 every 7 days can be given.

   For highest-risk patients, consider: EMA/EP or EP/EMA in those responded to EMA/CO but have plateauing low hCG levels or have developed re-elevation of hCG levels. Repeat every 2 weeks alternating EMA with EP/EP with EMA weekly through 6–8 weeks post-serologic remission) (EMA/EP: Etoposide, Methotrexate, Dactinomycin/Etoposide, Cisplatin; EP/EMA: Etoposide, Cisplatin/Etoposide, Methotrexate, Dactinomycin)
4. Response is monitored weekly by serum β-hCG till 3 consecutive values are normal and continued monthly for 12 months and contraception is advised for 24 months. In case of nonresponse/resistance, switch over to alternative regimen is done.

Reference

1. Gestational Trophoblastic Neoplasia, Version 1.2022, NCCN Clinical Practice Guidelines in Oncology

OSCE 18. A 33-year lady with one living issue presents to OPD with complaints of irregular vaginal bleeding. She gave history of molar pregnancy 6 months ago. She is taking progesterone only pills. Her reports after current evaluation are: β-hCG levels are 11932 mIU/mL, uterus size is normal, bilateral theca lutein cysts of 3 cm each, Chest X-ray shows two coin-shaped lesions.
1. What is her FIGO staging and risk score? How should pretreatment evaluation be done in this patient?
2. What is the role of surgery in GTN?
3. Describe dosage and route of methotrexate in low-risk GTN.
4. What is the mechanism of action of methotrexate? Describe its side effects and how these can be prevented.

Ans.

1. FIGO stage 1, Risk score 3, CBC, LFT, KFT, *blood type and antibody screen* urine protein, thyroid function tests, and quantitative serum hCG.
   S. Testosterone: If virilization is present, then pelvic ultrasound, chest radiograph.
2. Role of surgery in GTN cases is limited but important. Hysterectomy checks persistence of drug-resistant local disease and lessens duration and amount of chemotherapy.
   Indications of hysterectomy:
   - Uncontrolled vaginal bleeding
   - Salvage surgery to rectify chemo-resistant focus of disease.
   - Women with choriocarcinoma who do not desire future fertility.
   - Women with chemotherapy resistant disease particularly in placental site trophoblastic tumor
   - Presence of significant pelvic sepsis

3. Single agent chemotherapy, preferably inj. Methotrexate
   Methotrexate: 0.4 mg/kg/day (max 25 mg/day) IV (preferred) or IM daily × 5 days; repeat every 14 days or 1 mg/kg IM every other day × 4 days (Days 1, 3, 5, and 7) Alternating every other day with leucovorin 15 mg PO (preferred) on Days 2, 4, 6, and 8: repeat every 14 days.
4. Methotrexate is folic acid antagonist and inhibits enzyme folic acid reductase. Some common side effects are gastrointestinal mucositis, stomatitis, alopecia, and hepatotoxicity which can be reduced by use of folinic acid.

Reference
1. Gestational Trophoblastic Neoplasia, Version 1.2022, NCCN Clinical Practice Guidelines in Oncology.

OSCE 19. A 26-year, $P_1A_1L_0$ woman reported to the casualty with complaints of acute transient generalized tonic-clonic seizure for past 1 week. She had been experiencing hemoptysis also for the preceding 12 days, which had been diagnosed and managed as community acquired pneumonia. Her serum β-hCG level was 87,524 IU/L without evidence of pregnancy. She was diagnosed with GTN with lung, brain, and gum metastases.

1. Which treatment combination is most preferred in management of high-risk GTN?
2. Enumerate newer therapies in GTN.
3. What are the other options available for methotrexate-resistant high-risk GTN?
4. How should be the pregnancy after GTN be managed?

Ans.

1. *EMA/CO:* Etoposide, Methotrexate, Dactinomycin/Cyclophosphamide, Vincristine (Repeat every 2 weeks until hCG normalizes, then continue for an additional 6–8 weeks)
   - Etoposide 100 mg/m^2/day IV on Days 1 and 2.
   - Dactinomycin 0.5 mg IV push on Days 1 and 2.
   - Methotrexate 300 mg/m^2 IV infusion over 12 hours on Day 1.
   - Leucovorin 15 mg PO (preferred) or IM every 12 hours for 4 doses starting 24 hours after the start of methotrexate infusion.
   - Cyclophosphamide 600 mg/m^2 IV on Day 8.
   - Vincristine 0.8 mg/m^2 (maximum of 2 mg) IV over 5–10 minutes on Day 8.
2. High-dose chemotherapy with autologous stem cell transplant, immunotherapy (Pembrolizumab, Avelumab, Nivolumab), Gemcitabine, Capecitabine, and Fluorouracil.
3. Platinum-based compounds are used in cases of high-risk GTN resistant methotrexate like TP/TE (Paclitaxel, Cisplatin/Paclitaxel, Etoposide)
4. *Obstetric Management:*
   - First trimester USG—at 10 weeks POG—confirm normal gestational development.
   - Send placenta for HPE, if gross abnormality present.
   - hCG measurement 6 weeks after completion of pregnancy.
   - There are higher chances of spontaneous abortions, congenital malformations, pre-eclampsia, and preterm birth.

References
1. Gestational Trophoblastic Neoplasia, Version 1.2022, NCCN Clinical Practice Guidelines in Oncology.
2. Berek SJ, Hacker FN. Berek and Hacker's Gynaecologic Oncology, 7th edition, Wolters Kluwer Health, 2020.

OSCE 20. A 38-year-old woman, gestation 2, miscarriage 1, underwent a cesarean section because of fetal distress and gave birth to a healthy full-term girl in September 2023. There was no postpartum hemorrhage or puerperal fever during her postpartum period. The woman visited postpartum clinic for abnormal vaginal discharge 2 months after delivery. After clinical diagnosis of endometritis, she was prescribed antibiotics. The patient was not relieved, she made repeated follow-up visits and was intermittently treated with anti-inflammatory therapy, but the therapy was ineffective. After 6 months, her USG color Doppler pelvis showed a heterogeneous echo 21 mm × 15 mm in size in the uterine cavity which was not investigated. After 1 month, i.e., 9 months postpartum, a second pelvic color Doppler ultrasound indicated that the heterogeneous echo was 66 mm × 22 mm in size, and the patient's serum beta-human chorionic gonadotropin (β-hCG) level was 54.60 mIU/mL, compared to a normal level of lower than 5.4 mIU/mL. The patient subsequently underwent a hysteroscopy and endometrial curettage was done.

1. Give provisional diagnosis. Placental site trophoblastic tumor (PSTT) arises from_____ trophoblasts.
2. In PSTT, serum hCG levels are low but syncytiotrophoblasts secrete _____.
3. FIGO scoring for PSTT/ETT is _____. Treatment of choice in PSTT is _____.
4. PSTT comprises _____ percent of all GTN.
5. Metastasis occurs in _____ with the most common site being _____.

Ans.
1. PSTT, Intermediate
2. Human Placental Lactogen
3. Not valid, Hysterectomy with salpingectomy ± pelvic lymph node biopsy
4. One percent
5. 30–50%. Lungs

Reference
1. Gestational Trophoblastic Neoplasia, Version 1.2022, NCCN Clinical Practice Guidelines in Oncology.

CHAPTER 45

Hysterectomy

Nilanchali Singh, Nisha, Deepika Kashyap

OSCE 1.

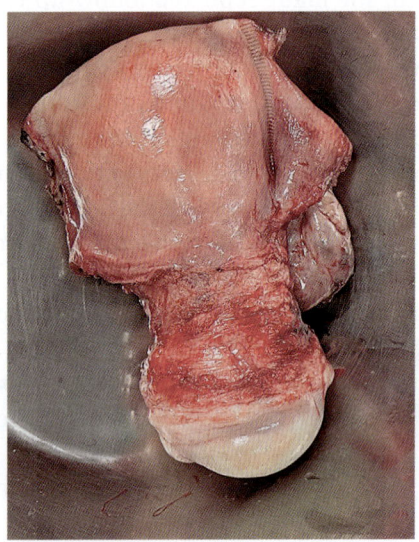

1. What is the procedure performed in above specimen?
2. What is the most common indication for this procedure?

Ans.

1. Total abdominal hysterectomy
2. Fibroid uterus

Reference

1. Te Linde's Operative Gynecology. 12th edition, 2019.

OSCE 2.

1. Identify the types of hysterectomy in the given diagram A, B, C.

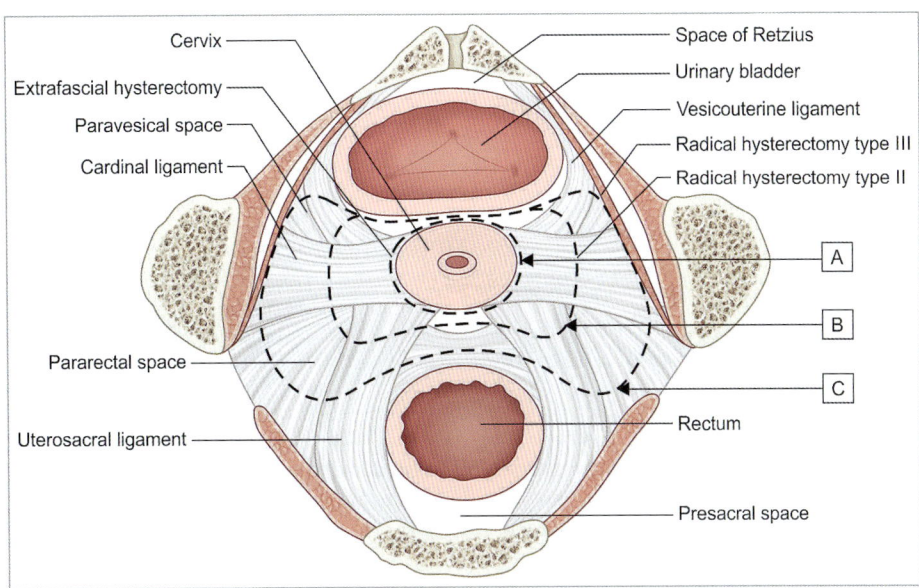

Ans.

1. A—Extrafascial hysterectomy, B—Modified radical hysterectomy (Wertheim's), C—Classical radical hysterectomy (Meig's).

   According to Piver-Rutledge and Smith classification (1974):

Class 1: Extrafascial hysterectomy	• Identify ureter • Uterosacral, cardinal ligament and uterine arteries incised close to uterus • No vaginal cuff removed
Class 2: Modified radical hysterectomy (Wertheim's)	• Ureters dissected in paracervical region • Uterine arteries ligated on medial side of ureter • Uterosacral ligaments resected midway • Medial 1/2 of cardinal ligaments removed • Removal of upper 1/3 vagina • Pelvic lymphadenectomy
Class 3: Classical radical hysterectomy (Meig's)	• Complete dissection of ureter till entry in bladder • Uterine vessels— at their origin from IIA • Uterosacral ligaments—at their sacral attachments • Cardinal ligaments resected at pelvic wall • Upper 1/2 vagina removed • Routine pelvic lymphadenectomy
Class 4	• Complete dissection of ureter from pubovesical ligament and superior vesicle artery sacrificed • Upper 3/4th of vagina removed
Class 5	• Excision of involved portion of distal ureter or bladder and reimplantation of ureter into bladder • Excision of involved portion of rectum

OSCE 3. A 48-year-old lady is planned for C1 radical hysterectomy for cervical carcinoma. According to Querleu and Morrow classification:
1. What is B1 and C1 radical hysterectomy?

Ans.

1.

B1	• Identical to B1 plus paracervical lymphadenectomy • No vascular structures/nerves resected	Partial excision of vesicouterine ligament	Partial resection of the rectouterine ligament and rectovaginal ligament along with uterosacral fold of peritoneum
C1	At level of internal iliac vessels transversally and caudal part is preserved	Excision of vesicouterine ligament at bladder and proximal part of vesicovaginal ligament (Bladder nerves are dissected and spared)	Excision of the rectouterine ligament at rectum (Hypogastric nerve is dissected and spared)

OSCE 4. A 42-year-old lady is planned for hysterectomy in view of abnormal uterine bleeding (AUB) not responding to medical management.
1. Which type of hysterectomy is the least invasive and is associated with a shorter recovery time?
2. How are robotic instruments unique and what extra advantage do they have over laparoscopic instruments?

Ans.

1. Laparoscopic hysterectomy
2. Robotic instruments have "wrists" that allow a larger range of complex movements than the human hand or laparoscopic instruments.

OSCE 5. A 51-year-old woman is planned for hysterectomy for endometrial hyperplasia. Examination reveals a 6 weeks size uterus which is mobile. Patient's blood type is A+ and is available in blood bank. A gynecologist who is well-versed in laparoscopic surgery plans to do a surgery.
1. Which factor is not typically considered when deciding the most appropriate type of hysterectomy for a patient, from the above information provided?

Ans.

1. *Patients' blood type:* The various factors determining choice of route of hysterectomy are:
   - Shape and size of uterus
   - Indication of surgery
   - Presence or absence of adnexal pathology
   - Pelvic adhesions

- Patient profile and surgical risks
- Surgeon's expertise and patient preference
- Availability of resources

Reference
1. Te Linde's Operative Gynecology. 12th edition, 2019.

OSCE 6.
1. Identify this instrument used in gynecology surgeries.

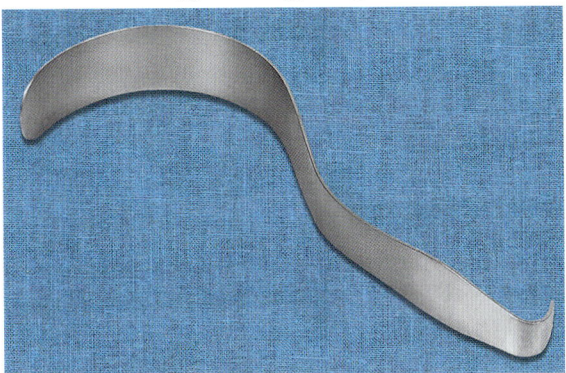

Ans.
1. *Deaver's retractor:* It is a large, handheld retractor which is used in retracting abdominal wall during hysterectomy. It has shape of question mark with thin, flat blade.

Reference
1. Berek and Novak's Gynecology. 18th edition.

OSCE 7.
A 46-year-old lady is planned for nondecent vaginal hysterectomy for adenomyosis and fibroid uterus. The uterus is of 18 weeks size. The surgeon decides to perform laparoscopic-assisted vaginal hysterectomy.

1. What is the purpose of a laparoscopic-assisted vaginal hysterectomy (LAVH) in this patient?

Ans.
1. To assist with visualization during vaginal hysterectomy.
   ELAVH enables the surgeon to convert most of the difficult abdominal hysterectomies into vaginal ones with all the benefits of a vaginal procedure. It is also a feasible and safe procedure in patients with previous abdominal surgery, large uterus and adnexal masses. The advantages of LAVH are lesser postoperative pain, shorter hospital stay, rapid return to normal activity and better body image.

Reference
1. Kapoor, et al. 2011.

OSCE 8.

1. **Name the gas used during total laparoscopic hysterectomy to create pneumoperitoneum.**

Ans.

1. Carbon dioxide
   - Almost ideal gas
   - Low cost/noninflammable/stable/high diffusion capacity
   - *Side effects:* Hypercapnia/acidosis/cardiac arrhythmia/tachycardia/pulmonary edema or peritoneal irritation which leads to postoperative pain

   Other gases: Helium/room air/N_2O—less soluble—more chances of gas embolism

Reference

1. American Association of Gynecologic Laparoscopists (AAGL) Guidelines.

OSCE 9.
A 45-year-old woman presents with heavy menstrual bleeding and dysmenorrhea. On examination, her uterus is enlarged, and ultrasound reveals multiple intramural fibroids.

1. **What is the most appropriate surgical management option?**

Ans.

1. *Total abdominal hysterectomy:* For a parous woman at 45 years with symptomatic multiple fibroid; the most appropriate management is hysterectomy because she has completed her family and it reduces need of daily drugs. Moreover, myomectomy may lead to recurrence of fibroids.

Reference

1. Berek and Novak's Gynecology. 18th edition.

OSCE 10.

1. **During hysterectomy, ureter inadvertently got cut near internal os. How lateral is the ureter from the internal os?**

Ans.

1. 1.5 cm lateral to internal os and passes beneath uterine artery
   Ureter course in pelvis:
   - Enters pelvis vertically downwards up to ischial spine and then course medial to internal iliac artery subsequently
   - At 1.5 cm lateral to internal os passes beneath uterine artery (water under bridge)
   - Passes through tunnel of cardinal ligament in paracervical tissues aka tunnel/web of Wertheim.
   - Once through this tunnel ureter passes medially over the vaginal fornix to enter trigone of bladder.

   At these points, during clamping of structures there is risk of ureteral injury.

Reference
1. Te Linde's Operative Gynecology. 12th edition, 2019.

OSCE 11. A 60-year-old woman underwent laparoscopic hysterectomy. In postoperative period she noticed paresthesia on the lateral side of leg and foot drop.
1. Injury to which nerve is likely to be responsible?

Ans.
1. *Common peroneal nerve:* Injury is due to the compression of common peroneal nerve between the lateral head of the fibula and stand holding the legs. Hence, special attention must be given during stirrup placement to avoid nerve compression.

Reference
1. Te Linde's Operative Gynecology. 12th edition, 2019.

OSCE 12. A 40-year-old woman had undergone laparoscopic hysterectomy in view of endometriosis. On postoperative day 3, she complained of fever and pain abdomen. There was decreased urine output and ascites.
1. What is the most likely diagnosis?

Ans.
1. *Ureteric injury:* It is confirmed with CT urogram and cystoscopy.

Reference
1. Te Linde's Operative Gynecology. 12th edition, 2019.

OSCE 13. In a patient undergoing a laparoscopic hysterectomy, bladder was suspected to be injured.
1. What is the next step?

Ans.
1. *Intraoperative cystoscopy should be performed:* Lower urinary tract injuries are a serious potential complication of laparoscopic hysterectomy. The risk of such injuries may be as high as 3%, and most, but not all, are detected at intraoperative cystoscopy. High-quality published data suggest a sensitivity of 80–90% for ureteral trauma. Among the injuries that may be missed are those related to the use of energy-based surgical tools that include ultrasound and radiofrequency electricity.

Reference
1. AAGL Practice Report: Practice guidelines for intraoperative cystoscopy in laparoscopic hysterectomy 2012.

OSCE 14. In a postoperative patient of hysterectomy, she was provided to wear well-fitting compression stockings and have intermittent pneumatic compression.

Multimodal analgesia was not adopted, intravenous fluids were terminated within 24 hours of surgery and regular diet was considered within 24 hours.

1. All are recommendations for postoperative care of hysterectomy patient, except.

Ans.

1. Multimodal analgesia should not be adopted
   Key postoperative components of ERAS with rationale:

Postoperative	
Avoidance of pelvic drains	Decreases infectious complications and improves the length of recovery
Goal-directed IV fluids, euvolemia	Improves pulmonary, bowel and diaphragmatic function. Avoids fluid disturbances
Wound infiltration with local anesthetic/local nerve blocks	Decreases surgical stress response, reduced narcotic needs, improves postoperative nausea and vomiting
Avoidance of nasogastric tube	Decreases infectious complications, improves the length of recovery
Avoidance of ileus	Encourages early oral nutrition, decrease catabolism, improves recovery
Prevention of postoperative nausea and vomiting	Encourages early oral nutrition, decrease catabolism, improves recovery
Multimodal analgesia	Improves organ function, improves mobilization, decrease catabolism, and improved overall recovery, reduce narcotic needs, improve postoperative nausea and vomiting
Early oral intake	Reduces catabolism and improves recovery
Nutritional supplements	Decrease infective complications, improves recovery and healing
Early mobilization, physical therapy	Decreases thromboembolic and pulmonary complications, decreases fatigue and loss of muscle
Thrombosis prophylaxis	Decreases the risk of thromboembolic and pulmonary complications

Reference

1. Guidelines for postoperative care in gynaecologic/oncology surgery: Enhanced Recovery after Surgery (ERAS®) Society recommendations—Part II 2016.

OSCE 15.

1. **Which imaging modality is most helpful in evaluating the extent of endometrial cancer before planning a hysterectomy?**

Ans.

1. *Magnetic resonance imaging (MRI):* Contrast-enhanced MRI—modality of choice in endometrial cancer for deciding surgical staging:

Contrast-enhanced MRI	Sensitivity	Specificity	Accuracy
Deep myometrial invasion	87%	57%	66%
Cervical stroma invasion	33%	95%	82%
Metastatic lymph nodes	59%	93%	90%

Reference

1. Leisby S, et al. Gynaecologic Oncology, 2013.

OSCE 16. A 29-year-old lady with one live issue has a 14 cm fibroid leading to dysmenorrhea and heavy menstrual bleeding. She does not want to undergo hysterectomy and all other medical methods of management have failed.
1. What are her options?

Ans.

1. Uterine artery embolization (UAE)
    - Safe and minimally invasive technique.
    - *Indications:* Menorrhagia, pelvic pain, pressure symptoms, fibroids with undiagnosed infertility, preoperative measure for large fibroids.
    - Myoma 50% shrinkage in 68% of patients.
    - Risk of re-intervention is almost 32%.
    - *Contraindications:* Contraindications to angiography, coagulopathy, severe renal insufficiency, pregnancy, active pelvic infection, prior pelvic radiation, connective tissue disease.
    - *Complications:* Postembolization syndrome, uterine artery dissection, sepsis, menopausal symptoms rarely.

Reference

1. Talshyn Ukybassova1, et al. Evaluation of Uterine Artery Embolization on Myoma Shrinkage: Results from a Large Cohort Analysis. Gynecol Minim Invasive Ther. 2019;8(4):165-71.

OSCE 17. A 30-year-old, multiparous lady comes with an ultrasound report showing uterine fibroid of 2.5 × 2.5 cm without any symptoms.
1. What will be the best management in her case?

Ans.

1. *Reassurance:* Asymptomatic fibroid less than 4 cm in size can be left with reassurance and proper counseling.

Reference

1. Berek and Novak's Gynecology. 18th edition.

OSCE 18. A 45-year-old lady is found to have 3rd degree uterovaginal prolapse.
1. What is the appropriate surgery to prevent recurrence?

Ans.

1. *Vaginal hysterectomy with McCall culdoplasty:* Vaginal hysterectomy and uterosacral suspension with McCalls Culdoplasty is generally seen as more successful than sacrospinous uteropexy.

Reference

1. Te Linde's Operative Gynecology. 12th edition, 2019.

OSCE 19.

1. Various trials are conducted on routes of surgery in cases of malignancy. LACE trial includes which gynecological cancer?

Ans.

1. *Endometrial cancer:* It is the most common gynecological malignancy in developed countries. The Laparoscopic Approach to Cancer of the Endometrium (LACE) trial was designed to assess equivalence of performing this in a total laparoscopic approach (TLH) to total abdominal hysterectomy. They found no difference in disease-free survival, recurrence, or overall survival in stage 1 endometrial cancer.

Reference

1. Janda M, et al. Total laparoscopic versus open surgery for stage 1 endometrial cancer: the LACE randomized controlled trial. Contemp Clin Trials. 2006;27(4):353-63.

OSCE 20.
A woman with endometroid adenocarcinoma of 1.5 x 2 cm with less than 50% myometrial invasion on MRI, along with enlarged lymph nodes.
1. What is best management?

Ans.

1. TAH + BSO + Sentinel lymph node biopsy
   Ca endometrium stage 1a:

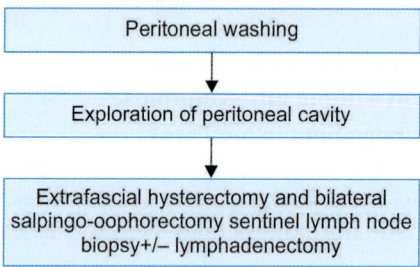

Reference

1. European Society of Gynaecological Oncology 2021.

CHAPTER 46

Menopause

Madhavi M Gupta, Ankita Chonla

OSCE 1.
1. What is the STRAW staging system?
2. What is the principal estrogen formed in a postmenopausal woman in peripheral tissue?
3. When should the annual screening mammography begin?

Ans.
1. STRAW staging system divides female lifespan into three broad phases: Reproductive phase, menopausal transition phase, postmenopausal phase.
2. Estrone
3. 40 years

OSCE 2. A 52-year-old lady has been presented with complaints of severe hot flushes, sweating and inability to sleep at night due to them. She underwent modified radical mastectomy 5 years back for carcinoma in her left breast. Currently, she is on tamoxifen for the same.
1. What drug will you prescribe her?
2. What is the dosage of that drug?

Ans.
1. Venlafaxine.
2. 37.5 mg/day to a maximum 75 mg/day

OSCE 3.
1. What are the changes in FSH, AMH and inhibin levels of a postmenopausal lady?
2. What is the cut-off level of FSH seen in postmenopausal females?

Ans.
1. FSH increases, inhibin decreases, AMH decreases
2. >40 IU/L

OSCE 4.
1. A 34-year-old lady underwent TAH + BSO for severe pelvic endometriosis. She now has complaints of severe hot flushes and sweating. What is the best treatment for her?

2. **What dose of ethinyl estradiol is roughly biologically equivalent to the typical postmenopausal dose of 625 mg of conjugated equine estrogen?**

Ans.

1. Combined continuous E (estrogen) + P (progesterone)
2. 0.005–0.010 mg

OSCE 5.

1. **A 45-year-old lady underwent TAH for Stage 1A endometrial cancer. She has debilitating menopausal symptoms after the surgery. What is the HT (hormone therapy) regimen you would prescribe? What is the rationale behind?**

Ans.

1. Combined E + P, due to potential protective action of the progesterone component of HT.

OSCE 6. A 52-year-old menopausal lady presented with complaints of hot flushes. Her T-score was –3 on DEXA scan.
1. What is the best drug for her management?
2. What is the rationale behind using the drug?
3. What is the dosage of the drug?

Ans.

1. Tibolone.
2. The metabolites of tibolone have estrogenic, androgenic, and progesterone properties. It treats menopausal symptoms as effectively as estrogen therapy. It has a beneficial effect on bones and prevents bone loss.
3. *Dose:* 2.5 mg daily orally.

OSCE 7. A 52-year-old lady has been presented with genitourinary symptoms and moderate hot flushes. You plan to start her on HT.
1. What are the factors that needed to be considered before starting HT?
2. What is the age criteria for initiating HT?
3. What is the standard recommended duration for use of HT?

Ans.

1. Patient's age, severity of symptoms, calculated risk of cardiovascular disease and breast cancer.
2. HT is safe for women who are within 10 years of menopause or less than 60 years of age who do not have any contraindications (WHI demonstrates adverse effects of HT in older postmenopausal females or who are more than 10 years since menopause).
3. 5 years

OSCE 8. A 52-year-old postmenopausal lady with a BMI of 36 kg/m² and history of diabetes mellitus presented with spotting per vaginum from past 1 week. She got a TVS done. The picture is shown below.

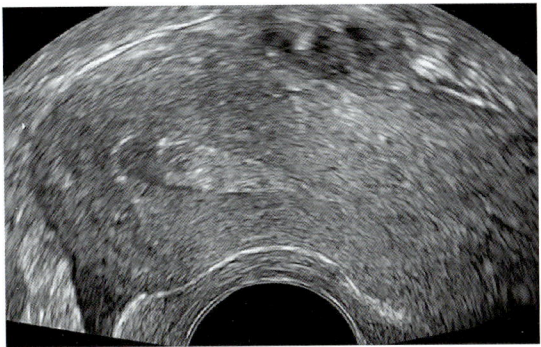

1. What is your interpretation?
2. What is the management?

Ans.

1. Thickened endometrial thickness
2. Endometrial biopsy to rule out endometrial hyperplasia/carcinoma.

OSCE 9.

1. A 50-year-old lady presents with severely debilitating vasomotor symptoms. She was diagnosed with HT by her physician as her mother had a history of stroke. She has no significant previous medical or surgical history. What would you prescribe her for the same?

Ans.

1. Transdermal E+P

OSCE 10. A 53-year-old woman presented with complaints of vaginal dryness, dyspareunia, and urinary urgency. On per speculum examination, the finding is as shown here:

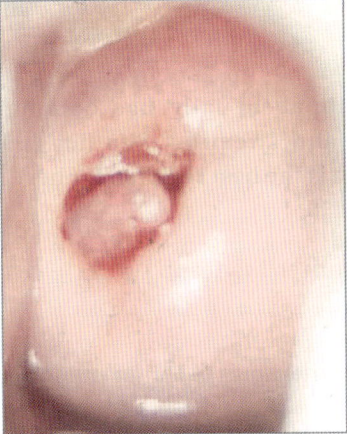

1. What is the treatment?
2. What is the dosage schedule for the above condition?

Ans.

1. Vaginal moisturizer and lubricants
2. Vaginal estrogen creams [CEE (Premarin) and Estradiol (Estrace)—1 g vaginally for 3 weeks and 1 week off, Estriol vaginal cream and Estradiol vaginal tablet—0.5 mg daily for 2 weeks followed by twice weekly.

Reference

1. Kelley C. Estrogen and its effect on vaginal atrophy in post-menopausal women. Urologic Nursing. 2007;27(1):40-5.

OSCE 11.

1. What is the incidence of hot flushes in surgically induced menopause?
2. How will you describe hot flushes?

Ans.

1. 90%

Reference

1. Tong, IL. Nonpharmacological treatment of postmenopausal symptoms. The Obstetrician & Gynecologist. 2013;15:19-25.
2. Peripheral vasodilation resulting from a direct LH action on sympathetic neurons.

OSCE 12.

1. What are the diagnostic criteria for primary ovarian insufficiency?
2. Which inborn error of metabolism is known to cause POI?

Ans.

1. Oligo/amenorrhea for at least 4 months, an elevated FSH level of >25 U/L on two occasions more than 4 weeks apart (Management of POI, ESHRE 2015).
2. Classic galactosemia

OSCE 13.

1. A 54-year-old, postmenopausal lady has complaints of recurrent episodes of bothersome flushing and sweating. She has itching in vulva, dyspareunia, and decreased libido. What is the best regimen for her?

Ans.

1. Oral E+P with vaginal moisturizer/lubricant

OSCE 14.

1. Enumerate four alternative therapies to HT for menopausal symptoms.

Ans.

1. a. Cognitive behavioral therapy
   b. Hypnosis

c. Stellate ganglion block
d. Hypnosis

OSCE 15.
1. **What type of stroke is associated with HRT?**
2. **What can be done to lower the risk?**

Ans.

1. As per the WHI study, there is a 31% increased risk of stroke in comparison to placebo. There is an increased risk of ischemic stroke but not hemorrhagic stroke.
2. Transdermal E+P preparations can be used as they have a lower incidence of stroke.

OSCE 16.
1. **What is the use of the drug shown below?**
2. **What is its mechanism of action?**

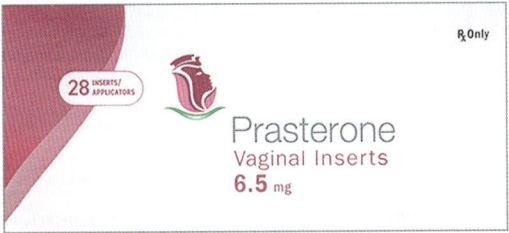

Ans.

1. Vaginal DHEA, used for vaginal dryness and dyspareunia.
2. Mechanism of action is aromatization to estrogen.

OSCE 17.
1. **A 60-year-old lady has presented with complaint of foul-smelling vaginal discharge. She had menopause 10 years back. Below is the per speculum examination finding. What is the next step of management?**

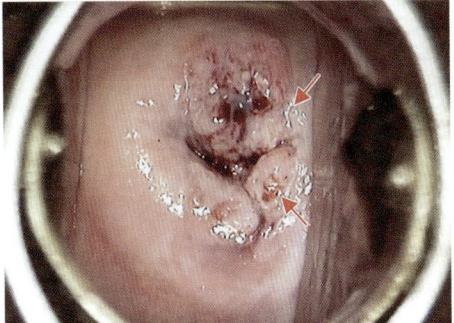

Ans.

1. Cervical biopsy

OSCE 18.

1. **What is KEEP study?**

Ans.

1. Kronos early estrogen prevention (KEEP) study. It was a trial in younger postmenopausal females which showed that four years of MHT (menopausal hormone therapy) had no overall effect on cognition in comparison to placebo.

OSCE 19.

1. **What is the use of the drug shown below in postmenopausal women?**
2. **What is the dosage?**

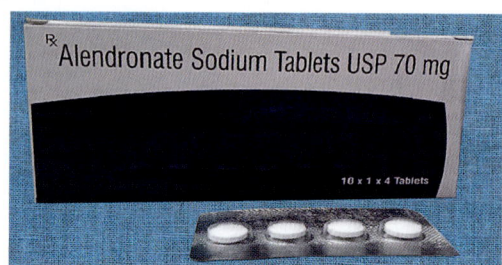

Ans.

1. It is a bisphosphonate approved for both prevention and treatment of osteoporosis.
2. 35–70 mg is given orally, weekly.

OSCE 20.

A 33-year-old lady comes with primary infertility of four years. She gives a history of irregular and infrequent menses. For the last 1-year, she bleeds only on hormone withdrawal. She has been amenorrheic for the last 4 months. Her TVS is shown below:

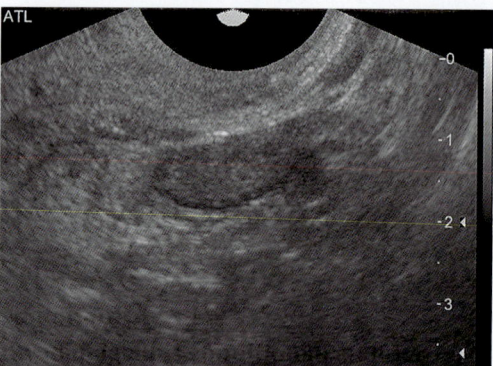

1. **Which test is further required now?**
2. **What is the provisional diagnosis?**

Ans.

1. Serum FSH
2. Primary ovarian insufficiency (TVS shows no follicles in the ovary).

CHAPTER 47

Urinary Incontinence and Vesicovaginal Fistula

Ajit Kumar Nayak

OSCE 1. A 27-year-old, P2L2, LCB (last childbirth) 1 year back, had previous two vaginal deliveries, history of instrumental delivery for prolonged second stage in last childbirth complaining of involuntary loss of urine while coughing and sneezing for last 2 months.
1. What is the diagnosis?
2. Mention one differential diagnosis of it.
3. Mention one conservative treatment for it.
4. Mention two surgical treatments for it.

Ans.
1. Stress urinary incontinence
2. Urge urinary incontinence
3. Kegel's pelvic floor muscle exercise
4. Burch colposupension and Sling operation

OSCE 2.

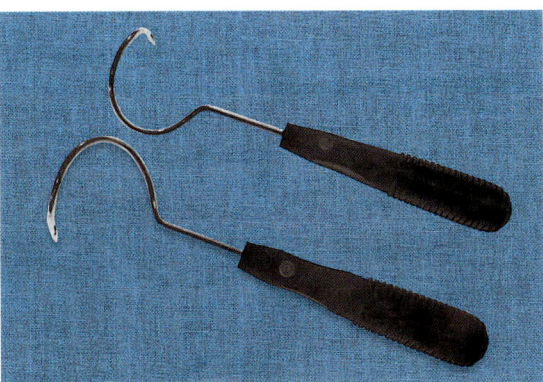

1. Identify the instrument.
2. What is the name of the medical condition where it is used?
3. Mention the name of the procedure in which it is used.
4. Mention two important complications of this surgical procedure.

Ans.
1. TOT needle

2. Stress urinary incontinence
3. Sling operation (Transobturator tap)
4. Mess erosion, bladder injury

OSCE 3.

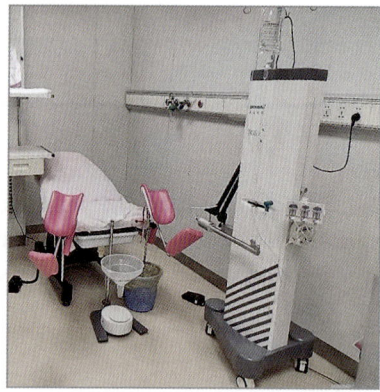

1. Identify the equipment.
2. It is used to diagnose which medical condition?
3. Mention three important components of urodynamic study.

Ans.

1. Urodynamometer
2. Stress or urge urinary incontinence, overactive bladder
3. Uroflowmetry, cystometry, and pressure-flow study

OSCE 4.

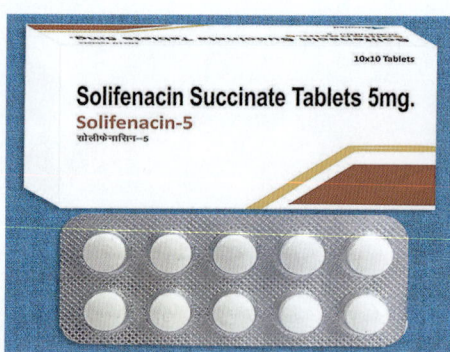

1. The above medicine belongs to which group of drugs?
2. It is used to treat which type of medical disease?
3. What is its dose?
4. Mention two other drugs used to treat such medical condition.

Ans.

1. Antimuscarinic drug

2. Overactive bladder with urinary incontinence, urgency, and frequency
3. 5 to 10 mg orally once daily
4. Tolterodine and Mirabegron

OSCE 5.

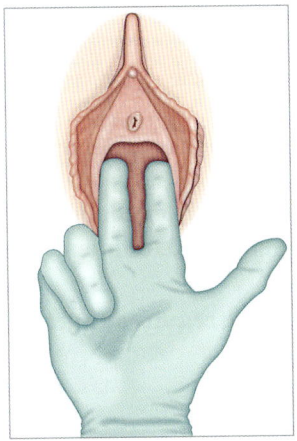

1. **Mention the name of this test.**
2. **This test is used to diagnose which medical disease?**
3. **Name one more test used for SUI.**
4. **Mention two causes of SUI.**

Ans.

1. Bonney's test
2. To anticipate the clinical effect of a suspension operation in SUI
3. Q-tip test
4. Urethral hypermobility and intrinsic sphincter defect

OSCE 6.

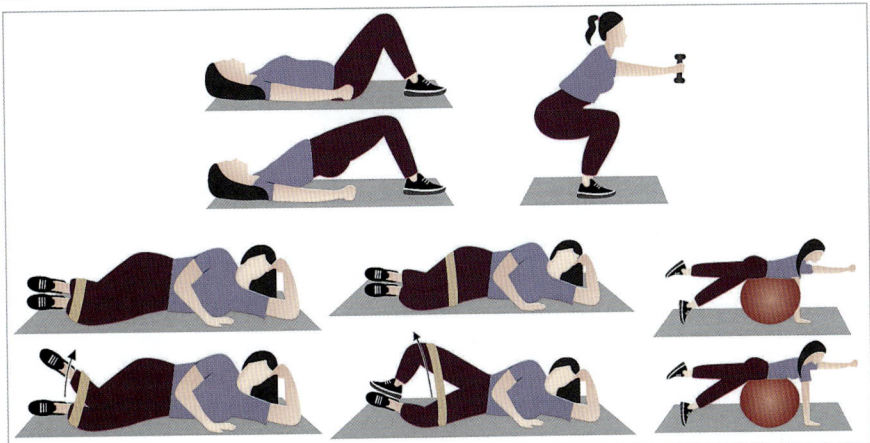

1. Mention the name of the exercise.
2. Name the muscles which are strengthened by this exercise.
3. Name one gynecological condition which is caused due to weakness of these muscles.
4. Mention two factors which lead to weakness of these muscles.

Ans.

1. Kegel's pelvic floor muscle exercise
2. Levator ani and other pelvic floor muscle
3. Pelvic organ prolapse
4. Multipara who had difficult vaginal delivery, menopausal state

OSCE 7. A 45-year-old, P2L2, suffering from diabetes and obesity, habituated to tea and coffee complaining of urinary urgency and frequency for last one month.
1. What is your diagnosis?
2. What behavioral modifications are required to get rid of these symptoms?
3. Mention one differential diagnosis.
4. Mention two treatment options.

Ans.

1. Urinary urge incontinence
2. Weight reduction, control of diabetes, avoid tea, coffee, stop smoking
3. Stress urinary incontinence
4. Behavioral techniques and anticholinergic drugs

OSCE 8.

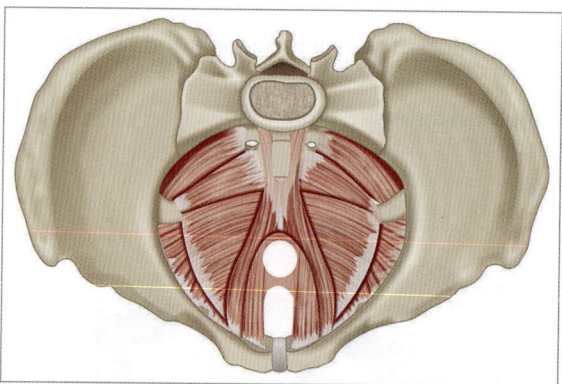

1. Identify the musculature in the pelvis.
2. Mention one important muscle of the pelvic floor.
3. What is its main function?
4. Name two medical conditions which occur due to weakness of this muscle.

Ans.

1. Muscles of the pelvic floor particularly levator ani
2. Pubococcygeus

3. To support the pelvic organs and constrictor or continence mechanism of the urethral, anal, and vaginal orifices
4. Pelvic organ prolapse and stress urinary incontinence.

OSCE 9. A 41-year-old, P2L2 with history of two instrumental vaginal deliveries, who is diabetic, complains of increased frequency of micturition, urinary urgency and dribbling of urine while sneezing and coughing since six months.
1. What is the diagnosis?
2. Name one special investigation required to differentiate urge incontinence from SUI.
3. Which type of incontinence should be treated first in the case of mixed incontinence before proceeding for surgery?
4. Name two drugs used for urge incontinence.

Ans.
1. Mixed urinary incontinence
2. Urodynamic study
3. Urinary urge incontinence
4. Solifenacin and Mirabegron

OSCE 10. A 24-year-old, P1L1 who had cesarean 1 month back for obstructed labor, complains of continuous passage of urine through vagina since 1 week.
1. What is the diagnosis?
2. In such a case, what could be the cause of urinary fistula?
3. When should it be repaired?
4. Mention two important causes of urinary fistula in a female.

Ans.
1. Urinary fistula (Vesicovaginal or ureterovaginal fistula)
2. Obstructed labor
3. Usually after 3–6 months
4. Obstructed labor and following hysterectomy operation.

OSCE 11.

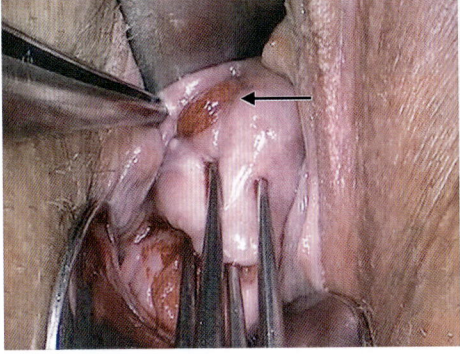
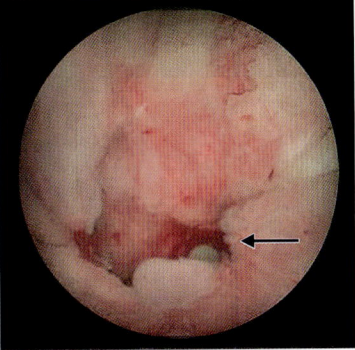

1. Spot the diagnosis.
2. Mention one clinical method to diagnose it.
3. Name one surgical procedure for VVF.
4. Name two surgical principles of VVF repair.

Ans.

1. Vesicovaginal fistula
2. Speculum examination with good light source and dye test
3. Vaginal approach by multiple layer method
4. Complete excision of fistulous tract, a tension-free, water-tight, multi-layered closure

OSCE 12. A 48-year-old lady who underwent laparoscopic hysterectomy for AUB-L two weeks back complains of continuous leakage of urine through vagina for 5 days.
1. What is the diagnosis?
2. What is the most possible cause for such a condition?
3. Mention one investigation to diagnose it.
4. Name two routes of surgical approach for such a urinary fistula.

Ans.

1. Urinary fistula (vesicovaginal or ureterovaginal fistula)
2. Injury to ureter or urinary bladder
3. Cystoscopy
4. Abdominal and vaginal route

OSCE 13.

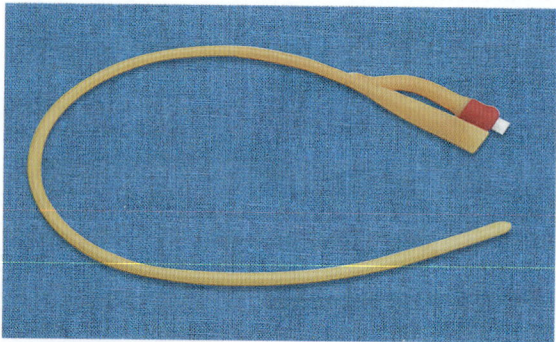

1. Identify it.
2. For how many days should it be kept for continuous bladder drainage following urinary fistula surgery?
3. What is the purpose of continuous bladder drainage following VVF repair?
4. Name two problems associated with prolonged catheterization.

Ans.

1. Foley's urinary catheter
2. Usually, 14 days

3. Keeps the bladder empty, so helps in healing the repair
4. Urinary tract infection and sometimes bladder atony

OSCE 14.

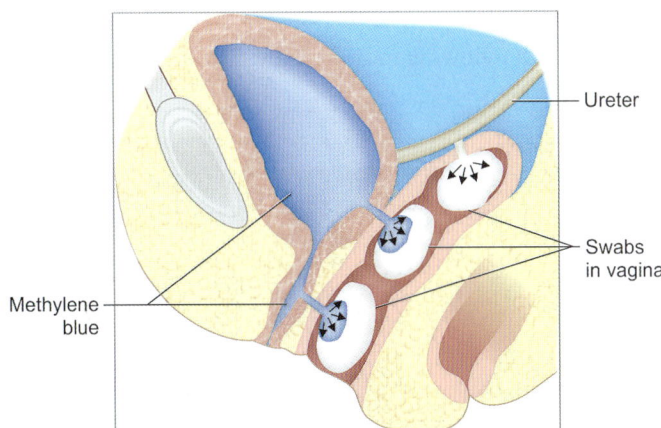

1. What is the name of this test?
2. What is the indication for this test?
3. How many cotton swabs are used in the test?
4. How is the test interpreted?

Ans.

1. Triple swab test
2. To differentiate between ureterovaginal, vesicovaginal, and urethra-vaginal fistula
3. Three
4. The uppermost swab is wet but not discolored—ureterovaginal fistula, upper swabs are wet with blue irrigant—vesicovaginal fistula, discoloration of only the lowest swab supports diagnosis of a low urethral fistula or urethral leakage.

OSCE 15.

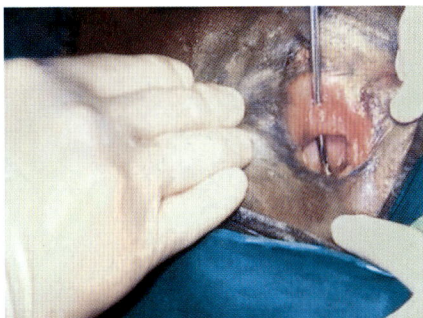

1. What is the diagnosis?
2. In the case of a single, very small opening between the urinary bladder and lower one-third of vagina, mention whether it is simple or complex fistula?
3. What is the size of a fistula in a complex urinary fistula?
4. Mention two criteria of a complex urinary fistula.

Ans.

1. Vesicovaginal fistula
2. Simple fistula
3. More than 2.5 cm
4. Failed fistula repair, fistula following radiotherapy, fistula following chronic diseases, and multiple fistulas.

OSCE 16.

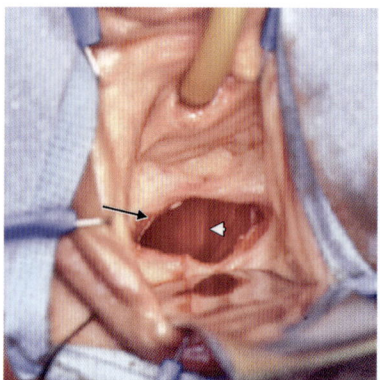

1. The size of this VVF is 3 cm which happened following difficult traumatic vaginal delivery in a case of obstructed labor, is it a simple or complex fistula?
2. Mention one point in favor of your diagnosis.
3. Name one cause of complex urinary fistula.

Ans.

1. Complex fistula
2. In complex, fistula size is more than 2.5 cm.
3. Fistula following radiotherapy.

OSCE 17.

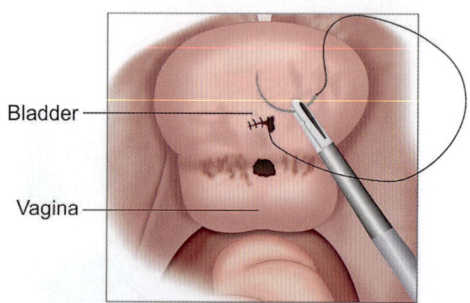

Closure of the bladder

1. This type of surgery is performed in which medical condition?
2. Mention one cause attributing to such a condition.
3. What are the routes for VVF repair?
4. Mention two criteria for abdominal route of VVF repair.

Ans.

1. Vesicovaginal fistula
2. Following hysterectomy operation
3. Abdominal and vaginal routes
4. High VVF and cases involving difficult vaginal access

OSCE 18.

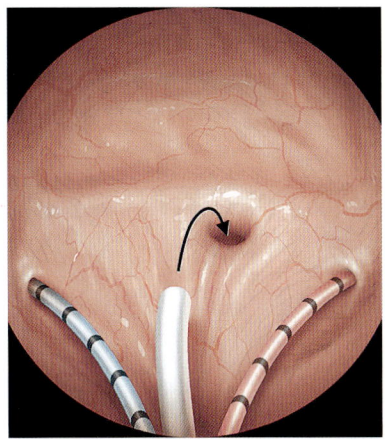

1. Spot the diagnosis.
2. What is the name of the instrument used to locate and diagnose it?
3. Is it a supratrigonal fistula? Answer as Yes/No.
4. Name two other modalities of investigations to diagnose and treat it.

Ans.

1. Vesicovaginal fistula
2. Cystoscopy
3. Yes
4. CT urogram, retrograde and voiding the cystourethrography.

OSCE 19.

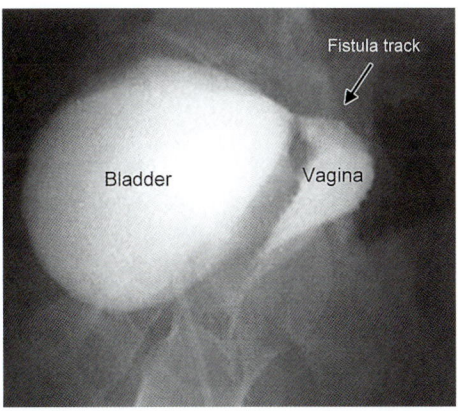

1. What is the diagnosis?
2. What is the imaging technique used to diagnose such a condition?
3. Which other investigation should be performed before proceeding for surgery?
4. Name two surgical procedures for VVF repair.

Ans.

1. Vesicovaginal fistula
2. Cystography
3. Ultrasonography of abdomen and pelvis including TVS and cystoscopy
4. Abdominal approach (O'Connor's technique) and vaginal approach using Martius interposition flap.

OSCE 20.

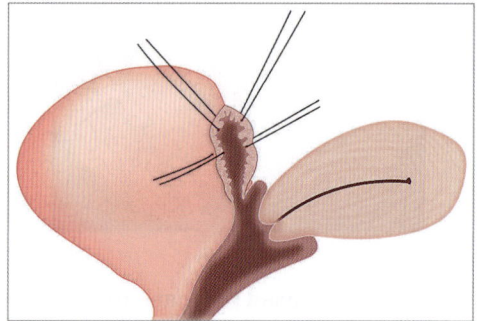

1. When should a VVF due to obstetric cause be repaired?
2. Name one criteria of VVF where vaginal route is preferred.
3. Name one classification of VVF.
4. Enumerate two complications of VVF repair.

Ans.

1. After 3–6 months in VVF due to obstetric cause
2. Simple and low VVF
3. Marion Sims classification
4. Recurrence of fistula, ureteric injury, or obstruction

CHAPTER 48

Gynecological Endoscopy

Aswath Kumar

OSCE 1.

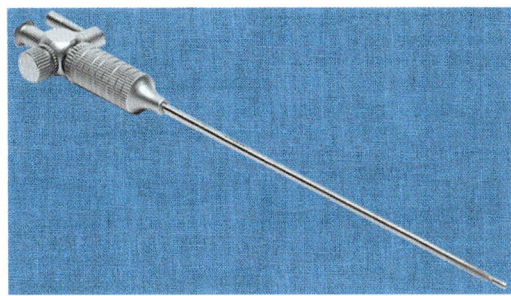

1. Identify the instrument.
2. What is it used for?
3. Enumerate four tests used to confirm the proper use of the instrument.

Ans.

1. Veress needle
2. For creating pneumoperitoneum
3. Tests for peritoneal entry (safety tests):
   - Hiss sound
   - Double click sound of Veress needle
   - Irrigation test (Syringe test)
   - Aspiration test (Palmer test)
   - Hanging drop of saline test
   - Insufflation of gas test
   - Needle movement test

OSCE 2.

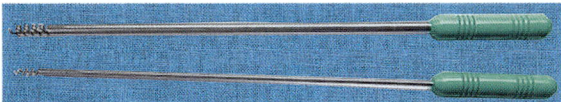

1. Identify the instrument.
2. What are the methods to decrease blood loss, in the surgery for which this instrument is most commonly used?

Ans.

1. Laparoscopic Myoma screw
2. Few methods used commonly are:
   - Intramyometrial vasopressin
   - Temporary occlusion of uterine artery (Shoelace knots)
   - Intravenous tranexamic acid.

OSCE 3.

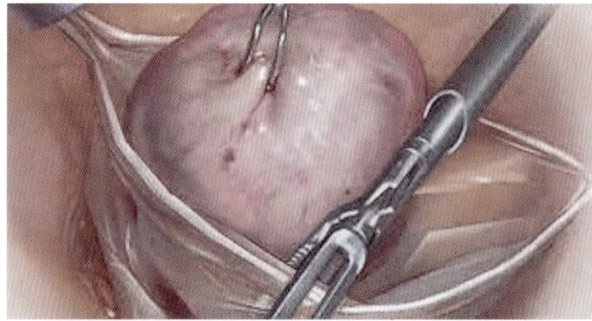

1. **Identify the procedure being done.**
2. **When is it done usually and why?**

Ans.

1. In bag placement of specimen (for retrieval or in bag morcellation)
2. Whenever spill of the contents to be removed can produce irritation/infection/spread of malignancy or in doubt of the same, specimens are removed in bag.

OSCE 4.

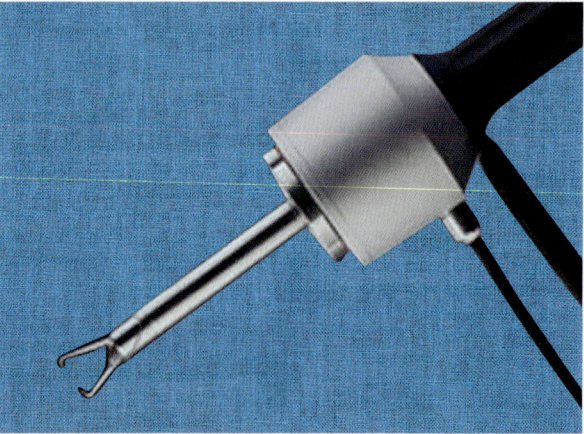

1. **Identify the instrument.**
2. **Why was it banned?**
3. **Is it still usable/any precautions to be taken while using?**

Ans.
1. Laparoscopic power morcellator.
2. It was banned, as one of the individuals on whom myoma morcellation done had leiomyoma sarcoma and the procedure disseminated the disease and was sued.
3. Power morcellation is now still used in India, but always done in bag.

OSCE 5.

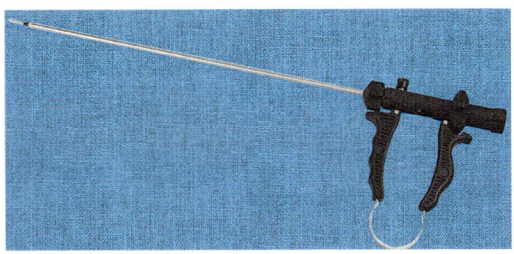

1. Identify the instrument.
2. What is the type of energy source used?
3. What is the difference from its counterpart and advantage over the same?

Ans.
1. Laparoscopic bipolar
2. It is a mode of electrosurgery and uses radiofrequency energy
3. It is the counterpart of monopolar, in bipolar only the tissue held in between the jaws of the instrument is included in the circuit, while in monopolar, the body (the point of touch of instrument to the pad attaching the leaving terminal) is included in the circuit. Also, lateral spread of thermal injury is much less compared in bipolar.

OSCE 6.

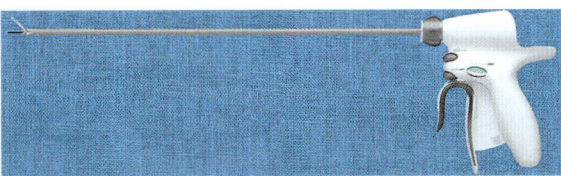

1. Identify the instrument.
2. What is the type of energy source used?
3. Enumerate two disadvantages?
4. Enumerate two of its advantages over traditional source of energy?

Ans.
1. Harmonic scalpel.
2. Uses ultrasound energy
3. Some of the disadvantages are:
   - Functioning blade is hot and will remain so after application. Contact with surrounding structures like bowel may result in injury.

- Cost of instrument
- Inability to coagulate vessels greater than 5 mm.

4. Advantages are:
   - Minimal thermal spread
   - No desiccation or charring of tissue
   - No risk of electrical injury
   - No smoke

OSCE 7.

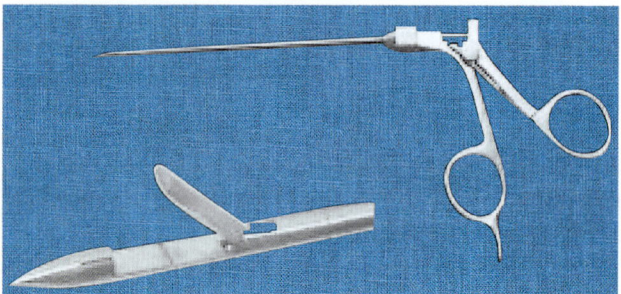

1. **Identify the instrument.**
2. **Mention the indication for its use?**

Ans.

1. Single jaw action suture carrier
2. For port closure (helps in preventing port site hernias especially in ports >1.5 cm)

OSCE 8.

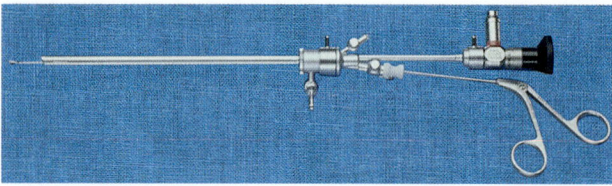

1. **Identify the instrument.**
2. **What is it used for?**
3. **Name the distending media used.**

Ans.

1. Operative hysteroscope
2. For hysteroscopic surgeries (hysteroscopic polypectomy, myomectomy, septal resection etc.)
3. Distending media generally used are:
   - CO_2 (carbon dioxide) (for office hysteroscopy)
   - 1.5% glycine (for operative hysteroscopy, monopolar energy can be used)

- 0.9% sodium chloride (ionizing solution so monopolar energy cannot be used)
- Sorbitol (alternative to glycine)
- 5% dextrose in water
- Dextran 70 (high viscosity fluid)

OSCE 9.

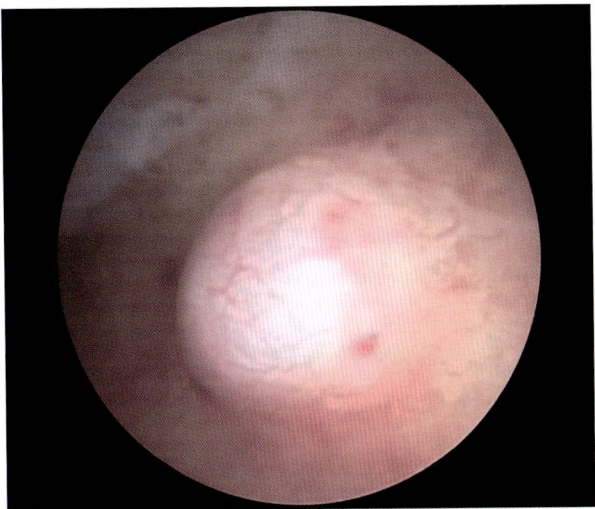

1. What procedure is being done here?
2. What does the image show?
3. What is STEP-W criteria?

Ans.

1. Hysteroscopic myomectomy
2. Submucous fibroid
3. STEP-W criteria:

	Size (cm)	Topography	Extension of the base	Penetration	Lateral wall	Total
0	<2	Low	<1/3	0	+1	
1	>2–5	Middle	>1/3–2/3	<50%		
2	>5	Upper	>2/3	>50%		
Score	+	+	+	+	+	

Score	Group	Complexity and therapeutic options
0–4	I	Low complexity hysteroscopic myomectomy
5–6	II	• High complexity hysteroscopic myomectomy. Consider GnRH use? • Consider two-step hysteroscopic myomectomy
7–9	III	Consider alternatives to the hysteroscopic technique

OSCE 10.

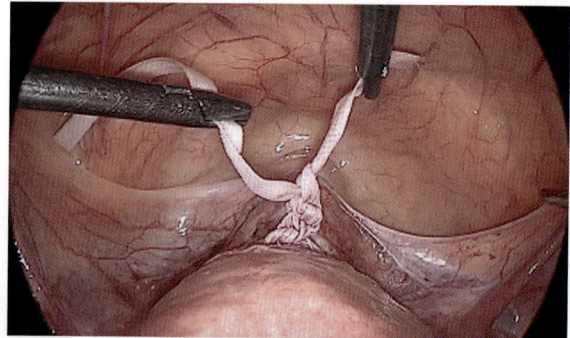

1. What is being done here?
2. Enumerate four indications for the same.
3. Enumerate two advantages of the same over traditional method?

Ans.

1. Laparoscopic encerclage
2. Indications of abdominal cerclage are:
   - Previously failed transvaginal cerclage
   - Extremely short (<15 mm) cervix
   - Congenitally deformed cervix
   - History of trachelectomy
   - Deeply lacerated or scarred cervix
   - Recurrent pregnancy loss with failed vaginal cerclage
   - Spontaneous preterm birth with intact vaginal cerclage.
3. Advantages of laparoscopic abdominal encirclage over traditional method are:
   - Lesser blood loss
   - Reduced postoperative pain and morbidity
   - Faster recovery

CHAPTER **49**

Infertility

Shikha Seth, Shristi Jaiswal

OSCE 1. A 28-year-old lady is admitted in casualty with severe abdominal pain and vomiting. She has been receiving fertility treatment. Her USG picture is showed below.

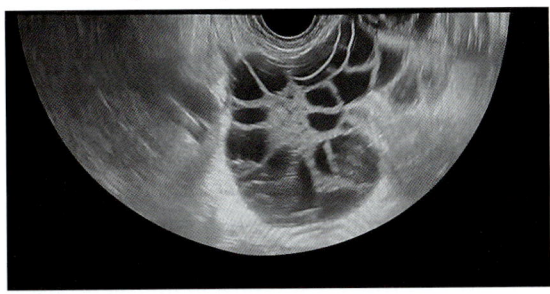

1. Identify the clinical condition shown in the sonogram.
2. Mention four risk factors for above condition.
3. How do you classify the given condition?
4. What investigations should be performed in such a case?

Ans.

1. *OHSS (Ovarian hyperstimulation syndrome):* The pathophysiology of OHSS is based on the damage in vascular endothelium leading to increased permeability, mediated by cytokines and interleukins derived from hyperstimulated ovaries under the effect of human chorionic gonadotropin (hCG). The major factor responsible for the vascular changes and extravasation of OHSS is vascular endothelial growth factor (VEGF).
2. Risk factors:
   - Age below 20 years (young)
   - Abnormal body mass index (low or high)
   - Polycystic ovary syndrome
   - Gonadotropins like FSH, LH, HMG-based stimulation
   - Past history of OHSS
   - More the number of follicles chances of OHSS increases.
3. OHSS has been classified based on symptom and biochemical severity:
   - Mild
   - Moderate
   - Severe
   - Critical

Category features:
- Mild OHSS has only clinical symptomatology of abdominal bloating, minimal abdominal pain and on USG, the ovarian size remains less than 8 cm^3.
- Moderate OHSS category has clinical symptomatology as nausea, vomiting, moderate abdominal persistent pain with presence of ascites on sonography and the ovarian size crosses 8 cm^3.
- Severe OHSS is confirmed based on clinical evidence of ascites, or hydrothorax, low urine output (<400 mL/day or 30 mL/hour)—oliguria, and laboratory changes as hematocrit greater than 0.45, hyponatremia (Na <135 mmol/L, hyperkalemia (K >5 mmol/L, hypoproteinemia (S. albumin <6 g/L) and ovarian size can be more than 12 mm^3
- Critical OHSS term is given when there is tense ascites, hematocrit is greater than 0.55 and total WBC count is greater than 25,000 /mL, kidney shut down, or thromboembolism or respiratory distress.

4. Required investigations for OHSS are:
   - Complete blood count (CBC)—white blood cells
   - Extravasation of fluid leads to hemoconcentration measured by packed cell volume (PCV).
   - Elevated fibrinogen and reduced antithrombin from the coagulation pathway.
   - C-reactive protein with raised value suggests severity of disease.
   - Renal function tests (RFT) serum creatinine and urea gets raised
   - Electrolytes as Na, K—for hyponatremia, hyperkalemia respectively.
   - Liver function tests as elevated enzymes (SGOT, SGPT, LDH and reduced albumin)
   - Chest X-ray—Posteroanterior view.
   - Ultrasound preferably transvaginal scan to assess the ovarian size, pelvic and abdominal free fluid (ascites). Possibility of torsion remains high due to enlargement and fluid collection, so ovarian Doppler should also be done if torsion is suspected by acute abdominal pain like features.

Reference
1. RCOG-GTG. The Management of Ovarian Hyperstimulation Syndrome (2016).

OSCE 2. A P1L0 32-year-old lady presents with secondary infertility. She has been trying to conceive since last 4 years. She gives history of cyclical premenstrual pain, dysmenorrhea, and deep dyspareunia. Serum progesterone (day 21) was 42 nmol/L while the FSH and LH levels were normal.
1. What is the most likely cause?
2. Which is the gold standard method for diagnosis of this condition?
3. How is it classified according to revised American Society for Reproductive Medicine (R-ASRM)?
4. What are the treatment options for stage 1–2 endometriosis associated with subfertility?
5. Define CPP (chronic pelvic pain).

Ans.

1. *Endometriosis:* Dysmenorrhea, deep dyspareunia, and secondary subfertility suggest endometriosis as the underlying cause.
2. *Diagnostic laparoscopy:* Surgical findings vary and may include discrete endometriotic lesions, endometrioma, or adhesions. Implants are typically found on pelvic organ serosa and pelvic peritoneum. Lesions are variably colored and can be red (red, red-pink, or clear), white (white or yellow-brown), and black (black or black-blue). White and red lesions most commonly correlate with the characteristic histologic findings of endometriosis (Jansen, 1986). Dark lesions are pigmented by hemosiderin deposition from trapped menstrual debris.
3. ESHRE has classified endometriosis into four categories as follows based on severity:
   - Stage I called as minimal
   - Stage II as mild disease
   - Stage III as moderate
   - Stage IV as severe most variety with almost frozen pelvis.
4. *Treatment:* The first two stages of endometriosis and associated subfertility can be treated by resection/excision of cysts if any with walls or ablation/fulguration of superficial or deep foci to improve outcome.
5. Definition of chronic pelvic pain as given by ACOG 2010.
   - A noncyclic, dull type, persistent pain for 6 or more months duration; localized to the pelvis, lower abdomen below umbilicus, and posteriorly at lumbosacral region.
   - Pain remains sufficiently severe to cause disability functional or often physical and require medical intervention.

Reference

1. William's Gynecology. 4th edition (2020).

American Society for Reproductive Medicine
Revised Classification of Endometriosis

Patient's Name_____ Date_____

Stage I (Minimal)   : 1–5
Stage II (Mild)   : 6–15
Stage III (Moderate): 16–40
Stage IV (Severe)   : >40
Total_____

Laparoscopy_____ Laparotomy_____ Photography_____
Recommended treatment_____
_____
Prognosis_____

	Endometriosis	<1 cm	1–3 cm	3 cm
Peritoneum	Superficial	1	2	4
	Deep	2	4	6
Ovary	R Superficial	1	2	4
	Deep	4	16	20
	L Superficial	1	2	4
	Deep	4	16	20
	Posterior cul-de-sac obliteration	Partial		Complete
		4		40
	Adhesions	<1/3 Enclosure	1/3–2/3 Enclosure	>2/3 Enclosure
Ovary	R Filmy	1	2	4
	Dense	4	8	16
	L Filmy	1	2	4
	Dense	4	8	16
Tube	R Filmy	1	2	4
	Dense	4*	8*	16
	L Filmy	1	2	4
	Dense	4*	8*	16

*If the fimbriated end of the fallopian tube is completely enclosed, change the point assignment to 16. Denote appearance of superficial implant types as red [(R), red, red-pink, flamelike, vesicular blobs, clear vesicles], white [(W), opacifications, peritoneal defects, yellow-brown], or black [(B) black, hemosiderin deposits, blue]. Denote percent of total described as R____%, W____% and B____%. Total should equal 100%

Additional endometriosis:_____

Associated pathology:_____

To be used with normal tubes and ovaries

To be used with abnormal tubes and/or ovaries

Chapter 49: Infertility

OSCE 3. A 35-year-old lady presents with primary infertility. She has been trying to conceive for the last 5 years but has not been successful. She also complains of hot flushes and irritability for the last 3 months. Her FSH is 60 IU/mL.
1. What is your provisional diagnosis?
2. What are the diagnostic criteria for above condition?
3. Write WHO classification of ovulation disorder. In which class does above condition fall?
4. What are the options in her case to yield the best pregnancy rate?

Ans.

1. *Premature ovarian failure (POF):* POF is defined as loss of oocytes and the surrounding support cells prior to age 40 years. Around 5–10% of women will have sporadic ovulation and therefore should be advised to use contraception to avoid pregnancy if they have already completed their family.
   Causes of premature ovarian failure:
   - Idiopathic
   - Autoimmune
   - Congenital—chromosomal, metabolic
   - Immunologic
   - Iatrogenic causes include surgery, radiotherapy, and chemotherapy
2. The diagnostic criteria of POF as per GDG:
   - Oligomenorrhea or amenorrhea lasting for at least 4 months, and raised FSH level greater than 25 IU/L on two occasions at least 4 weeks apart.
   - Raised FSH and low estrogen levels are the hallmark of POF.
   - Careful evaluation is mandatory as the diagnosis, differentiation from natural menopause and effective treatment may have implications on women's psychologic, sexual, cardiovascular, and bone health.
   - In most cases, a definitive etiology of POF is not determined
3. WHO ovulation disorder classification:
   - Hypogonadotropic hypogonadism, WHO class-I (hypothalamic amenorrhea)
   - Normogonadotropic normogonadism, WHO class-II (PCOS)
   - Hypergonadotropic hypogonadism WHO class-III (primary ovarian failure)
   Hypergonadotropic hypogonadism: When ovaries have failed and not producing adequate steroid that is estrogen and due to absent negative feedback, pituitary continues to form and release high levels of FSH and LH: This group implies primary ovarian dysfunction.
4. a. Oocyte donation
   b. Embryo donation
   c. Adoption
   Chances of fertility in women with premature ovarian failure: Only 5–10% women experience spontaneous resolution and return of menses in POF. There are no clear-cut factors defined for assessing the clinical outcome in form of menses of pregnancy. The oral contraceptives often fail to suppress the raised FSH values characteristic of premature ovarian failure. For those young couples who actively desire to be parents,

the options are either the adoption or oocyte or embryo donation. In donation cycles, the foremost important aspect is to prepare the endometrium for implantation via the exogenous estrogen therapy and estradiol valerate, from 2–6 mg is preferred way and builds up over a 2-week period, followed by progesterone support (vaginal pessary 400 mg) as there is no endogenous hormones. Both exogenous estrogen and progesterone are required to make endometrium receptive to embryo implantation. Ovulation induction is not useful in POF cases.

References
1. William's Gynecology. 4th edition (2020).
2. ESHRE: Management of women with premature ovarian insufficiency (2015).

OSCE 4. A 29-year-old lady is referred to the infertility clinic. The couple is seen together in the clinic. She is reviewed with the following investigations:
- Mid cycle progesterone—65 ng/mL
- Normal day 3 follicle-stimulating hormone (FSH) and luteinizing hormone (LH)
- Normal hysterosalpingo-contrast-sonography (HyCoSy) scan
- Normal thyroid function
- Normal serum prolactin
- Transvaginal scan—Normal
- Semen analysis—Azoospermia

1. When should semen analysis be repeated if there is any abnormality?
2. Write WHO semen analysis criteria.
3. Enlist causes of azoospermia.
4. What is the treatment option?

Ans.

1. *The semen analysis should be repeated after 3 months:* Ideally the semen analysis be repeated at 3 months interval after the initial poor report to allow time for the complete cycle of fresh spermatogenesis. However, in cases of azoospermia or severe oligozoospermia, the repeat test may be undertaken as soon as possible to confirm the diagnosis.
2. WHO semen analysis criteria, 2010.

Variables	Cut-off marks
Sperm volume	More than 1.5 mL
Liquefaction time	30 minutes
Sperm concentration/mL	More than 15 million/mL
Total sperm count in ejaculate	More than 39 million
Sperm motility (A + B) rapid progressive and linear	More than 32%
Sperm morphology	More than 4% abnormal forms
Sperm DNA fragmentation	Less than 30%
Nonsperm cells-round cells	Less than 1 million/mL

3. a. Azoospermia is defined as total absence of sperms in semen and its causes are divided into three major sections obstructive, nonobstructive, and testicular failure.
   b. Prior vasectomy or pathological ejaculatory duct obstruction secondary to infection leads to obstructive azoospermia which may have chances of surgical correction while congenital bilateral absence of the vas deferens (CBAVD) is one of the common reasons of azoospermia not surgically treatable. CBAVD cases, testicular sperm extraction (TESE) is the option to collect the sperms followed by ICSI and IVF.
   c. *Genetic abnormalities like* Klinefelter syndrome (47, XXY) or balanced translocation; deletion of part of Y chromosome are responsible for nonobstructive azoospermia or testicular failure.
4. Intracytoplasmic sperm injection (ICSI) is the only option for azoospermic cases with sperm collection above the obstruction or directly from epididymis or testicles.

References
1. William's Gynecology. 4th edition (2020).
2. NICE—Fertility problems: assessment and treatment (2017).

OSCE 5. A 38 years woman married at 35 years of age presents with primary infertility and informs that they are trying to conceive since 3 years and having regular unprotected intercourse. Male partner's semen report is normal as per the WHO criteria. Her hormonal profile, ultrasound scan are within normal limits. Hysterosalpingogram shows normal cavity uterus with bilateral tubal patency. Premenstrual endometrial biopsy suggested secretory changes.
1. What is the cause of infertility in above case?
2. What is the treatment option?
3. Mention four predictors of IVF success.
4. What treatment should be given for luteal phase support?

Ans.
1. Unexplained infertility.
2. *Assisted reproductive technology stepwise going from level-I to IVF*: As the age increases, chances of fertility decreases. Hence, once all factors like ovarian, uterine, tubal and male factors have been evaluated and found to be normal, the woman should be checked for ovarian hyperstimulation followed by inducing ovulation with timed intercourse or intra-uterine insemination of processed sperms.
3. Predictors of IVF success are:
   - *Age* (maternal and paternal) quality of gametes falls with increasing age in both genders.
   - *Number of previous ovarian hyperstimulation or induction cycles.*
   - *Previous pregnancy history*: Previous normal spontaneous conception is a positive predictor for IVF treatment success.
   - *Body mass index categorizing obesity*: Ideal BMI for best reproductive outcome is in the range 19–28 before commencing assisted reproduction.

   Junk diet and sedentary lifestyle reduces the success rate—alcohol, smoking, tea, or caffeine addiction is associated with poor outcome.

Section 2: Gynecology

4. Progesterone (preferably natural micronized one and prevaginal route) is required for luteal phase support after IVF treatment.

Reference
1. NICE—Fertility problems: assessment and treatment (2017).

OSCE 6. A 34 years P2L1 woman with a BMI of 30 kg/m², presented with secondary infertility. She had a 3rd degree perineal tear during her first childbirth at peripheral hospital and had postpartum massive hemorrhage during her second delivery, received three units of blood transfusion with early neonatal death. She wants to conceive again but is still having amenorrhea since her last childbirth.
1. What is the diagnosis?
2. It belongs to which category of WHO ovulatory disorder?
3. Mention four important hormonal tests for diagnosis of this case.
4. What is the next line of management of infertility in this case?

Ans.

1. *Sheehan's syndrome:* Panhypopituitarism is common after massive PPH and a complete multiorgan symptomatology is defined under the term 'Sheehan syndrome'. The sudden, speedy, severe hypotension created at time of massive obstetric hemorrhage leads to pituitary ischemia and necrosis (stated by Kelestimur, 2003). Women with severe form often develop shock due to pituitary infarction/apoplexy characterized by headache, nausea, visual deficits, and hormonal dysfunction. Loss of gonadotropic activity from anterior pituitary leads to anovulation and subsequent amenorrhea. Depending upon the affection of area of pituitary (anterior or posterior) clinical presentation differs patient to patient. Failure of lactation, loss of sexual and axillary hair, and hypothyroidism or adrenal insufficiency are other symptoms.
2. *WHO Type 1 ovulatory disorder:* Sheehan syndrome is pituitary necrosis and loss of gonadotrophic support leads to poor steroidogenesis form gonads (ovaries) so term hypogonadotropic hypogonadism has been given in relation to hypothalamic-pituitary axis. As a result, poor gonadotropin stimulation of the ovaries leads to impaired follicular development. Generally, in these patients, LH and FSH levels, although low, will still be in the detectable range (<5 mIU/mL).
3. a. ACTH (Adrenocorticotropic hormone)
   b. TSH (Thyroid-stimulating hormone)
   c. Growth hormone
   d. FSH (Follicle-stimulating hormone)
   e. LH (Luteinizing hormone)
   f. Prolactin (PRL)
4. Hypothalamopituitary Type 1 ovulatory disorder can be treated with either pulsatile GnRH or Gonadotrophins with LH/hCG activity should be given—Sheehan's syndrome.

Chapter 49: Infertility

References
1. William's Gynecology. 4th edition (2020).
2. NICE—Fertility problems: assessment and treatment (2017).

OSCE 7. A 30-year lady reports to the infertility clinic AIIMS, Gorakhpur with a history of oligomenorrhea since last 6 months. She is obese with BMI of 30 kg/m^2 and trying to conceive since last 3 years. Her hormonal profile is normal, patent tubes demonstrable on Sonosalpingography and husband's semen analysis (HAS) is within normal limits. She is planned for ovulation induction.
1. Which is the drug of choice for ovulation induction?
2. Write dose, route of administration and duration of use of above-mentioned drug.
3. Enumerate two complications of ovulation induction.
4. What is advantage of aromatase inhibitor (letrozole) over clomiphene citrate?

Ans.

1. Letrozole or Clomiphene citrate (CC) is the initial ovulation inducing agents for most anovulatory infertility cases.
   - Clomiphene formula is chemically similar to tamoxifen, and is competitive binder for the estrogen receptors. It gets bind to pituitary and hypothalamic estrogen receptor and prevents the negative feedback that is normally produced by estrogen. Thus they continue to release gonadotropin-releasing hormone (GnRH) secretion as well as FSH respectively. The resulting increase in follicle-stimulating hormone (FSH) levels, in turn, drives ovarian follicular hyperstimulation.
   - Letrozole another ovulation induction agent is more preferred and considered first-line now a days. It works as inhibitor of enzyme aromatase and thus inhibits peripheral conversion of androgens to estrogen, thus decreasing the negative feedback to hypothalamopituitary axis.
2. a. Clomiphene (CC) dose is 50–250 mg/day, oral, for 5 days from D2 to D6
   b. Letrozole is 2.5–5 mg/day oral for 5 days from D2 to D6
   c. Prior to therapy, sonography should be done to exclude residual follicular cysts. Doses are increased by a 50 mg increment in Clomiphene cycle and 2.5 mg in Letrozole in subsequent cycle until ovulation is induced. The dose of CC should not be increased if normal ovulation is confirmed in further cycles. The effective dose of CC ranges from 50 to 250 mg/d, although doses in excess of 100 mg/d are associated with risks and complications.
3. Complications of ovulation induction are:
   - OHSS (ovarian hyperstimulation syndrome)
   - Multifetal gestation
4. Advantage of Aromatase inhibitor (letrozole) over Clomiphene citrate:
   - Higher pregnancy rate
   - Lesser side-effects

Section 2: Gynecology

Reference
1. William's Gynecology. 4th edition (2020).

OSCE 8. A 39 years obese women (BMI of 32) presents to infertility clinic with oligomenorrhea and infetility. Husband's semen and tubal patency test are normal. She had 5 cycles of clomiphene citrate induction at increasing dosage with follicular monitoring but cycles remained anovulatory.
1. What do you understand by 'clomiphene resistant' and 'clomiphene failure'?
2. In above scenario, what is the next line of management?
3. Enumerate two side-effects of metformin.
4. What is the mechanism of laparoscopic ovarian drilling and enumerate two complications of this procedure.

Ans.
1. a. *Clomiphene resistance*: Failure to ovulate after receiving 150 mg of CC daily for 5 days per cycle, for at least 3 cycles.
   b. *Clomiphene failure*: Failure to conceive with clomiphene citrate despite successful regular ovulation for 6–9 cycles.
2. Women with WHO Group-II normogonadotropic ovulation disorders who are resistant to clomiphene citrate, following second-line treatments be tried depending on clinical findings and the woman's preference:
   - *Ovarian drilling:* Laparoscopically preferred (LOD) or
   - *Combined therapy:* Clomiphene citrate/Letrozole with metformin if not already offered as first-line treatment or
   - Gonadotrophins as FSH, or HMG.
3. *Side-effects of metformin*: Nausea, vomiting, gastrointestinal disturbances
4. Mechanism of laparoscopic ovarian drilling (LOD):
   - It destroys ovarian androgen-producing tissue and reduces peripheral conversion of androgens to estrogens. There is fall in serum levels of androgens and LH and an increase in FSH levels.
   - In LOD, four to five punctures are made on the antimesenteric surface of both the ovaries symmetrically. Drilling should be avoided on the lateral surfaces of the ovaries as it may lead to adhesion formation to the pelvic sidewall. Drilling should be avoided at the ovarian hilum to limit bleeding risks and reduction in ovarian vascularity. Depth of drilling should be of 4–8 mm to cover the hyperechoic ovary. Controlled electrical current be applied for just 4 seconds and after the drilling the ovarian surface should be irrigated with saline.

   Complications:
   - Postoperative adhesion formation
   - Diminished ovarian reserve
   - Premature ovarian failure

References
1. NICE—Fertility problems: assessment and treatment (2017).

2. Brown J, Farquhar C, Beck J, Boothroyd C, Hughes E. Clomiphene and anti-oestrogens for ovulation induction in PCOS. Cochrane Database Syst Rev. 2009;(4):CD002249. doi: 10.1002/14651858. CD002249.pub4. Update in: Cochrane Database Syst Rev. 2016 Dec 15;12 : CD002249. PMID: 19821295.

OSCE 9. A 23 years lady, married for 2 years presents to the OPD. She has been trying to conceive since 2 years. Her obstetric formula is P0L0A1. Her hormonal profile is normal and luteal phase progesterone is ovulatory. Her pelvic ultrasound scan suggests a septate uterus but is otherwise normal. She is very anxious to conceive.

1. What is the next line of investigation in her case?
2. Write other investigations to evaluate uterine factors for infertility.
3. What is the management in above case?
4. Name one important drug to be given in postoperative period.
5. Write classification of Müllerian anomalies.

Ans.

1. Hysteroscopy with laparoscopic chromopertubation
2. Evaluation of uterine factors:
   - Hysterosalpingography (HSG)
   - Transvaginal sonography (TVS) with saline-infusion sonography (SSG)
   - Sonocontrast hysterography (HyCoSy)
   - Magnetic resonance imaging (MRI)
3. Hysteroscopic-guided septum excision is an effective and safe method to treat women with complete or partial septate uterus. Operative hysteroscopy with concurrent laparoscopic supervision reduces the risk of uterine perforation.
4. Estradiol—2 mg, orally for 30 days, helps endometrial proliferation and reduces the risk of adhesion reformation after resection. Conception should be delayed for 2–3 months following septum resection. Second look hysteroscopy is the option if septum resection suspected incomplete in primary surgery or women ends into repeated miscarriage or presents with amenorrhea suggesting formation of adhesions. Hysterosalpingography (HSG) is the first choice.
5. Classification of Müllerian anomalies
   A. *Segmental Müllerian hypoplasia or agenesis*
      - Vaginal
      - Cervical
      - Uterine
      - Tubal
      - Combined
   B. *Unicornuate uterus*
      - Rudimentary communicating horn with cavity
      - Rudimentary noncommunicating horn with cavity
      - Rudimentary horn without cavity
      - Unicornuate uterus without a rudimentary horn
   C. *Uterine didelphys*

Section 2: Gynecology

   D. *Bicornuate uterus*
      - Complete bifurcation (bicollis)
      - Partial bifurcation (unicollis)
   E. *Septate uterus*
      - Complete septa
      - Partial septa
   F. *Arcuate uterus*
   G. *Diet/stilbestrol-related anomalies*

Reference
1. William's Gynecology. 4th edition (2020).

OSCE 10. A 28-year-old lady presents with secondary amenorrhea since 6 months. She is short statured with height approx. 10 cm below her mid-parental height. UPT was negative. She started menarche at 18 years of age with oligohypomenorrhea. She wants to discuss about her chances of conception.
1. What is the most probable diagnosis?
2. What are the routes to parenthood for her?
3. Menton two ways of ovarian preservation in an 18-year female planned for radiation therapy.
4. How do you see ovarian response to gonadotropin stimulation in IVF?

Ans.

1. *Turner's syndrome (XO):* Short stature with amenorrhea should prompt a diagnosis of Turner's syndrome. It can occasionally present with secondary amenorrhea.
2. Routes to parenthood for women with Turner syndrome:
   - ART (assisted reproductive techniques)
   - Use of donor oocytes or embryos
   - Surrogacy
3. Chemotherapy or radiotherapy can give rise to ovarian failure. Ovarian follicular damage can be reduced by:
   - Gonadal shielding at time of X-ray or radiotherapy.
   - Surgical ovarian transposition to areas out of radiation zone.
   - Ovarian suppression by gonadotrophin-releasing hormone
   - Ovulation induction and cryopreservation of oocyte, embryo or ovarian tissue.
4. Ovarian response in IVF is measured by:
   - *Total antral follicle count (AFC):* On day 2–3 of menstrual cycle less than 4 follicles of less than or equal to 5 mm on TVS suggest poor ovarian reserve while more than 16 follicles of 2–10 mm on day 3 suggests high response.
   - Anti-Müllerian hormone (AMH) values of less than 5.4 pmol/L is suggestive of a low response and more than 25 pmol/L for a high response.
   - Follicular-stimulating hormone of more than 10 IU/L and less than 4 IU/L suggest low response.
   - A low response is defined as less than four oocytes or cancellation of cycle while more than 20 oocyte yield is termed as high response.

Chapter 49: Infertility

References
1. NICE—Fertility problems: assessment and treatment (2017).
2. RCOG TOG article (2019): Routes to parenthood for women with Turner syndrome.

OSCE 11. An nulliparous lady came to hospital with history of infertility complaining of menorrhagia, dysmenorrhea, and constipation. On per abdominal examination, there is mass arising from pelvis palpable up to 20 weeks size of pregnant uterus, nontender.
1. What is the possible cause of her infertility?
2. Which investigation would you like to do for diagnosis and planning management?
3. What is STEP-W classification of fibroids for Hysteroscopic myomectomy?
4. Mention two methods to control blood loss during abdominal myomectomy.

Ans.

1. Fibroid uterus
2. Investigations
   - *USG:* Well-defined hypoechoic lesions. Peripheral calcification with distal shadowing in old fibroids. To differentiate from adenomyosis/adenomyoma by diffuse/focal lesion, less echodense, disordered echogenicity and loss of endomyometrial junction.
   - *Saline infusion sonography*: To differentiate polyps and submucous myomas from intramural fibroids
   - *MRI:* Most accurate imaging modality for diagnosis of fibroid and differentiating from adenomyoma. It does precise fibroid mapping and characterization like number, size shape, type, position, cavity distortion and bulge, etc. Detects all fibroids accurately.
   - *Hysteroscopy:* Submucous fibroids/polyps (preferred if small suggested in cavity)
3. *Classification of fibroids (STEP-W):* For suitability of hysteroscopic surgery

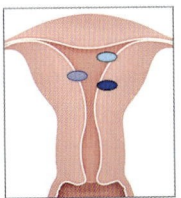 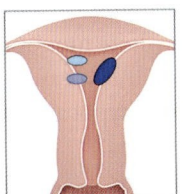 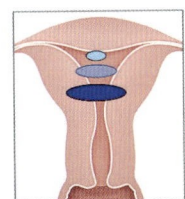 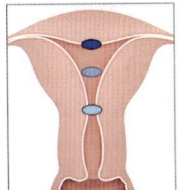

| | Degree of penetration of the myoma into myometrium | The extension of the base of the nodule with respect to the wall of the uterus | Size of the nodule—up to 2 cm between 2 and 5 cm and more than 5 cm | Topography—in the lateral wall an extra point is added |

STEP-W classification	Size (cm)	Topography	Extension of the base	Penetration	Lateral wall	Total
0	<2	Low	<1/3	0		
1	2–5	Middle	1/3–2/3	<50%	+1	
2	>5	Upper	>2/3	>50%		

Score	Group	Complexity and therapeutic options
0–4	I	Low complexity hysteroscopic myomectomy
5–6	II	High complexity hysteroscopic myomectomy. Consider GnRH use. Consider two-step hysteroscopic myomectomy
7–9	III	Consider alternatives to the hysteroscopic technique

○ = Score 0
● = Score 1
● = Score 2

4. Medical or mechanical means to control blood loss
   - Bonney's myomectomy clamp be used to compress uterine A. flow
   - Rubber tourniquet at isthmus and uterine cornua
   - Vasopressin infiltration 10–20 units diluted in 100 mL saline before uterine incision.

OSCE 12.

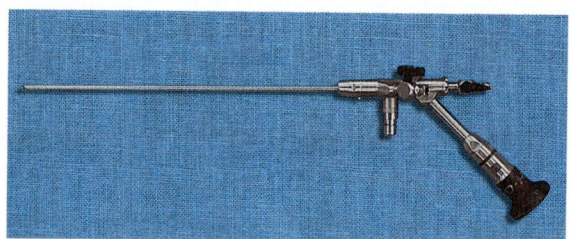

1. Identify the instrument shown in above figure.
2. Write five distension media used during hysteroscopy and their preference.
3. Write five indications of diagnostic hysteroscopy in infertility.
4. Write five indications of operative hysteroscopy in infertility.
5. What are the safe limits of fluid deficit in hysteroscopy and basic management plan?

Ans.

1. Hysteroscope (rigid)
2. Use of distending media for the uterus is dependent on the incision technique or energy source and includes:
   a. CO_2 (not preferred now a days as vision gets affected in bleeding)
   b. Isotonic Saline (most frequently used media except in cases where monopolar current need to be used.) Bipolar electrosurgical systems can utilize saline
   c. Glycine 1.5% is hypotonic (operative cases where monopolar cautery needs to be used)
   d. Sorbitol 3% is a hypotonic sugar solution and if excessive intravasation of sorbitol occurs, it can also lead to hyperglycemia and hypocalcemia.
   e. Mannitol.
3. Indications of diagnostic hysteroscopy in infertility:
   - Abnormal HSG
   - Unexplained infertility
   - Recurrent spontaneous abortions
   - Suspected Müllerian anomalies
   - Suspected intrauterine cavitary lesion
   - Infertility with AUB
4. Indications of operative hysteroscopy in infertile women:
   - Hysteroscopy directed biopsy
   - Resection of submucous myoma
   - Removal of uterine polyp
   - Excision of uterine septum
   - Adhesiolysis of uterine synechiae
   - Tubal cannulation for proximal tube occlusion and falloposcopy

5. Fluid overload and deficit safe limits
   - A maximum allowed fluid deficit limit is 1000 mL using a hypotonic solution in a healthy lady and surgery should be stopped if achieved.
   - For Isotonic solution use deficit of 2500 mL can be allowed in a healthy woman and surgery be stopped at this cutoff
   - Lesser fluid deficit threshold should be considered in the elderly, those with comorbidities like cardiovascular, renal or pulmonary pathologies. In such cormorbid situations suggested safe upper limits should be 750 mL for hypotonic solutions and 1500 mL for isotonic solutions.

   Management plan of suspected fluid overload:

Acute hypervolemic hyponatremia	Management
Hyponatremia with sodium levels ≥120 mmol/L and Asymptomatic	Fluid be restricted to less than 1 liter/day and diuretics as Furosemide, e.g., 20–40 mg be added.
Hyponatremia with sodium levels below 20 mmol/L or symptomatic	Hypertonic saline (3%) is better option for severe hyponatremia which has 513 mmol/L NaCl compared to 154 mmol/L in normal saline along with supplementation of oxygen, Input output strict monitoring with Foley's catheterization and multidisciplinary team involvement

References

1. http://www.rcog.org.uk/womens-health/clinical-guidance/development-rcog-green-top-guidelines-policies-andprocesses.
2. BSGE/ESGE guideline of fluid management in operative hysteroscopy.

OSCE 13.

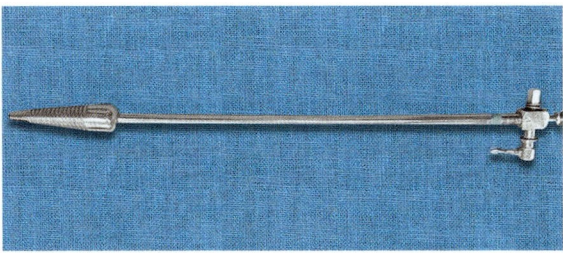

1. Identify the instrument.
2. Name the procedure where it is used.
3. Enumerate two contraindications for the procedure.
4. Define the causes of tubal factor infertility in our country and best management options for the same.

Ans.

1. Leech Wilkinson cannula
2. Hysterosalpingography (HSG) to push the radio-opaque contrast media.

Section 2: Gynecology

3. Laparoscopic chromopertubation to push in methylene blue dye
   Contraindications to HSG:
   - Acute pelvic infection
   - Active uterine bleeding
   - Pregnancy
   - Iodine allergy
   - Active tuberculosis
4. Causes of tubal infertility:
   - Endometriosis causing edema, peritubal adhesions and kinking
   - PID—internal tubal blockage
   - Genital TB
   - Salpingitis

   Best management options are:
   - Tubal surgeries preferred in hydrosalpinx with distal blocks or
   - ART-IVF

OSCE 14. A 26 years lady with history of vaginal discharge and lower abdomen pain for which was treated. She could not conceive after 2 years of married life. On per vaginal examination there are bilateral adnexal masses. She has bilateral hydrosalpinx on pelvic ultrasound. Rest work-up of both partners were satisfactory.
1. What is the most probable cause of her infertility?
2. How does hydrosalpinx affect fertility?
3. What is her management?
4. Write treatment options for tubal blockage at various sections of fallopian tube.

Ans.

1. *Tubal Factor:* Probably hydrosalpinx
2. Hydrosalpinx fluid include microorganism, endotoxin, cytokines, oxidative stress, and hence embryotoxic and a mechanical hindrance for the implantation.
3. Women with hydrosalpinx should be offered salpingectomy, preferably by laparoscopy before IVF treatment because this improves the chance of life birth.
4. Surgical options with proper counseling:
   - *Proximal tubal blockage:* Tubal cannulation
   - *Midsegment block:* Resection and microsurgical reanastomosis
   - *Distal tubal blockage:* Laparoscopic neosalpingostomy and fimbrioplasty or
   - Laparoscopic salpingectomy or Tubal clipping followed by assisted reproductive technique.

References
1. William's Gynecology. 4th edition (2020).
2. Chanelles O, Ducarme G, Sifer C, Hugues JN, Touboul C, Poncelet C. Hydrosalpinx and infertility: what about conservative surgical management? Eur J Obstet Gynecol Reprod Biol. 2011;159(1):122-6.

OSCE 15.

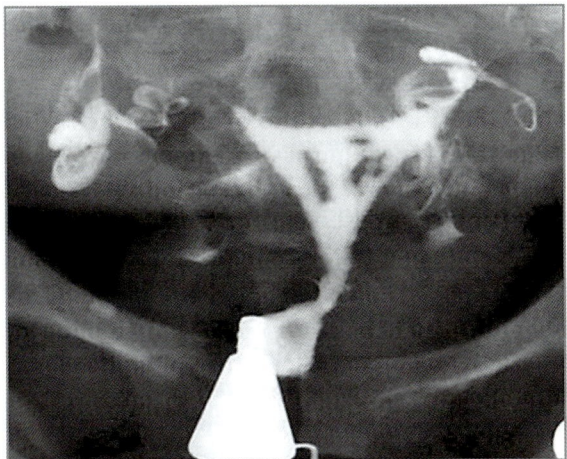

A 29 years lady presented with secondary amenorrhea and infertility since 1.5 years. She had dilatation and curettage (D and C) done twice previously in view of unplanned pregnancy in a private clinic. Her HSG findings are shown in the figure above.

1. What is the most probable diagnosis?
2. Enumerate two etiological factors which can lead to this condition.
3. What is the gold standard diagnostic modality?
4. What is the basis of treatment?

Ans.

1. This is most probably a case of Asherman's syndrome, intrauterine adhesions or intrauterine synechiae (IUS) as history of D&C, amenorrhea are there to support this.
2. Vigorous or repeated dilatation and curettage. Other causes are genital tuberculosis, Retained placenta, postmyomectomy, endometritis, endometriosis.
3. Hysteroscopy is considered to be as gold standard modality of investigation and simultaneous treatment. Saline sonohysterography is also a good screening modality for such cases of suspected IUS as it is OPD procedure and avoids the adversities of contrast and X-rays.
4. Amenorrhea and intrauterine adhesions should be offered a hysteroscopic adhesiolysis and measures be taken to keep the walls apart and reformation of adhesions, with hormone therapy (estrogen) to develop the endometrium for restoration of menstruation and possibility of fertility (placement of intrauterine, uterine inert devices, balloon, Foley's catheter).

References

1. Smikle C, Yarrarapu SNS, Khetarpal S. Asherman Syndrome. In: StatPearls [Internet]. Treasure Island (FL): StatPearls Publishing; 2023 [cited 2023 Dec 7]. Available from: http://www.ncbi.nlm.nih.gov/books/NBK448088/
2. Asherman's Syndrome - an overview | ScienceDirect Topics [Internet]. [cited 2023 Dec 7]. Available from: https://www.sciencedirect.com/topics/medicine-and-dentistry/ashermans-syndrome

Section 2: Gynecology

3. Nahirniak P, Tuma F. Adhesiolysis. In: StatPearls [Internet]. Treasure Island (FL): StatPearls Publishing; 2023 [cited 2023 Dec 7]. Available from:http://www.ncbi.nlm.nih.gov/books/NBK563219/

OSCE 16. A 26 years lady, known case of PCOS, presents to the fertility clinic. She is trying for conception since 2 years. Her BMI is 28 kg/m². Her hormonal profile was normal. Tubes are patent bilaterally and husband's semen analysis was normal. She has been given Clomiphene citrate for ovulation induction for 5 days starting from D2 of cycle.

1. How will monitor for growth of follicles and ovulation?
2. The above test is started from which day of cycle?
3. Name three signs of ovulation on USG.
4. Define the Clomiphene-based ovulation induction protocol.
5. Name another indication of Clomiphene in infertile cases.
6. Enumerate two other drugs used for ovulation induction.

Ans.

1. TVS (Transvaginal sonography)—Follicular monitoring
2. Ideally be started from base line D2-D3 scan, then Day 10 of cycle and followed every alternate day according to the growth of the developing follicle.
3. Signs of ovulation on USG are:
   - Size of follicle suddenly decreases—crumpled with peripheral hypervascular follicle seen.
   - Fluid in POD which was not there earlier
   - Trilaminar appearance of the endometrium disappears.
4. Start with 50 mg/day for 5 days in the early follicular phase. If ovulation does not occur, or the optimal follicular size is not attained, the dose is increased by 50 mg from the next cycle. Prefer progesterone-induced withdrawal bleeding. Treatment can be repeated for up to six cycles. A low dosage or treatment duration is explicitly recommended for patients with PCOS to prevent ovarian hyperstimulation syndrome. Injection hCG (2000–5000) is given when follicle reaches 20 mm in size in the clomiphene-induced cycle.
5. Clomiphene is used also for the spermiogenesis in male partners who have oligozoospermia. The regimen is 25 mg daily (half of a tablet) for 25 days, off for 5 days.
6. Letrozole, Clomiphene, HMG, FSH, purified forms, etc.

Reference

1. William's Gynecology. 4th edition (2020).

OSCE 17.

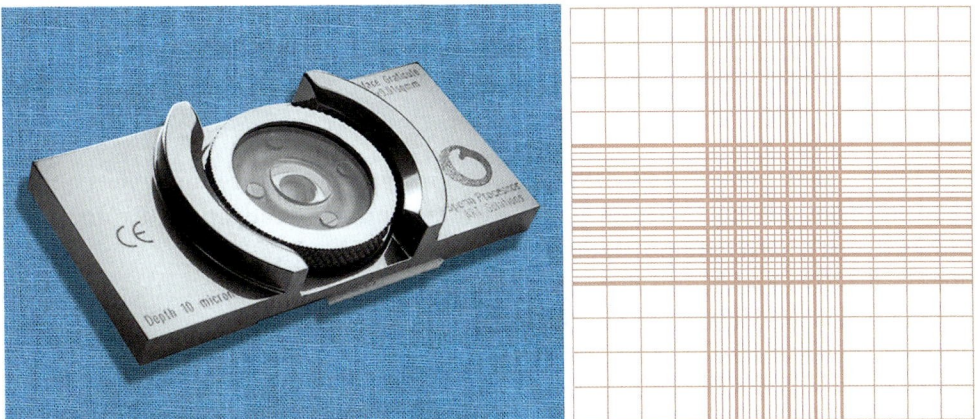

1. Identify the items shown and define its role.
2. What is the alternative method in modern era against it?
3. How do you counsel the couple for semen testing?
4. How can one differentiate between the dead or immotile sperm?
5. Define the sperm functions utilized to fertilize the ova stepwise.
6. Name five sperm function tests.

Ans.

1. Makler's sperm counting chamber and Neubauer's chamber grid
   Makler's sperm counting chamber is used for rapid and accurate sperm count, motility and morphology evaluation, from undiluted specimen.
2. CASA computer-assisted semen analysis
3. Counseling points
   - Inform about the utility of the test for infertility workup.
   - Information about the basic procedure required for the test.
   - Duration of abstinence should be strictly 3–5 days. Small and long interval can affect the results.
   - Sample should be given in the lab itself or submitted to lab so that processing should start in 1 hour of collection
   - Specimen should be collected properly in wide mouth container without any chemical
4. *Immotile and dead sperm* can be differentiated by sperm vitality test—HOST, i.e., hypo-osmotic swelling test—sperms are incubated in hypo-osmotic saline for some time and if living and membrane enzymes are active, they imbibe the fluid because of which swelling and coiling or mid-piece or tail is noted. Dead sperm does not show this phenomenon.
5. Motility, capacitation, zona binding, acrosome reaction, zona penetration, fusion with oolemma. These are not reflected in conventional semen analysis.
6. Sperm function tests
   - HOST—vitality test, MAR test—immunological test
   - Sperm penetration assay (in vivo sperm is checked to penetrate the Ham's egg)

- Sperm DNA integrity tests:
    - SCSA sperm chromatin structural assay—used in unexplained infertility with normal semen parameters especially in recurrent early pregnancy loss cases.
    - TUNEL—test for nuclear DNA fragmentation
    - COMET test

OSCE 18. A young couple visits OPD for preconceptional counseling where on basic workup, husband is found to be HIV positive while all other investigations are normal.
1. How will you counsel them—Mention the counseling points.
2. What will be your advice for them to get healthy pregnancy and neonatal outcome.
3. Define sperm preparation methods and their principles.
4. Write three indications of donor insemination.

Ans.

1. *Information*: Couple counseling is a must. HIV is sexually transmitted as well as maternal to child transmission is also possible. Need to confirm the present HIV status of the wife after the pretest counseling. Couple must use barrier method to avoid male-to-female transmission of disease. Male partner clinical disease status stage has to be tested and accordingly, if required ART (antiretroviral therapy) needs to be started.
   For pregnancy, intrauterine insemination is one option that avoids the risk of HIV disease transmission. Intrauterine insemination (IUI) is a procedure in which processed and concentrated motile sperm are placed directly into the uterine cavity to increase the likelihood of conception. The procedure is timed with ovulation, which may be natural or a result of ovarian hyperstimulation.
2. Consider unstimulated intrauterine insemination with partner sperm as a treatment option in the following groups as an alternative to vaginal sexual intercourse:
    - If husband's semen analysis is very poor, donor sperm can also be the option.
3. Sperm preparation methods:
    - *Swim-up technique:* Spermatozoa selected on their ability to swim, performed by layering culture medium over the liquefied semen in the tilted syringe or tube creating a greater interphase. Motile active spermatozoa swim up into the culture medium. The upper part of the layered medium is then carefully removed for insemination purpose.
    - *Gradient technique:* Multiple gradient media are layered one over other creating a density column and the semen sample is pipetted on the top of the density column. This layered tube is centrifuged which separates spermatozoa according to their density. The motile, active, morphologically normal spermatozoa in the solution with the highest concentration of gradient, which is aspirated for further use (WHO, 1999). Sperm preparation with the use of density gradient centrifugation has been suggested as best and standard technique in assisted reproductive techniques.
    - *Wash technique:* The semen sample is mixed with a sperm wash medium and centrifuged. The pellet (the bottom part after centrifugation) has the spermatozoa. It is resuspended in a small amount of fresh medium and incubated until the time of insemination.

Chapter 49: Infertility

4. Indications for donor insemination
    - Obstructive azoospermia
    - Nonobstructive azoospermia
    - Severe deficits in semen quality in couples who do not wish to undergo intracytoplasmic sperm injection (ICSI).

References
1. Boomsma CM, Cohlen BJ, Farquhar C. Semen preparation techniques for intrauterine insemination. Cochrane Database Syst Rev. 2019;10(10):CD004507. doi: 10.1002/14651858.CD004507.pub4. PMID: 31612995; PMCID: PMC6792139.
2. NICE—Fertility problems: assessment and treatment (2017).

OSCE 19.

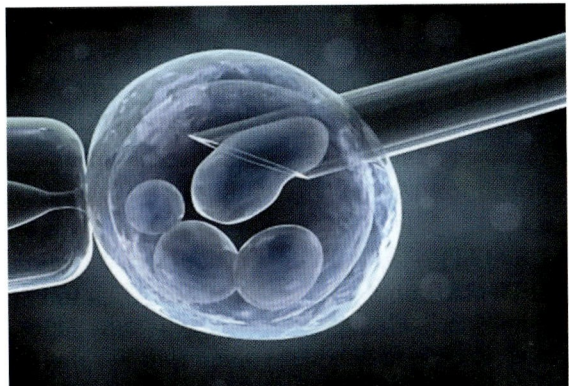

1. Identify the procedure being shown in the figure.
2. What is its role?
3. What time is it done?
4. Name two indications for this procedure.
5. What is the difference between PGS and PGD?

Ans.

1. Biopsy of the embryonic cell done for preimplantation genetic diagnosis (PGD) Day three cleavage stage blastomere biopsy.
2. It is done to identify the genetic abnormalities of the developing embryo before it is implanted inside the uterus. It's a screening test where cells extracted from embryo (trophoblastic or inner cell mass) and tested for aneuploidy. On embryos developing in the IVF laboratory prior to transfer to the uterus.
   It's a diagnostic test that identify if embryo carries:
    - A single gene disorder (Cystic fibrosis, Tay Sachs disease, sickle cell disease and myotonic dystrophy)
    - Aneuploidy screening (high maternal paternal age)
    - Chromosome abnormalities (inherited as structural rearrangements, such as translocations, inversions, or duplications/deletions)

Section 2: Gynecology

In high-risk couple for, that may lead to failed implantation, miscarriage or the birth of a child with a mental, physical or developmental disability. Can be used to select sex of embryo to avoid the X-linked disorder affection.

3. *Timings:* Polar body biopsy, Day 3 blastomere biopsy, Day 5 trophectoderm biopsy
4. *Indications:*
   - Good for those couples who had recurrent abortions
   - Those who have family history of hereditary transmittable disorder (e.g., Thalassemia)
   - Repeated IVF failures, advanced maternal age
5. As the name suggests preimplantation genetic screening (PGS) analyzes biopsied cells from the embryo to screen for potential genetic abnormalities in cases when there is no known potentially inherited disease while the preimplantation genetic diagnosis, uses the same process to detect a specific known familial disorder that has a high probability of being parent to child transmission.

Reference

1. Stern HJ. Preimplantation Genetic Diagnosis: Prenatal Testing for Embryos Finally Achieving Its Potential. J Clin Med. 2014;3(1):280-309. doi: 10.3390/jcm3010280. PMID: 26237262; PMCID: PMC4449675.

OSCE 20.

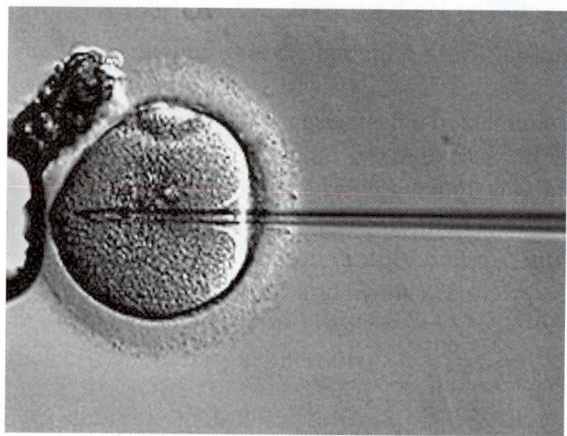

1. Identify the procedure shown in the figure.
2. **Name the various possible sources of sperm for above procedure in male factor infertility.**
3. What is ROSI?
4. Name two risks associated with the above procedure.

Ans.

1. Intracytoplasmic sperm injection (ICSI)—direct insertion of single sperm cell into the cytoplasm of an oocyte by micropuncture through a manipulator.
2. Possible sources of sperm for ICSI in severe male infertility:
   - Normal ejaculated sperm

- MESA (Microsurgical epididymal sperm aspiration)—in cases of vasa block epididymal collection is offered—Obstructive azoospermia
  - PESA (Percutaneous epididymal sperm aspiration)
  - TESE (Testicular sperm extraction)—for nonobstructive azoospermic cases
  - TESA (Testicular sperm aspiration)
3. *Round spermatid injection (ROSI):* A technique of assisted reproduction where round spermatid collected from the testes is injected in the oocyte cytoplasm. It is tried for genetic fatherhood in cases where there is azoospermia and even TESE fails to provide normal spermatid.
4. Risks
   - Increased risk of congenital abnormalities (including hypospadias)
   - Autosomal and chromosomal aneuploidy from meiotic errors
   - Endocrine abnormalities
   - Epigenetic imprinting affects and influences gene expression and transmission like Angelman and Beckwith-Wiedemann syndrome
   - Developmental delay and impaired neurological status
   - Multiple gestation and preterm labor

Reference

1. Alukal JP, Lamb DJ. Intracytoplasmic sperm injection (ICSI)—what are the risks? Urol Clin North Am. 2008;35(2):277-88.

Index

A

Abacavir, side effects of 227
Abdomen
    magnetic resonance imaging of 404
    ultrasonography of 590
Abdominal cervical cerclage 136, 348, 351
Abdominovaginal method 45
Abnormal biophysical score 239
Abortion 49, 330, 334, 339, 362
    incomplete 333, 338, 422
    inevitable 334
    missed 49, 338, 422
    recurrent spontaneous 610
    septate 308, 330, 332
    threatened 331, 422
    tubal 432
    types of 49
Abruptio placentae 364
    severe 249
Abruption, placental 53, 92, 218, 249, 300
Acanthosis nigricans 470
Accredited Social Health Workers 319
Acetone 140
Acidemia, metabolic 303
Acidosis 117
    metabolic 312
Acrania 75
Acriflavine 479
Acupressure therapy 142
Acute respiratory distress syndrome 315
Acyclovir 449, 462
Adenomatoid malformation, congenital pulmonary 79
Adenomyoma 347
Adenomyomectomy 347
Adenomyosis 397, 403, 404, 408-410, 415, 417, 501
    diffuse 399
Adhesiolysis, laparoscopic 414
Adhesions 407
    formation 509
Adnexal mass, benign 388
Adnexal tenderness 422, 457
Adrenal cortical tumor 521
Adrenocorticotropic hormone 604
Agenesis 77, 607
AIDS 231, 325
Airway 165
Alcohol 127, 138
Alkalosis, metabolic 293
Alobar holoprosencephaly 75
Amenorrhea 467, 517, 578, 613
    functional hypothalamic 390
    primary 517, 518
Amino acid damage 130
Amniocentesis 73, 74, 78, 80, 82, 84, 86, 362
Amnioreduction 215
Amniotic cavities 214
Amniotic fluid 265
    embolism 92
    index 81, 95, 265, 267
Amniotomy 229
Ampicillin 330
Ampulla 50, 335, 432
Amsel's criteria 455
Anal wink reflex 485
Analgesia, epidural 98, 182
Analgesics 407
Anastrozole 421
Androgen insensitivity syndrome 388, 522, 525
Android pelvis 22, 97
Anemia 112, 147, 151, 203, 397
    correction of 401
    cut-off for 10
    fetal 202
    maternal 149
    microcytic hypochromic 147, 148
    nutritional 149
    physiological 10, 152
    refractory 145
    severe 198
    sideroblastic 147
    treatment of 393
Anencephaly 21, 260, 360
Anesthesia
    general 182
    spinal 134
Aneuploidy 77
Aneurysm, aortic 491
Anorectal discharge 461
Anovulation 520
Anovulatory cycles 391
Anoxia, fetal 99
Antenatal anti-D prophylaxis 208
Anterior abdominal wall defects 75
Anthropoid pelvis 22
Antibiotics 130, 131, 308
Antibody 199, 227
    quantification 205
Anticholinergic drugs 584
Anticoagulant 178
Anti-D binds 201
Anti-D immunoglobulin 245
Anti-D prophylaxis 333
Antigen 227
Anti-human globulin 199
Antihypertensive 165, 166, 222
    drugs 243
Anti-Müllerian hormone 608
Antimuscarinic drug 582
Antiretroviral therapy 228
    active 226
    principles of 226
Antiseptic 479
Antispasmodics 407
Antiviral therapy 223
Antral follicle count 475
    total 608
Aorta
    abdominal 412
    severe coarctation of 175
Aortic dilatation 175
Aortic stenosis 182
APLA syndrome 347
Apoptosis, placental 262
Arcus tendineous fascia pelvis 480
Aromatase inhibitor 514
    advantage of 605
Arrhythmias 174
    cardiac 506
Arterioarterial anastomosis 214
Aseptic bone necrosis 148
Asherman's syndrome 346, 466, 510, 613
Aspiration
    follicular 514
    pneumonitis 261
    test 591
Aspirin 514

Index

Assisted reproductive technology 603
Asthma, bronchial 166
Asynclitism 30
Atosiban 129
Atresia, urethral 75
Atrial fibrillation 179
Atrophy, postmenopausal 491
Autism 353
Autosomal recessive condition 148
Ayres spatula 542
AYUSH 320
Azithromycin 449, 451, 461
Azoospermia 603
    nonobstructive 617
    obstructive 505, 617

B

Bacteroides 332, 455
Bakri balloon 90, 310
Balloon
    mitral valvuloplasty,
        percutaneous 180
    tamponade 276
Bandl's ring 99
    upper uterine segment,
        pathological 99
Bariatric surgery 151
    cut-off BMI for 476
Bartholin gland abscess 392
Bartter syndrome 86
Basal crepitations,
        auscultation for 167
Basophilia, punctate 146
Beckwith-Wiedemann syndrome 84
Benson and Durfee's abdominal
        method 343
Benzathine penicillin 461, 463
Beta-blocking agents 182
Beta-human chorionic
        gonadotrophin 555
Beta-hydroxy butyrate 140
Betamethasone 131, 177, 242
Betamimetics 129
Beta-thalassemia 149
Bicarbonate 193, 312
Biguanides 191
Bile acid 220
    concentration 221
Bilirubin, serum 205
Bimastoid diameter 17
Biochemical tests 477
Biophysical profile
    modified 260
    types of 267
Biopsy 404, 479
    cervical 579
    directed 610
    endometrial 400, 406, 529, 577

Biparietal diameter 17
Birth
    asphyxia 91, 115, 127, 132, 261
    canal 272
    injuries 191
    premature 22
    preterm 127
Bisacromial diameter 35
BISHOP score 111, 241
    components of 100
Bisphosphonates 419
Bite cells 144
Bitemporal diameter 17
Black lesion 409
Bladder
    injury 443, 486, 582
    mild enlargement of 76
    pressure necrosis of 99
    repair of 487
    wall interruption 244
Bleeding 443
    anovulatory 49, 398, 399, 405
    irregular 493
    per vaginum, mild 197
    postcoital 405
Blighted ovum 50
Blindness 159
Blood 153
    arterial gases 193
    count, complete 436, 598
    fresh gush of 95
    glucose
        capillary 193
        level 192
    group 205
    investigations 477
    loss 438
    pressure 162
        apparatus 156
        monitoring 165
    sampling, fetal 203
    smear, peripheral 10, 144, 404
    sugar
        fasting 191
        level 186, 471
        low 222
    transfusion 121, 145
        autologous 154
B-Lynch suture 277, 315
Body
    fat percentage 476
    mass index 377
        categorizing obesity 603
    stalk anomaly 75
Bone 16
    loss 419
Bonney's myomectomy clamp 610
Bonney's test 583
    positive 481

Bowel
    injury 441
    obstruction 82
Brachial plexus
    impairment 105
    injury 91
Brachytherapy uterine
        applicators 548
Bradycardia 166
Brain natriuretic peptide 170
Breast 5
    cancer 418
    modified sebaceous glands of 5
Breastfeeding 223, 401, 425
    considerations 230
Breathlessness, progressive 170
Breech presentation 91, 92, 217
Broad ligament 417
Bronchopulmonary sequestration 79
Burch colposuspension 581
Burns–Marshall
    method 36
    technique 119

C

Caffeine 138
Calcifications, periventricular 78
Calcium
    infusion 514
    metabolism 14
Caldwell–Moloy classification 110
Calvarium, partial absence of 187
Calymmatobacterium
        granulomatis 449
Cancer
    endometrial 368, 402, 471, 574
    genome atlas studies 529
    ovarian 368
    stomach 470
Candida albicans 445, 454
Candidal infection 454
Candidiasis 445
Caput
    importance of 19
    succedaneum 100
Carbetocin 274
Carbon dioxide 570
Carboprost 115, 167
Carcinoma 577
    cervical 537
    cervix 49
    endometrial 404, 418, 526
Cardiac defects 66, 73, 80
Cardiac disease 170, 172, 173, 183
    fetal complications of 175
    maternal complications of 175
    pregnancy associated 183

Cardiac failure 171, 179
   congestive 83, 166, 175
Cardiac transplantation
      recipients 177
Cardinal ligament, level of 487
Cardiomyopathy, peripartum 180
Cardiopulmonary exercise
      testing 170
Cardiotocography 264, 265
Cardiovascular anomaly 364
Cardiovascular computed
      tomography 170
Carotene, low dietary intake of 550
Carpel tunnel syndrome 7
Carvallo's sign 179
Catecholamine 182
Caudal regression 187
   sequence 364
Cefazoline 177
Cefixime 461, 462
Cefotaxime 332
Ceftriaxone 177
   intramuscular 446
Centchroman pills 367
Central nervous system
      malformation 139, 187
Cephalic-breech 217
Cephalohematoma 19, 100
Cephalopelvic disproportion 41, 42
Cerclage
   indications of 62
   operations, types of 130
Cerebral palsy 132
Cervarix 448, 544
Cervical
   amputation 496
   barrier, interruption of 458
   canal 430
   cerclage 356, 430
   changes 9
   consistency 111
   dilatation 94, 95, 100, 343
   dilation 126
   discharge 461
   ectopic pregnancy 429
   elongation 481
   erosion 49
   funneling 61
   incompetence 361, 486
   insufficiency 61
   involvement 528
   length, assessment of 61
   motion tenderness 422, 457
   mucus 10
   polyp 49, 246
   somite anomalies 390
   spine dislocation 91
   tear 278

Cervicitis 462
Cervix 61, 218, 263, 367
   absence of 481
   length of 100
   position of 111
   shapes of 135
Cesarean delivery 218, 219, 223, 268
   elective 229
Cesarean scar
   ectopic pregnancy 430, 431
   pregnancy, classification of 431
Cesarean section 3, 134, 183, 214,
      241, 251, 365
   emergency 98, 248
   indications for 243
Chance 452
Chancroid 448
Chemoradiation therapy 546
Chemotherapy 445
   high-dose 564
Chest
   pain 170
   X-ray 13, 555
Chhaya 367
   benefits of 367
Chignon 100
Chlamydia 232, 447, 457, 461, 462
   trachomatis 330, 450, 457,
      460, 465
Chloasma 4
Cho square suture 315
Chocolate
   agar 446
   cyst 409
Cholecystitis 140
Choriocarcinoma 558, 562
Chorionic peak sign 53
Chorionic villi 553, 554
Chorionicity 51, 211
Choroid plexus cyst 65
   bilateral 65
Chromopertubation 505
   laparoscopic 607
Chromosomal abnormalities 54, 56,
      66, 68, 69, 84
Chromosomal testing 67, 68, 71
Ciprofloxacin 332
Cirrhosis 223
Cisplatin 546
Clamp pedicle 411
Cleavage, timing of 209
Cleft
   lip 353
   palate 353
Clindamycin 330
Clitoris 511
Cloacal exstrophy 84

Clomiphene 605
   citrate 605
   failure 606
   resistance 606
Clonus 159
Clostridium 330, 332
Clotrimazole 454
Clue cells 455
Coagulation
   abnormalities of 120
   defects 272
   disorder 405
   screen 221
Coagulopathy, consumptive 301
Coelomic metaplasia theory 416
Cognitive behavioral therapy 578
Collin's knife 442
Colloid infusion 514
Color Doppler examination 413
Colpoperineorrhaphy 500
Colporrhaphy 499
   anterior 495
Colposcope 539
Colpotomy 459
Coma 506
Combined hormonal
      contraception 377, 419
Combined oral contraceptive 377,
      399, 475
   contraindications of 368
   pills 474
Complex fistula 588
Conception
   products of 289
   retained products of 119
Condom 447
   promotion 447
Condyloma acuminata 464
Condylomata lata 449
Confusion 506
Congenital anomaly 58, 127, 186
Congenital malformation 73, 191
Conjoined twins 214, 217
Contraception 365
   emergency 373, 398
Contraceptive 231
   advice 194, 393
   hormonal 231, 474
   oral 447
   patch 381
   precautions 379
Controlled cord traction 95
Convulsions 165, 506
Coombs test
   direct 205
   indirect 197, 199
Copper 327
   intrauterine device 372

Index

Cord
    blood sample 202
    clamping, early 202
    compression 261, 265
    insertion 84
    presentation 250
    prolapse 91, 108, 218, 249
        chance of 39
Cordocentesis 203
Cornual block, bilateral 468
Corpus callosum, agenesis of 77
Corpus luteal cyst 423
Corticosteroid, antenatal 225
COVID-19 vaccination 232
Crampy lower abdominal pain 393
Crown rump length 236
Cryoprecipitate 247
Cryptomenorrhea 394
Crystalloid 168, 312
    infusion 120
Cul-de sac 417, 426
    obliteration 407
Culdocentesis 426
Cusco's speculum 411, 541
Cushing's syndrome 5, 471, 521
Cyclophosphamide 564
Cyst, blue domed 409
Cystectomy 410
    endometriotic 418
    ovarian 388
Cystic degeneration 403
Cystic teratoma, benign 389
Cystitis, interstitial 409
Cystocele 499
Cystography 590
Cystometry 582
Cystoscopy 487, 586, 589
    intraoperative 571
Cytobrush 542
Cytokine 357
    mitigation of 130
Cytomegalovirus infection, fetal 78

D

Dactinomycin 561, 564
Dawn phenomenon 192
Deafness 132
Death 506
    fetal 92, 99, 139
Deaver's retractor 569
Decidua
    basalis 11, 364
    capsularis 11, 48
    parietalis 11, 48
    types of 11
    vera 11
Decubitus ulcer 493
    biopsy of 493

Deep transverse arrest 32
    causes of 32
Deep vein thrombosis 356
Defibrillator 313
Deflexion 18
    moderate 33
    severe 33
Dehydration 137, 140
    maternal 112
Delivery 224
    methods of 123
    mode of 195, 214, 219
    preterm 133
    timing of 181
Deltoid muscle 200
Denonvillier's fascia 484
Dense abdominal adhesions 426
Depot medroxyprogesterone
    acetate 377
Dermal papilla, enzyme of 474
Dermoid cyst 516
Desogestrel 373, 475
Dexamethasone 131, 177, 242
    suppression test 471
Dextran 595
Diabetes mellitus 189, 363, 400, 404, 406, 445, 470
    control of 584
    gestational 86, 188
    maternal 262
Diabetic ketoacidosis 140, 193, 316
    diagnosis of 193
Dichorionic 211
    diamniotic 212
    twins 216
Dichorionicity 212
Dilutional coagulopathy 301
Dinoprostone 181
Diphenhydramine 142
Discordant 215
    twin 215
Disseminated intravascular
    coagulation 120
Distal tubal
    blockage 612
    obstruction 468
Dizogotic 210, 211
    twin 209
Donor
    oocyte 505
    semen 512
Donovan bodies 449
Donovanosis 449
Dopamine agonists 514
Doppler studies 159
Doppler transthoracic
    echocardiography 170
Double bleb sign 48

Double decidual sign 48
Double-balloon catheter 111
Down syndrome 64, 65, 68, 69, 86
Doxycycline 450, 451, 461, 462, 465
Doxylamine 139
Drospirenone 373, 475
Dry mucous membrane 141
Ductus venosus 60, 72, 177
Duodenal atresia 86
Dyschezia 416
Dyslipidemia, risk of 378
Dysmaturity syndrome 257
Dysmenorrhea 367, 416, 433, 467
    congestive 414
    severe 397, 403
    spasmodic 409
Dyspareunia 493
    deep 416
Dyspnea 170
    paroxysmal nocturnal 170
Dystocia, cervical 99
Dysuria 416

E

Echocardiography 170
Echogenic intracardiac focus 65
Eclampsia 157, 221, 359, 363
Ecosprin 347
Ectocervix 538
Ectoderm 389
Ectopic pregnancy 49, 50, 200, 422, 423, 427
    chronic 432
    management of 51, 424
    persistent 428
    previous 423
    risk factors of 423
    ruptured 392
    unruptured 427, 429
Edema 9
    cerebral 169
    pathological 8
    pulmonary 167, 169, 175, 179, 183, 304
Efavirenz 227, 228
Efferent ductules 511
Eflornithine 474
Elagolix, oral 419
Elbows 470
Electrolyte
    disturbances, correction of 316
    imbalance 137, 438
Elliptocyte 144
Embolus, migration of 282
Embryo
    cryopreservation 506
    reduction 52, 53
    transfer 415

Embryonic cell, biopsy of 617
Embryonic urogenital structures 511
Emergency exploratory
    laparotomy 557
Encephalitis 449
Encerclage, laparoscopic 596
Endocarditis, infective 176
Endocervical canal 430
Endocervix 538
Endoduplication 552
Endometrial biopsy 400, 406, 529, 577
    cannula 395
Ehyperplasia 395, 401, 404, 476, 577
Endometrial hyperplasia
    persistent 406
    risk of 471
Endometrial intraepithelial
    neoplasia 398, 401, 406
Endometrioma 408, 416, 417
    ovarian 408
    ruptured 421
Endometriosis 407-409, 414, 415,
    417-420, 423, 459, 516, 599
    deep infiltrating 420
    laparoscopic excision of 420
    moderate 415
    severe 415
    site of 419
Endometriotic lesions,
    excision of 419
Endometriotic tissues
    lymphatic of 409
    vascular spread of 409
Endometritis 282, 330
    chronic 460, 461
    clinical features of 290
Endometrium 354
    thickened 400
Endomyometritis 330
Endopelvic fascia 482
Enterocele 485
    formation 484
Enterococcus faecalis 461
Enzyme-linked immunosorbent
    assay 340
Epidural analgesia 98, 182
    use of 106, 117
Episiotomy
    extension of 88
    scissors 122
    suturing 122
Epithelioid trophoblastic tumor 558
Epsilon sign 52
Epulis gravidarum 12
    course of 12
Erb-Duchenne palsy 105
Ergometrine 167, 182
Erosions 493

Erythromycin 450, 451
Estranes, nonethylated 381
Estrogen 5, 421
    maternal 387
Estrone 575
Ethambutol 228
Ethinyl estradiol 367
Etonogestrel
    implants 378
    releasing subdermal implant 418
Etoposide 564
Euploid pregnancies 64
Exercise, aerobic 194
Exomphalos 67
External cephalic version 41, 92, 219

F

Face mask 302
Facial anomalies 71
Fallopian tubes 408, 417, 466, 511
    patency of 504
    surgery 423
Falloposcopy 610
Family Planning Logistics
    Management Information
    System 369
Fasting insulin level 471
Fasting lipid
    panel 471
    profile 476
Fat, subcutaneous 257
Ferning 10
Ferritin, serum 146, 147, 154
Fertility 496
    chances of 601
    sparing 496
Fertilization, time of 506
Fetal anomalies 57
Fetal arterial wave 60
Fetal biometry 59, 233
    chart 162
Fetal complications 53, 175, 191,
    255, 292
Fetal distress 97
    intrapartum 218
    signs of 421
Fetal echo 80
Fetal face 68
Fetal fibronectin 128
Fetal gender 212
Fetal growth restriction 77, 158, 160,
    162, 175, 233, 553, 554
    complications of 237
    severe 91
Fetal head
    deceleration 264, 265
    delivery of 190

different stations of 24
    monitoring 193
    rate tracing 264, 265
    severe moulding of 18
    station of 100
Fetal hydrops 206
    diagnosis for 206
Fetal maxilla, development of 70
Fetal monitoring, tests for 112
Fetal nuchal translucency 66
Fetal skull 15-17
    transverse diameters of 17
Fetal sleep 117
Fetal surveillance, methods of 240
Fetal ultrasound monitoring 203
Fetal urinary bladder 68
Fetal weight, estimated 236
Feticide, selective 215
Fetus 123
    complete structural
        evaluation of 65
    in utero, position of 96
    malformed 256
Fever 441
Fibrinogen 120, 318
Fibroids 441
    anterior wall 436
    cervical 443
    classification of 434, 502, 609
    location of 436
    pieces, dissemination of 441
    polyp, endometrial 404
    size, shrinkage of 401
    submucous 595
    type of 433
    uterus 403, 436, 437, 566, 609
First trimester scan 54, 66
    advantages of 55
Fistula 588
    recurrence of 590
    ureterovaginal 585, 586
Fistulous tract, complete
    excision of 586
Fitz-Hugh-Curtis syndrome 458,
    460, 462
Flexion
    incomplete 18
    point, importance of 89
Flow cytometry tests 201
Fluconazole 461
Fluid
    overload syndrome 183, 506, 611
    replacement 193
    responsiveness 308
Folate deficiency 145
Foley's catheter 111, 123, 586
Folic acid 21, 149, 326, 360
    consumption 491

Follicle, accessibility of 421
Follicle-stimulating
hormone 604, 608
low-dose 184
Forceps delivery 37, 88
Fothergill modification 496
Fothergill operation 496
Fracture 91
Fresh frozen plasma 251, 293
Frog eye sign 260
Fulguration 410
Furosemide 182

G

Ganzoni formula 147
Gardasil quadrivalent 544
Gardnerella vaginalis 455, 457
Gas test, insufflation of 591
Gastric mucosa 327
Gastroschisis 84
Gelhorn pessary 483
Genetic syndromes 66
Genital herpes 448, 452, 453
Genital herpetic vesicles 464
Genital tract
 bleeding 401
 injury 120
Genital tuberculosis 393, 457
 female 467
 treatment of 468
Genital ulcer disease 461
Genital warts, external 448
Gentamicin 330, 332
Gestation 162
 multiple 52, 216
 period of 6
Gestational age 60
 large for 262
 preterm 134
Gestational diabetes mellitus 86, 188
 increased risk of 222
 management of 194
Gestational sac 47, 48, 430
Gestational trophoblastic
 neoplasia 550
Gestodene 475
Girth, abdominal 6
Glands
 duct, obstruction of 392
 sebaceous 5
Glans penis 511
Globular uterus 501
Glomerular filtration rate 13
Glucocorticoids 474, 514
Glucose challenge test 190
Glutamate 363
Gluteal artery, superior 285

Glyburide 191
Glycerine 479
Gonorrhea 232, 446, 447, 457, 461, 462
 pelvic manifestation of 446
Graham Steel murmur 179
Gram staining 455
Grand multipara 272
Granulocyte colony-stimulating factor 357
Granuloma inguinale 449, 452, 453
Granulosa cells 511
Gravidogram 235
Groin 470
Groove sign 465
Growth
 hormone 604
 restriction 139
Gubernaculum testis 511
Guedel airway 165
Gut 67
Gynecoid pelvis 22, 110
Gynecological endoscopy 591

H

Hair
 terminal 473
 types of 473
Halban's theory 409
Hanging drop preparation 456
Hayman suture 277
Head
 delivery of 36, 38
 engagement of 36
 entrapment 108
 measurement of 18
 sagittal suture of 32
Headache 304, 506
 severe 159
Heart
 change, size of 14
 defect, congenital 174
 disease 171
  acquired 172
  congenital 172, 177, 353
 rate 14
  control 182
Hegar dilator 335
Helicobacter pylori 137
HELLP syndrome 53, 221, 225
 diagnostic features of 164
 management of 224
Helmet cells 144
Hematoma, size of 287
Hemochromatosis 151
Hemodilution, hypervolemia-
 induced 5

Hemoglobin 436
 artificially modified 155
 based oxygen carriers 155
Hemoglobinopathy 146
 inherited 148
 maternal 201
Hemolytic disease 198, 205
Hemoperitoneum
 blood indicates 426
 spontaneous 421
Hemoptysis 170
Hemorrhage 269, 400
 active 293
 acute 153
 antepartum 244
 atonic postpartum 269, 276
 early pregnancy 49
 fetomaternal 197, 198, 200, 202
 intracranial 91
 intraventricular 237
 obstetric 271
 postpartum 95, 189, 269
 primary 269
 retroplacental 337
 secondary postpartum 289
 subchorionic 333
 traumatic postpartum 278
Hemorrhagic manifestations 251
Hemosiderosis 151
Hemostatic forceps 122
Hepatic calcifications 78
Hepatitis 140
 B
  vaccine, dose of 224
  virus, mother-to-child
   transmission of 223
 C 221
  infection 224
Hernia
 congenital diaphragmatic 79
 repair 499
Herniation, physiological 84
Heterotaxy 80
Hirsutism 469, 473, 474
 causes of 473
Hiss sound 591
HIV 226
Holoprosencephaly 71
Hormonal vaginal ring 379
Hormone 4, 8
 free interval 373
Hot flashes 401
Howell Jolly bodies 146
Human chorionic gonadotropin 597
Human papilloma virus 448, 464
Human placental lactogen 565
Hyaline 403
Hybrid fibroid 437

Hydatidiform mole 7, 49, 140
  complete 550
Hydralazine therapy 168
Hydramnios 215
Hydrocephalus 21, 22
  acquired 22
Hydronephrosis 81
Hydrops
  fetalis 205
    causes of 206
    nonimmune 206
Hydrosalpinx 508
  fluid 612
Hydroureteronephrosis 394
Hydroxy urea 149
Hydroxyethyl starch 121
Hygroscopic solution 479
Hymenotomy 394, 519
Hyperandrogenism 354, 470, 521
Hyperemesis 53
  gravidarum 137-139, 220
Hyperglycemia 242
Hyperosmolar glucose 425
Hyperplasia, endometrial 395, 401, 404, 476, 577
Hyperprolactinemia 354
Hypersensitivity 151, 367
Hypertension 156, 304, 306, 404
  chronic 156
  gestational 194
  management of 243
  pulmonary artery 175, 182
  severe 169
Hyperthyroidism 140
Hypertrichosis 474
Hypnosis 578, 579
Hypochromic microcytic anemia 10
Hypoestrogenic symptoms 419
Hypoglycemia 127, 132, 237
  neonatal 191
  risk of 195
Hypogonadism,
    hypergonadotropic 601
Hypokalemia 139, 193
Hyponatremia 139, 506
Hypoplastic nasal bone 64
Hypotension 9, 96, 112, 177
Hypothermia 127, 237
Hypothyroidism 339, 354, 404, 478
Hypovolemia
  signs of 90
  symptoms of 90
Hypoxia 112
  fetal 117
Hysterectomy 406, 411, 430, 498, 499, 566
  abdominal 403, 412
  extrafascial 567

  indications of 563
  laparoscopic 568
  operation 585
  total abdominal 566, 570
  vaginal 439, 487, 493, 574
Hysterosalpingography 505, 607, 611
  abnormal 610
Hysteroscope 610
Hysteroscopic
  adhesiolysis 346, 442, 510
  isthmocele repair 442
  morcellator device 440
  resection 431
  septal resection 344, 350, 442, 503
  tubal cannulation 504
Hysteroscopy 184, 404, 528, 607, 609, 610, 613

I

Ileal atresia 86
Iliac fossa 25
Iliopectineal lines 43
Imiquimod 465
Immotile 615
Immunodeficiency 425
Immunosuppression 445
Imperforate hymen 519, 522
Implantation bleeding 49
Implants, removal of 379
In vitro fertilization 505
In vitro maturation 514
Incomplete breech 91, 108
Indomethacin 129
Indwelling catheterization 487
Infant respiratory distress
    syndrome 191
Infections 189, 400, 499
  bacterial 447
  enterococcus 177
  fetal 78
  genitourinary 444
  severe 332
  signs of 130
Infertility 415, 416, 597, 610
  causes of 466
  primary 467
  secondary 467
  unexplained 603, 610
Inflammation, perihepatic 446
Influenza 149
Infundibulum 50
Inguinal bubo 461
Injury
  fetal 88
  interstitial 459
  ureteric 443, 571, 590
  visceral 412

Insulin
  morning dose of 192
  sensitizers 472, 474
Internal iliac artery 72, 282
  branches of 285
Interspinous diameter 28
Intra-abdominal organ damage 91
Intra-abdominal pressure 498
Intracardiac shunts 182
Intracavitary lesions 355
Intracellular gram-negative
    bacterium 449
Intracorporeal morcellation 437
Intracytoplasmic sperm
  injection 603, 617, 618
  insemination 513
Intramyometrial vasopressin 592
Intranuclear bodies 466
Intraoperative cell salvage 155
Intrauterine blood transfusion 203
Intrauterine cavitary lesion 610
Intrauterine contraceptive device 176, 231, 379, 447
  postpartum 365
Intrauterine death 191
Intrauterine fetal death 224, 247
Intrauterine insemination 508
  catheter 508
Intrauterine synechia 282, 613
  formation of 466
Intrauterine transfusion 82, 359
Intravascular coagulation
    syndrome 300
Intrinsic sphincter defect 583
Invasive mole 558
Iodine allergy 612
Iron 151, 326
  absorption, enhancers of 149
  binding capacity, total 154
  deficiency 151
    anemia 10, 147, 154
    evolution of 154
  requirement 147
  serum 146, 147
  stores 154
  sucrose 152
  therapy 151
Irrigation test 591
Irritable bowel syndrome 417, 459
Ischial spine 24, 43, 487
  importance of 24
  plane of 24
Ischiococcygeus 482
Ischiopubic rami 29
Isoniazid 228
Isotonic solutions 438
Isthmus 50

Index

J

Janani Sishu Suraksha Karayakaram 319
Janani Suraksha Yojna 319
Jarisch-Herxheimer reaction 453
Jaundice 127, 132
Junk diet 603

K

Kabuki syndrome 74
Kallmann syndrome 522
Kangaroo nutrition 132
Kangaroo support 132
Karman's cannula 338, 553
Karyotype 388
Kegel's exercise 486, 494, 581, 584
Kelly's plication 481
Ketosis, signs of 140
Ketotic breath smell 141
Key-hole signs 81
Kidney
    injury, acute 168
    size of 13
Kiwi cup pump 102
    parts of 102
Klebsiella 332
    granulomatis 449
Kleihauer-Betke test 201, 248
Klinefelter's syndrome 518, 603
Knee 470
    chest position 394
    hammer 159
Kocher's hemostatic clamp 411
Kronos Early Estrogen Prevention Study 580

L

Labia minora 511
Labor 88, 189
    abnormalities 105
    care guide, components of 114
    first stage of 153
    induction of 99, 266
    mechanism of 38
    obstructed 189, 585
    painful 182
    premature 175
    preterm 331
    room quality improvement initiative 325
    second stage of 153
    third stage of 103, 153, 288
Lactation 224, 367
Lactobacillus 444
Lambda sign 51, 70
Lambdoid sutures 15
Lamivudine 227, 325
Landon vaginal retractor 486
Lanugo 257
    hair 473
Laparoscopic conservative surgery 413
Laparoscopic myoma screw 592
Laparoscopic ovarian drilling 470, 475, 509
    mechanism of 606
Laparoscopy 184, 335, 407, 410, 419, 599
Laparotomy 335, 410, 431
Laryngeal papillomatosis 448
Le Fort's partial procedure, modified 497
Least pelvic dimension, plane of 28
Leech Wilkinson cannula 505, 611
Leg ulcers 148
Leiomyoma 408, 410, 417
Leiomyomatosis, diffuse peritoneal 441
Leiomyosarcoma, dissemination of 437, 441
Leishman stain 449
Leopard skin appearance 468
Lethargy 251
Letrozole 421, 475, 605
Leucovorin 564
Leukorrhea 493
Leuprolide acetate 401
Levator ani 486, 584
Levonorgestrel 367
    intrauterine device 399, 418
Liberal episiotom 133
Limb
    defects 362
    reduction defects 75
Linea nigra 4
Liquefaction time 602
Liquid chromatography 148
Liver
    cirrhosis 8
    disease 220
    disease, chronic 425
    enzymes, elevated 164
    function test 158, 598
L-ornithine decarboxylase 474
Loveset's maneuver 108, 118
Lower abdominal pain 414, 461, 467
    differential diagnosis of 458
Lung ultrasound 167
Luteinizing hormone 604
Lymph node
    involvement 528
    paracervical 545
Lymphatic metastases 416
Lymphogranuloma venereum 449, 450, 452, 453, 465
Lynch syndrome 531, 532

M

MacKenrodt ligament 488
Macrosomia 7, 189-191, 262
    fetal 192, 268
Magnesium sulphate 129, 130, 159, 165, 166, 243, 309, 359
    dose of 159
    toxicity, monitoring of 159
Magnetic resonance imaging 572, 607
Makler's sperm counting chamber 615
Malabsorption syndromes 151
Malignancy 409
Mallory Weiss tear 139
Malnutrition 139
Manchester operation 496
Mandibular gap 70
Manual vacuum aspiration 333
    syringe 336
Marfan syndrome 175, 491
Marion Sims classification 590
Martius interposition flap 590
Mass, abdominal 490, 491
Massive blood transfusion 314
Maternal death 92, 322
Mauriceau-Smellie-Veit maneuver 119
Mayer-Rokitansky-Küster-Hauser syndrome 390, 524
McCall culdoplasty 482, 487, 574
    external 484
    internal 484
McDonald operation 136
McDonald's vaginal cerclage, elective 361
McRobert's maneuver 104
Meclizine 142
Meconium
    aspiration 237, 257, 258, 261, 268
    passage 261
    stained amniotic fluid 222
Medical nutritional therapy 188
Medroxyprogesterone 400, 404
    acetate 148, 366, 534
    cyclical 405
Megacystis 68, 75
Melanocyte-stimulating hormone 5
Membranes
    artificial rupture of 181
    rupture of 130
Menarche 393
Menopause 409, 575
Menorrhagia 367, 403, 405
Menses 409
Menstrual bleeding, heavy 397, 433
Menstrual cycle 409
    regularization of 368

Menstrual hygiene, poor 458
Menstruation, retrograde 409
Mersilene tape 349
Mesh
   erosion 487, 499
   removal of 487
Metabolic syndrome 391, 476
Metastatic theory 416
Metformin 191, 472, 475, 514
   side effects of 606
Methemoglobinemia 304
Methotrexate 335, 425, 430, 564
   contraindications of 425
   induced photosensitivity
      skin rash 425
Methylergometrine 115
Metoclopramide 141
Metronidazole 330, 332, 446, 455, 462
Micro-immunofluorescence 450
Microsurgical epididymal sperm
      aspiration 512, 619
Microsurgical testicular sperm
      extraction 512
Mid diastolic murmur 179
Mid-trimester anomaly scan 57
Migraine 401
Miliary tubercles 460
Mirabegron 583, 585
Mirror syndrome 207
Miscarriage 49
   risk of 74
   threatened 333, 337
Misoprostol 115, 181
Mission Parivar Vikas 323, 370
Mitral stenosis 179
   characteristic clinical diagnostic
      signs of 179
   severe 175
Mitral valve 179
   prolapse 491
Molar pregnancy, complete 556
Mole, partial 551
Molluscum contagiosum 464, 466
Monitor growth discordant twins 216
Monoamniotic twins 213, 216
Monochorionic diamniotic
      pregnancy 215
Monochorionic monoamniotic 212
Monochorionicity 212
Monogenic gene defect 363
Morning sickness 138
Morphological uterine sonographic
      assessment 501
Morris waste space 29
Moth-eaten appearance 468
Mother to child tracking system 320
Motile spirochete *Treponema*
      pallidum 452

Mouth gag 165
Müllerian agenesis 522, 525
Müllerian anomalies 610
   classification of 607
Müllerian aplasia 390
Müllerian hypoplasia, segmental 607
Müllerian uterine malformation 349
Multigravida 98
Multiple pregnancy 7, 52, 90, 137,
      209, 222
   assessment of 51
Multiple vertical suture 277
Muscle fibers, arrangement of 6
MusQan initiative 321
Myasthenia gravis 309
Mycoplasma 461
   genitalium 457
   hominis 455
Myohyperplasia 399
Myoinositol 472
Myoma
   base, extension of 435
   intramural 502
   screw 400, 438
Myomectomy 403, 411, 436, 439
   hysteroscopic 433, 438, 442, 595
   laparoscopic 440
   myoma screw for 400
Myometrial invasion 528
Myometrium 291

N

Narcotic analgesics, use of 117
Nasal bone 68
   absent 64, 73
National AIDS Control
      Programme 325
National Ambulance Service 320
National Deworming Day
      Programme 326
National Iron Plus Initiative 320
National Mobile Medical Units
      Service 320
National Population Stabilization
      Fund 382
National PPTCT Programme 325
National Quality Assurance
      Standards 325
Nausea 163, 304, 506
Nayi Pahel Kits 332
Necrotizing enterocolitis 237, 242
Needle movement test 591
Neisseria 462
   gonorrhoeae 330, 446, 457, 460
Neoplasm 449
Nerves, para-sympathetic 287
Neubauer's chamber grid 615

Neurectomy, presacral 414
Neuroprotection 157
Neurosonogram, complete 65
Neutrophils 145
Neville Barnes forceps 119
Nevirapine 228
Nickel 380
Nifedipine 129, 222
Nitabuch's layer 11
Nitroglycerine 129
Noninvasive prenatal testing 353
Noninvasive ventilation mask 305
Non-Müllerian origin 342
Non-nucleoside reverse transcriptase
      inhibitors 227
Non-pneumatic antishock
      garment 298
Nonsperm cells 602
Nonstress test 159, 166, 260, 267
Noonan syndrome 74
Noradrenaline 311
Norethisterone enanthate 377
Norgestimate 475
Normal vagina, pH level of 444
Nosocomial pneumonia 306
Nuchal fold thickness,
      measurement of 174
Nuchal translucency, raised 55
Nucleoside reverse transcriptase
      inhibitors 227
Nugent's score 455
Nulliparity 137

O

O'Connor's technique 590
Obesity 5, 127, 189, 260, 261, 404,
      445, 469, 470
   apple-type 475
   maternal 137
Obstetric score index 296
Obstetrical pelvis axis 27
Obstetrics forceps, application of 119
Obstruction 392, 590
   intestinal 459
Oligo-anovulation 469
Oligoasthenozoospermia 415
Oligohydraminos 91, 214, 239, 261,
      264, 265, 268, 364
Oligomenorrhea 467, 469
Omentum 408
Omphalocele 84
Oocyte cryopreservation 506
Oophoritis 466
Operative hysteroscopy, indications
      of 610
Opioid 21
Organ dysfunction 300

Index

Orthopnea 170
Ovarian carcinoma, epithelial 418
Ovarian cyst 459
    clamp pedicle of 412
    decreases formation of 368
Ovarian cystectomy, bilateral 415
Ovarian endometriosis, bilateral 394
Ovarian epithelial tumor, benign 388
Ovarian failure, premature 601
Ovarian hyperstimulation syndrome 184, 472, 511, 597, 605
    moderate 513
Ovarian insufficiency, primary 580
Ovarian remnant syndrome 408, 410
Ovarian tumor, clamp pedicle of 412
Ovary 417, 511
    endometriosis of 409
    torsion of 516
Ovulation
    induction, complications of 605
    time of 506
Ovulatory dysfunction 403
Oxygenation 169
Oxytocin 90, 103, 115, 120, 167, 270, 275
    augmentation 229
    drip 98
    infusion of 181
    low cost of 275

P

Page's classification 247
Pain 409, 427
    abdomen
        severe 443
        sudden onset 441
    acute abdominal 421
    acyclical 409
    burning 409
    chronic 148
    cramp-like 409
    cyclical 409
    functional 459
    severe abdominal 251, 597
    type of 414
    upper abdomen 159, 163
Palmar erythema 220
Palmer test 591
Palpitation 177
Panicker's vacuum suction 297
Pap smear 246
Parabasal cells predominate 444
Paracervical fascia 484
Paradidymis 511
Paramesonephric ducts 511
Parathyroid hormone 14
    levels, oral 14

Parietal bone, posterior 31
Passive leg raising test 308
Patellar reflex 157
Patwardhan technique 115
Pelvic
    abscess 462
        drainage of 459
    adhesions 426, 568
    axis 28
    brim 25
    devascularization 314
    endometriosis 399, 407, 410, 419
    floor
        distress inventory 482
        impact questionnaire 482
        muscle 486, 584
        repair 499
    infection, acute 612
    inflammatory disease 380, 408, 417, 423, 446, 460
        complications of 458
        stages of 459
    inlet
        axis of 27
        longest diameter of 27
    masses 460
    mesh 499
    organ prolapse 479, 488, 584
        Q classification 492
        Q system 481
        sling surgeries 499
    pain 467
        chronic 408, 420
    peritonitis 458
    tenderness 422
    ultrasound 408, 417
Pelvicalyceal system 13
Pelvis 42, 555
    assessment of 43, 110
    contracted 42
    false 25
    female 22
    inclination of 25
    magnetic resonance imaging of 404
    oral 15
    ultrasound 333, 522, 524
Penicillin 361
    allergic 177
Percutaneous epididymal sperm aspiration 505, 512, 619
Perinatal asphyxia 237
Perineal injuries, chances of 33
Perineal tear 280
    grade of 280
Peripheral calyceal dilatation 81
Peritoneal cavity, free fluid in 422

Peritonitis, acute 418
Peroneal nerve 571
Phocomelia 141
Phosphate 14, 151
Phytates 151
Pinard's living ligature 6
Pinard's maneuver 118
Pipelle suction curette 527
Piper's forceps 119
Piver-Rutledge classification 567
Placenta 11, 62, 209, 244
    accreta 314
        spectrum 244
    delivery of 365
    grading of 262
    increta 314
    mature 262
    percreta 256, 314
    previa 92, 253
    removal 103
    structural abnormalities of 11
    variants of 62
Placental alpha-macroglobulin 128
Placental site
    nodule, atypical 558
    trophoblastic tumor 558
Platelets 293
    count 158
Platypelloid pelvis 22
Pneumonitis, chemical 258
Pneumoperitoneum 591
Podophyllotoxin 448
Polar bodies 506
Polycystic ovarian syndrome 189, 350, 469, 471, 511
    diagnosis of 472
Polycystic ovary morphology 469
Polyhydramnios 7, 41, 189, 203, 214
Polyp 499
    endometrial 396
Polypectomy, hysteroscopic 442
Polypropylene mesh 499
Postabortion intrauterine contraceptive device 365
Posterior reversible encephalopathy syndrome 169
Posthysterectomy 480
Postmaturity syndrome 257, 259, 268, 364
Povidone-iodine 479
Powder burn 409
Pox virus 464
Prader orchidometer 516
Pradhan Mantri Sushrakshit Matritivya Abhiyaan 324
Preconceptional folic acid supplementation 187

Preeclampsia 53, 160, 169, 183, 189, 268
  increased risk of 222
  prevention of 158
  severe 164
    features of 163
Pregnancy 4-6, 8, 14, 65, 170-174, 202, 220, 226, 367, 395, 401, 421, 445, 459, 612
  ailment of 7
  anembryonic 49, 50
  asymptomatic bacteriuria of 13
  cervical eversion of 9
  cholestasis of 220
  ectopic 49, 50, 200, 422, 423, 427
  failure, early 49
  first trimester 4
  gingivitis of 12
  heterotopic 422
  hypertensive disorder of 156, 160, 242
  intrahepatic cholestasis of 221, 358
  late 260
  late-term 259, 261
  lordosis of 14
  loss, recurrent 344, 352
  medical termination of 554
  molar 140, 200, 207, 338, 555, 558, 560
  morbidity 340
  multifetal 209
  multiple 7, 52, 90, 137, 209, 222
  partial molar 554
  post-term 258-262, 264, 265, 268
  scan, early 47
  second trimester 4
  termination of 242, 243, 306, 458
  therapeutic termination of 200
  third trimester 4
  tissue 351
  triplet 216
Prehysterectomy 481
Prematurity, retinopathy of 132
Prenatal tests 56
Prerna scheme 329
Preterm labor 331
  diagnosis of 130
Primigravida 193, 197, 201, 260, 261
Primipara 224
Procidentia 480
  case of 480
Proctitis 451
Proctocolitis 451
Progesterone 5, 129, 130, 444, 604
  cyclical 406
  effect of 10
  high-dose 406

levels, elevated 194
  only pills, combination of 176
Progestin monotherapy 419
Progestogen 419, 421
  only pill 373
Prolactin 471, 604
Prolapse, stages of 483
Promethazine 141
Prophylactic vaginal progesterone 134
Prostaglandin 100, 181, 182, 266, 267
Prostatic utricle 511
Prosthetic cardiac valve 176
Protease inhibitors 227
Proteinuria 158
Proximal tubal blockage 504, 612
Prune Belly syndrome 68
Pseudomonas 332
Puberty 405
Pubic arch 43
Pubic rami, inferior 44
Pubis delivery, face of 32, 33
Pubocervical fascia defect 495
Pubococcygeus 482, 584
Pulmonary edema 167, 169, 175, 179, 183, 304
  risk of 168
Pulse
  periodic monitoring of 193
  waveform 60
Punch biopsy forceps 546
Pyrazinamide 228
Pyridoxine 139
  administration 139

Q

Q-tip testing 481, 583
Quadruplet 53
Quintero staging 215

R

Radical hysterectomy
  classical 567
  modified 567
Raltegravir 232
Rashtriya Bal Swasthya Karyakaram 320
Rashtriya Kishor Swasthya Karyakaram 320
Rectal misoprostol 167
Rectal wall, anterior 548
Rectocele 484, 485, 500
Rectovaginal septum, bowel 420
Red blood cells 293
Red cell 146
  units, selection of 121

Reflex, bulbocavernous 485
Refractory anemia 145
  diagnosis of 145
Regurgitation, pulmonary 179
Renal function test 158, 164
Residual ovary syndrome 410
Respiratory distress syndrome 127, 237, 242
Reticulocyte count 205
Retroperitoneal lymph-node dissection 402
Retroplacental hypoechoic zone, loss of 244
Rhabdomyomas 83
Rhabdomyosarcoma, embryonal 392
Rhesus
  antigens 196
  D genotyping 196
  isoimmunization 359
Rheumatoid arthritis 8
Rifampicin 228
Right ovarian endometriotic cyst 516
Rilpivirine 228
Ring of fire sign 423
Ring pessary 487, 493
Rogi Kalyaan Samiti 319
Rosette appearance 468
Rotterdam criteria 520
Round ligament 282, 408
Round spermatid injection 619
Routine antenatal prophylaxis 197, 208
Rudimentary horn 109

S

Saarthi 323, 382
Saas Bahu Sammelan 323, 382
Sacral agenesis 187
Sacrococcygeal joint 43
Sacrocotyloid diameter 27
Sacrosciatic notch 43
Sacrospinous fixation 482, 498
Sacrotuberous ligament 29
Sacrum 43
Saline infusion
  sonography 607, 609
  sono-salpingography 396
Saline test, hanging drop of 591
Salphingo-oophrectomy, unilateral 411
Salpingectomy 508
  bilateral 403
Salpingo-ophorectomy, bilateral 402
Salpingo-ovariolysis 410
Salpingostomy 427
Salpingotomy 427
Sampson's theory 409, 416

Index

Santushti scheme 329
Sarcoma botryoides 392
Sarcoptes scabiei 466
Saturated fats 188
Scar 8
Schizophrenia 353
Sclerosis, tuberous 83
Scrotum 511
Secnidazole 461
Seizure disorder, pre-existing 306
Selective estrogen receptor
    modulators 419
Selective progesterone receptor
    modulator 398
Semen
    analysis 380, 408, 602, 605
    quality 617
Seminiferous tubules 511
Sentinel node 533
    biopsy 533
Sepsis 99, 127, 493
    pre-existing 183
Septal resection 341
Septicemia 458
Septostomy 215
Serological test 452
Sertoli cells 511
Serum alkaline phosphatase 220
Sex cords 511
Sexual dysfunction 497
Sexually transmitted infections 458
Sheehan's syndrome 522, 604
Shirodkar's abdominal sling 496
Shirodkar's cervical cerclage 337
Shock
    hypovolemic 421
    neurogenic 287
    septic 308
    signs of 153
Shoelace knots 592
Shoulder 34
    dystocia 104, 191, 363
Sickle cell 148
    anemia 148
Sim's speculum 122, 486, 541
Single fertilized ovum 210
Single gene disorder 84
Sinus formation 499
Sinusoidal pattern 250
Skeletal abnormalities 74
Sliding sign 49, 50
Sling operation 487, 581, 582
Smith classification 567
Snowstorm appearance 140
Sodium 312
Solifenacin 585
Somatotypes 144

Somogyi phenomenon 192
Sonocontrast hysterography 607
Sonography, transvaginal 333,
    607, 614
Soonawala sling 496
Speculum examination 586
Sperm 618
    concentration 602
    count, total 602
    dead 615
    DNA fragmentation 602
    function tests 615
    morphology 602
    motility 602
    preparation methods 616
    retrieval techniques 512
    volume 602
Spermatozoa 511
Spherocytes 144
Spider angioma 4, 8
Spina bifida 22, 491
Spironolactone 474
Spur cells 144
Staphylococcus 332
Stellate ganglion block 579
Stenosis 180
STEPW submucous fibroid
    classification 503
Sterilization 176
Steroids 130, 131, 243
    prophylaxis 242
Stillbirth 268
    chances of 222
Strassman metroplasty 346, 350
Strawberry cervix 446, 456
Streptococcus 330, 332, 461
Stress 127, 582
    test 170
    urinary incontinence 481, 581,
    582, 584
Stroke 159
Submucous myoma 502
    resection of 610
Suburethral diverticulum 492
Succinylated gelatin 121
Sulfamethoxazole 450
Sulfonylurea 191
Superfecundation 210
    consequence of 210
Superfetation 210
Superficial cells 444
Superovulation 184
Supine hypotension syndrome 9
Suprapubic pressure 104
Surgery, role of 563
Surgical approach preferred
    method 175

Suture 122
Swellings, labioscrotal 511
Swim-up technique 616
Swyers syndrome 519
Symphysis pubis
    lower border 29
    posterior surface of 43
    upper border of 26
Syncope 9
Syndactyly 553
Syntometrine 270
Syphilis 232, 447, 452, 453, 463
    infection, oral 361
    primary 449, 452
    secondary 449
Syringe test 591

T

Tachycardia 9, 177
Tamponade 430
Tampons use 458
Target cell 146, 148
Tenderness, lower abdominal 457
Tennessee classification system 143
Tenofovir 227, 325
    disoproxil fumarate 223
Teratoma, mature 516
Terbutaline 129
Testicular sperm
    aspiration 505, 512, 619
    extraction 603, 619
Testis 511
    appendix of 511
Testosterone 471
Thalassemia 10, 146, 147
Thalidomide 141
Thayer-Martin agar 446
Thiamine 138
Thrombin 120
Thromboelastometry, rotational 318
Thromboembolic complications 179
Thromboembolism 399
    arterial 378
Thrombosis, risk of 378
Thyroid
    function test 405, 471
    gland 4
    stimulating hormone 604
        normal range of 4
Thyrotoxicosis 8
Tibolone 419, 576
Tissue 119
    embryonic 432
    forceps 122
Titanium 380
Tobacco-pouch appearance 468

Tocolytics 130
    administration of 183
Tolterodine 583
Toluidine blue 449
Topography 595
Torsion 389
Total bile acid concentration,
    raised 221
Toxoplasmosis 358
Trachelectomy 545
Tracheo-esophageal fistula 86
Tranexamic acid 273, 400, 478
    intravenous 592
Transobturator tap 582
Transvaginal method 342
Transvaginal scan 508
Transverse lie 92, 107, 219
Transverse vaginal septum 519,
    522, 523
Trauma 120
Treponema pallidum 463
Trichomonas vaginalis 446, 456
Tricuspid flows 69
Triflupromazine 141
Trimethoprim 450
Triple swab test 587
Triploid 553
Trisomy 57, 67, 71, 73, 75
Trophoblastic disease 137
Tubal infertility, causes of 612
Tubal ligation 176
Tubal occlusion 468, 508
Tubal wall edema 460
Tuberculosis 461, 466
    active 612
    cutaneous 449
    extrapulmonary 468
    genital 393, 457
    pulmonary 468
Tubo-ovarian abscess 393, 457-460
    ruptured 459
Tumor cells, spindle shaped 392
Turner's syndrome 517, 519, 608
Turtle sign 190, 363
Twins 215
    fetuses 210
    fraternal 210
    gestation 51
    growth, sonographic
        monitoring of 216
    locked 217
    monochorionic 216
    oligopolyhydraminos
        sequence 214
    peak sign 51, 53
    pregnancy 60, 210, 213, 216, 217
    vanishing 51, 53

Twin-twin transfusion
    syndrome 214
    diagnosis of 215

U

Ulcer
    decubitus 493
    development of 479
    treatment of 479
    type of 452
Ultrasonography
    transabdominal 403, 471
    transvaginal 403, 413, 422, 526
Ultrasound
    obstetric 158, 159
    transducer 64
Umbilical artery 177
    Doppler 216
    study 160
    resistance, degree of 160
Umbilical cord entanglement 84
Upper paravaginal fibromuscular
        connective tissue 484
Ureaplasma 461
Uremia 140
Ureter 586
Ureteric stone 409
Urethral caruncle 492
Urethral dilatation 5
Urethral discharge 461
Urethral hypermobility 481, 583
Urethral valve, posterior 75, 81
Urethrocele 492
Urinary bladder 263, 417, 586
Urinary fistula 585, 586
Urinary incontinence 581
    mixed 585
Urinary retention 394
Urinary tract
    dilatation 81
    infection 459, 587
    involvement 449
    obstruction, lower 68
Urinary urge incontinence 495, 581,
        582, 584, 585
Urination 445
Urine
    analysis 141
    dipstick test 140, 162
    ketones 193
    protein creatinine ratio 162
Urodynamometer 582
Uroflowmetry 582
Urogenital folds 511
Uropathies, obstructive 81
Ursodeoxycholic acid 358

Uterine
    abnormality 291, 402
    artery 72, 115
        abnormal 72
        embolization 430
        ligation, left-sided 282
        temporary occlusion of 592
    atony 88, 90, 189, 271, 272
    bleeding
        abnormal 395, 467
        active 612
    cavity 430, 468
        distorted 401
        honey-comb appearance
            of 468
    compression suture 277
    contraction 130, 264, 265
        abnormalities of 119
    descent 495
    didelphys 607
    displacement 311
    empty 430
    endometrium, persistent
        inflammation of 461
    factors, evaluation of 607
    fibroid 397, 399, 403, 433
        management of 398
    hyperstimulation 266, 267
    incision, extension of 115
    inversion 95, 287
    isthmus 3
    malformation 99
    musculature, arrangement of 6
    polyp, removal of 610
    rupture 92, 100, 109, 291
        causes of 291
        signs of 109
    segment, lower 3
    septum, excision of 610
    serosa 244
    synechiae, adhesiolysis of 610
    tachysystole 266, 267
    wall 435
Uteroplacental insufficiency 112
Uterosacral ligament 408, 417,
        484, 488
    endometriosis of 409
    level of 487
    support failure 481
Uterosacral nerve ablation,
        laparoscopic 414, 420
Uterotonic 273
    agent, administration of 90, 96
Uterovaginal prolapse, recurrent 485
Uterus 6, 11, 408, 466, 511
    arcuate 608
    asymmetrical enlargement of 397

Index

bicornuate 345, 346, 349, 608
dextrorotation of 5
empty 422
infection of 330
instrumentation of 458
overdistended 90
prolapse of 499
rupture 248, 249, 291
septate 341, 344, 345, 349, 503, 608
strengthening supports of 494
symmetrical enlargement of 403
transvaginal ultrasound of 424
unicornuate 345, 607
unscarred 109

V

Vagina, upper 511
Vaginal bleeding, active 130
Vaginal cerclage
    failed 349
    pervious failed 351
Vaginal cuff, leading edge of 481
Vaginal delivery 32, 181, 192, 219, 229, 241, 321, 338, 499, 584
Vaginal discharge 461, 483
    abnormal 467
Vaginal estrogen creams 578
Vaginal examination 39, 40, 104, 105, 417
Vaginal itching 445
Vaginal lubricants 578
Vaginal micronized progesterone 356
Vaginal moisturizer 578
Vaginal pH 455
Vaginal progesterone 348
Vaginal ring pessary 494
Vaginal route 129, 586, 589
Vaginal tampons 479
Vaginal wall 480
    defect, anterior 480
Vaginitis 461
Vaginosis, bacterial 444, 455, 458, 462

Valaciclovir 449
    oral 78
Varicose veins 12
Vas deferens, congenital bilateral absence of 505, 603
Vasa previa 249, 250
Vascular endothelial growth factor 597
Vascular injury 412
Vascular thrombosis 340
Vasectomy, failure rate of 380
Vasopressin 400
    infiltration 610
    injection 438
Vasovagal reaction 376
Vault prolapse 485, 498
Vellus hair 473
Venipuncture 120
Venlafaxine 575
Ventouse delivery 89
    trial of 89
Ventricular fibrillation 313
Ventricular septal defect 187
Ventricular tachycardia 313
Ventriculomegaly, severe 77
Veress needle 591
    double click sound of 591
Vernix 257
Vesicovaginal fistula 99, 483, 581, 585, 586, 588-590
Vesicovaginal septum, bladder 420
Village Health Sanitation and Nutrition Committee 319
Vincristine 564
Virilism 474
Virkud sling 496
Vision, blurring of 506
Visual scotomata 159
Vitamin
    A 327
        deficiency 550
    B_1 138, 141
    B_{12} 141, 327
        deficiency 145

    B_6 138, 141
    B_9 deficiency 21
    C 12, 138, 141, 149, 151
    supplementation 12
Vomiting 137, 251, 304, 506, 597
    intractable 140
von Willebrand's disease 478
Vulval hematoma 286

W

Waist circumference 476
Ward-Mayo's vaginal hysterectomy 482
Warfarin 178
Wash technique 616
Weight
    gain 401
    lifting 491
Weight reduction 584
Wernicke's encephalopathy 138, 139
Whiff test 444
Wrigley's outlet forceps 101
Wurm stitch 343

X

X-ray hysterosalpingogram 504

Y

Y chromosome microdeletion 515
Yeast 461
Yolk sac 47, 48

Z

Zinc, deficiencies of 327
Zona basalis 11
Zona functionalis 11
    components of 11
Zygosity 51, 52
    types of 211
Zygote splitting 209